Endocrine Surgery in Children

Daniel J. Ledbetter · Paul R.V. Johnson
Editors

Endocrine Surgery in Children

Springer

Editors
Daniel J. Ledbetter
Seattle Children's Hospital
Seattle, WA
USA

and

University of Washington
Seattle, WA
USA

Paul R.V. Johnson
Academic Pediatric Surgery Unit, Nuffield Department of Surgical Sciences
John Radcliffe Hospital
Oxford
UK

and

University of Oxford
Oxford
UK

ISBN 978-3-662-54254-5 ISBN 978-3-662-54256-9 (eBook)
DOI 10.1007/978-3-662-54256-9

Library of Congress Control Number: 2016963608

Printed on acid-free paper

This Springer imprint is published by Springer Nature
The registered company is Springer-Verlag GmbH Germany
The registered company address is: Heidelberger Platz 3, 14197 Berlin, Germany

To Sunny, Kelly, and Brian—the greatest joys of my life.

Daniel J. Ledbetter

To Hilary, Thomas, and Tilly—for your unconditional love, support, and patience during the preparation of this book.

Paul R.V. Johnson

Foreword

Endocrine conditions requiring surgery in children are extremely rare. Surgeons undertaking this surgery need to be specifically trained and exposed to a large volume of cases in order to maintain their expertise. Therefore, it is clear that the surgery needs to be concentrated in designated regional centers and carried out by a select number of pediatric surgeons. In addition, a close working relationship with the pediatric endocrinologists is essential for the overall well-being of the child.

While management of many of these conditions must remain within the armamentarium of the pediatric surgeon, for example neuroblastoma, hyperinsulinism, adrenal tumors, and gonadal conditions, there is a tendency to engage adult endocrine surgeons with specific expertise in a particular organ, such as thyroid, parathyroid, pituitary, to perform the procedures in conjunction with the pediatric surgeons. In the latter situation, it is important that the overall care of the child should remain firmly in the province of the pediatric specialist.

This book devoted to the surgery of endocrine disorders in children fills a major gap in the pediatric surgical literature and brings together the full range of endocrine conditions encountered in the pediatric age range. The last publication devoted to the surgery of endocrine disorders in children was part of the Progress in Pediatric Surgery series (now discontinued) published in 1991.

This publication includes contributions from international authorities in pediatric surgery and endocrinology, mainly from the United Kingdom and North America and should be viewed as the standard text for many years to come.

Lewis Spitz
MD, Ph.D., FRCS(Edin, Eng, I), FRCHCP, FAAP, FCS(SA), FACS
Emeritus Nuffield Professor of Paediatric Surgery
Institute of Child Health, University College, London
Honorable Consultant Paediatric Surgeon
Great Ormond Street Hospital NHS Trust
London, UK

Preface

Endocrine surgical conditions during childhood are relatively rare. However, they represent an interesting and challenging group of conditions that all pediatric surgeons will encounter sometime during their careers. This book is one of the first to provide a specific overview of the range of different endocrine surgical conditions encountered in children, together with their management. It is aimed at any surgeon operating on endocrine conditions in children and adolescents.

The book is divided into sections based on the different endocrine organs. Each section begins with a chapter outlining the embryology, anatomy, and physiology of that organ, before subsequent chapters address the different surgical conditions that occur, together with their diagnosis, management, and outcomes. Basic science and state-of-the-art research perspectives are included as they relate to surgical decision-making and optimal clinical care. We have intentionally chosen a diverse group of authors who have experience and expertise in caring for children with endocrine surgical conditions in North America and the UK. The authors include endocrinologists, adult endocrine surgeons, and pediatric surgeons, and represent many who are at the forefront of both clinical care and cutting-edge research. One of the key messages that comes out throughout the book is that rare endocrine surgical conditions require a collaborative multidisciplinary team approach to ensure that the children receive the very best management resulting in the most favorable outcomes.

It is our hope that this international, multidisciplinary perspective will give surgeons caring for children with endocrine conditions requiring surgery, additional insights that will lead to a better understanding of the conditions and ultimately improved patient care.

Seattle, USA — Daniel J. Ledbetter
Oxford, UK — Paul R.V. Johnson

Acknowledgements

We want to thank the many people who have directly and indirectly contributed to this book. First, we would like to thank our mentors who stimulated our interests in pediatric endocrine surgery. These include late David Tapper and the late Nick Dudley, both of whom demonstrated excellence in the operative care of children. Next, Diana Farmer, who persuaded the American College of Surgeons that a panel discussion of endocrine problems in children deserved a place on the program of its annual Clinical Congress. That panel discussion was the primary inspiration for this book.

Next, we would like to thank Springer, who supported this book through its long gestation to publication. In particular we would like to thank Margaret Burns who guided the book throughout its development to the point of completion.

We would also like to thank all the contributing authors. They have shown remarkable patience throughout the production of the book and without them this book would clearly not have been possible.

We would like to thank all our excellent clinical colleagues in Anesthesia, Surgery, Pathology, Radiology, Endocrinology, and Oncology at both Seattle Children's Hospital and the Children's Hospital in Oxford who have helped care for the many and varied patients with endocrine problems who have needed surgery. This includes pediatric surgical colleagues in the Division of Pediatric General and Thoracic Surgery in Seattle (Robert Sawin, John Waldhausen, Pat Healey, Adam Goldin, Ken Gow, John Meehan, George Drugas, Jeff Avansino, Patrick Javid, and Kim Riehle) and in the Department of Paediatric Surgery, Endocrinology, and Endocrine Surgery in Oxford (Hugh Grant, Kokila Lakhoo, Silke Wagener, Alex Lee, Ian Willetts, Rosa Romero, Radu Mihai, Fiona Ryan, and Taffy Makayer). Finally, we would like to thank all the surgical trainees including residents, fellows, core trainees, and registrars who do much of the work in the hospital, but more importantly, ask many of the most important questions that inspire everyone to discover new and better ways to care for children.

Contents

Contributors

Roger Ackroyd Department of General Surgery, Northern General Hospital, Sheffield, South Yorkshire, UK

Michael S.D. Agus Department of Pediatrics, Harvard Medical School, Boston Children's Hospital, Boston, MA, USA

Geoffrey K. Blair Division of Pediatric Surgery, British Columbia's Children's Hospital, Vancouver, BC, Canada

Mary L. Brandt Department of Pediatric Surgery, Texas Children's Hospital, Houston, TX, USA

Samuel R. Browd Department of Neurological Surgery, University of Washington, Seattle, WA, USA

Antonio Bruni 5-040 Li Ka Shing Health Research, Edmonton, AB, Canada

Jocelyn Burke Department of Surgery, University of Wisconsin School of Medicine and Public Health, Madison, WI, USA

Darius J. Bägli Department of Surgery, Division of Urology, The Hospital for Sick Children, University of Toronto, Toronto, ON, Canada

Herbert Chen Department of Surgery, University of Wisconsin School of Medicine and Public Health, Madison, WI, USA

Daniel W. Colliver Department of Paediatric Surgery and Urology, Queens Medical Centre, Nottingham, UK

Mehul T. Dattani Section of Genetics and Epigenetics in Health and Disease, Genetics and Genomic Medicine Programme, UCL GOS Institute of Child Health and Great Ormond Street Hospital for Children, London, UK

Jennifer E. Dietrich Department of Pediatric and Adolescent Gynecology, Texas Children's Hospital, Houston, TX, USA

Patricia K. Donahoe Pediatric Surgical Research Laboratories, Massachusetts General Hospital, Boston, MA, USA

Yaser El-Hout American University of Beirut Medical Center, Riad El Solh, Beirut, Lebanon

Anne C. Fischer Pediatric Surgery, West Palm Beach, FL, USA

Joseph Fusco Department of Pediatric Surgery, Children's Hospital of Pittsburgh, Pittsburgh, PA, USA

George K. Gittes Department of Pediatric Surgery, Children's Hospital of Pittsburgh, Pittsburgh, PA, USA

Tim Goodacre Nuffield Department of Surgery, University of Oxford, Headington, Oxford, UK

Ankush Gosain Department of Surgery, University of Wisconsin School of Medicine and Public Health, Madison, WI, USA

Kenneth W. Gow Department of General and Thoracic Surgery, Seattle Children's Hospital and the University of Washington, Seattle, WA, USA

Keith Holmes Department of Paediatric Surgery, St. George's Hospital, London, UK

Khalid Hussain Department of Paediatrics, Division of Endocrinology, Sidra Medical and Research Centre, Doha, Qatar

John Hutson Department of Paediatrics, University of Melbourne, Melbourne, AustraliaDepartment of Urology, Royal Children's Hospital, Melbourne, AustraliaDouglas Stephens Surgical Research Laboratory, Melbourne Royal Children's Hospital, Murdoch Children's Research Institute, Parkville, VIC, Australia

Thomas H. Inge Akers Chair in Pediatric Surgery, Division of Pediatric Surgery, Adolescent Metabolic and Bariatric Surgery, Children's Hospital Colorado, Aurora, CO, USA

A.M. James Shapiro , Edmonton, AB, Canada

Paul R.V. Johnson Academic Pediatric Surgery Unit, Nuffield Department of Surgical Sciences, John Radcliffe Hospital, University of Oxford and Oxford Islet Transplant Programme, Oxford, UK

Stephen Kennedy Nuffield Department of Obstetrics and Gynaecology, University of Oxford, Oxford, UKJohn Radcliffe Hospital, Oxford, UK

Mansoor Ali Khan Department of Surgery and Trauma, Imperial College London, London, UK

Kokila Lakhoo Department of Paediatric Surgery, Children's Hospital Oxford, Oxford Radcliffe Hospitals NHS Trust, Headington, UK

Daniel J. Ledbetter Seattle Children's Hospital, Seattle, WA, USA

Monica E. Lopez Division of Pediatric Surgery, Texas Children's Hospital, Houston, TX, USA

Michael McCall 5-040 Li Ka Shing Health Research, Edmonton, AB, Canada

Gavin McCoubrey Salisbury NHS Foundation Trust, Salisbury, UK

Betty Panayota Messazos Department of Paediatric Endocrinology, Oxford Children's Hospital, Oxford University Hospitals NHS Trust, Headington, Oxford, UK

Jennia Michaeli Department of Obstetrics and Gynaecology, Hadassah Medical Center and Hebrew University-Hadassah Medical School, Jerusalem, Israel

Radu Mihai Department of Surgery, Churchill Cancer Centre, Oxford, UKDepartment of Surgery, John Radcliffe Hospital, Oxford, UK

Shireen A. Nah The Surgery Unit2, UCL Institute of Child Health, Great Ormond Street Hospital for Children, NHS Trust, University College London, London, UK

Toba Niazi Department of Clinical Neurological Surgery and Pediatrics, University of Miami, Miami, FL, USA

Oluyinka O. Olutoye Division of Pediatric Surgery, Texas Children's Hospital, Houston, TX, USATexas Children's Fetal Center, Texas Children's Hospital, Houston, TX, USA

Eduardo A. Perez Division of Pediatric Surgery, The Dewitt Daughtry Family Department of Surgery, University of Miami, Miller School of Medicine, Miami, FL, USA

Rafael V. Pieretti Department of Pediatric Surgery, MassGeneral Hospital for Children, Boston, MA, USA

Agostino Pierro Department of Pediatric General and Thoracic Surgery, Hospital for Sick Children, Toronto, ON, Canada

Clare M. Rees Department of Paediatric Surgery, Children's Hospital Oxford, Oxford Radcliffe Hospitals NHS Trust, Headington, UK

Ariel Revel Department of Obstetrics and Gynaecology, Hadassah Medical Center and Hebrew University-Hadassah Medical School, Jerusalem, Israel

P.G. Roy Churchill Hospital, Oxford, UK

Fiona Jane Ryan Department of Paediatric Endocrinology, Oxford Children's Hospital, Headington, Oxford, UK

Gregory P. Sadler Department of Endocrine Surgery, John Radcliffe Hospital, Oxford, UK

Michael Skinner Department of Pediatric Surgery, University of Texas Southwestern Medical Center Children's Medical Center, Dallas, TX, USA

Nancy Sokkary Department of Pediatrics, UNM Children's Hospital, The University of New Mexico, Albuquerque, NM, USA

Michael J. Stechman Department of Endocrine Surgery, University Hospital of Wales, Cardiff, UK

David F.M. Thomas Department of Paediatric Urology, Leeds Teaching Hospitals, University of Leeds, Leeds General Infirmary, Leeds, UK

Vaitsa Tziaferi Department of Paediatric Endocrinology, Great Ormond Street Hospital, London, UK

Sanjeev Vasudevan Department of Pediatric Surgery, Texas Children's Hospital, Houston, TX, USA

Gerard V. Walls Royal Lancaster Infirmary, University Hospitals of Morecambe Bay NHS Foundation Trust, Lancaster, UK, Consultant General and Endocrine Surgeon, University Hospitals of Morecambe Bay NHS Foundation Trust, Royal Lancaster Infirmary, Lancaster, UK

Ari J. Wassner Department of Pediatrics, Harvard Medical School, Boston Children's Hospital, Boston, MA, USA

Part I
Thyroid

Thyroid Gland Embryology, Anatomy, and Physiology

1

Gerard V. Walls and Radu Mihai

Thyroid Gland—Embryology, Anatomy, and Physiology

This chapter reviews the embryology, anatomy, and physiology of the thyroid gland with special emphasis on how these topics relate to surgical conditions and surgical decision-making. First, thyroid development is reviewed since it is the essential foundation to understand thyroid anatomy. Next, the anatomy of the thyroid, its blood supply and its relationship to nearby nerves are reviewed to understand the conduct of thyroid operations and the risks and complications of those operations. Finally, the details of the thyroid gland's principle function—the synthesis and secretion of thyroid hormones—are considered. Understanding these normal physiologic functions and their control provides insight into the diagnostic evaluation and treatment of thyroid diseases. Parathyroid gland embryology, anatomy, and function are reviewed in Chap. 5.

G.V. Walls
Royal Lancaster Infirmary, University Hospitals of Morecambe Bay NHS Foundation Trust, Ashton Road, Lancaster LA1 4RP, UK
e-mail: gerard.walls@nds.ox.ac.uk

R. Mihai (✉)
Department of Surgery, Churchill Cancer Centre, Oxford OX3 9DU, UK
e-mail: radumihai@doctors.org.uk; radu.mihai@ouh.nhs.uk

Embryology of the Thyroid Gland

At embryonic day 20, a portion of the endoderm in the ventral midline of the primitive pharynx begins to differentiate into what will become the thyroid gland. This thyroid primordium forms a diverticulum cephalad to the respiratory diverticulum at the level of the second pharyngeal arch. The origin of this diverticulum will later be recognized as the *foramen caecum* at the junction of the anterior two-thirds and posterior one-third of the tongue. The thyroid diverticulum migrates caudally from the pharyngeal floor by day 24, then passes through or in front of the hyoid bone, and by day 50 reaches its final position in front of the trachea shaped like the mature thyroid gland with two lateral lobes joined by a small, anterior isthmus (Fig. 1.1). The descending diverticulum of the developing thyroid usually disappears but about 50% of people will have a midline pyramidal lobe of variable length that extends from the thyroid isthmus towards the hyoid bone. In addition, scattered cellular remnants of the diverticulum may persist and explain thyroid scan activity after total thyroidectomy. Finally, larger remnants of the thyroid diverticulum may persist and form thyroglossal duct cysts and sinuses which are discussed in more detail in section, "Embryological anomalies of the thyroid with clinical significance".

Follicles appear within the thyroid gland at the beginning of the second month of gestation and most follicles are formed by the end of the fourth month of gestation. Even though it is the first endocrine gland to form, the foetal thyroid does not produce thyroid hormones until 18–20 weeks

D.J. Ledbetter and P.R.V. Johnson (eds.), *Endocrine Surgery in Children*,
DOI 10.1007/978-3-662-54256-9_1

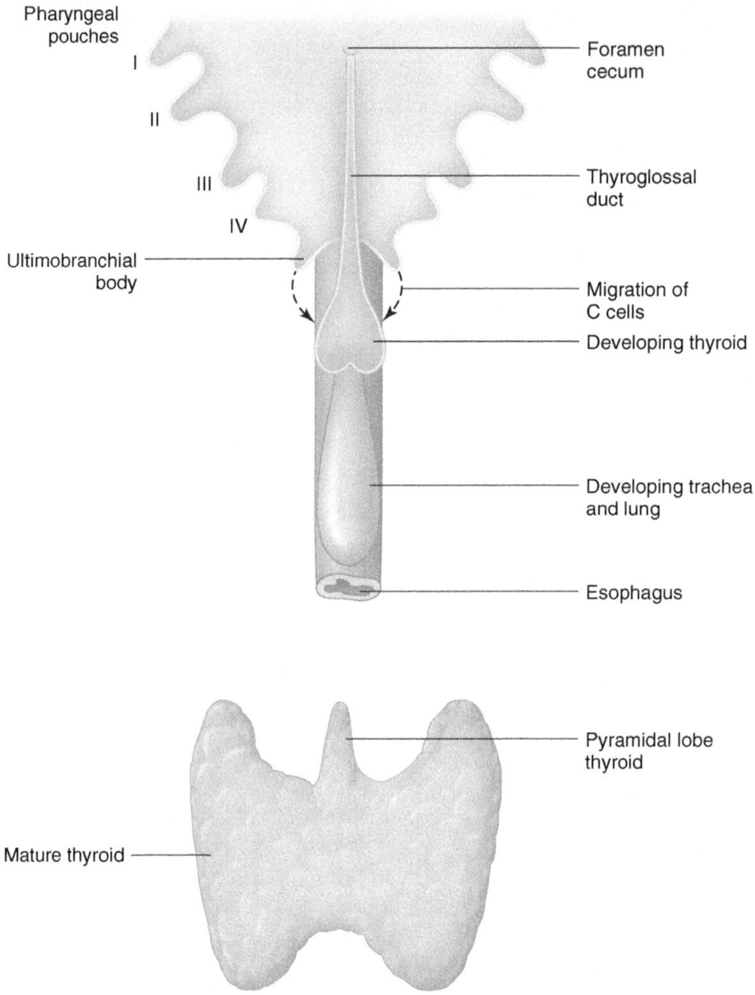

Fig. 1.1 Thyroid development—anterior view. The thyroid originates at the foramen cecum in the midline embryonic pharynx and descends as the thyroid diverticulum to the lower neck to its final position anterior to the trachea. Parafollicular C cells originate from the ultimobranchial bodies adjacent to the 4th pharyngeal pouches and join the developing median thyroid during its migration

of gestation. Therefore, for the first half of gestation the foetus is dependent on maternal thyroid hormones that cross the placenta. This supply of maternal thyroid hormone is especially critical for early neurological development. Maternal hypothyroidism can lead to marked neurodevelopmental compromise of the child [1].

In addition to thyroid hormone-producing follicular cells another group of hormonally active cells in the thyroid are the calcitonin-producing parafollicular C cells. Parafollicular C cells originate from the neuroectoderm of the fifth pharyngeal pouch, the ultimobranchial bodies. They migrate from their lateral origins to merge with the midline developing thyroid. C cells are scattered throughout the mature thyroid gland but are concentrated near the embryologic merger point at the central posterior portion of the upper third of each thyroid lobe.

The molecular genetics of thyroid embryology has been investigated and many transcription factors such as FGF10, FOXE1, HHEX, HOXA3, NKX2-1 AND PAX8 have been identified that are essential for normal thyroid development [2]. For example, heterozygous mutations in PAX8 are associated with thyroid hemiagenesis. Furthermore, gene mutations and copy number gains in key pathways occur in thyroid tumours. Examples of such abnormalities include the RET (rearranged during transfection)-Ras-BRAF-MEK and RET-beta-catenin pathways in medullary thyroid carcinoma in Multiple Endocrine Neoplasia 2A and 2B, FAP (familial adenomatous polyposis) and TRK-PI3K-Akt in papillary thyroid carcinoma, and MDM-p53-PTEN (phosphatase and tensin homolog) pathway in follicular thyroid carcinoma in Cowden syndrome [3]. Another mechanism of papillary thyroid tumourigenesis results from rearrangement of genes encoding receptors with tyrosine kinase activity such as *RET* rearrangements with *H4, PRKAR1A, ELE1, PCM1, RFG5, TIF1A*, and *TIF1G*, known as RET/PTC1-7 and *NTRK1* rearrangements with *TPM3, TPR* and *TFG*. Autonomous activation of these tyrosine kinase receptors stimulates growth of follicular thyroid and anaplastic thyroid carcinomas via the PI3 K/Akt and MAPK pathways [4]. As a consequence, tyrosine kinase inhibitors are being investigated as a potential treatment for advanced thyroid cancer.

Embryological Anomalies of the Thyroid with Clinical Significance

Thyroid dysgenesis is the term used to describe abnormalities of thyroid gland development and includes a spectrum of conditions including **thyroid agenesis** (complete absence of thyroid tissue), thyroid **hypoplasia** (less than the normal amount of thyroid tissue), and **thyroid ectopia** (thyroid tissue in abnormal locations). Agenesis of the thyroid gland is a very rare anomaly and like thyroid hypoplasia is a cause of congenital hypothyroidism that must be recognized and treated with thyroid hormone replacement in early infancy to prevent neurodevelopmental compromise. One form of hypoplasia is **hemiagenesis** when one lobe does not develop. In this rare condition the left lobe is more commonly absent.

A **thyroglossal duct cyst** is a remnant of the diverticulum that forms along the migration path of the thyroid primordium from the foramen caecum at the base of the tongue to the thyroid gland's final position in front of the trachea. This

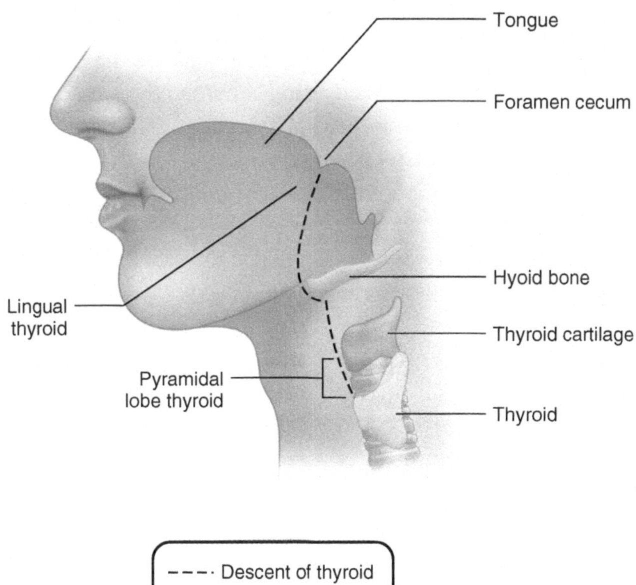

Fig. 1.2 Thyroid development—midline sagittal view of the path of thyroid descent in mature human. Ectopic thyroid can be present anywhere along the path such as in the midline posterior tongue where it is known as a lingual thyroid or attached to the thyroid isthmus as the pyramidal lobe. Remnants of the thyroid diverticulum known as thyroglossal duct cysts or sinuses can occur anywhere along the path, most commonly in the midline neck between the hyoid bone and thyroid

diverticulum usually begins to involute during the 5th week of development but incomplete involution may result in ectopic thyroid tissue that is typically located in the midline or just off the midline between the hyoid bone and the thyroid isthmus (Fig. 1.2). Thyroglossal duct cyst is the most common congenital neck mass found in children and it can also present later in life in the same location. Thyroglossal duct cysts may enlarge, become infected or rarely undergo malignant transformation. The treatment of a thyroglossal duct cyst is surgical excision of the cyst and (to reduce the chance of recurrence) the entire course of the thyroglossal duct including the middle third of the hyoid bone. This is known as the Sistrunk procedure [5].

Failure of the thyroid migration results in a **lingual thyroid** which is the most common form of complete thyroid ectopia. Lingual thyroid is a relatively rare condition that is more prevalent in women and in the majority of cases it is associated with an absence of a normal cervical thyroid. It is generally presents incidentally as an asymptomatic mass at the back of the tongue (Fig. 1.2). If large, a lingual thyroid can produce obstructive symptoms such as dysphagia, dysphonia, or dyspnoea. When a lingual thyroid is suspected based by clinical findings the diagnosis can be confirmed by radioisotope scanning which also confirms the absence of other thyroid tissue in the neck.

Thyrothymic thyroid rests are ectopic collections of thyroid follicular cells often connected to the lower lobes of the thyroid but sometimes completely separate. In either case, they descend in the anterior or posterior mediastinum and may cause symptoms if they enlarge. This abnormally located thyroid tissue can present similarly to the more common retrosternal goitre which is an exuberant growth of normally located thyroid lobes down into the mediastinum.

Struma ovarii, also known as thyroid goitre of the ovary, is an ovarian teratoma that contains mostly thyroid tissue. The teratoma is a developmental anomaly of foetal gonadal tissue. This exceedingly rare condition is usually an unexpected histological finding in patients who have excision of an ovarian mass.

Embryology of the Recurrent Laryngeal Nerve

The recurrent laryngeal nerve (RLN) is a branch of the vagus nerve going to the larynx and its final path is linked to developmental changes in the aortic arches. By the 6th–7th week, the lowest persisting aortic arch on each side pulls the respective RLN downwards. On the left, the RLN passes around the 6th aortic arch which in the foetus becomes the ductus arteriosus that normally closes postnatally and becomes the ligamentum arteriosum. It then travels upwards in the tracheo-oesophageal groove. On the right, the 5th and 6th aortic arches disappear and the RLN passes around the 4th aortic arch which becomes the right subclavian artery. From this position the right RLN then ascends more obliquely than the left RLN (Fig. 1.3). As a consequence, the left RLN is longer than the right RLN and, during intraoperative nerve monitoring there is a slightly longer latency of the signal obtained during stimulation of the vagus on the left side compared with the right side.

An embryological vascular anomaly (present in 0.5–1% of people) leads to a **non-recurrent laryngeal *nerve*** and illustrates the close connection between the developing RLN and aortic arches. When the 4th aortic arch on the right does not develop an aberrant right subclavian artery originates from the left side of the aortic arch, distal to the origins of the right carotid, left carotid and left subclavian artery. From this origin it passes upwards and to the right behind the oesophagus. Occasionally this retro-oesophageal location is associated with esophageal compression and dysphagia explaining its designation as *arteria lusoria.* Since there is no embryological right aortic arch to pull the right RLN downwards the nerve goes straight from the vagus into the larynx and is therefore "non-recurrent" (Fig. 1.3). This unusual vascular anomaly can be demonstrated on Doppler ultrasound, which in some centres is part of routine preoperative investigation before thyroid surgery. The use of intraoperative neuromonitoring may also identify patients with this anatomical anomaly [6] when stimulation of the distal vagus nerve does not produce a RLN signal while stimulation

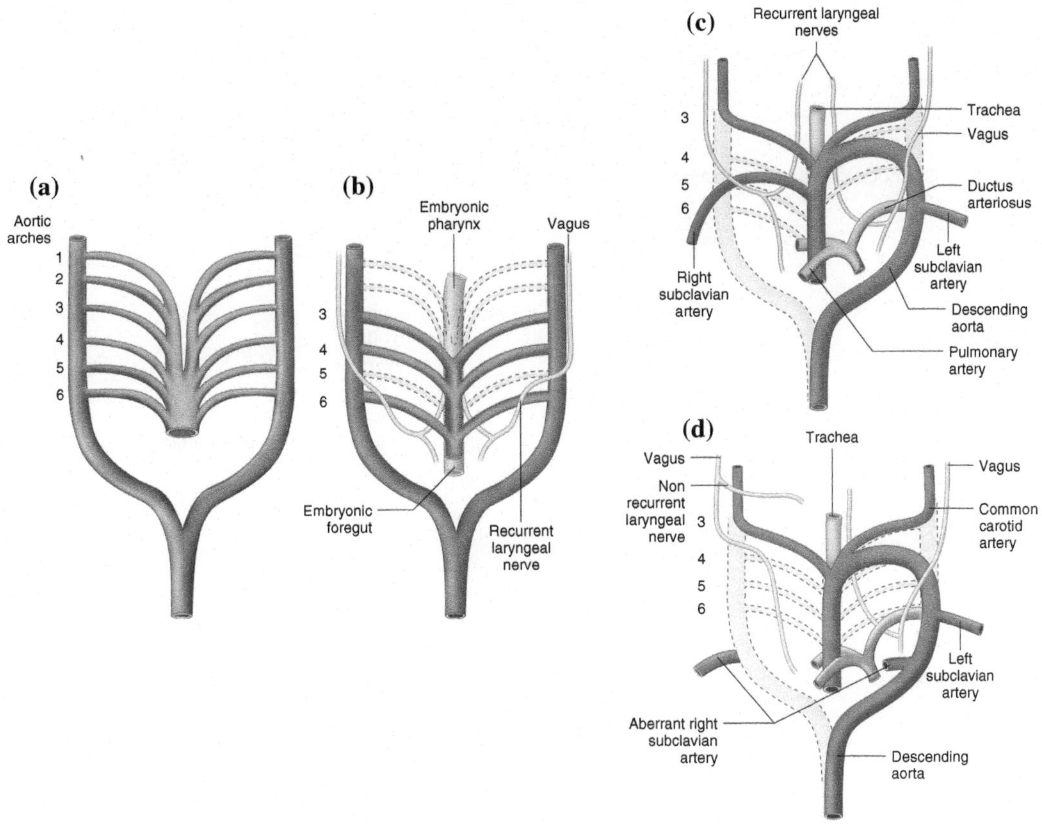

Fig. 1.3 Aortic arch development and recurrent laryngeal nerve. **a** Embryonic paired aortic arch vessels, also known as pharyngeal arch arteries correlating to developing pharyngeal arches. **b** Embryonic paired aortic arches with recurrent laryngeal nerve (RLN). The RLN loops around the lowest (6th) aortic arch on each and then goes to the larynx. In this depiction the 1st, 2nd, and 5th aortic arches have already regressed. **c** As normal development proceeds the right 6th aortic arch regresses so that the right RLN loops around the lowest remaining arch, the 4th aortic arch which becomes the right subclavian. The left RLN passes around the persisting 6th aortic arch which in the foetus becomes the ductus arteriosus and postnatally normally closes to becomes the ligamentum arteriosum. **d** When the right 4th aortic arch does not develop then an aberrant right subclavian artery originates from the aortic arch distal to the right carotid, left carotid and left subclavian artery and passes to the right upwards and behind the oesophagus. With no embryological right aortic arch to pull it downward, the right RLN nerve goes straight from the vagus into the larynx and is therefore "non-recurrent"

proximal to the origin of the non-recurrent RLN generates the correct signal [7]. The diagnosis can be confirmed postoperatively by ultrasound identification of the vascular anomaly or by a barium swallow showing the retroesophageal artery as an extrinsic compression of the posterior oesophagus. On the left side the non-recurrent RLN is exceptionally rare with only a few cases reported. A more common finding is a false non-recurrent RLN which is seen when a large anastomotic branch of the cervical sympathetic chain joins a normal RLN.

Anatomy of the Thyroid Gland

Gross Anatomy

The normal adult thyroid weights 20–30 g and has two lobes measuring approximately 5 cm in length and 3 cm in width. The thyroid gland lies between the anterior borders of the sternocleidomastoid (SCM) muscles in the anterior triangle of the neck in front of the trachea caudal to the cricothyroid membrane and the thyroid cartilage ("Adam's apple"), with the isthmus overlying the second to fourth tracheal rings. A pyramidal lobe

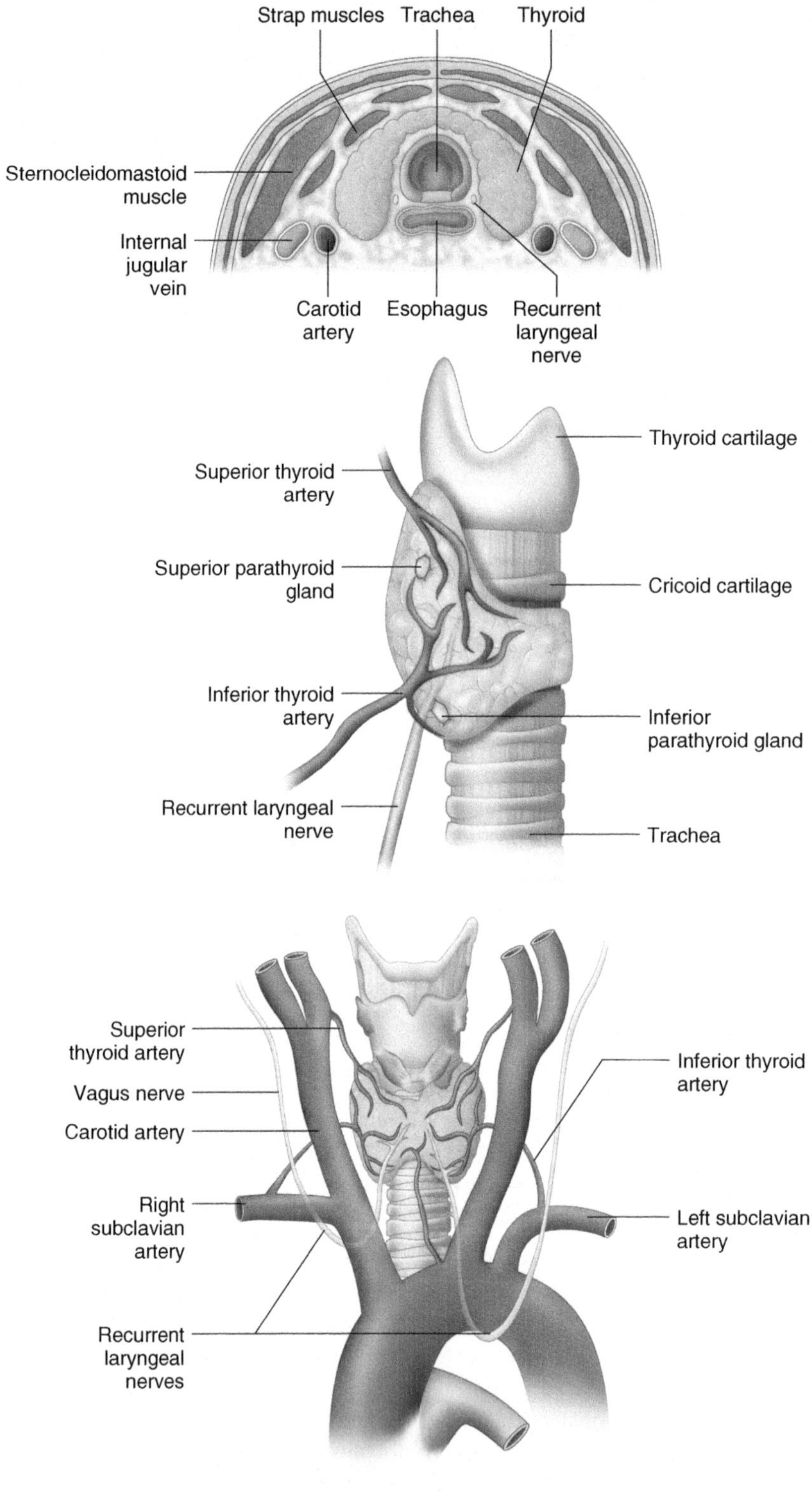

Fig. 1.4 Thyroid anatomy. Anterior, lateral, and cross-sectional

can be observed in some 50% of patients as an extension of thyroid tissue from the isthmus towards the hyoid bone (Fig. 1.4).

A midline mass situated at or above the thyroid cartilage is usually not the thyroid gland but more likely a thyroglossal cyst or an enlarged lymph node. A mass visible along the edge or just under the SCM is more likely to be a branchial cyst. A mass visible lateral to SCM (i.e. in the posterior triangle) is more likely to be an enlarged lymph node.

Surgical Anatomy of Classical Thyroidectomy (in the Order Encountered During the Operation)

1. The **skin** incision follows Langer's lines or the wrinkle lines in the neck overlying the thyroid isthmus. Kocher was the first to describe the transverse collar incision [8].
2. The **subcutaneous fat** contains numerous small blood vessels.
3. The **platysma muscle** is a broad and very thin muscle layer extending from the deep fascia of the upper pectoralis muscle to the mandible and lower face. The platysma muscle may be incomplete with bands of muscle separated by subcutaneous fat in the lower part of the neck and therefore might not be seen with short incisions. Immediately beneath the platysma are the **anterior jugular veins**.
4. The **deep cervical fascia** is a poorly defined layer in front of the strap muscles that splits and passes anterior and posterior to the sternocleidomastoid muscle. The **anterior jugular veins** are immediately superficial to this fibrous layer.
5. **Strap muscles** are thin, flat muscles overlying the thyroid and deeper neck structures. Strap muscles encountered during thyroidectomy include the narrow **sternohyoid** muscle that extends from the hyoid bone to the back of the sternoclavicular joint. Beneath the sternohyoid is the **sternothyroid** muscle, a wider muscle stretching between the oblique line of the thyroid cartilage to the posterior surface of the manubrium of the sternum. There is a clear plane between sternohyoid and sternothyroid muscles that may be extended laterally to the internal jugular vein. On the lateral edge of the strap muscles the **ansa cervicalis**, a branch of the cervical plexus, is readily apparent and can be misinterpreted as a non-recurrent RLN. Intraoperative nerve stimulation of this nerve branch triggers contraction of the strap muscles. This nerve branch has been used as a graft to reconstruct a damaged RLN (although with only limited success).
6. **Thyroid veins**. The **middle thyroid vein** is seen after mobilization of the straps muscles. A dominant middle thyroid vein is present in about 50% of patients as a large branch travelling laterally from the thyroid and crossing in front of the carotid artery before draining into the internal jugular vein. **Inferior thyroid veins** form either a plexus in front of the trachea or occur as distinct branches that drain into the brachiocephalic veins. The **superior thyroid vein** is close to the superior thyroid artery and is occasionally very prominent, especially in the presence of an enlarged lobe. The superior thyroid vein drains into the jugular vein or the facial vein.
7. The **superior thyroid artery** is the first branch of the external carotid or occasionally slightly more centrally from the common carotid. As the artery approaches the gland it splits into anterior and posterior branches that should be ligated separately during thyroidectomy. This surgical technique makes it less likely to injure the superior laryngeal nerve (vide infra).
8. **Superior laryngeal nerve** (SLN). Close to its origin from the vagus nerve, the SLN divides into an internal and external branch. The internal branch passes through the thyrohyoid membrane and provides sensation to the larynx proximal to the vocal cords. The external branch (EBSLN) innervates the cricothyroid muscle, which rocks the articulation between the thyroid and cricoid cartilages and pulls the front of the cricoid upwards increasing tension in the vocal ligaments and allowing the pitch of the voice to rise. Damage to this nerve has a major impact on voice quality and hence protecting the EBSLN is important. However, the nerve is small and the course variable. Identification of the EBSLN is easier

when its course is superficial to the inferior constrictor (Friedman classification type I) and is impossible if the EBSLN travels its entire course beneath the inferior constrictor (Friedman classification type III) [9]. It is also easier to protect the EBSLN when it crosses the trunk of the superior thyroid artery more than 1 cm proximal to its branches (Cernea classification type I) rather than in between its branches (Cernea classification type III) [10].

9. The **inferior thyroid artery** is a branch of the thyrocervical trunk that divides into an inferior branch going to the lower pole and a superior branch which travels on the posterior aspect of the thyroid lobe and may contribute to vascularization of the superior parathyroid gland. Ligation of the main inferior thyroid artery laterally was done in the past but it is now discouraged as it increases the risk of compromising the blood supply to the parathyroid glands with resulting postoperative hypoparathyroidism. About 10% of patients have an inferior artery called **arteria thyroidea ima** arising directly from the aortic arch, the right brachiocephalic artery or the right common carotid artery. It represents a persistent embryonic vessel that disappears in most people.
10. **Recurrent laryngeal nerve** (RLN). Identification of the RLN is an integral part of a safe technique for thyroid surgery. The left RLN loops around the aortic arch and ascends in the tracheo-oesophageal groove in a fairly vertical direction. Most commonly the nerve is identified at the lower pole of the thyroid, in the area medial to the carotid artery, lateral to the oesophagus and below the inferior thyroid artery.

    The right RLN loops around the subclavian artery and enters the neck more obliquely from behind the carotid artery. The RLN relationship to the inferior thyroid artery is variable. In about 50% of patients it is posterior to the inferior thyroid artery while in the other 50% the nerve is either between branches of the artery or anterior to the artery. Before entering the larynx the RLN is in close proximity to the **ligament of Berry** usually passing just lateral and posterior to the tough, white connective tissue band attaching the thyroid gland to the trachea. Branching of RLN can occur before entering the larynx and some consider that the anterior (or medial) branch contains most of the motor fibres while the posterior (or lateral) branch is mainly sensory [11, 12]. An ascending branch can anastomose with the SLN through the **nerve of Galen**.
11. **Lymphatic drainage**. Lymphatic drainage in the neck can be described by the anatomic location or by more defined regions or "levels" (see Chap. 4 for a more detailed description of neck lymph node levels). The lymph nodes closest to the thyroid and most often the site of metastatic spread of thyroid cancer are in the central compartment also known as level VI. Level VI is defined anatomically by the hyoid bone superiorly, the medial borders of the carotid arteries laterally and the sternal notch and origin of the carotids inferiorly. It includes lymph nodes situated both in front of the RLN (level VIa) and posterior to the nerve (level VIb). The superior poles and the isthmus drain into the Delphian or prelaryngeal lymph nodes in level VI and jugular lymph nodes (levels II–IV). The lateral part of the lobe drains along the middle thyroid vein through the central compartment (level VI) and towards the jugular lymph nodes (levels II–IV). The inferior part of the lobe drains towards pretracheal/paratracheal lymph nodes (level VI), mediastinal lymph nodes (level VII) and lower jugular lymph nodes (level IV). In recent years, it has become common practice to remove the central compartment lymph nodes in patients with thyroid cancer.

Histology of the Thyroid Gland

The thyroid consists of a large number of spherical follicles surrounded by a capsule. A follicle consists of a single layer of thyroid follicular epithelial cells surrounding a cavity (the follicular lumen) that contains colloid (see Fig. 1.5). Colloid is an amorphous liquid

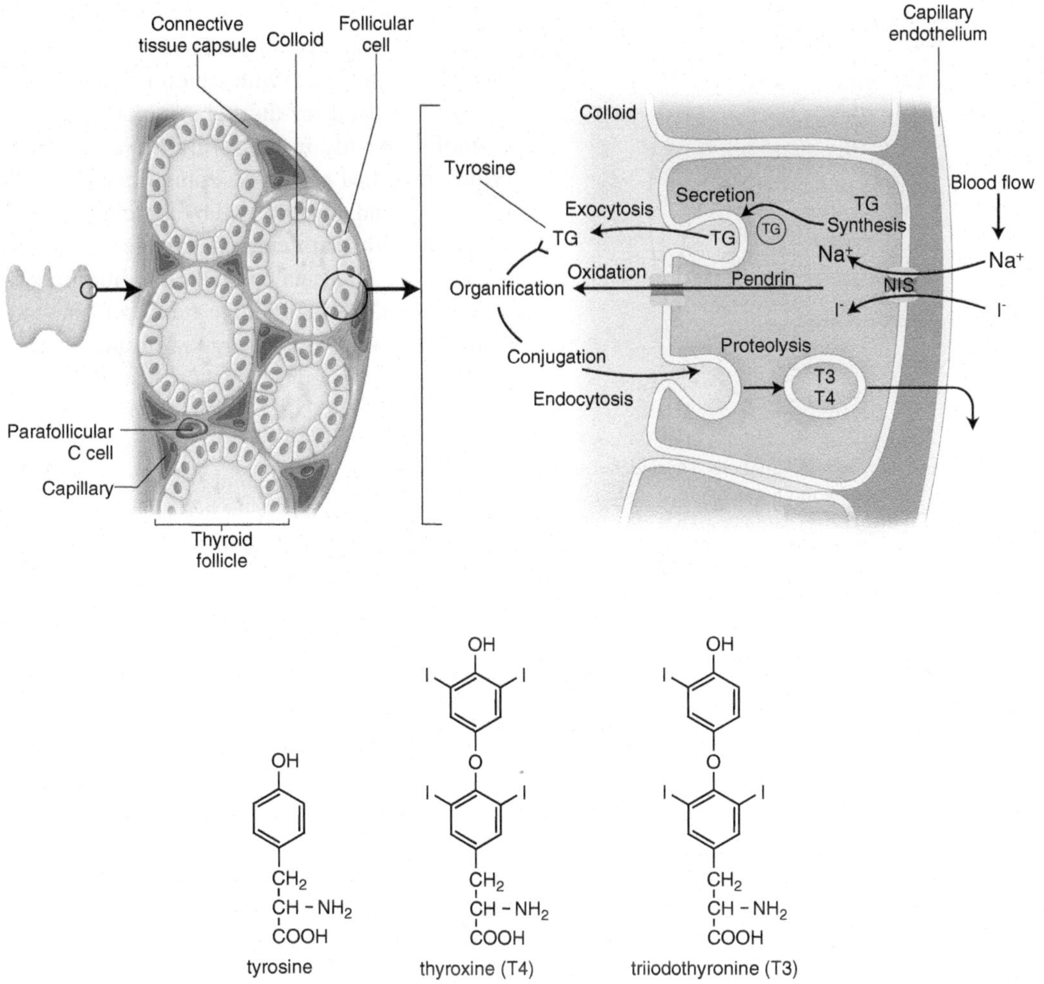

Fig. 1.5 **a** Histology thyroid follicle. **b** Thyroid hormone synthesis. I^-, Iodide; NIS, sodium-iodide symporter or "iodine trap" concentrates iodine in follicular cells. Pendrin transports iodide from follicular cells into colloid TG, thyroglobulin (TG), a large glycoprotein rich in tyrosine; **Organification** iodide oxidized to a very reactive form that links to tyrosine in TG mediated by the enzyme thyroperoxidase (TPO). Organification generates monoiodotyrosine (MIT) and diiodotyrosine (DIT) within TG. **Conjugation** TPO mediates the coupling of iodinated tyrosine residues to form thyroid hormones T3 and T4

substance that serves as a reservoir for thyroglobulin, a large protein to which iodinated thyroid hormones are bound. Small amounts of colloid are engulfed into follicular cells via pinocytosis. These ingested vesicles of colloid fuse with lysosomes, allowing T3 (triiodothyronine) and T4 (thyroxine) hormones to be released from thyroglobulin. Scattered between follicles are occasional parafollicular cells that are also known as "C cells" because they secrete the hormone calcitonin. They are more apparent in cases of C-cell hyperplasia, such as is found in patients with MEN-2.

Thyroid Physiology

The main function of the thyroid gland is to produce thyroid hormones and release them into the systemic circulation where they affect almost every cell in the body. Thyroid hormone levels are regulated by thyroid stimulating hormone

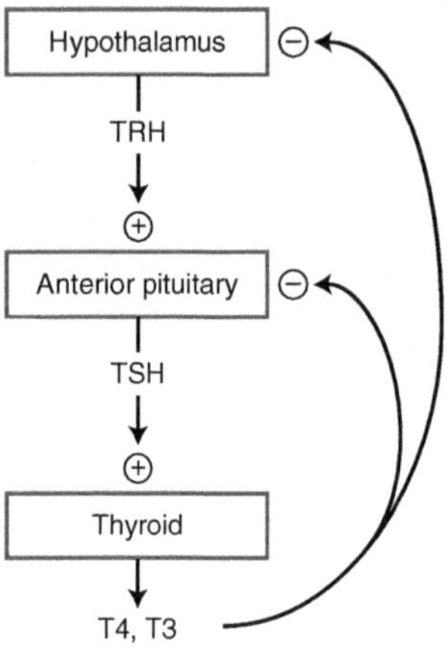

Fig. 1.6 Control of thyroid function. Thyroid hormone secretion is controlled by the hypothalamus and anterior pituitary. The hypothalamus produces TRH (thyrotropin releasing hormone) which acts on the anterior pituitary to produce thyroid stimulating hormone (TSH). TSH stimulates the thyroid to produce thyroid hormones T4 and T3. Circulating thyroid hormones are sensed by the anterior pituitary and hypothalamus and decrease the production of TRH and TSH creating a negative feedback loop

(TSH) from the pituitary in a reverse feedback loop via hypothalamus secretion of thyrotropin releasing factor. The overall regulation of thyroid hormone production is outlined in schematic form in Fig. 1.6. In addition to thyroid hormone production from follicular cells the thyroid gland also produces the hormone calcitonin from the parafollicular C cells. Calcitonin is not essential to calcium homeostasis in humans but calcitonin levels are increased and serve as a serum marker in pathologic states of C-cell hyperplasia and the C-cell malignancy known as medullary carcinoma of the thyroid.

Thyroid Hormone Synthesis

Thyroid hormone is produced in the thyroid follicle by incorporation of iodide into tyrosine residues of thyroglobulin (see Fig. 1.5b). The production of thyroid hormones is critically dependent on iodine that comes from the dietary sources. Deficient dietary intake of iodine can lead to endemic goitre, hypothyroidism, and even cretinism, a state of marked physical and neurodevelopmental impairment resulting from a lack of foetal thyroid hormone during development. Cretinism is usually caused by severe maternal hypothyroidism. Excess iodine intake is associated with autoimmune thyroid disease and papillary thyroid carcinoma.

Iodine, mainly in the form of iodide, is efficiently absorbed by the gastrointestinal tract and is taken up and concentrated by thyroid follicular cells through an energy-dependent process mediated by a plasma membrane **sodium-iodide symporter** (**NIS**) or "iodine trap". NIS activity results in iodide concentration inside thyroid follicular cells 40 times higher than circulating levels. NIS is regulated by circulating TSH and iodine concentrations.

TSH binding to follicular cells increases NIS transcription and leads to increased iodide uptake. When TSH is absent then membrane NIS moves into the cell and iodide uptake decreases. Iodide levels also effect NIS expression and iodide uptake. A rapid increase in blood iodide levels leads to a shutdown of iodide incorporation and the decrease of iodide incorporation leads to decreased thyroid hormone production. This time-limited response is known as the **Wolff–Chaikoff effect** and it protects against iodine overload. The Wolff–Chaikoff effect can be used to therapeutic advantage in patients with Graves' disease whose thyroid hormone production can be temporarily controlled by administering exogenous iodide. For example, when a patient with Graves' disease develops an allergic reaction that requires discontinuation of their antithyroid medication they can be given iodide to block thyroid hormone production while being prepared for urgent thyroidectomy. Another example of a medical benefit of the Wolff–Chaikoff effect is the prophylactic intake of potassium iodide to prevent thyroid uptake of environmental radioactive iodide after a nuclear accident.

From within follicular cells, iodide is transported into the colloid of the follicular lumen by pendrin, a membrane protein also known as iodide–chloride transporter. Mutations of the pendrin gene, SLC26A4, are associated with the autosomal recessive Pendred syndrome of congenital goitre and deafness. Once in the follicular lumen iodide is joined to thyroglobulin forming the precursors of thyroid hormones.

Thyroglobulin (TG) is a large glycoprotein made only by follicular cells. Thyroglobulin is rich in tyrosine. Within follicular cells TG is incorporated into vesicles that migrate to the apical (colloid-facing) pole and are extruded by exocytosis into the colloid of the follicular lumen. In the colloid follicle iodide is oxidized to a very reactive form of that links to tyrosine residues of TG. This process is called **organification** and is mediated by the enzyme thyroperoxidase (TPO). Organification generates monoiodotyrosine (MIT) and diiodotyrosine (DIT) residues within TG. Next, in a process called **conjugation** TPO mediates the coupling of these iodinated tyrosine residues to form thyroid hormones. MIT and DIT are linked forming either triiodothyroxine (T3) which is an active thyroid hormone or reverse triiodothyroxine (rT3), an inactive form. When two DITs link together then thyroxine (T4) is formed. Each TG molecule contains 10-20 times more T4 than T3 and similarly higher proportions of T4 are eventually released into the circulation. From the colloid in the follicular lumen thyroglobulin containing thyroid hormones is taken back into thyroid follicle cells by endocytosis and after proteolysis T4, T3 and rT3 are released into the systemic circulation.

Antithyroid drugs, such as carbimazole and propylthiouracil, inhibit enzymes involved in thyroid hormone synthesis. Lithium inhibits the release of thyroid hormone and has been used as an adjunct to radioactive iodine treatment for thyroid cancer to increase the intracellular concentration of radioactive iodine.

Table 1 Physiologic effects of thyroid hormones

- Metabolic
  - Increases basal metabolic rate
    Increases heat production
  - Increases oxygen consumption
  - Increases sensitivity to catecholamines
    Increase lipolysis
    Increase gluconeogenesis
    Increase glycogenolysis
- Development
  - Essential for normal musculoskeletal growth
  - Essential for normal brain development of foetus and newborn
    Synaptogenesis
    Neuronal maturation
    Myelination
    Cell migration
- Specific organ system effects
  - Cardiovascular system
    Increase heart rate
    Increase contractility
    Increase cardiac output
    Increase vasodilation
  - Central nervous system
    Anxiety
    Restlessness
  - Reproductive system
    Essential for fertility

Circulating Thyroid Hormones

More than 99% of circulating T4 and T3 is protein bound. Most (75%) T4 and T3 is bound to thyroid binding globulin (TBG). Another 15% is bound to thyroid binding prealbumin (TBPA) and the final 10% is bound to albumin. Only 0.02% of circulating T4 and 0.4% of circulating T3 is free (not protein bound) and biologically active. The large proportion of T4 and T3 bound to proteins and variable amounts of binding proteins explains why measurements of total thyroxine can be misleading. For example, pregnancy and oral contraceptives increase the synthesis of binding proteins and result in higher levels of total of T4 and T3 but normal free T4 and T3 levels. The higher percentage of bound T4 explains its longer half-life (7 days) compared to T3 (12–24 h) as the bound form is protected from cellular uptake and metabolism.

Cellular Effects of Thyroid Hormones

Thyroid hormones effect almost every cell in the body. Thyroid hormones (both T3 and T4) enter cells by several carrier mediated processes rather than simple diffusion. Many cell types have unique thyroid hormone transporters. The ratio of intracellular T4 to T3 is controlled by the enzymes that generate T3 from T4. Once inside cells T4 is either converted to the active T3 by tissue specific 5′-deiodinases (DI) or else metabolized to inactive forms. All these enzymes require selenium for their action, hence lack of selenium leads to abnormal thyroid function. The balance between the activating and deactivating enzyme systems can change intracellular levels of active thyroid hormone. For example, during intense stress a decrease in deiodinase activity and an increase in T4 deactivating enzyme activity will decrease intracellular T3 and lead to a lower metabolic rate in target cells. Within cells, T3 binds to nuclear thyroid receptors (TR) to act with thyroid responsive elements (TRE) at promoter sites of target genes. This process induces enhancement or inhibition of target gene expression and produces the physiologic effects of the thyroid hormone (Table 1).

Control of Thyroid Function by TSH

Thyroid stimulating hormone (TSH) is a glycoprotein secreted by pituitary thyrocytes through a negative feedback loop with T4/T3 levels (Fig. 1.6). The control cascade starts with TRH (thyrotropin releasing hormone) produced in the paraventricular nucleus of the hypothalamus and released through the hypothalamic–pituitary circulation to reach the anterior pituitary. In the pituitary TRH stimulates the thyrotroph cells to produce TSH that is released into the systemic circulation. Circulating TSH acts on specific TSH receptors on follicular cell membranes and stimulates adenylate cyclase to produce cyclic AMP, leading to increased activity of NIS that stimulates iodine uptake and also leading to increased activity of intracellular enzymes involved in thyroid hormone synthesis resulting in increased synthesis of TG and increased iodination of tyrosine resides on TG. Persistent elevated TSH levels lead to an increase in the size of the gland.

Mutations in TSH receptor structure can lead to autonomous stimulation and a toxic adenoma, also known as a Plummer's adenoma. This unregulated production of thyroid hormone suppresses TSH secretion. The overactive nodule is able to incorporate iodine tracer without the need for circulating TSH and appears "hot" on an I^{123} scan, while the rest of the gland does not incorporate iodine tracer since NIS activity is absent when TSH is suppressed and it appears "cold". Activating autoantibodies against the TSH receptors are present in Graves's disease and lead to unregulated thyroid hormone secretion and hyperthyroidism (see Chap. 2).

Calcitonin

Calcitonin is a 32-amino acid peptide secreted from parafollicular C cells in response to rising serum calcium levels. Calcitonin decreases osteoclast activity and bone resorption, decreases gastrointestinal absorption of calcium and increases renal excretion of calcium. All of these actions tend to decrease serum calcium and explain the physiological rationale for using calcitonin to treat osteoporosis, Paget's disease of bone, and hypercalcemia although there is limited clinical efficacy. The role of calcitonin in human biology remains unclear. There are no known ill effects or impact on calcium homeostasis of either low calcitonin levels or very high levels seen in patients with medullary thyroid carcinoma. Calcitonin belongs to a larger group of related peptides, the calcitonin family peptides, that have a wide variety of effects in the brain and gastrointestinal tract that are still being characterized.

References

1. de Escobar GM, Obregón MJ, del Rey FE. Maternal thyroid hormones early in pregnancy and fetal brain development. Best Pract Res Clin Endocrinol Metab. 2004;18:225–48.
2. Fagman H, Nilsson M. Morphogenesis of the thyroid gland. Mol Cell Endocrinol. 2010;323:35–54.
3. Kouniavsky G, Zeiger MA. Thyroid tumorigenesis and molecular markers in thyroid cancer. Curr Opin Oncol. 2010;22(1):23–9.
4. Liu Z, Hou P, Ji M, Guan H, Studeman K, Jensen K, Vasko V, El-Naggar AK, Xing M. Highly prevalent genetic alterations in receptor tyrosine kinases and phosphatidylinositol 3-kinase/akt and mitogen-activated protein kinase pathways in anaplastic and follicular thyroid cancers. Clin Endocrinol Metab. 2008;93(8):3106–16.
5. Sistrunk WE. The surgical treatment of cysts of the thyroglossal tract. Ann Surg. 1920;71:121–4.
6. Thomusch O, Sekulla C, Walls GV, Machens A, Dralle H. Intraoperative neuromonitoring of surgery for benign goiter. Am J Surg. 2002;183:673–8.
7. Brauckhoff M, Walls GV, Brauckhoff K, Thanh PN, Thomusch O, Dralle H. Identification of the non-recurrent inferior laryngeal nerve using intraoperative neurostimulation. Langenbeck's Arch Surg. 2002;386:482–7.

8. Dunhill TP. Removal of intrathoracic tumours by the trans-sternal route. Br J Surg. 1922;10:4–14.
9. Friedman M, LoSavio P, Ibrahim H. Superior laryngeal nerve identification and preservation in thyroidectomy. Arch Otolaryngol Head Neck Surg. 2002;128:296–303.
10. Cernea CC, Ferraz AR, Nishio S, Dutra A, Hojaij FC, dos Santos LRM. Surgical anatomy of the external branch of the superior laryngeal nerve. Head and Neck. 1992;14(5):380–3.
11. Kandil E, Abdelghanis S, Friedlander P, Alrasheedi S, Bellows CF, Slakey D. Motor and sensory branching of the recurrent laryngeal nerve in thyroid surgery. Surgery. 2011;150(6):1222–7.
12. Serpill JW, Yeung MJ, Grodski S. The motor fibers of the recurrent laryngeal nerve are located in the anterior extralaryngeal branch. Ann Surg. 2009;294 (4):648–52.

Hyperthyroidism

2

Betty Panayota Messazos, Radu Mihai
and Fiona Jane Ryan

This chapter reviews the pathophysiology, clinical manifestations, diagnosis and treatment of hyperthyroidism. Hyperthyroidism has multiple and often dramatic clinical manifestations because thyroid hormones control the basal metabolic rate, affect cardiovascular function by increasing the sensitivity of beta-receptors to catecholamines, and profoundly influence growth, sexual maturation, and neurological and cognitive development [1, 2]. "Hyperthyroidism" refers to excessive activity of the thyroid gland resulting in overproduction of thyroid hormones while "thyrotoxicosis" describes the clinical features of the hypermetabolic state associated with excess levels of circulating free thyroid hormones. In practice, the two terms are often used less precisely and interchangeably. There are several challenges in the diagnosis and management of hyperthyroidism in children including biological, psychosocial, and environmental issues [3, 4]. However, despite these challenges the vast majority of pediatric patients with hyperthyroidism have an excellent prognosis.

Pathophysiology

A brief review of the normal mechanisms of thyroid hormone production, control and action is necessary before considering the abnormal state of hyperthyroidism. Please see Chap. 1 for further details.

Thyroid hormone production depends on an adequate supply of iodine. Dietary inorganic iodide is absorbed by the intestine into the circulation and then actively transported into follicular cells by an iodide transporter, the iodide pump (sodium iodide symporter or NIS, a transmembrane glycoprotein), that efficiently concentrates iodide in the thyroid gland. Then via a process called organification, thyroid peroxidase converts iodide into reactive iodine that is incorporated into tyrosine residues in the thyroglobulin molecule forming either monoiodothyronine (MIT) or diiodothyronine (DIT). These iodinated tyrosines are then coupled. MIT may combine with DIT to form triiodothyronine (T3) or its isomer, reverse T3, or two DITs can combine to form tetraiodothyronine (T4 or thyroxine). T3, reverse T3, and T4 remain attached to thyroglobulin that is stored in the follicular lumen. Thyroglobulin returns to the follicular cell by endocytosis and in the follicular

B.P. Messazos
Department of Paediatric Endocrinology, Oxford Children's Hospital, Oxford University Hospitals NHS Trust, Headley Way, Headington, Oxford OX39DU, UK
e-mail: betty.messazos@rch.org.au

R. Mihai
Department of Surgery, John Radcliffe Hospital, Oxford OX3 9DU, UK
e-mail: radumihai@doctors.org.uk; radu.mihai@ouh.nhs.uk

F.J. Ryan (✉)
Department of Paediatric Endocrinology, Oxford Children's Hospital, Headley Way, Headington, Oxford OX3 9DU, UK
e-mail: fiona.ryan@ouh.nhs.uk

D.J. Ledbetter and P.R.V. Johnson (eds.), *Endocrine Surgery in Children*,
DOI 10.1007/978-3-662-54256-9_2

cell free T3 (fT3) and free T4 (fT4) are cleaved from thyroglobulin by hydrolysis and released into the circulation. T3 is the active form of thyroid hormone and is 3 or 4 times more potent than T4 [1].

The synthesis of T4 and T3 is controlled by a complex feedback mechanism influenced by stimulatory and inhibitory factors via the hypothalamic–pituitary–thyroid axis. Thyrotrophin-releasing hormone (TRH) is secreted by the hypothalamus and stimulates the anterior pituitary gland to secrete thyroid stimulating hormone (TSH). Circulating TSH binds to specific TSH receptors on thyroid follicular cells. The TSH receptor is a G-protein coupled receptor and activates thyroid hormone production via a second messenger system, ultimately leading to the release of T4 and a lesser amount of T3. Raised circulating levels of T3 act as a negative feedback stimulus for the hypothalamus and anterior pituitary, resulting in decreased TSH production [5].

All T4 is produced by the thyroid gland but 85% of T3 is derived from peripheral conversion of T4 to T3 by deiodination. Most of the T3 and T4 circulating in the blood is bound to transport proteins such as thyroxine binding globulin (TBG) and albumin and only a small amount is unbound and biologically active. T3 and T4 act by binding to receptors in peripheral tissues. T3 acts by binding to nuclear receptors and regulates the transcription of various cellular proteins that affect metabolism. Any process that causes an increase in the peripheral circulation of unbound thyroid hormone can cause signs and symptoms of hyperthyroidism. Disturbances of the normal homeostatic mechanism can occur at the level of the pituitary gland, the thyroid gland, or in the periphery. Regardless of aetiology, the result is an increase in transcription in cellular proteins causing an increase in the basal metabolic rate and the other effects of hyperthyroidism.

Aetiology and Incidence

More than 95% of children and adolescents with thyrotoxicosis suffer from Graves' disease [6]. The aetiology is still unclear but a likely combination of hereditary, immunological and environmental factors. Other rare conditions that cause hyperthyroidism in childhood are listed in Table 2.1 [5, 7–9].

Graves' disease is caused by thyroid stimulating immunoglobulins that activate TSH receptors on thyroid follicular cells resulting in thyroid hormone overproduction. Note that the clinical aspects of this syndrome, including the

Table 2.1 Causes of hyperthyroidism in children

• Graves' disease (95% of cases)
• Thyroiditis
– Chronic lymphocytic thyroiditis (Hashimoto's thyroiditis)—transient
– Subacute thyroiditis
• Autoimmune neonatal thyrotoxicosis (placental passage of maternal thyroid hormone receptor antibodies)—transient
• Autonomous functioning lesions
– Toxic thyroid adenoma
– Activating mutation of the TSH receptor gene
– Activating mutation of Gsα (McCune–Albright syndrome)
– Hyperfunctioning papillary or follicular carcinoma
• Isolated pituitary resistance to thyroid hormone
• TSH secreting pituitary adenoma
• Exogenous causes
– Excessive thyroid hormone replacement therapy
– Iodine induced hyperthyroidism

goitre, ophthalmopathy, and palpitations were described in the late eighteenth and early nineteenth centuries independently by several physicians from Great Britain and continental Europe including Parry, Graves, Basedow and Flajani. All of their names, either singly or in various combinations, have been attached to this common clinical condition. We will use the name "Graves' disease" because it is commonly recognised in the English medical literature.

Although Graves' disease is common in adults it is uncommon in children with a frequency of 0.1–3 per 100,000 children [10]. The incidence increases throughout childhood, with the peak incidence in children aged 10–15 years. The majority (60%) of patients being postpubertal [11]. As with most autoimmune diseases, Graves' disease in children is more common in girls than boys, at a ratio of 5–6:1 [12]. Other causes of hyperthyroidism do not show a male or female preponderance. For example, the hyperthyroidism of McCune–Albright syndrome is not more common in girls even though the associated precocious puberty is more common in girls than in boys [13].

Graves' disease is often associated with other autoimmune diseases and there is often a strong family history of thyroid and non-thyroid autoimmune problems [14] such as systemic lupus erythematous, rheumatoid arthritis, myasthenia gravis, vitiligo, immune thrombocytopenic purpura, and pernicious anaemia. In addition, there are several lines of evidence suggesting a genetic component or predisposition to the disease. Some studies suggest that up to 80% of the susceptibility to Graves' is determined by genetic factors [9]. Graves' disease has been linked with human leukocyte antigen (HLA)-B8 and (HLA)-DR3 and with abnormalities in chromosomes 6p21 and 2q33 [15]. It is also more common in children with Trisomy 21 [16]. Overall, genetic susceptibility is thought to have a polygenic inheritance, although monozygotic twin studies suggest interplay between environmental and genetic factors.

Evaluation

The diagnosis of hyperthyroidism is often challenging due to the large spectrum of physical and psychological complaints [17]. However, a focused history and physical examination can usually select patients for lab tests and imaging studies that will confirm the diagnosis. The following discussion of the evaluation of patients with hyperthyroidism will focus on Graves' disease and only briefly mention the other rare causes of hyperthyroidism in children.

History

The symptoms of Graves' disease in children and adolescents can develop insidiously over months but can also have an abrupt onset. The most common symptoms are behaviour changes such as increased anxiety and hyperactivity. These symptoms are often similar to those of attention deficit hyperactivity disorder (ADHD), [18] and a high degree of clinical suspicion is necessary to pursue the diagnosis of Graves' disease in this situation. Individuals with Graves' disease invariably have an altered mental status with increased irritability, emotional lability, and outbursts which understandably create distress for themselves and their families. Other early symptoms of hyperthyroidism in children include deterioration of school performance and changes in handwriting.

Children with hyperthyroidism may fatigue easily and this usually manifests as exercise intolerance. In severe cases they may have difficulty climbing up stairs as a result of muscle weakness. Sleep disturbances are common as is weight loss despite a good appetite. Hyperthyroidism can also cause idiopathic intracranial hypertension (also known as benign intracranial hypertension or pseudotumor cerebri) in children and present with headache and even nausea and vomiting [19]. Symptoms of hyperthyroidism caused by autonomic nervous system disturbances include tremor, heat intolerance, sweating, diarrhoea and palpitations. In girls, menstrual cycle irregularities, including amenorrhoea, are common symptoms. Finally, parents may report that the child has a growth spurt that results from the increased height velocity associated with hyperthyroidism [20].

In addition to hyperthyroidism, Graves' disease may be associated with eye abnormalities that are the result of autoimmune attack of soft tissue in the orbit. The full array of signs and symptoms in Graves' ophthalmopathy describes the triad of exophthalmos, chemosis and diplopia. Patients may complain of persistent visual blurring secondary to optic neuropathy or severe eye pain secondary to corneal ulceration. When these symptoms of congestive ophthalmopathy are present then urgent referral to an ophthalmologist for an eye assessment is necessary. Compared to adults, thyroid eye disease is usually mild in children.

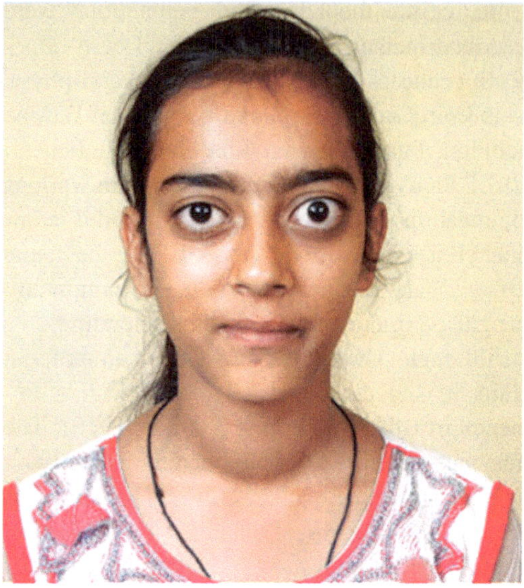

Fig. 2.1 A 14-year-old girl with Graves' disease who had diffuse goitre and asymmetrical proptosis (From Bhansali et al. [47], with permission.)

Physical Examination

Vital signs of children with hyperthyroidism usually reveal tachycardia and less commonly hypertension. Height and weight are important to evaluate because hyperthyroidism may cause increased linear growth velocity and weight loss. General examination may reveal sweatiness, facial flushing, a tremor or, rarely, choreiform movements [21]. Further to the symptoms described above the eye signs such as eyelid retraction, proptosis, periorbital oedema, optic neuropathy, corneal ulceration, and rarely ophthalmoplegia may be present in Graves' disease (Fig. 2.1). Importantly, the eye changes sometimes present before signs of thyrotoxicosis. All children with Graves' disease should be referred to ophthalmology for formal assessment since the eye findings may be subtle but potentially serious.

Pubertal stage should be assessed as part of the evaluation of associated menstrual irregularity and to evaluate the uncommon possibility of McCune–Albright syndrome which could present with precocious puberty and cafe au lait pigmentation. Additional skin signs of Graves' disease include the uncommon finding of pretibial myxoedema which represents an unusual autoimmune dermopathy.

The examination of the neck for thyroid abnormalities is essential in the assessment of hyperthyroidism. A goitre or diffuse enlargement of the thyroid is almost always present in Graves' disease even though it may not have been noticed by the patient or family. Thyroid nodules are less commonly present. Examination of the thyroid is usually done with the neck slightly extended. Swallowing will elicit movement of the thyroid and potentially clarify the identity of a midline neck swelling. Examination of the thyroid is often best performed by standing behind the patient. As with any swelling or mass, evaluation and description of a thyroid goitre or nodule's size, site, symmetry, consistency and tenderness is essential. The increased blood flow to a hyperfunctioning thyroid sometimes results in a thyroid bruit.

Laboratory Tests

In the evaluation of hyperthyroidism the pivotal investigation is to measure thyroid function tests

—particularly the TSH, fT4 and fT3. In primary hyperthyroidism, when the thyroid gland is producing excessive thyroid hormones, TSH is suppressed and fT4 and fT3 are elevated. In addition, there is preferential conversion of fT4 to fT3 so usually the fT3 will be relatively more elevated. In contrast to the low TSH in primary or thyroid hyperthyroidism, the TSH is elevated in secondary or pituitary hyperthyroidism when there is production of TSH from the pituitary that is not responsive to the normal control mechanisms. When evaluating and managing hyperthyroidism fT3 and fT4 are usually better tests than total T3 and total T4 because total T3 and total T4 measure the much larger pool of protein-bound thyroid hormones in addition to the unbound, free forms. Therefore measurement of total T3 and T4 may be misleading in situations with abnormal serum protein levels or when there are changes in protein binding. Free T3 is relatively more important than free T4 in the diagnosis of hyperthyroidism since fT3 rises before fT4 in thyrotoxicosis. Rarely the fT4 levels can be normal but the fT3 is raised in "T3-toxicosis".

Other thyroid tests can confirm the aetiology of hyperthyroidism. The diagnosis of Graves' disease can be confirmed by the detection of stimulatory TSH receptor antibodies. Thyroid peroxidase antibodies are elevated in autoimmune thyroiditis that may present with hyperthyroidism as well as the more common presentation of hypothyroidism. Graves' disease may also have thyroid ophthalmological immunoglobulin associated with eye signs and thyroid growth immunoglobulins associated with thyroid enlargement.

Other Investigations

Although history, physical examination and thyroid function tests are the critical components of the evaluation of hyperthyroidism other imaging investigations are occasionally useful. Thyroid ultrasound can be useful to confirm the suspicion of a diffuse thyroid goitre and screen for thyroid nodules. See Chap. 3 for further discussion of the evaluation and management of thyroid nodules.

Radioactive iodine (RAI) uptake and scanning may be used when the aetiology of hyperthyroidism is still unclear after laboratory evaluation. In Graves' disease, RAI uptake is elevated and the scan shows diffuse uptake.

Management

Current treatment options include antithyroid medications that block thyroid hormone production and radioactive iodine and thyroidectomy that eliminate thyroid hormone producing follicular cells. None of the current treatment options are ideal and there is controversy regarding the best therapy for children with hyperthyroidism. In view of the lack of clinical trials to guide treatment decisions, our current opinion is to tailor treatment based on the individual patient's needs while considering the risks and benefits of each treatment [22]. Medical treatment is the first option for treating hyperthyroidism and maybe the only treatment necessary. It is rare that children require hospital admission at diagnosis, however, if there are marked hyperdynamic cardiovascular symptoms then admission maybe necessary until beta-blockers have controlled these symptoms. Two-thirds of patients relapse following medical treatment and in these individuals, radioiodine or surgery are the second-line options [21]. The outcome from both is excellent. Although the patient will be hypothyroid and need lifelong thyroxine treatment this is easy to manage and results in clinically euthyroid individuals. The risk of relapse decreases with a longer primary course of antithyroid medication [9].

Despite the management challenges, prognosis in the majority of children with hyperthyroidism is good when treatment is timely and appropriate [23]. It is important to remember that long-term consequences of hyperthyroidism can result from both the disease and the treatment used [2]. Stratifying patients according to risk of relapse after medical management with antithyroid medication by identifying predictive factors early has led to improvement in overall management. Factors include young age, severity of hyperthyroidism at diagnosis and the presence or absence of other autoimmune conditions are important to consider.

Medical Management

If the individual is very symptomatic then propranolol (or another beta blocker) is used to control the symptoms of sympathetic overdrive, such as tremor and tachycardia, until definitive therapy. Propranolol is usually begun orally at 0.25–0.5 mg/kg/dose, two to four times daily and the dose is titrated for symptom relief. Propranolol can be stopped when the thyroid hormone levels fall into the normal range. Propranolol should be avoided in patients with asthma but a more selective beta-blocker can be used in this circumstance.

Antithyroid drugs are usually considered first-line treatment of hyperthyroidism in children [24]. Antithyroid drugs are known as thionamides and include propylthiouracil (PTU), carbimazole and the active metabolite methimazole. They inhibit thyroid hormone synthesis by interfering with the organification process by which iodine attaches to the tyrosine moieties in thyroglobulin, i.e. the thyroid peroxidase mediated iodination. PTU and methimazole are available in the United States and much of the rest of the world. Methimazole is preferred to PTU because PTU is associated with a risk of severe liver damage (PTU induced hepatitis) and production of cytoplasmic anti-neutrophil autoantibodies. Antibody-positive vasculitis is exceptionally rare. PTU can block the conversion of T4 to T3 whereas methimazole cannot [9, 25]. The United States Food and Drug Administration (FDA) recommend that PTU should be used in children only if other treatment options are unavailable. Another antithyroid drug is carbimazole. Carbimazole is metabolised by the patient into methimazole. Carbimazole is widely used in the United Kingdom, Europe, and the countries of the former British Commonwealth. Carbimazole, methimazole and propylthiouracil have side effects that range in severity from a transient rash to agranulocytosis and neutropenia. Allergic-type reactions with fever, rash, urticaria, gastrointestinal symptoms and arthralgia occur in 1–5% of patients. These reactions are usually transient and can be treated with antihistamines without discontinuing therapy. Agranulocytosis and neutropenia is a rare but serious side effect. Although it is not necessary to check regular complete blood counts it is important to communicate to the family and child that they should immediately report symptoms of easy bruising, sore throat, mouth ulcers, or fever and a complete blood count performed urgently to ensure immunocompetency. It is important to provide the family with verbal and written instructions that specify what symptoms mandate urgent reporting and the need to stop medications. Clear documentation of these discussions and instructions is essential. Even when the patient suffers a serious side effect of an antithyroid drug it is often possible to switch to an alternative antithyroid drug with careful monitoring.

The recommended dose of carbimazole for children less than 12 years is 0.25 mg/kg/dose three times per day. For children between 12 and 18 years the dose is 10 mg three times per day. The dose for propylthiouracil is 25 mg three times per day for children 1–5 years, 50 mg three times per day for children 5–12 years and 100 mg three times per day for adolescents 12–18 years. The conversion between these two antithyroid drugs is 1 mg of carbimazole equates to approximately 10 mg of propylthiouracil.

There are two main antithyroid drug treatment strategies, (1) block and replacement or (2) dose titration. In block and replacement the thyroid gland is first “blocked” or “switched off” with antithyroid drugs, suppressing T4 and T3 and rendering the patient virtually hypothyroid. The “block” is accomplished using relatively higher doses of any of the antithyroid drugs. With this strategy it usually takes 2 weeks or more of treatment before the patient becomes euthyroid. When T4 and T3 levels have fallen and stimulate the patient’s TSH into the normal range then “replacement” with exogenous thyroxine commences. Some of the possible advantages of the "block and replace" regimen include having less blood tests, improved stability and possibly higher remission rates [5, 26–28]. The higher doses of antithyroid drugs used in "block and replacement therapy" provides better control of thyroid hyperfunction and may be responsible for a higher remission rate. Compliance with taking the needed thyroxine replacement can be increased by direct observation of treatment by parents or providing a pill box. The best routine with the most effective pharmacokinetic action is to take thyroxine in the morning on an empty stomach.

The second antithyroid drug strategy is "dose titration therapy" which uses lower doses of antithyroid drugs so that within 1–2 months of starting antithyroid treatment the fT4 and fT3 fall and the TSH remains suppressed. When fT3 and fT4 are within the lower half of the normal range, which can take up to 3 months with this option, the antithyroid drug dose is reduced and "titrated" to keep the fT3 and fT4 in the normal range without the need for exogenous thyroxine treatment. A potential advantage of the "dose titration" strategy may be better compliance with the monotherapy of an antithyroid drug alone rather than an antithyroid drug and thyroid hormone replacement. In addition, the lower doses of antithyroid drugs may result in fewer side effects. More blood tests may be necessary in the "titration" phase and this is a disadvantage of the dose titration therapy, especially in children.

It is not clear which treatment strategy is superior. Part of the controversy exists due to the variability of patient response to antithyroid drugs and the limited data available about definitive therapy in prepubertal children [29]. A recent study reports that the relapse risk was higher for children of nonwhite ethnic origin with high serum levels of TSH receptor autoantibodies and T4 at diagnosis. However, children who were older at disease onset and had a longer duration of antithyroid treatment had a lower relapse risk [29, 30]. Ongoing trials by the British Society of Paediatric Endocrinology and Diabetes may provide information as to the ideal method of antithyroid drug treatment of Graves's disease in children.

Antithyroid drugs have been associated with a lower remission rate in children with Graves' disease compared to adults and a longer duration of therapy is required in prepubertal patients [11]. Treatment with antithyroid drugs should be for a minimum of 2 years as this has been shown to decrease the risk of relapse [9, 31]. Most clinicians report a remission rate of less than 25%, with approximately two-thirds of patients relapsing either on treatment or after stopping treatment. The decision to stop antithyroid drug treatment is planned around the age and particular circumstances of a patient. It should not be stopped in adolescents going through puberty or during important exam times in their life. A cautious reduction of treatment and close monitoring over summer holidays is recommended. Once relapsed, individuals will need further medical management to regain control before definitive treatment is undertaken with radioactive iodine or surgery [24].

Methods identifying the likelihood of remission would greatly improve patient management [9, 32]. There are very few studies evaluating the long-term outcome of the relationship between duration of antithyroid treatment and remission rates. Some studies have evaluated age, goitre size, severity of hyperthyroidism at onset measured by thyroid hormone receptor antibodies (TRAb) levels at onset and at end of antithyroid treatment as well as duration of treatment as predictive markers of Graves' relapse. Absence of goitre at diagnosis is associated with better outcome. TRAb levels which normalise within a year are also predictive of positive outcome as well as levels that are less than 2.5 times the upper reference limit at diagnosis [33]. A recent multicentre study has shown that serum TRAb levels are a sensitive, specific and reproducible biomarker for pediatric Graves' and that is correlates well with disease severity [34]. Furthermore, recent studies have concluded that antithyroid medication could be offered up to 10 years before definitive management in cases with good compliance and with no major adverse effects secondary to antithyroid medication. [9] Regardless of the mode of treatment it does not seem to impact on the health associated quality of life. However, this would be important to study specifically in children in order to evaluate the emotional, behavioural and neuropsychological long-term outcomes. Certainly large prospective randomised trials in children would address these management dilemmas.

Radioactive Iodine Treatment

Radioactive iodine therapy is increasingly viewed as a safe and effective treatment in the management of hyperthyroidism in children [6, 28, 35–37]. The goal of radioiodine treatment is to ablate thyroid follicular cells to the extent that results in the patient becoming hypothyroid [15]. There have always been concerns around giving radioiodine therapy to children due to the long-term risk of thyroid cancer and certainly there are rare cases. However, thyroid cancer is also more common in patients with untreated Graves' disease so the magnitude of risk after radioiodine treatment is unclear. Radioiodine is not considered first-line treatment in paediatrics but reserved for children who either relapse while being treated with antithyroid drugs or following discontinuation of antithyroid drugs. It is also indicated for individuals who cannot tolerate antithyroid drugs or who will not comply with the prescribed treatment. The cure rate for radioiodine is up to 50% and the incidence of hypothyroidism around 40% [35]. The efficacy of radioiodine therapy is dose related. High cure rates without an associated higher risk of thyroid cancer are reported when using appropriate doses of radioiodine. Due to the theoretical risk of thyroid cancer in children treated with radioiodine, it is considered best to use a high dose of radioiodine in order to minimise the thyroid tissue that remains and is at long-term risk of neoplastic change. It has been shown that at least 300 microCi/g are needed in order to ensure ablation of thyroid tissue [2, 37]. In 85–90% of patients, a single dose of radioiodine is sufficient to cure hyperthyroidism but even when a moderately high initial dose of radioiodine is used a second dose maybe necessary [36]. Of 48 patients treated with radioiodine, 89% became hypothyroid after the initial dose, whilst the remaining 11% needed a second dose. [15].

In the United Kingdom, only patients over 10 years of age are generally offered radioiodine treatment. In circumstances of significant eye involvement radioiodine is not recommended because it may cause marked deterioration although this is not a universal observation [36]. Long-term follow-up studies have been reassuring so far but more are required.

Surgical Management of Hyperthyroidism

Indications for Operative Management of Hyperthyroidism

Thyroidectomy as treatment for hyperthyroidism is generally indicated when there is failure of medical therapy, intolerance of medical treatment (such as adverse drug reactions), severe thyrotoxicosis, severe ophthalmopathy, large glands producing obstructive or compressive symptoms, coexistence of a thyroid nodule, or patient preference. As mentioned previously, radioactive iodine is not indicated in children younger than 10 years of age so those patients should be referred for surgical treatment. An important additional benefit of surgical treatment is that it can allow for detection and treatment of clinically occult malignancies that may coexist in up to 5% of children [38].

Access to thyroid surgery for children is limited because of a vicious cycle. Most surgeons have limited experience since few children are referred for thyroidectomy and physicians are reluctant to refer children for thyroidectomy because they unlikely to have access to a surgical unit with sufficient experience. For example, the national audit maintained by the British Association of Endocrine and Thyroid Surgeons (http://www.baets.org.uk) showed that 52 surgeons performed 151 thyroid operations in children <17 years, with only 6 surgeons performing more than five such operations over the lifetime of the database. In the financial year 2009 only seven thyroidectomies for Graves' disease in children were recorded. Though these data might be incomplete, it is undoubted that most surgeons rarely perform thyroidectomy for Graves' disease in children. This has a negative impact on availability of this service and partially explains the reticence to recommend surgery in these patients.

Preoperative Preparation

All patients undergoing thyroidectomy for hyperthyroidism have to be fully controlled on medication and biochemically euthyroid at the time of the operation. Those who do not tolerate antithyroid drugs (e.g. those with agranulocytosis induced by carbimazole) can be controlled acutely using high dose iodine (either from Lugol solution or from potassium iodine) for 7–10 days before proceeding with the operation. Beta-blockers (e.g. propranolol) can also be added to control the heart rate and decrease the peripheral conversion of T3 in T4. The operation must be done in a narrow time-window because the acute inhibition of the thyroid with iodine fails after 10–14 days and a severe, rebound thyrotoxicosis can ensue.

Perioperative Anaesthesia Considerations

The current medical practice of good preoperative medical control of thyrotoxicosis has eliminated the much feared perioperative complication of "thyroid storm". Routine monitoring of cardiac rhythm is maintained during the perioperative period but it is unlikely to demonstrate severe changes during the procedure.

There is increasing evidence that the use of an endotracheal tube with electrodes touching the vocal cords may be beneficial. Such tubes allow the use of intraoperative nerve monitoring (IONM), whereby during the operation the surgeon has the possibility of using a stimulating electrode to demonstrate normal conductibility of the current through the recurrent laryngeal nerve (RLN). Guidelines and standards for the use of IONM have been published and can easily be adopted in children. In short, the vagus nerve is identified at the beginning of the procedure and successful stimulation of the vagus nerve demonstrates that the circuit is functional. Thereafter, any anatomical structure thought to be the RLN during the dissection may be stimulated to test for RLN function. At the end of the procedure, the vagus is stimulated once more to check whether the latency or amplitude of the current has changed (i.e. whether there is any electrophysiological evidence of injury to the nerve).

Choice of Operation for Hyperthyroidism

There is an on-going debate on which surgical procedure provides best outcomes for children with Graves' disease. Total thyroidectomy is the preferred surgical treatment for Graves' disease in adults in the United Kingdom. Those who favour total thyroidectomy argue that it is the only operation that essentially eliminates the risk of relapse and has an increased efficacy in patients with severe ophthalmopathy [39]. The fact that it leads to permanent hypothyroidism which requires a lifelong replacement therapy is of minimal medical and financial consequence in the western world. In areas of the world where access to medication is limited the argument will be different.

Subtotal thyroidectomy has fewer advocates but is the standard treatment of thyrotoxicosis in Japan. It can be performed either as a bilateral subtotal resection (bilateral remnants of $\sim$3 g) or lobectomy plus subtotal lobectomy (Dunhill procedure, unilateral remnant of $\sim$5–7 g). Some suggest the remnant size of 3–4 g provides an optimal balance between low relapse rate (4% recurrence after 2–3 years) and acceptable complication rate in both pediatric and adult population [40]. The argument against subtotal resection is the high risk of recurrence of hyperthyroidism ranging between 1.2 and 16.2% (9) to 30% [41]. Though similar comparative studies have not been undertaken in children, one can safely assume that subtotal thyroidectomies in children would have an even higher risk of recurrent disease compared with adults. Near-total thyroidectomy with a total thyroid remnant of 2–4 g may minimise risk of relapse and at the same time may prevent permanent hypothyroidism.

Most published series report the results of traditional thyroidectomy and there is minimal data available on minimally invasive video-assisted thyroidectomy (MIVAT) in children. In a small study of children undergoing MIVAT, the cosmetic results were better and postoperative recovery was shorter than after open thyroidectomy and no complications were recorded [42] but this technique is seldom available. No reports have been published regarding the use of robotic transaxillary thyroidectomy in children.

Whatever the surgical approach is, there is evidence that an individual surgeon's experience is associated with of better treatment outcomes. Higher volumes of thyroidectomies performed result in lower complication rates and shorter hospital stay [43] therefore it seems reasonable to refer this group of patients to national referral centres where surgeons with adequate level of experience can deal with this relatively rare condition.

Postoperative Care

Patients should be able to drink fluids immediately after surgery. Patients with RLN injury may have difficulty swallowing and are at risk for aspiration so when there is a clinical suspicion of RLN injury they should be observed when attempting to drink water for the first time after the operation.

Development of a neck haematoma that can lead to airway compromise is the most severe complication of thyroidectomy. The risk is highest in the first 6 h postoperatively but it remains a possible risk for the first 24 h. Close monitoring by nursing staff and early assessment and treatment by clinicians with appropriate experience is mandatory. Most such haematomas can be dealt with conservatively but some require emergency removal of the sutures and return to the operating theatre for evacuation of haematoma and control of bleeding.

The morning after the operation calcium and PTH levels should be checked. If hypocalcaemia is present (<2.0 mmol/l) or if patient is symptomatic, oral calcium supplements should be instituted. It is desirable to avoid development of severe hypocalcaemia that needs administration of intravenous calcium.

Voice should be assessed within few weeks after the operation. If there are changes suggestive of laryngeal nerve injury, further evaluation is necessary and referral to a specialised voice clinic may be beneficial.

Results of Thyroidectomy for Hyperthyroidism

Published series from the Mayo Clinic (1986–2003, 78 children) [44] Japan (1989–1998, 74 children) [45], Chicago (2000–2007, 12 children) [46] show no recurrent hyperthyroidism after total thyroidectomy and definite recurrence risk (4–10%) after less-than total thyroidectomy.

With the limited published data on the outcomes of treatment of children with hyperthyroidism, it is necessary to balance the pros and cons for each of the methods available to choose the treatment that is be offered to an individual patient (Table 2.2). Clinicians have to balance not only the published data and the experience of individual surgeons but also the other resources available, parent and child preferences, and the family's cultural and social beliefs. Surgeons involved in the care of these children should work as part of a multidisciplinary team that includes pediatric endocrinologists and anesthesiologists, pediatricians, nuclear medicine physicians and pathologists to afford children the best clinical outcomes.

Table 2.2 Pros and cons of methods available for treatment of Graves' disease in children (see text for details)

Treatment	Pro	Con
Antithyroid drugs	• Controls thyrotoxicosis • Ambulatory treatment • Long-term remission in up to a third of patients	• High relapse rates (60–80% long term) • Hypothyroidism • Minor side effects (25%) – Pruritus, hives, myalgia, elevated liver enzymes, leukopenia • Major side effects (0.5%) – Liver failure, bone marrow failure, death • Need for monitoring and follow-up
Radioactive iodine	• Cost effective • Ambulatory treatment • Remission rate 95% • No clear increased risk of thyroid malignancy • No increased risk of malignancy in off-spring	• No long-term follow-up data after high dose radioactive iodide • Possible increased risk of malignancy (thyroid, brain, stomach, kidney) • Potential to induce hyperparathyroidism and benign thyroid nodules • Transient hypocalcaemia (6%) • Hypothyroidism (27–92%) • Recurrent hyperthyroidism (0–40%) • Nausea and vomiting (0–12%) • Transient pain over the thyroid • Worsening ophthalmopathy • Radiation thyroiditis (0–33%)
Thyroidectomy	• Appropriate for children <5 years of age • High cure rate (97–100%) • Low complication rate, in experienced hands (1–3%) • Ophthalmopathy improvement (up to 85%) • Controls compressive symptoms • Avoids non-compliance of medical treatment • Detection of occult malignancy (up to 5%)	• Risks related to surgical expertise and experience • Higher cost • Lifelong hypothyroidism with total thyroidectomy • Risk of recurrent hyperthyroidism if less than a total thyroidectomy – 30% for subtotal thyroidectomy – 5% in near-total thyroidectomy • RLN palsy/paralysis (0–2%) • Transient hypocalcaemia (6–71%) • Permanent hypoparathyroidism (0–7%) • Neck haematoma (0.2–2%) • Keloid scar (0–12%) • Postoperative pain (100%)

References

1. Gaon P. Paediatric exams: a survival guide. 2nd ed. Elsevier: St Louis; 2005.
2. Segni M, Gorman CA. The aftermath of childhood hyperthyroidism. J Pediatr Endocrinol. 2001;14(5): 1277–82 (discussion 1297–8).
3. Amer KS. Advances in assessment, diagnosis, and treatment of hyperthyroidism in children. J Pediatr Nurs. 2005;20(2):119–26.
4. Brown RB, Huang S. The thyroid and its disorders. In: Brook C, Clayton P, Brown R, editors. Brook's clinical pediatric endocrinology. 5th ed. Hoboken: Blackwell Publishing; 2005.
5. Raine JE, Donaldson MDC, Gregory JW, et al. Practical endocrinology and diabetes in children. 2nd ed. Hoboken: Blackwell Publishing; 2006.
6. Rivkees SA, Szarfman A. Dissimilar hepatotoxicity profiles of Propylthiouracil and methimazole in children. J Clin Endocrinol Metab. 2010;95(7) (Epub 2013 July 02).
7. Acosta Gordillo L, Cormenzana Carpio M, Espino Aguilar R, et al. Toxic adenoma as cause of hyperthyroidism in childhood. Diagnosis and treatment. Rev Esp Pediatr. 2009;65(2).
8. Fisher D. Disorders of the thyroid in the newborn and the infant. In: Pediatric endocrinology, 1st ed. Saunders: Sperling; 1996.
9. Leger J, Carel JC. Hyperthyroidism in childhood: causes, when and how to treat. J Clin Res Pediatr Endocrinol. 2013;5(1):50–6.
10. Lazar L, Kalter-Leibovici O, Pertzelan A, et al. Thyrotoxicosis in prepubertal children compared with pubertal and postpubertal patients. J Clin Endocrinol Metab. 2000;85:3678–82.

11. Poyrazoğlu S, Saka N, Bas F, et al. Evaluation of diagnosis and treatment results in children with Graves' disease with emphasis on the pubertal status of patients. J Pediatr Endocrinol Metab. 2008;21 (8):745–51.
12. Lavard L, Ranlov R, Perrild H, et al. Incidence of juvenile thyrotoxicosis in Denmark, 1982–1988, a nationwide study. Eur J Endocrinol. 1994;130: 565–8.
13. Mastorakos G, Mitsiades NS, Doufas AG, et al. Hyperthyroidism in McCune-Albright syndrome with a review of thyroid abnormalities sixty years after the first report. Thyroid. 1997;1997(7):433–9.
14. Vaidya B, Kendall-Taylor P, Pearce SH. The genetics of autoimmune thyroid disease. J Clin Endocrinol Metab. 2002;87:5385–97.
15. McCormack S, Mitchell DM, Woo M. Radioactive iodine for hyperthyroidism in children and adolescents: referral rate and response to treatment. Clin Endocrinol. 2009;71(6):884–91.
16. Severinski S, Banac S, Severinski NS, et al. Epidemiology and clinical characteristics of thyroid dysfunction in children and adolescents with type 1 diabetes. Coll Antropol. 2009;33(1):273–9.
17. McKeown NJ, Tews MC, Gossain VV et al. Hyperthyroidism. Emerg Med Clin North Am. 2005; 23 (3):669–85, viii.
18. Suresh PA, Sebastian S, George A, et al. Subclinical hyperthyroidism and hyperkinetic behavior in children. Pediatr Neurol. 1999;20(3):192–4.
19. Merkenschlager A, Ehrt O, Muller-Felber W, et al. Reversible benign intracranial hypertension in a child with hyperthyroidism J Pediatr Endocrinol. 2008;21 (11):1099–101.
20. Iranmanesh A, Lizarralde G, Johnson ML, et al. Nature of altered growth hormone secretion in hyperthyroidism. J Clin Endocrinol Metab. 1991; 72:108–15.
21. Mokhashi MH, Desai U, Desai MP. Hyperthyroidism in children. Indian J Pediatr. 2000; 67(9):653–6.
22. Hung W, Sarlis NJ. Autoimmune and non-autoimmune hyperthyroidism in pediatric patients: a review and personal commentary on management. Pediatr Endocrinol Rev. 2004;2(1): 21–38.
23. Bandgar TR, Shah NS. Thyroid disorders in childhood and adolescence. J Indian Med Assoc. 2006;104(10):580–2.
24. Godoy CC, Acevedo MM, Barrera NA, et al. Hyperthyroidism in children and adolescents. Rev Chil Pediatr. 2009;80(1):21–9.
25. Rivkees SA, Szarfman A. Dissimilar hepatotoxicity profiles of propylthiouracil and methimazole in children. J Clin Endocrinol Metab. 2010;95 (7):3260–7 (Epub 02 July 2013).
26. Birrell G, Cheetham T. Juvenile thyrotoxicosis; can we do better? Arch Dis Child. 2004;89:745–50.
27. Grutters A. Treatment of Graves' disease in children and adolescents. Horm Res. 1998;49:255–7.
28. Iagaru A, McDougall R. Treatment of thyrotoxicosis. J Nucl Med. 2007;48:379–89.
29. Kaguelidou F, Alberti C, Castanet M, et al. Predictors of autoimmune hyperthyroidism relapse in children after discontinuation of antithyroid drug treatment. J Clin Endocrinol Metab. 2008;93(10): 3817–26.
30. Huang SA. Can hyperthyroidism relapse after antithyroid drug treatment be predicted in children with Graves disease? Nat Clin Pract Endocrinol Metab. 2009;5(2):74–5.
31. Lippe BM, Landaw EM, Kaplan SA. Hyperthyroidism in children treated with long term medical therapy: twenty-five percent remission every two years. J Clin Endocrinol Metab. 1987;64:1241–5.
32. Glaser NS, Styne DM. Predictors of early remission of hyperthyroidism in children. J Clin Endocrinol Metab. 1997;82:1719–26.
33. Gastaldi R, Poggi E, Mussa A, et al. Graves disease in children: thyroid-stimulating hormone receptor antibodies as remission markers. J Pediatr. 2014;164 (5):1189–94 (E pub ahead of print).
34. Diana T, Brown R, Bossowski A, et al. Clinical relevance of thyroid-stimulating autoantibodies in pediatric graves' disease—a multicentre study. J Clin Endocrinol Metab. 2014;99(5):1648–55. (Epub ahead of print).
35. Chao M, Jiawei X, Guoming W, et al. Radioiodine treatment for pediatric hyperthyroid Grave's disease. Eur J Pediatr 2009;168(10):1165–69.
36. Cheetham TD, Wraight EP, Hughes IA, et al. Radioiodine treatment of Graves' disease in young people. Horm Res. 1998;49:255–9.
37. Rivkees SA, Cornelius EA. Influence of iodine-131 dose on the outcome of hyperthyroidism in children. Pediatrics 2003;111(4 Pt 1):745–9.
38. Sherman J, Thompson GB, Lteif A, Schwenk WF II, van Heerden J, Farley DR, Kumar S, Zimmerman D, Churchward M, Grant CS. Surgical management of Graves disease in childhood and adolescence: an institutional experience. Surgery. 2006;140: 1056–62.
39. Spinelli C, Bertocchini A, Lima M, Miccoli P. Graves-Basedow's disease in children and adolescents: total vs subtotal thyroidectomy. Pediatria Medica e Chirurgica 2002;24(5):383–6.
40. Sugino K, Ito K, Nagahama M, Kitagawa W, Shibuya H, Ito K. Surgical management of Graves' disease—10-year prospective trial at a single institution. Endocr J. 2008;55(1):161–7.
41. Wilhelm SM, McHenry CR. Total thyroidectomy is superior to subtotal thyroidectomy for management of Graves' disease in the United States. World J Surg. 2010;34:1261–4.
42. Spinelli C, Bertocchini A, Donatini G, Miccoli P. Minimally invasive video-assisted thyroidectomy: report of 16 cases in children older than 10 years. J Pediatr Surg 2004;39(9):1312–15.
43. Sosa JA, Bowman HM, Tielsch JM, Powe NR, Gordon TA, Udelsman R. The importance of surgeon experience for clinical and economic outcomes from thyroidectomy. Ann Surg. 1998;228(3):320–30.

44. Sugino K, Ito K, Mimura T, Fukunari N, Nagahama M, Ito K. Surgical treatment of Graves' disease in children. Thyroid. 2004;14(6):447–52.
45. Raval MV, Browne M, Chin AC, Zimmerman D, Angelos P, Reynolds M. J Pediatr Surg. 2009;44:1529–33.
46. Breuer C, Tuggle C, Solomon D, Sosa JA. Pediatric thyroid disease: when is surgery necessary, and who should be operating on our children? J Clin Res Pediatr Endocrinol. 2013;5(1):79–85.
47. Bhansali A, Aggarwal A, Parthan G, et al. Thyroid disorders in children. In: Clinical Rounds in Endocrinology. Springer Science+Business Media; 2016. p. 71–107.

Thyroid Nodules in Children

3

Geoffrey K. Blair and Daniel J. Ledbetter

This chapter will review thyroid nodules in children. Nodular disease of the thyroid, as with other thyroid disorders, is much less common in children than in adults but it is a regular occurrence in regional centers that provide comprehensive care for children and adolescents. The major clinical concern of thyroid nodules in both children and adults is the risk of malignancy. Since the risk of a thyroid nodule being malignant seems to be higher in children than adults, children presenting with thyroid nodules deserve the same organized approach to their evaluation that adults receive. This chapter will present one approach to the evaluation and management of thyroid nodules in children.

The care for these young patients with thyroid nodules is best done by a team of experienced pediatricians and pediatric-trained specialists, including endocrinologists, radiologists, oncologists, pathologists, and surgeons. Even in the largest pediatric centers, the role of the pediatric thyroid surgeon should be designated to one or two specific surgeons, for the cases are not frequent and the occasional pediatric thyroid surgeon can be a menace.

Incidence and Epidemiology

Palpable nodularity of the thyroid is found in roughly 5% of adults [1]. The incidence of thyroid nodules detected by an ultrasound exam of the thyroid is much higher [2]. Nodules not appreciated on physical examination and seen only with imaging are sometimes called "incidentalomas" but since they have a risk of malignancy as high as palpable nodules they should be managed in the same ways as palpable nodules [3]. These nodules are sonographically discrete areas within the thyroid that look different from the surrounding gland and they do not always correlate with physical exam findings but correlate well with pathologic findings [4]. Because of its accuracy, precision, reproducibility, and ease of use ultrasound is now the gold standard for diagnosis of thyroid nodules [5].

Although less common than in adults, thyroid nodules are not rare in children. In a large screening program to detect thyroid abnormalities in children with possible radiation exposure in the American Southwest almost 2% of school-aged children were found to have palpable thyroid nodularity [6, 7]. Other estimates of the incidence of thyroid nodules in children range between 1.0 and 1.5%—less common than in adults but not a rare problem by pediatric standards [8].

G.K. Blair (✉)
Division of Pediatric Surgery, British Columbia's Children's Hospital, Room K0-106 BC Children's Hospital, 4480 Oak St., Vancouver, BC V6H 3V4, Canada
e-mail: gblair@cw.bc.ca

D.J. Ledbetter (✉)
Seattle Children's Hospital, 4800 Sand Point Way NE, PO Box 5371/M/S OA.9.220, Seattle, WA 98105, USA
e-mail: dan.ledbetter@seattlechildrens.org

D.J. Ledbetter and P.R.V. Johnson (eds.), *Endocrine Surgery in Children*,
DOI 10.1007/978-3-662-54256-9_3

In adults, thyroid nodules are much more common in women than in men [9]. In pediatric patients thyroid nodules are also more common in girls but there is not such an overwhelming preponderance of females who are afflicted, especially in particularly in the pre-pubescent age group [10, 11].

Etiology

Nodules may be solitary or multiple and may be associated with a wide spectrum of thyroid disorders including multinodular goiter, autoimmune thyroiditis, Hashimoto's disease, or Graves' disease [8]. The most worrisome risk is that a thyroid nodule may represent a thyroid neoplasm and this risk seems to be higher in nodules in children compared to nodules in adults [8, 12, 13].

Evaluation of Thyroid Nodules

Thyroid nodules are usually asymptomatic and the most common reason to evaluate them further is the concern for thyroid malignancy. A clinical pathway guideline or algorithm can strategically acknowledge the protean presentations of the child with a "thyroid nodule." Several of practice guidelines for the evaluation and management of thyroid nodules have been published [5, 12–15]. New guidelines appear regularly and one of the most recent is from the American Thyroid Association Task Force on Pediatric Thyroid Cancer—"Management Guidelines for Children with Thyroid Nodules and Differentiated Thyroid Cancer" [16].

As with any clinical guideline, they must be applied intelligently to individual patient variability, needs, preferences, and to the practice setting. Figure 3.1 represents a modified algorithm of management generated through an iteration and expert consensus among the pediatric surgeons, endocrinologists, pathologists/cytologists, and radiologists engaged in the Canadian Thyroid Nodule Study (CaPTNS) group [7]. The following text provides further explanation.

History and Physical Examination of the Child with a Thyroid Nodule

The evaluation of a child with a thyroid nodule begins with a history and physical examination. Most thyroid nodules are asymptomatic but symptoms of neck pain, difficult or painful swallowing, difficult or noisy breathing, or hoarseness suggest the possibility of local invasion or compression of the airway, esophagus, or recurrent laryngeal nerve. The rate of growth should be assessed. Rapid growth of a thyroid mass classically would suggest anaplastic thyroid cancer or thyroid lymphoma; however, both of these tumors are rare in children. In addition, although most patients with thyroid cancer are euthyroid it is necessary to ask about symptoms of hyper and hypothyroidism [9].

In addition to the history of the thyroid nodule and the state of thyroid function, it is important to ask about a personal history of radiation exposure or thyroid disease and about any family history of thyroid disease, thyroid cancer, or tumors common in familial tumor syndromes.

Physical examination should look for signs of hyper or hypothyroidism and for any of the signs seen in syndromes with a risk of thyroid cancer (see Chap. 4 for specific examples of syndromes with a risk of thyroid cancer). The characteristics of the thyroid nodule—its size, character, tenderness, mobility, and fixation—should be noted. Finally, it is very important to examine for associated cervical lymphadenopathy. However, although a complete history and physical examination is important and necessary to provide optimal care of the patient, by itself it is usually unreliable in making a diagnosis of malignancy [9, 12]. After the history and physical examination the next steps in evaluation of a child with a thyroid nodule are to obtain basic laboratory tests of thyroid function and an ultrasound of the thyroid.

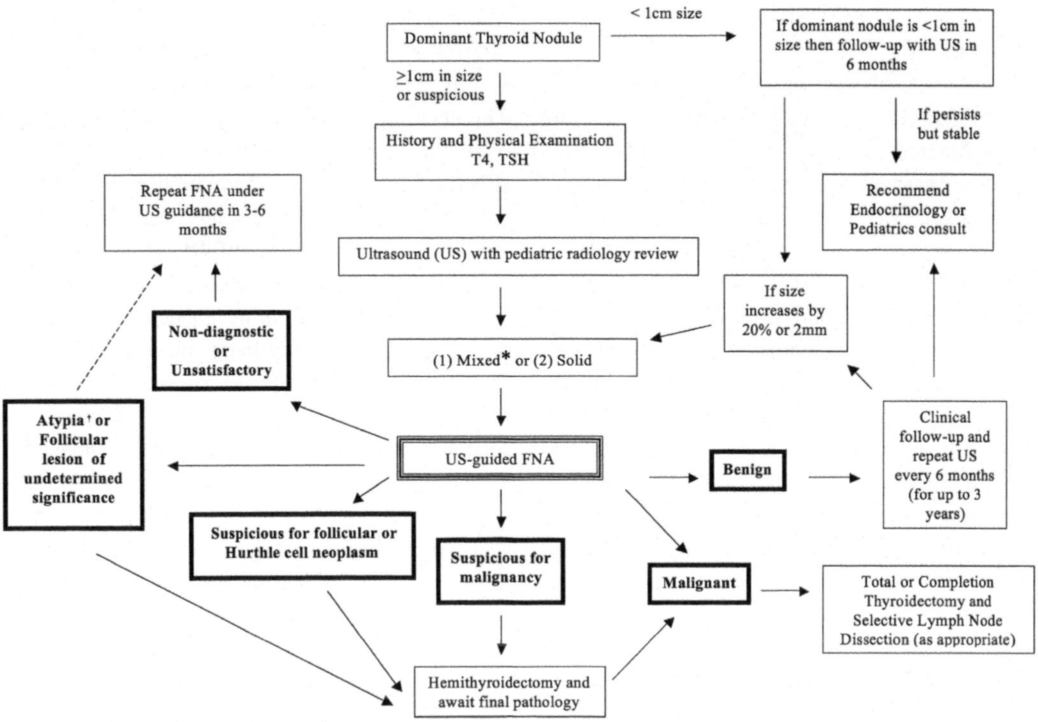

Fig. 3.1 Pathway for pediatric thyroid nodules. *Purely cystic lesions, i.e., no solid component, are not managed using this guideline. Surgical consultation may be considered. Recommend external expert review if atypia of undetermined significance occurs on repeat FNA

Laboratory Tests to Evaluate Thyroid Nodules

Serum thyroid stimulating hormone (TSH) levels as a measure of thyroid function are indicated in patients with diffuse or focal enlargement of the thyroid gland [5]. When the TSH is lower than normal then a thorough evaluation for hyperthyroidism should be performed including radionuclide thyroid scanning. Radionuclide scanning will identify nodules as "cold" (uptake less than surrounding thyroid), "warm" (uptake equal to surrounding thyroid), or "hot" (uptake greater than surrounding thyroid). "Hot" nodules are hyperfunctioning. Hyperfunctioning thyroid nodules are usually not malignant [5, 9] but patients with laboratory and clinical hyperthyroidism require treatment for the hyperthyroidism that could include surgical excision with a thyroid lobectomy of the hyperfunctioning nodule. When TSH levels are higher than normal (or even in the high normal range) then the thyroid nodule has an increased risk of being malignant [17].

Other laboratory tests have been used in the evaluation of patients with thyroid nodules but there is no consensus about their routine use. Serum thyroglobulin levels can be elevated in patients with differentiated thyroid cancer but similar elevations are found in other, nonmalignant thyroid diseases. Therefore, serum thyroglobulin is neither sensitive nor specific for thyroid cancer and not useful during the evaluation of a thyroid nodule [18]. Serum calcitonin levels have been advocated in the evaluation of thyroid nodules to detect medullary thyroid cancer although this has not been the standard practice in the United States, and probably not warranted as a routine test in childhood thyroid nodules, unless, of course there is a family history of Multiple Endocrine Neoplasia Type 2 or Familial Medullary Cancer syndromes [19–21].

Imaging in the Evaluation of Thyroid Nodules

Ultrasound (US) should be the first imaging study obtained for a thyroid nodule and is often the only imaging study needed during the evaluation [22]. US can identify the number of nodules, their size, and whether they are solid or cystic. In addition, more subtle characteristics such as nodule regularity, vascularity, and the presence of calcifications can be assessed. Ultrasonographic findings suggesting malignancy include nodules with increased peripheral vascularity, irregular, "infiltrative" margins, and microcalcifications [23]. Additional features suggesting malignancy include nodules that are hypoechoic compared to surrounding thyroid and nodule dimensions that are taller than wider in the transverse viewing plane [24, 25]. None of these features is diagnostic for malignancy but may be useful to risk stratify nodules that require biopsy [5]. Some ultrasound features argue against malignancy. For example, pure cystic nodules are rarely malignant [26] and would not typically require further evaluation by biopsy although they might need intervention for their mass effect alone.

The objective of ultrasound in evaluating thyroid nodules is to identify nodules that need further evaluation with a biopsy. The major criteria used to decide if biopsy is needed are size and character of the nodule. As a general rule, thyroid nodules 1 cm or larger in diameter that have solid components should be biopsied [5]. Certain aspects of the patient's history and physical exam (e.g., a history of radiation exposure [27] or family history of thyroid cancer [28], or exam findings suggesting a syndrome with an increased risk of thyroid cancer) or the finding of ultrasound characteristics of malignancy might cause suspicion and lead to biopsy of nodules smaller than 1 cm. Finally, biopsy is indicated when lesions are seen to be enlarging or especially when they are associated with enlarged cervical lymph nodes [5].

Fine Needle Aspiration of Thyroid Nodules

The technique of biopsy of thyroid lesions to evaluate for malignancy is fine needle aspiration (FNA) [29]. This technique has been used extensively in adults and it has been shown to be equally useful in children [30]. FNA should be performed in children under ultrasound guidance, to ensure proper sampling especially when the nodule has cystic components or when it is small [31]. One unique aspect of FNA in children when compared to adults is the increased need for sedation or even general anesthesia since children are not always as cooperative as adults with even minor procedures.

FNA requires an experienced pathologist to interpret the biopsy specimens and clearly report the findings to the physicians and surgeons caring for the patient. Since biopsy findings are critical to the diagnosis of malignancy and surgical treatment there have been efforts to standardize the reporting of FNA. One standard reporting scheme was the outcome of the National Cancer Institute sponsored thyroid FNA "State of the Science" conference in 2007. Based on these discussions and using the Bethesda System for reporting cervical cytology interpretations as "inspiration," the National Cancer Institute's Bethesda System for Reporting Thyroid Cytopathology was developed [32].

This system defines six different categories to describe FNA results:

- Nondiagnostic/Unsatisfactory,
- Benign,
- Atypia of Undetermined Significance or Follicular Lesion of Undetermined Significance,
- Follicular Neoplasm or suspicious for a Follicular Neoplasm,
- Suspicious for malignancy,
- Malignant.

When initial FNA yields an unsatisfactory or nondiagnostic sample then close follow-up with a repeat FNA under US guidance in 3–6 months is recommended and often provides a more definitive answer [33, 34]. Persistently unsatisfactory or nondiagnostic samples, especially when the nodule is solid, when it is growing, or in patients with risk factors for malignancy should lead to the consideration of hemithyroidectomy (lobectomy + isthmusectomy) to obtain a definitive diagnosis and relieve family uncertainty [35].

The other categories of FNA findings have increasing risks of malignancy. The lowest risk of malignancy is for nodules classified as benign where there is a small, but real risk of a false-negative result. Close follow-up of these patients is required [36, 37]. Follow-up should include repeat US and if the nodule is growing then a repeat FNA [2]. Similar to purely cystic nodules, when nodules that are predominantly cystic are benign by FNA and then again accumulate cystic fluid and are symptomatic then hemithyroidectomy can be considered [5]. Another option for treatment of symptomatic, benign cystic nodules that has been described in adults is ablation by injection of ethanol [38].

There is a spectrum malignancy risk among FNAs of indeterminate cytology. Those reported as "atypia" or "follicular lesion of undetermined significance" (AUS/FLUS) have a relatively low (5–10%) risk of malignancy in adulthood [32]. However, the reported rates of malignancy in lesions where the FNA results show AUS/FLUS in childhood is significantly higher and argument can be made to proceed to hemithyroidectomy [39]. Alternatively, with care and selection, these lesions may be observed closely and a repeat FNA done in 3–6 months.

FNAs reported as "suspicious for follicular or Hürthle cell neoplasm" the risk may be as high as 20–30% although the exact risk debatable and may be lower in certain patients. It is impossible to distinguish follicular adenomas from follicular carcinomas because the diagnostic criteria for malignancy are not cytological but rather evidence of capsular or vascular invasion, which requires examination of the whole lesion. Because of the higher risk of malignancy hemithyroidectomy for a definitive diagnosis is recommended [12]. In a meta-analysis of the utility of FNA in children, the issue of finding follicular cells on cytology recognized the difficulty in differentiating benign follicular adenomas from follicular carcinomas. They concluded that the finding of follicular cells on FNA in a child should be viewed as "suspicious for malignancy" and that surgery should proceed [30].

The highest risk of malignancy is in those FNA samples that are read as "suspicious for malignancy" or "malignancy" and those patients should be prepared for surgery. Where the FNA cytology indicates "malignancy" the patient should have a total thyroidectomy and, where indicated, the appropriate zonal cervical lymph node dissection [40, 41].

References

1. Tunbridge WM, Evered DC, Hall R, Appleton D, Brewis M, Clark F, Evans JG, Young E, Bird T, Smith PA. The spectrum of thyroid disease in a community: the Whickham survey. Clin Endocrinol. 1977;7:481–93.
2. Tan GH, Gharib H. Thyroid incidentalomas: management approaches to nonpalpable nodules discovered incidentally on thyroid imaging. Ann Intern Med. 1997;126:226–31.
3. Hagag P, Strauss S, Weiss M. Role of ultrasound-guided fine-needle aspiration biopsy in evaluation of nonpalpable thyroid nodules. Thyroid (official journal of the American Thyroid Association). 1998;8:989–95.
4. Marqusee E, Benson CB, Frates MC, Doubilet PM, Larsen PR, Cibas ES, Mandel SJ. Usefulness of ultrasonography in the management of nodular thyroid disease. Ann Intern Med. 2000;133:696–700.
5. American Thyroid Association Guidelines Taskforce on Thyroid N, Differentiated Thyroid C, Cooper DS, Doherty GM, Haugen BR, Kloos RT, Lee SL, Mandel SJ, Mazzaferri EL, McIver B, Pacini F, Schlumberger M, Sherman SI, Steward DL, Tuttle RM. Revised American Thyroid Association management guidelines for patients with thyroid nodules and differentiated thyroid cancer. Thyroid (official journal of the American Thyroid Association). 2009;19:1167–1214.
6. Rallison ML, Dobyns BM, Keating FR Jr, Rall JE, Tyler FH. Thyroid nodularity in children. Jama. 1975;233:1069–72.
7. Rallison ML, Dobyns BM, Meikle AW, Bishop M, Lyon JL, Stevens W. Natural history of thyroid abnormalities: prevalence, incidence, and regression

of thyroid diseases in adolescents and young adults. Am J Med. 1991;91:363–70.
8. Josefson J, Zimmerman D. Thyroid nodules and cancers in children. Pediatr Endocrinol Rev PER. 2008;6:14–23.
9. Hegedus L. Clinical practice. The thyroid nodule. New Engl J Med. 2004;351:1764–71.
10. Farahati J, Bucsky P, Parlowsky T, Mader U, Reiners C. Characteristics of differentiated thyroid carcinoma in children and adolescents with respect to age, gender, and histology. Cancer. 1997;80:2156–62.
11. Harach HR, Williams ED. Childhood thyroid cancer in England and Wales. Br J Cancer. 1995;72:777–83.
12. Canadian Pediatric Thyroid Nodule Study G. The Canadian Pediatric Thyroid Nodule Study: an evaluation of current management practices. J Pediatr Surg. 2008;43:826–30.
13. Wiersinga WM. Management of thyroid nodules in children and adolescents. Hormones. 2007;6:194–9.
14. Gharib H, Papini E, Paschke R, Duick DS, Valcavi R, Hegedus L, Vitti P, Nodules AAETFoT. American Association of Clinical Endocrinologists, Associazione Medici Endocrinologi, and European Thyroid Association medical guidelines for clinical practice for the diagnosis and management of thyroid nodules. J Endocrinol Inv. 2010;33:1–50.
15. Niedziela M. Pathogenesis, diagnosis and management of thyroid nodules in children. Endocr Relat Cancer. 2006;13:427–53.
16. Francis GL, Waguespack SG, Bauer AJ, Angelos P, Benvenga S, Cerutti JM, Dinauer CA, Hamilton J, Hay ID, Luster M, Parisi MT, Rachmiel M, Thompson GB, Yamashita S. Management guidelines for children with thyroid nodules and differentiated thyroid cancer. Thyroid (official journal of the American Thyroid Association). 2015;25:716–59.
17. Boelaert K, Horacek J, Holder RL, Watkinson JC, Sheppard MC, Franklyn JA. Serum thyrotropin concentration as a novel predictor of malignancy in thyroid nodules investigated by fine-needle aspiration. J Clin Endocrinol Metab. 2006;91:4295–301.
18. Pacini F, Pinchera A, Giani C, Grasso L, Doveri F, Baschieri L. Serum thyroglobulin in thyroid carcinoma and other thyroid disorders. J Endocrinol Invest. 1980;3:283–92.
19. Cheung K, Roman SA, Wang TS, Walker HD, Sosa JA. Calcitonin measurement in the evaluation of thyroid nodules in the United States: a cost-effectiveness and decision analysis. J Clin Endocrinol Metab. 2008;93:2173–80.
20. Costante G, Meringolo D, Durante C, Bianchi D, Nocera M, Tumino S, Crocetti U, Attard M, Maranghi M, Torlontano M, Filetti S. Predictive value of serum calcitonin levels for preoperative diagnosis of medullary thyroid carcinoma in a cohort of 5817 consecutive patients with thyroid nodules. J Clin Endocrinol Metab. 2007;92:450–5.
21. Elisei R, Bottici V, Luchetti F, Di Coscio G, Romei C, Grasso L, Miccoli P, Iacconi P, Basolo F, Pinchera A, Pacini F. Impact of routine measurement of serum calcitonin on the diagnosis and outcome of medullary thyroid cancer: experience in 10,864 patients with nodular thyroid disorders. J Clin Endocrinol Metab. 2004;89:163–8.
22. Hegedus L. Thyroid ultrasonography as a screening tool for thyroid disease. Thyroid (official journal of the American Thyroid Association). 2004;14:879–80.
23. Papini E, Guglielmi R, Bianchini A, Crescenzi A, Taccogna S, Nardi F, Panunzi C, Rinaldi R, Toscano V, Pacella CM. Risk of malignancy in nonpalpable thyroid nodules: predictive value of ultrasound and color-Doppler features. J Clin Endocrinol Metab. 2002;87:1941–6.
24. Cappelli C, Castellano M, Pirola I, Cumetti D, Agosti B, Gandossi E, Agabiti Rosei E. The predictive value of ultrasound findings in the management of thyroid nodules. QJM (monthly journal of the Association of Physicians). 2007;100:29–35.
25. Moon WJ, Jung SL, Lee JH, Na DG, Baek JH, Lee YH, Kim J, Kim HS, Byun JS, Lee DH, Thyroid Study Group KSoN, Head, Neck R. Benign and malignant thyroid nodules: US differentiation-multicenter retrospective study. Radiology. 2008;247:762–70
26. Frates MC, Benson CB, Doubilet PM, Kunreuther E, Contreras M, Cibas ES, Orcutt J, Moore FD Jr, Larsen PR, Marqusee E, Alexander EK. Prevalence and distribution of carcinoma in patients with solitary and multiple thyroid nodules on sonography. J Clin Endocrinol Metab. 2006;91:3411–7.
27. Schneider AB, Ron E, Lubin J, Stovall M, Gierlowski TC. Dose-response relationships for radiation-induced thyroid cancer and thyroid nodules: evidence for the prolonged effects of radiation on the thyroid. J Clin Endocrinol Metab. 1993;77:362–9.
28. Hemminki K, Eng C, Chen B. Familial risks for nonmedullary thyroid cancer. J Clin Endocrinol Metab. 2005;90:5747–53.
29. Pitman MB, Abele J, Ali SZ, Duick D, Elsheikh TM, Jeffrey RB, Powers CN, Randolph G, Renshaw A, Scoutt L. Techniques for thyroid FNA: a synopsis of the National Cancer Institute Thyroid Fine-Needle Aspiration State of the Science Conference. Diagn Cytopathol. 2008;36:407–24.
30. Stevens C, Lee JK, Sadatsafavi M, Blair GK. Pediatric thyroid fine-needle aspiration cytology: a meta-analysis. J Pediatr Surg. 2009;44:2184–91.
31. Izquierdo R, Arekat MR, Knudson PE, Kartun KF, Khurana K, Kort K, Numann PJ. Comparison of palpation-guided versus ultrasound-guided fine-needle aspiration biopsies of thyroid nodules in an outpatient endocrinology practice. Endocrine Pract (official journal of the American College of Endocrinology and the American Association of Clinical Endocrinologists). 2006;12:609–14.
32. Baloch ZW, LiVolsi VA, Asa SL, Rosai J, Merino MJ, Randolph G, Vielh P, DeMay RM, Sidawy MK, Frable WJ. Diagnostic terminology and

morphologic criteria for cytologic diagnosis of thyroid lesions: a synopsis of the National Cancer Institute Thyroid Fine-Needle Aspiration State of the Science Conference. Diagn Cytopathol. 2008;36: 425–37.
33. Alexander EK, Heering JP, Benson CB, Frates MC, Doubilet PM, Cibas ES, Marqusee E. Assessment of nondiagnostic ultrasound-guided fine needle aspirations of thyroid nodules. J Clin Endocrinol Metab. 2002;87:4924–7.
34. Braga M, Cavalcanti TC, Collaco LM, Graf H. Efficacy of ultrasound-guided fine-needle aspiration biopsy in the diagnosis of complex thyroid nodules. J Clin Endocrinol Metab. 2001;86:4089–91.
35. de los Santos ET, Keyhani-Rofagha S, Cunningham JJ, Mazzaferri EL. Cystic thyroid nodules. Dilemma Malignant Lesions Arch Intern Med. 1990;150:1422–7.
36. Carmeci C, Jeffrey RB, McDougall IR, Nowels KW, Weigel RJ. Ultrasound-guided fine-needle aspiration biopsy of thyroid masses. Thyroid (official journal of the American Thyroid Association). 1998;8:283–9.
37. Ylagan LR, Farkas T, Dehner LP. Fine needle aspiration of the thyroid: a cytohistologic correlation and study of discrepant cases. Thyroid (official journal of the American Thyroid Association). 2004;14:35–41.
38. Bennedbaek FN, Hegedus L. Treatment of recurrent thyroid cysts with ethanol: a randomized double-blind controlled trial. J Clin Endocrinol Metab. 2003;88:5773–7.
39. Norlen O, Charlton A, Sarkis LM, Henwood T, Shun A, Gill AJ, Delbridge L. Risk of malignancy for each Bethesda class in pediatric thyroid nodules. J Pediatr Surg. 2015;50:1147–9.
40. Gharib H, Goellner JR, Johnson DA. Fine-needle aspiration cytology of the thyroid. A 12-year experience with 11,000 biopsies. Clin Lab Med. 1993;13:699–709.
41. Raval MV, Bentrem DJ, Stewart AK, Ko CY, Reynolds M. Utilization of total thyroidectomy for differentiated thyroid cancer in children. Ann Surg Oncol. 2010;17:2545–53.

Thyroid Cancer in Children

4

Daniel J. Ledbetter

This chapter reviews thyroid cancer in children. It concentrates on differentiated thyroid cancer that arises from thyroid follicle cells, especially papillary thyroid cancer. The other major differentiated thyroid cancer, follicular cell carcinoma, is also discussed but other thyroid cancers are only briefly mentioned. Medullary carcinoma of the thyroid is discussed in Chap. 31, Multiple Endocrine Neoplasia Type 2.

Discussions of thyroid cancer in children are often dominated by extrapolations of data from adults because thyroid cancer is so much more common in adults than children. But thyroid cancer in children is not the same as thyroid cancer in adults. There are different etiologies, risk factors, clinical presentations, and natural histories. The unique aspects of thyroid cancer in children have been recognized and in 2015 the American Thyroid Association published specific recommendations regarding the evaluation and management of thyroid cancer in children 18 years of age and younger [1]. This chapter will review some of those recommendations.

As for many surgical conditions, the lack of controlled trials for patients with thyroid cancer has led to treatment recommendations that are largely based on upon the consensus of experts [1, 2]. As a general rule, treatment of thyroid cancer typically consists of initial operation to remove gross disease in the neck and then radioactive iodine (I-131) is given to patients who have residual disease or to patients who are at a significant risk for recurrent disease [3, 4]. Unlike many other childhood cancers, chemotherapy and external beam radiation are generally not effective against thyroid cancer.

Incidence

Thyroid cancer is an example of a common clinical scenario in pediatric surgery—it is not a rare problem in children, but the absolute number of children affected is small when compared to the number of adults. A report examining more than 30 years of data from the Surveillance, Epidemiology, and End Results (SEER) registry identified 1753 patients younger than 20 years old with thyroid carcinoma and calculated the annual incidence in this age group to be 0.5 cases per 100,000 people [5]. Over the duration of the study, the incidence of thyroid cancer in children steadily increased by 1.1% per year. This increasing incidence in children is consistent with the findings that the overall incidence of thyroid carcinoma has more than doubled from 1975 to 2001 [6].

The relatively low incidence of the thyroid cancer in children can be considered from different perspectives. First, when looking at all patients with thyroid cancer, children are a definite minority, with patients under 20 years of age accounting for less than 2% of patients with a new

D.J. Ledbetter (✉)
Seattle Children's Hospital, 4800 Sand Point Way NE, PO Box 5371/M/S OA.9.220, Seattle, WA 98105, USA
e-mail: dan.ledbetter@seattlechildrens.org

D.J. Ledbetter and P.R.V. Johnson (eds.), *Endocrine Surgery in Children*,
DOI 10.1007/978-3-662-54256-9_4

diagnosis of differentiated thyroid cancer [1, 4]. However, from the perspective of malignancy in the young, thyroid cancer is an important problem.

Among young people the risk of thyroid cancer is directly related to increasing age. Thyroid cancers make up less than 1% of malignant tumors in children younger than 10 years of age but they are much more common in adolescents. In children aged 15–19 years thyroid cancer accounts for 7.5% of all cancers making it the 8th most common malignancy in that age group (and the second most common in girls) and in young adults 20–24 years old thyroid cancer accounts for 10.5% of all cancers making it the third most common cancer in that age group [5, 7].

These incidence figures translate to between 300 and 400 young people with new diagnoses of thyroid cancer each year in the United States. When compared to the roughly 500 new cases of Wilms tumor each year it is apparent that thyroid cancer is a relatively common pediatric tumor requiring surgery [4]. However, the relative frequency that patients with thyroid cancer are seen at any individual pediatric center varies widely depending upon referral patterns and the number of adolescents cared for by that center.

Epidemiology

As with adults, pediatric patients diagnosed with thyroid carcinoma are more likely to be female than male [8, 9]. This female gender predominance is more marked with increasing age. Children younger than 10 years of age with thyroid cancer are only slightly more likely to be female with a gender distribution of 1.2–1.6 girls: 1 boy, while for children aged 10–14 years the ratio is 3.3 girls: 1 boy, and for those aged 15–19 years old the gender distribution is 5.2 girls: 1 boy [10]. Although the data is not as robust in children there are differences in the racial distribution of thyroid carcinoma in adults indicating a higher frequency of diagnosis in Non-Hispanic whites relative to African-Americans [11, 12].

Etiology

Although the cause of most thyroid cancers is unknown, there is an increased risk of thyroid cancer with radiation exposure and in some genetic syndromes.

Risk of Thyroid Cancer After Radiation Exposure

Radiation exposure is the best-known environmental risk factor for developing thyroid cancer. The majority of thyroid cancers that develop after radiation exposure are papillary carcinomas [13]. The magnitude of the risk of thyroid malignancy after radiation exposure is related to the age of the patient at the time of the exposure, the radiation dose, and associated conditions and treatments.

The sensitivity of the thyroid gland to irradiation is higher in younger patients [13–15] and the increased risk is especially marked with radiation doses at or above 20–29 Gy [16].

Radiation exposure can be classified as either low- or high dose. Low-dose exposures include [1] therapeutic irradiation for benign conditions such as hemangiomas, enlarged tonsils, or thymic hyperplasia and [2] living in the vicinity of nuclear accidents such as Chernobyl or in areas impacted by atomic bombs. High-dose exposure occurs with radiation treatment for malignancy. The risk of malignancy is higher with higher radiation doses.

Although the cumulative incidence of thyroid malignancy following medical treatment is low, the incidence of thyroid cancer was found to be higher than expected in cohort analyses of survivors of other childhood cancer [17]. The increased risk of thyroid cancer in individuals who have had radiation exposure to their thyroid during childhood has led to recommendations for long-term thyroid ultrasound surveillance of these patients to detect thyroid nodules [18].

The age-dependent sensitivity of the thyroid to the carcinogenic effects of radiation has also been noted with exposure to I-131. In adults treated with I-131 there seems to be a minimally increased risk of future thyroid cancer, whereas children and even adolescents seem to have an increased risk. The risk is even more substantial if the child was younger than 10 years at the time exposure [19]. The clinical relevance of this increased risk was demonstrated by the epidemic of papillary thyroid cancer among children exposed to I-131 after the Chernobyl nuclear reactor accident in 1986 [20]. Even though radiation-related papillary thyroid cancers look more aggressive histologically and have higher recurrence rates, the overall patient survival with these tumors is similar to tumors not associated with radiation exposure [21].

Risk of Thyroid Cancer in Syndromes

Thyroid cancers are associated with several genetic syndromes including multiple endocrine neoplasia, familial adenomatous polyposis, PTEN hamartoma tumor syndromes, the Carney complex, DICER1 syndrome, and familial non medullary thyroid carcinoma (FNMTC).

Multiple endocrine neoplasia (MEN) type IIA, MEN IIB, and familial medullary thyroid cancer, are autosomal dominant syndromes caused by mutations in the RET proto-oncogene. These syndromes are associated with a very high risk of medullary carcinoma of the thyroid. These syndromes and medullary thyroid carcinoma are discussed in more detail is in Chap. 31.

The autosomal dominant syndrome of familial adenomatous polyposis (FAP) is caused by mutations in the adenomatous polyposis coli (APC) gene. The subset of patients with FAP who have extraintestinal manifestations of their APC mutation are often labeled as having Gardner syndrome. Patients with FAP/Gardner syndrome are at increased risk of developing thyroid cancer at a relatively young age. The thyroid cancer is usually papillary carcinoma and the mean age at diagnosis is 33 years. Because of their relatively high risk of developing thyroid cancer it is recommended that patients with FAP/Gardner syndrome have regular ultrasound screening for thyroid nodules [22].

Mutations in the protein tyrosine phosphatase and tensin (PTEN) gene are associated with a group of rare conditions known as PTEN hamartoma tumor syndromes. The best-described PTEN hamartoma tumor syndrome is Cowden syndrome, which is an autosomal dominant syndrome of macrocephaly, multiple hamartomas, and characteristic skin abnormalities such as trichilemmomas. Patients with Cowden syndrome have an increased risk of differentiated thyroid cancer that can present in childhood. This risk has led to ultrasound screening for thyroid abnormalities [23–25].

The Carney complex is an autosomal dominant syndrome of abnormal skin pigmentation (lentigenes and blue nevi) and an increased risk of endocrine and nonendocrine tumors. The most common endocrine tumor in Carney complex is primary pigmented nodular adrenocortical disease (PPNAD), which can cause Cushing's syndrome. Patients with the Carney complex also have an increased risk of thyroid adenomas and carcinomas [26].

DICER1 syndrome is a rare, autosomal dominant syndrome that increases the affected individuals' risk of developing a variety of unusual benign and malignant tumors at a young age. The most common tumor that develops in DICER1 syndrome is pleuropulmonary blastoma, which usually presents before 6 years of age [27]. Patients with DICER1 are also at risk for including ovarian sex cord stromal tumors, cystic nephroma, multinodular goiter, and differentiated thyroid cancer [28]. Most patients with DICER1 do not develop tumors.

A child with a sibling or a parent with a differentiated thyroid cancer has an increased risk of developing a differentiated thyroid cancer. These patients with familial non-medullary thyroid cancer (FNMTC) may account for up to 5% of all patients with differentiated thyroid cancers [29]. There is probably more than one genetic pathway to explain the increased risk of differentiated thyroid cancer within certain families and it is an area of ongoing investigation [30]. Although controversial, patients with FNMTC seem to be more likely to present with multifocal, bilateral, disease and to present with lymph node involvement at diagnosis [31].

Pathology

The pathologic classification and histologic definition of types of thyroid cancers is from the World Health Organization (WHO) and is the same in children and adults [32]. The overwhelming majority of thyroid tumors in children are differentiated thyroid cancers that arise from thyroid follicular cells. In the SEER registry report mentioned previously, more than 90% of the 1753 children and adolescents had differentiated thyroid cancers and most of those were papillary thyroid cancer (Table 4.1) [5]. Other series from around the world suggest that papillary thyroid cancer accounts is even more prevalent that the SEER report suggests with 90–95% of childhood thyroid cancer [33–35]. The other major differentiated thyroid cancer, follicular cancer, accounts for most of the rest of thyroid cancers [5]. Other thyroid cancers including medullary thyroid cancer and poorly differentiated or anaplastic thyroid cancer are rare.

Papillary Thyroid Cancer

Pathologic features of papillary thyroid cancer include psammoma bodies and nuclear ground glass appearance, longitudinal grooves, and inclusions [32]. Histologic subtypes of papillary thyroid cancer seen in children include classic, solid, follicular, and diffuse sclerosing variants. The diffuse sclerosing variant is important to consider because it is more common in children, especially younger children, than in adults and it has a unique clinical presentation of enlargement of an entire thyroid lobe or the entire gland rather than as a nodule within the gland [36]. The relative prevalence of this variant has led to the recommendation that children presenting with diffusely enlarged thyroid glands or lobes have ultrasound imaging to evaluate for findings of malignancy [1].

Table 4.1 Histologic types of thyroid cancers in children from SEER registry report

83% papillary
60% papillary
23% follicular variant of papillary
10% follicular thyroid cancer
5% medullary
2% other

From Ref. [5], with permission

Papillary thyroid cancer is often multifocal (30–60%) and bilateral (30%) and neck lymph node metastases are present in at least 30–60% of children at diagnosis [37–40]. Pulmonary metastases are also common (10–25%) in children at diagnosis, usually when neck lymph nodes metastases are present [41, 42]. Overall, at the time of diagnosis, children with papillary thyroid cancer are more likely than adults to have tumor extending beyond the capsule of the thyroid, regional lymph node metastases, and pulmonary metastases, even when controlled for tumor size and histology [37–39, 41, 42]. But despite having more advanced disease at the time they present, children with papillary thyroid cancer have an excellent prognosis.

Follicular Thyroid Cancer

Follicular thyroid cancer is relatively rare [5] and it is usually seen in adolescents rather than younger children. Unlike papillary cancer there is less of a female preponderance [41] and its incidence seems to be decreasing rather than increasing [43]. The risk factors for developing follicular thyroid cancer are different than the risk factors for developing papillary thyroid cancer with iodine deficiency related to follicular thyroid cancer but not papillary cancer [44, 45] and radiation exposure related to papillary thyroid cancer but not follicular cancer [37]. Follicular thyroid cancers are common thyroid tumors in the PTEN syndromes so patients with follicular thyroid cancers should be closely evaluated for PTEN syndromes [25].

Follicular neoplasms are typically encapsulated. The cytological features of follicular thyroid cancers and benign follicular adenomas are identical and it is only possible to make the diagnosis of malignancy when there is tumor invasion through the capsule or into blood vessels. This explains why FNA can only identify a follicular tumor and not a follicular malignancy. Histologic subtypes of follicular thyroid cancer include Hürthle cell, clear cell, and insular variants. These less differentiated variants are all rare in children [46] and tend to be associated with more aggressive disease and a worse prognosis in adults [47].

The clinical presentation and behavior of follicular thyroid cancer are distinct from the more common papillary thyroid cancer with fewer neck lymph metastases but rather a propensity for hematogenous spread and lung metastases. Follicular and papillary thyroid cancers have the same excellent prognosis [5].

Other Thyroid Cancers

Other, non-differentiated thyroid cancers in children include medullary and anaplastic thyroid cancer and lymphomas. Medullary thyroid cancer derives from parafollicular C cells that produce calcitonin rather than follicular cells that produce thyroid hormones. This tumor is reviewed in Chap. 31.

Anaplastic thyroid cancer accounts for <2% of thyroid cancers of all ages. It is mainly a disease of the elderly with the large majority of afflicted patients more than 60 years of age. Anaplastic thyroid cancer is very rare in children. Histologically, it is undifferentiated and similar to non-Hodgkin lymphoma, medullary thyroid carcinoma, the insular variant of follicular thyroid carcinoma, and poorly differentiated carcinoma that has metastasized to the thyroid. Modern immunohistochemistry techniques should make diagnostic confusion less likely. Anaplastic thyroid cancer is also functionally primitive and it does not concentrate iodine so radioactive iodine is not useful for treatment. Anaplastic thyroid cancer grows rapidly, invades locally, and often presents with symptoms such as dysphagia and hoarseness. More than 40% of patients have distant metastatic disease when they present. It is a deadly disease with more than 80% of patients dead within a year of diagnosis and most are dead within 6 months [48].

Lymphoma of the thyroid is rare in adults and children. It usually presents as a relatively rapidly enlarging neck mass in a patient with a history of Hashimoto's thyroiditis. Pathologically, lymphomas of the thyroid are usually large B-cell lymphomas, but other types of lymphoma are possible. The diagnosis of lymphoma can be made by fine-needle aspiration biopsy by an experienced pathologist. Surgery is limited to the biopsy and treatment consists of chemotherapy and radiation depending upon the type of lymphoma [49].

Clinical Presentations of Thyroid Cancer

Thyroid cancer usually presents as a thyroid nodule or an enlarged thyroid gland that may be noticed by the patient or the patient's family or is found on routine physical exam. Thyroid nodules may not be visible or palpable and only be discovered on imaging studies done for screening purposes or for other reasons. Significant thyroid nodules are usually evaluated by fine needle aspiration (FNA) that allows for risk stratification that defines a risk of malignancy. For more on the evaluation of thyroid nodules see Chap. 3.

Thyroid cancer may also be discovered in the surgical specimen after resection of part or all the thyroid gland done for diagnosis of a thyroid nodule or for a benign disease. Finally, thyroid cancer can present with a neck lymph node metastasis or even distant metastatic disease. As noted previously, children and especially younger children are more likely than adults to present with advanced disease [37, 41, 50].

Evaluation

The preoperative evaluation (or staging) of a patient with thyroid cancer usually begins during the evaluation of a patient's thyroid nodule (see Chap. 3). A full history and physical examination should be done with directed questioning about symptoms of hoarseness, voice change, dysphagia, neck pain, and the onset and rapidity of growth of any neck mass. Any history of radiation exposure and family history of thyroid cancer or any malignancy should be noted. A full physical exam should be done with special attention to the thyroid gland and neck lymph nodes. If not already done, thyroid function tests should be obtained.

Critical for preoperative staging is a high-quality ultrasound of the thyroid gland and the entire neck with the goal of identifying cervical lymph node metastases that would dictate the performance of a neck dissection at the time of thyroid resection. If there is bulky lymphadenopathy or if there are any concerns about local invasion of the trachea, esophagus, or recurrent laryngeal nerve then more detailed imaging of the neck should be done with either a CT scan with contrast or MRI [1]. The potential disadvantage of a CT scan with (iodinated) contrast is that the iodine load given could delay postoperative staging and treatment with radioactive iodine. When abnormal lymph nodes are seen on imaging then FNA should be done to confirm the presence of metastases.

Nuclear medicine thyroid scans are not usually indicated preoperatively, except in the early evaluation of an undiagnosed thyroid nodule in a patient with a low TSH. If there is cervical lymph node metastases then a chest X-ray or a chest CT scan could be considered, although any lung metastases would probably be identified on the postoperative radioactive iodine scan.

Treatment

Children with thyroid cancer have been treated by a variety of methods over the last 50 years with very high survival rates, even though recurrent disease and persistent is relatively common. The goal of current treatment is to maintain the very low disease-specific mortality that has been has been obtained in the past while minimizing the complications and morbidity associated with treatment. The treatment of children with thyroid cancer is best done by an experienced, multidisciplinary team of medical and surgical specialists working in an environment with all the resources and personnel to care for children [1]. The team approach is essential in all phases of treatment because the evaluation, surgical treatment, medical treatment, and long-term follow-up are closely linked and interdependent.

In brief, the treatment of children with thyroid cancer begins surgery to remove all gross disease in the neck—usually total thyroidectomy [51] and compartmental excision of any involved cervical lymph nodes. Postoperative staging follows surgical resection. Patients found to have persistent local disease or distant metastatic disease and patients who are thought to be at high risk for recurrent disease are treated with radioactive iodine for [3, 4]. The goal of the combination of surgical resection and radioactive iodine is to eliminate all disease that can be detected by diagnostic whole-body radioactive iodine scanning and serum thyroglobulin.

Surgical Treatment

The operations done for treatment of thyroid cancer should be done by a surgeon experienced in thyroid surgery [1], although how these surgeons should be identified is a matter of ongoing debate. The initial operation for a known thyroid cancer is usually a total or near-total thyroidectomy (near-total thyroidectomy defined as preserving 1–2% of the thyroid gland that is adjacent to the recurrent laryngeal nerve or blood supply to the superior parathyroid gland). Total thyroidectomy is now favored over the previously commonly done thyroid lobectomy because of the high risk for bilateral disease (noted previously in Section "Papillary Thyroid Cancer") and the higher risk of local recurrence and later surgical procedures when less than a total thyroidectomy is performed [40, 52, 53]. Total thyroidectomy also makes postoperative follow-up with diagnostic radioactive iodine scans and serum thyroglobulin easier and more reliable. Unilateral thyroid lobectomy is sometimes favored for very small tumors, especially when there is no evidence of disease outside the thyroid gland and future radioactive iodine imaging and treatment is not likely. The anatomic principles of total thyroidectomy are discussed in detail in Chap. 1.

The most serious complications after total thyroidectomy include hypoparathyroidism and recurrent laryngeal nerve injury. Postoperative hypoparathyroidism with resulting hypocalcemia is caused by resection or devascularization of the parathyroid glands [54]. If devascularization is recognized then the parathyroid gland can be autotransplanted into the sternocleidomastoid muscle [55]. Transient hypocalcemia requiring postoperative treatment with calcitriol (the active form of vitamin D) and calcium is a relatively common problem after total thyroidectomy that can prolong hospitalization while the serum calcium levels stabilize. There are different strategies to deal with this problem including intraoperative monitoring of the parathyroid hormone (PTH) [56] and initiating early, prophylactic treatment of all patients with calcitriol and calcium [57]. Efforts to prevent recurrent laryngeal nerve injury have been concentrated on methods of nerve monitoring which although technically possible have not been found to reliably decrease the risk of nerve injury [58].

Surgery for follicular neoplasms usually consists of an initial thyroid lobectomy. Frozen section may be useful to look for unexpected papillary thyroid cancer but will not be able to differentiate a benign from a malignant follicular tumor. When the follicular neoplasm is benign then no further surgery is needed. When the follicular tumor is malignant then careful consultation with pathology, endocrinology, oncology, and nuclear medicine experts is needed to decide if completion thyroidectomy is needed or if lobectomy will be sufficient resection. Smaller tumors that have minimal evidence of invasion may potentially be treated by lobectomy alone while larger tumors and those that are more invasive histologically are probably best treated by completion thyroidectomy. The usual lack of neck lymph metastases means that neck lymph node dissections are typically not part of surgical treatment of follicular cancer.

The frequent spread of papillary thyroid cancer to neck lymph nodes and the treatment goal of removing gross disease lead to the frequent performance of lymph node resections [40]. These procedures can be therapeutic, prophylactic, unilateral, or bilateral. It is optimal that any lymph node resection be done at the time of the thyroid operation, which is why preoperative assessment of the neck lymph nodes is so important.

When lymph nodes are removed it should be done as "compartment dissection" rather than as "berry-picking", the removal of only obvious, enlarged lymph node [59]. The definition and reporting terminology of neck dissections for thyroid cancer have been standardized [60, 61]. The central neck or anterior compartment is immediately adjacent to the thyroid gland and is designated level VI. Level I is also central but higher in the neck in the submental area (level IA) and submandibular area (level IB). Levels in the lateral neck are II through V. Levels IIA and IIB are the upper jugular group with IIA being anterior (medial) and IIB being posterior (lateral to the spinal accessory nerve). Level III is the middle jugular area from the hyoid bone superiorly to the cricoid cartilage inferiorly. Level IV is the lower jugular area from the cricoid cartilage to the clavicle and Level V is the posterior triangle area (Fig. 4.1).

Papillary thyroid cancer most commonly metastasizes to the central area, level VI, on the same side as the tumor. When there is preoperative evidence of abnormal lymph nodes in the central neck (or in the lateral neck) then central neck dissection is recommended [1, 60]. Unfortunately, neck ultrasound is less reliable at identifying abnormal lymph nodes in the central neck than in the lateral neck [62]. Also, it is not clear if ultrasound size criteria of the tumor or the lymph node that have been used for adults to identify patients at high risk for metastatic disease are applicable to children [63]. Central neck lymph node dissections increase the risk of recurrent laryngeal nerve injury and permanent hypoparathyroidism so there is considerable debate on when and how (unilateral or bilateral) they should be performed [64, 65].

Lateral neck dissections are those compartmental lymph node resections beyond the central

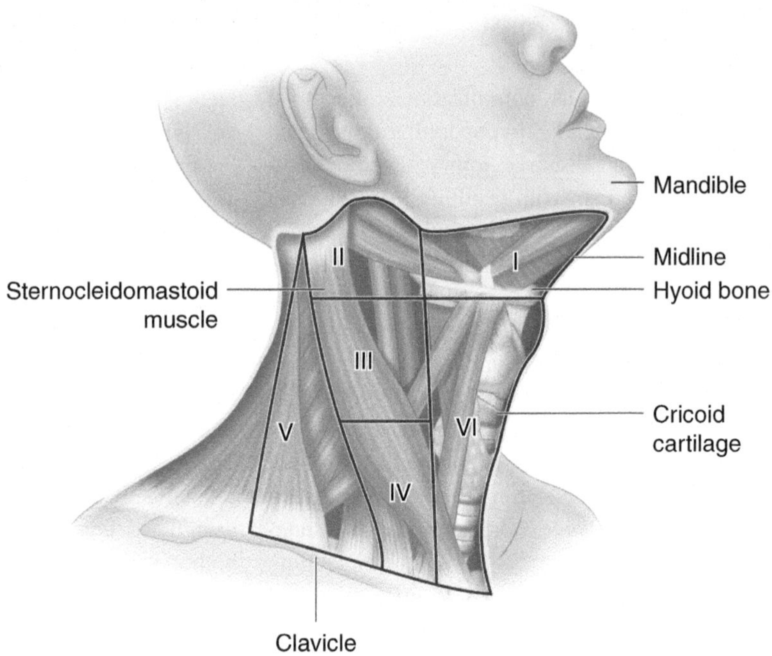

Fig. 4.1 Neck lymph node levels (see text for descriptions)

compartment (level VI). Lateral neck dissections are recommended when there is preoperative evidence of lymph node metastases in those compartments to decrease the chance of persistent and recurrent disease [37, 40]. The dissection can be tailored based on the preoperative staging but often involves levels III, IV, V, and II [66].

Although thyroid surgery in adults is increasingly being done on an outpatient basis, most children, especially younger children and those undergoing a total thyroidectomy with or without neck dissection are admitted after their operation. They are observed for potential bleeding, airway compromise, recurrent laryngeal nerve injury, and hypocalcemia due to hypoparathyroidism. Operative complications are directly related to younger ages and the extent of the operation with recurrent laryngeal nerve injury reported in 3.8% of children 6 years and under, in 1.1% of children 7–12 years, and in 0.6 of patients 13–17 years of age [67]. TSH usually stimulates differentiated thyroid cancer so after surgery thyroid hormone replacement is given to suppress TSH with the target TSH level being lower in patients at higher risk [1].

Postoperative Staging

After the initial operation postop evaluation (staging) is done to identify patients who would benefit from postoperative radioactive iodine treatment and to help define the intensity of follow-up care needed. This staging is dependent upon the surgical pathology, a postoperative diagnostic whole-body radioactive iodine scan, and serum thyroglobulin level [1]. Staging is best done within 12 weeks of surgery.

Pathologic staging for children is a modification of the adult method by the American Thyroid Association that is designed to better risk stratify patients [1]. There are three risk groups—Low, Intermediate, and High [1]. The Low risk group has either no neck lymph node metastases or only microscopic metastases to a small number of central (level VI) lymph nodes. Low-risk patients have a low risk of distant metastases but some risk of recurrent or persistent disease in the neck lymph nodes. Intermediate risk patients have extensive central neck lymph node metastases or minimal lateral compartment neck lymph node metastases. They are also at a low risk for distant metastases but have an increased risk (compared to Low risk patients) of recurrent or persistent disease in the neck lymph nodes. High-risk patients have locally invasive disease, extensive metastases to lateral compartment lymph nodes, or distant metastases. They have the highest risk of recurrent or persistent regional or distant disease [1].

The staging for Low-risk patients consists of serum thyroglobulin levels while they are euthyroid; i.e., when their TSH is suppressed by their thyroid hormone replacement. Thyroglobulin is a glycoprotein made by follicular cells and follicular cell malignancies and its presence correlates well with the presence and magnitude of metastatic disease in patients who have had their normal thyroid removed [68]. This value can then be followed in the future to observe trends. If the thyroglobulin is initially low and increases over time then it would indicate recurrent disease.

Staging for patients who are Intermediate and High Risk consists of serum thyroglobulin levels when their TSH levels are elevated (the TSH will tend to stimulate any persistent disease) and diagnostic whole-body radioactive iodine (RAI) scans, although some Intermediate risk patients may not need diagnostic scanning [1]. Diagnostic radioactive iodine scans are done with either I-123, which is ideal but more expensive, or I-131, which is the same isotope, used for treatment.

Postoperative Radioactive Iodine Treatment

Radioactive iodine treatment is given to treat known residual or metastatic disease and to prevent recurrent disease [69]. Enthusiasm for its routine use has been tempered by the observation that when children with differentiated thyroid cancer are followed for a very long time that those treated with radioactive iodine have an increase in all-cause mortality compared to those not treated with radioactive iodine. This increased mortality is mainly due to an increased risk second malignancy in those treated with radiation [52, 70].

Radioactive iodine may be given for diagnostic scans (see above) or may be given for treatment. Treatment is with I-131. Radioactive iodine is effective because iodine is markedly concentrated in cells of differentiated thyroid cancers as well as normal thyroid tissue. This concentration of iodine is most pronounced when TSH (thyroid stimulating hormone or thyrotropin) is present at relatively high levels. This requires that the patient either be hypothyroid, raising endogenous TSH levels, or receive recombinant human TSH (rhTSH). In addition, the patient must be in a state of relative iodine deficiency with no recent iodinated contrast and often a low iodine diet [4].

The dosing of radioactive iodine in children requires either an empiric determination based on the patient's size or a more specific determination with calculation of the theoretical maximum dose that will avoid bone marrow toxicity. This specific calculation is known as dosimetry [4]. Radioactive iodine toxicities are mainly to tissues incorporating iodine and consist of—sialadenitis (salivary gland inflammation), xerostomia (dry mouth), dental caries, stomatitis (inflammation of the mouth), dry eyes, and nasolacriminal duct obstruction [71]. Decreased spermatogenesis has been observed in post pubertal males, so sperm banking should be offered.

Outcomes/Complications

Even though children present with more advanced disease than adults they have a better survival. Even with advanced local disease or metastatic disease children with differentiated thyroid cancer have an excellent survival. In the SEER data base study of 1753 children with thyroid cancer those with papillary thyroid cancer had survivals of 98, 97, and 91% at 5, 15, and 30 years [5]. In the same study the survival with follicular thyroid cancer was 96, 95, and 92% at 5, 15, and 30 years [5]. Many series report nearly 100% disease specific survival over 10 and 20 and more years [37, 41, 52]. Even with tumor recurrence and lung metastases prognosis is good.

Recurrences are relatively common and the most important risk factor for disease free survival is the extent of the original operation [40, 52]. Recurrence in the neck can be treated with surgical resection of gross disease if technically possible. Radioactive iodine treatment is given when operation is not deemed to be effective or safe. Pulmonary metastases are treated with radioactive iodine and even though it is persistent the disease may not progress.

References

1. Francis GL, Waguespack SG, Bauer AJ, Angelos P, Benvenga S, Cerutti JM, Dinauer CA, Hamilton J, Hay ID, Luster M, Parisi MT, Rachmiel M, Thompson GB, Yamashita S. Management guidelines for children with thyroid nodules and differentiated thyroid cancer. Thyroid. 2015;25:716–59.
2. American Thyroid Association Guidelines Taskforce on Thyroid N, Differentiated Thyroid C, Cooper DS, Doherty GM, Haugen BR, Kloos RT, Lee SL, Mandel SJ, Mazzaferri EL, Mciver B, Pacini F, Schlumberger M, Sherman SI, Steward DL, Tuttle RM. Revised American Thyroid Association management guidelines for patients with thyroid nodules and differentiated thyroid cancer. Thyroid. 2009;19:1167–214.
3. Rivkees SA, Mazzaferri EL, Verburg FA, Reiners C, Luster M, Breuer CK, Dinauer CA, Udelsman R. The treatment of differentiated thyroid cancer in children: emphasis on surgical approach and radioactive iodine therapy. Endocr Rev. 2011;32:798–826.
4. Parisi MT, Mankoff D. Differentiated pediatric thyroid cancer: correlates with adult disease, controversies in treatment. Semin Nucl Med. 2007;37:340–56.
5. Hogan AR, Zhuge Y, Perez EA, Koniaris LG, Lew JI, Sola JE. Pediatric thyroid carcinoma: incidence and outcomes in 1753 patients. J Surg Res. 2009;156:167–72.
6. Davies L, Welch HG. Increasing incidence of thyroid cancer in the United States, 1973–2002. JAMA. 2006;295:2164–7.
7. Wu XC, Chen VW, Steele B, Roffers S, Klotz JB, Correa CN, Carozza SE. Cancer incidence in adolescents and young adults in the United States, 1992–1997. J Adolesc Health. 2003;32:405–15.
8. Siegel R, Ward E, Brawley O, Jemal A. Cancer statistics, 2011: the impact of eliminating socioeconomic and racial disparities on premature cancer deaths. CA Cancer J Clin. 2011;61:212–36.
9. Bleyer A, Viny A, Barr R. Cancer in 15- to 29-year-olds by primary site. Oncologist. 2006;11:590–601.
10. Cramer JD, Fu P, Harth KC, Margevicius S, Wilhelm SM. Analysis of the rising incidence of thyroid cancer using the surveillance, epidemiology and end results national cancer data registry. Surgery. 2010;148:1147–52 (discussion 1152–3).
11. Enewold L, Zhu K, Ron E, Marrogi AJ, Stojadinovic A, Peoples GE, Devesa SS. Rising thyroid cancer incidence in the United States by demographic and tumor characteristics, 1980–2005. Cancer Epidemiol Biomarkers Prev. 2009;18:784–91.
12. Aschebrook-Kilfoy B, Ward MH, Sabra MM, Devesa SS. Thyroid cancer incidence patterns in the United States by histologic type, 1992–2006. Thyroid. 2011;21:125–34.
13. Ron E, Lubin JH, Shore RE, Mabuchi K, Modan B, Pottern LM, Schneider AB, Tucker MA, Boice JD Jr. Thyroid cancer after exposure to external radiation: a pooled analysis of seven studies. Radiat Res. 1995;178:AV43-60.
14. Schonfeld SJ, Lee C, de Gonzalez AB. Medical exposure to radiation and thyroid cancer. Clin Oncol (R Coll Radiol). 2011;244–50.
15. Ron E, Saftlas AF. Head and neck radiation carcinogenesis: epidemiologic evidence. Otolaryngol Head Neck Surg. 1996;115:403–8.
16. Ronckers CM, Sigurdson AJ, Stovall M, Smith SA, Mertens AC, Liu Y, Hammond S, Land CE, Neglia JP, Donaldson SS, Meadows AT, Sklar CA, Robison LL, Inskip PD. Thyroid cancer in childhood cancer survivors: a detailed evaluation of radiation dose response and its modifiers. Radiat Res. 2006;166:618–28.
17. Taylor AJ, Croft AP, Palace AM, Winter DL, Reulen RC, Stiller CA, Stevens MC, Hawkins MM. Risk of thyroid cancer in survivors of childhood cancer: results from the British Childhood Cancer Survivor Study. Int J Cancer. 2009;125:2400–5.
18. Schneider AB, Bekerman C, Leland J, Rosengarten J, Hyun H, Collins B, Shore-Freedman E, Gierlowski TC. Thyroid nodules in the follow-up of irradiated individuals: comparison of thyroid ultrasound with scanning and palpation. J Clin Endocrinol Metab. 1997;82:4020–7.
19. Jacob P, Goulko G, Heidenreich WF, Likhtarev I, Kairo I, Tronko ND, Bogdanova TI, Kenigsberg J, Buglova E, Drozdovitch V, Golovneva A, Demidchik EP, Balonov M, Zvonova I, Beral V. Thyroid cancer risk to children calculated. Nature. 1998;392:31–2.
20. Tronko MD, Howe GR, Bogdanova TI, Bouville AC, Epstein OV, Brill AB, Likhtarev IA, Fink DJ, Markov VV, Greenebaum E, Olijnyk VA, Masnyk IJ, Shpak VM, McConnell RJ, Tereshchenko VP, Robbins J, Zvinchuk OV, Zablotska LB, Hatch M, Luckyanov NK, Ron E, Thomas TL, Voilleque PG, Beebe GW. A cohort study of thyroid cancer and other thyroid diseases after the Chornobyl accident: thyroid cancer in Ukraine detected during first screening. J Natl Cancer Inst. 2006;98:897–903.

21. Schneider AB. Radiation-induced thyroid tumors. Endocrinol Metab Clin North Am. 1990;19:495–508.
22. Herraiz M, Barbesino G, Faquin W, Chan-Smutko G, Patel D, Shannon KM, Daniels GH, Chung DC. Prevalence of thyroid cancer in familial adenomatous polyposis syndrome and the role of screening ultrasound examinations. Clin Gastroenterol Hepatol. 2007;5:367–73.
23. Ngeow J, Mester J, Rybicki LA, Ni Y, Milas M, Eng C. Incidence and clinical characteristics of thyroid cancer in prospective series of individuals with Cowden and Cowden-like syndrome characterized by germline PTEN, SDH, or KLLN alterations. J Clin Endocrinol Metab. 2011;96:E2063–71.
24. Smith JR, Marqusee E, Webb S, Nose V, Fishman SJ, Shamberger RC, Frates MC, Huang SA. Thyroid nodules and cancer in children with PTEN hamartoma tumor syndrome. J Clin Endocrinol Metab. 2011;96:34–7.
25. Hall JE, Abdollahian DJ, Sinard RJ. Thyroid disease associated with Cowden syndrome: a meta-analysis. Head Neck. 2013;35:1189–94.
26. Stratakis CA, Courcoutsakis NA, Abati A, Filie A, Doppman JL, Carney JA, Shawker T. Thyroid gland abnormalities in patients with the syndrome of spotty skin pigmentation, myxomas, endocrine overactivity, and schwannomas (Carney complex). J Clin Endocrinol Metab. 1997;82:2037–43.
27. Doros L, Schultz KA, Stewart DR, Bauer AJ, Williams G, Rossi CT, Carr A, Yang J, Dehner LP, Messinger Y, Hill DA. DICER1-related disorders. In: Pagon RA, Adam MP, Ardinger HH, Wallace SE, Amemiya A, Bean LJH, Bird TD, Ledbetter N, Mefford HC, Smith RJH, Stephens K (eds) GeneReviews (R), Seattle, WA; 1993.
28. de Kock L, Sabbaghian N, Soglio DB, Guillerman RP, Park BK, Chami R, Deal CL, Priest JR, Foulkes WD. Exploring the association between DICER1 mutations and differentiated thyroid carcinoma. J Clin Endocrinol Metab. 2014;99:E1072–7.
29. Bonora E, Tallini G, Romeo G. Genetic predisposition to familial nonmedullary thyroid cancer: an update of molecular findings and state-of-the-art studies. J Oncol. 2010;2010:385206.
30. Gara SK, Jia L, Merino MJ, Agarwal SK, Zhang L, Cam M, Patel D, Kebebew E. Germline HABP2 mutation causing familial nonmedullary thyroid cancer. N Engl J Med. 2015;373:448–55.
31. Moses W, Weng J, Kebebew E. Prevalence, clinicopathologic features, and somatic genetic mutation profile in familial versus sporadic nonmedullary thyroid cancer. Thyroid. 2011;21:367–71.
32. Delellis RA. Pathology and genetics of thyroid carcinoma. J Surg Oncol. 2006;94:662–9.
33. Harness JK, Thompson NW, Mcleod MK, Pasieka JL, Fukuuchi A. Differentiated thyroid carcinoma in children and adolescents. World J Surg. 1992;16:547–53 (discussion 553–4).
34. Halac I, Zimmerman D. Thyroid nodules and cancers in children. Endocrinol Metab Clin North Am. 2005;34:725–44, x.
35. Gupta A, Ly S, Castroneves LA, Frates MC, Benson CB, Feldman HA, Wassner AJ, Smith JR, Marqusee E, Alexander EK, Barletta J, Doubilet PM, Peters HE, Webb S, Modi BP, Paltiel HJ, Kozakewich H, Cibas ES, Moore Jr FD, Shamberger RC, Larsen PR, Huang SA. A standardized assessment of thyroid nodules in children confirms higher cancer prevalence than in adults. J Clin Endocrinol Metab. 2013;98:3238–45.
36. Koo JS, Hong S, Park CS. Diffuse sclerosing variant is a major subtype of papillary thyroid carcinoma in the young. Thyroid. 2009;19:1225–31.
37. Demidchik YE, Demidchik EP, Reiners C, Biko J, Mine M, Saenko VA, Yamashita S. Comprehensive clinical assessment of 740 cases of surgically treated thyroid cancer in children of Belarus. Ann Surg. 2006;243:525–32.
38. Zimmerman D, Hay ID, Gough IR, Goellner JR, Ryan JJ, Grant CS, McConahey WM. Papillary thyroid carcinoma in children and adults: long-term follow-up of 1039 patients conservatively treated at one institution during three decades. Surgery. 1988;104:1157–66.
39. Savio R, Gosnell J, Palazzo FF, Sywak M, Agarwal G, Cowell C, Shun A, Robinson B, Delbridge LW. The role of a more extensive surgical approach in the initial multimodality management of papillary thyroid cancer in children. J Pediatr Surg. 2005;40:1696–700.
40. Jarzab B, Handkiewicz Junak D, Wloch J, Kalemba B, Roskosz J, Kukulska A, Puch Z. Multivariate analysis of prognostic factors for differentiated thyroid carcinoma in children. Eur J Nucl Med. 2000;27:833–41.
41. Chow SM, Law SC, Mendenhall WM, Au SK, Yau S, Mang O, Lau WH. Differentiated thyroid carcinoma in childhood and adolescence-clinical course and role of radioiodine. Pediatr Blood Cancer. 2004;42:176–83.
42. Vassilopoulou-Sellin R, Klein MJ, Smith TH, Samaan NA, Frankenthaler RA, Goepfert H, Cangir A, Haynie TP. Pulmonary metastases in children and young adults with differentiated thyroid cancer. Cancer. 1993;71:1348–52.
43. Otto KJ, Lam JS, Macmillan C, Freeman JL. Diminishing diagnosis of follicular thyroid carcinoma. Head Neck. 2010;32:1629–34.
44. McHenry CR, Phitayakorn R. Follicular adenoma and carcinoma of the thyroid gland. Oncologist. 2011;16:585–93.
45. Woodruff SL, Arowolo OA, Akute OO, Afolabi AO, Nwariaku F. Global variation in the pattern of differentiated thyroid cancer. Am J Surg. 2010;200:462–6.
46. Yusuf K, Reyes-Mugica M, Carpenter TO. Insular carcinoma of the thyroid in an adolescent: a case

report and review of the literature. Curr Opin Pediatr. 2003;15:512–5.
47. Lopez-Penabad L, Chiu AC, Hoff AO, Schultz P, Gaztambide S, Ordonez NG, Sherman SI. Prognostic factors in patients with Hurthle cell neoplasms of the thyroid. Cancer. 2003;97:1186–94.
48. Kebebew E, Greenspan FS, Clark OH, Woeber KA, McMillan A. Anaplastic thyroid carcinoma. Treatment outcome and prognostic factors. Cancer. 2005;103:1330–5.
49. Stein SA, Wartofsky L. Primary thyroid lymphoma: a clinical review. J Clin Endocrinol Metab. 2013;98:3131–8.
50. Lazar L, Lebenthal Y, Steinmetz A, Yackobovitch-Gavan M, Phillip M. Differentiated thyroid carcinoma in pediatric patients: comparison of presentation and course between pre-pubertal children and adolescents. J Pediatr. 2009;154:708–14.
51. Raval MV, Bentrem DJ, Stewart AK, Ko CY, Reynolds M. Utilization of total thyroidectomy for differentiated thyroid cancer in children. Ann Surg Oncol. 2010;17:2545–53.
52. Hay ID, Gonzalez-Losada T, Reinalda MS, Honetschlager JA, Richards ML, Thompson GB. Long-term outcome in 215 children and adolescents with papillary thyroid cancer treated during 1940 through 2008. World J Surg. 2010;34:1192–202.
53. Machens A, Lorenz K, Nguyen Thanh P, Brauckhoff M, Dralle H. Papillary thyroid cancer in children and adolescents does not differ in growth pattern and metastatic behavior. J Pediatr. 2010;157:648–52.
54. Ritter K, Elfenbein D, Schneider DF, Chen H, Sippel RS. Hypoparathyroidism after total thyroidectomy: incidence and resolution. J Surg Res. 2015;197:348–53.
55. Lo CY. Parathyroid autotransplantation during thyroidectomy. ANZ J Surg. 2002;72:902–7.
56. Puzziello A, Gervasi R, Orlando G, Innaro N, Vitale M, Sacco R. Hypocalcaemia after total thyroidectomy: could intact parathyroid hormone be a predictive factor for transient postoperative hypocalcemia? Surgery. 2015;157:344–8.
57. Antakia R, Edafe O, Uttley L, Balasubramanian SP. Effectiveness of preventative and other surgical measures on hypocalcemia following bilateral thyroid surgery: a systematic review and meta-analysis. Thyroid. 2015;25:95–106.
58. Pisanu A, Porceddu G, Podda M, Cois A, Uccheddu A. Systematic review with meta-analysis of studies comparing intraoperative neuromonitoring of recurrent laryngeal nerves versus visualization alone during thyroidectomy. J Surg Res. 2014;188:152–61.
59. Musacchio MJ, Kim AW, Vijungco JD, Prinz RA. Greater local recurrence occurs with "berry picking" than neck dissection in thyroid cancer. Am Surg. 2003;69:191–6 (discussion 196–7).
60. American Thyroid Association Surgery Working G, American Association of Endocrine S, American Academy of OH, Neck S, American H, Neck S, Carty SE, Cooper DS, Doherty GM, Duh QY, Kloos RT, Mandel SJ, Randolph GW, Stack BC, Jr, Steward DL, Terris DJ, Thompson GB, Tufano RP, Tuttle RM, Udelsman R. Consensus statement on the terminology and classification of central neck dissection for thyroid cancer. Thyroid. 2009;19:1153–8.
61. Stack BC, Jr, Ferris RL, Goldenberg D, Haymart M, Shaha A, Sheth S, Sosa JA, Tufano RP, American Thyroid Association Surgical Affairs C. American Thyroid Association consensus review and statement regarding the anatomy, terminology, and rationale for lateral neck dissection in differentiated thyroid cancer. Thyroid. 2012;22:501–8.
62. Solorzano CC, Carneiro DM, Ramirez M, Lee TM, Irvin GL, 3rd. Surgeon-performed ultrasound in the management of thyroid malignancy. Am Surg. 2004;70:576–80 (discussion 580–2).
63. Farahati J, Reiners C, Demidchik EP. Is the UICC/AJCC classification of primary tumor in childhood thyroid carcinoma valid? J Nucl Med. 1999;40:2125.
64. Giordano D, Valcavi R, Thompson GB, Pedroni C, Renna L, Gradoni P, Barbieri V. Complications of central neck dissection in patients with papillary thyroid carcinoma: results of a study on 1087 patients and review of the literature. Thyroid. 2012;22:911–7.
65. Machens A, Elwerr M, Thanh PN, Lorenz K, Schneider R, Dralle H. Impact of central node dissection on postoperative morbidity in pediatric patients with suspected or proven thyroid cancer. Surgery. 2016;160:484–92.
66. Sturgeon C, Yang A, Elaraj D. Surgical management of lymph node compartments in papillary thyroid cancer. Surg Oncol Clin N Am. 2016;25:17–40.
67. Sosa JA, Tuggle CT, Wang TS, Thomas DC, Boudourakis L, Rivkees S, Roman SA. Clinical and economic outcomes of thyroid and parathyroid surgery in children. J Clin Endocrinol Metab. 2008;93:3058–65.
68. Eustatia-Rutten CF, Smit JW, Romijn JA, Van der Kleij-Corssmit EP, Pereira AM, Stokkel MP, Kievit J. Diagnostic value of serum thyroglobulin measurements in the follow-up of differentiated thyroid carcinoma, a structured meta-analysis. Clin Endocrinol (Oxf). 2004;61:61–74.
69. Hung W, Sarlis NJ. Current controversies in the management of pediatric patients with well-differentiated nonmedullary thyroid cancer: a review. Thyroid. 2002;12:683–702.
70. Brown AP, Chen J, Hitchcock YJ, Szabo A, Shrieve DC, Tward JD. The risk of second primary malignancies up to three decades after the treatment of differentiated thyroid cancer. J Clin Endocrinol Metab. 2008;93:504–15.
71. Fard-Esfahani A, Emami-Ardekani A, Fallahi B, Fard-Esfahani P, Beiki D, Hassanzadeh-Rad A, Eftekhari M. Adverse effects of radioactive iodine-131 treatment for differentiated thyroid carcinoma. Nucl Med Commun. 2014;35:808–17.

Part II
Parathyroid

Parathyroid Gland Embryology, Anatomy and Physiology

5

Gerard V. Walls and Radu Mihai

This chapter reviews the embryology, anatomy and physiology of the parathyroid glands with emphasis on surgical conditions and surgical decision making. First, parathyroid development is considered as it is the basis to understand normal and abnormal parathyroid anatomy. Next, parathyroid anatomy is examined because knowledge of parathyroid location, blood supply and relationship to the recurrent laryngeal nerve and thyroid are essential to understand parathyroid operations and the potential risks and complications of those operations. Finally, we will review the parathyroid gland's role in calcium homeostasis which explains the clinical findings of hypo and hyperparathyroidism. Additional information regarding the embryology and anatomy of the adjacent thyroid gland and recurrent laryngeal nerve are discussed in detail in Chap. 1 (Thyroid gland embryology, anatomy and physiology).

Parathyroid Embryology

Paired inferior and superior parathyroid glands originate from the endoderm of the dorsal part of third and fourth pharyngeal pouches in gestational weeks 5–6 and then migrate to their final position with the primordia of the thymus and thyroid glands. The inferior parathyroid glands originate from the third pharyngeal pouch (hence their designation P-III) and by week 7 of gestation move caudally and medially with the thyroid and thymus (Fig. 5.1). Roughly, half of inferior parathyroid glands eventually end up on the dorsal surface of the thyroid while the other half migrate further caudally into the thyrothymic ligament or thymus. The superior parathyroid glands originate from the fourth pharyngeal pouch (hence their designation P-IV) and by week 7 of gestation move caudally away from the pharynx with the thyroid gland (Fig. 5.1). The superior parathyroid glands migration path is shorter and their final position more constant than the inferior parathyroid glands with the majority of superior glands ending up on the posterior surface of the thyroid.

During the descent of the parathyroid glands, the P-IVs are crossed by the P-IIIs and occasionally the superior and inferior glands fuse. The final position of fused (or near fused) glands is usually close to the inferior thyroid artery. Parathyroid gland fusion during development may lead to the two separate glands being mistaken for a single bi-lobed gland which would give a false impression of an unidentified gland

G.V. Walls
Consultant General and Endocrine Surgeon, University Hospitals of Morecambe Bay NHS Foundation Trust, Royal Lancaster Infirmary, Ashton Road, Lancaster LA1 4RP, UK
e-mail: gerard.walls@nds.ox.ac.uk

R. Mihai (✉)
Department of Surgery, Churchill Cancer Centre, Oxford OX3 9DU, UK
e-mail: radumihai@doctors.org.uk; radu.mihai@ouh.nhs.uk

D.J. Ledbetter and P.R.V. Johnson (eds.), *Endocrine Surgery in Children*,
DOI 10.1007/978-3-662-54256-9_5

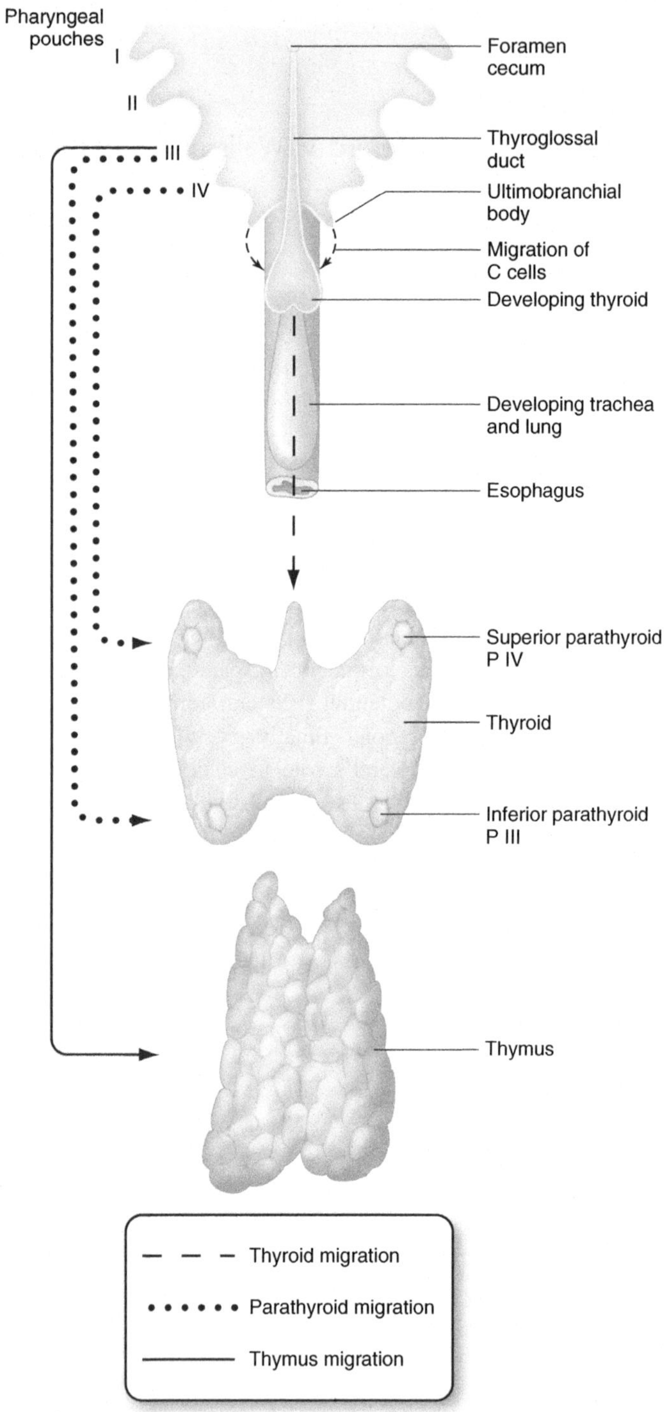

Fig. 5.1 Development of Parathyroid Glands. Superior parathyroid glands originate from fourth pharyngeal pouch and are designated as P-IVs. Their migration path is shorter and final position more reliable than inferior parathyroid glands. Inferior parathyroid glands originate from third pharyngeal pouch and are designated as P IIIs. Their migration path is longer and final position is more variable than superior parathyroid glands. The thymus also originates from the third pharyngeal pouch and the final position of the inferior parathyroids is often adjacent to or even within the thymus

during parathyroid exploration. This misinterpretation can be avoided by close inspection of the blood supply to the parathyroid. Each gland will have a unique blood supply so even an enlarged single gland has a single arterial pedicle while a bilobed gland has two separate arterial pedicles.

Supernumerary parathyroid glands can occur in up to 15% of population [1]. They are most often found in the thymus, but they have also been described in the middle mediastinum at the level of the aortopulmonary window and lateral to the jugulo-carotid axis. Intravagal parathyroid tissue has also been reported. Such locations are thought to be due to fragmentation of the foetal superior parathyroid during development.

Human foetal parathyroid glands can synthesize parathyroid hormone (PTH) from as early as 10 weeks of gestation [2]. Foetal parathyroid hormone is essential for foetal calcium homeostasis [3] as intact maternal PTH does not cross the placenta. Maternal serum calcium crosses the placenta and may influence foetal PTH secretion.

The embryological development of the parathyroid gland requires the coordinated expression of many transcription factors including GCMB, SHH, GATA3, TBCE, Six1/4, Eya1, Hoxa3, Tbx1, Sox3, Pax1 and Pax9. Studies in a mouse knockout model demonstrated that loss of GATA3 expression or its target GCM2, a parathyroid-specific transcription factor, resulted in abnormal third and fourth pharyngeal pouch morphology and the absence of parathyroid glands, although some PTH was produced by the thymus gland [4]. Deletion of the homeobox gene *Hoxa3* resulted in lack of both thymus and parathyroid glands [5]. Parathyroid hyperplasia or tumours develop in several familial conditions noted in Table 5.1.

Parathyroid Anatomy

As predicted by embryology, most people have four parathyroid glands, two on each side of the neck: a superior parathyroid gland (derived from the fourth pharyngeal pouch) and an inferior parathyroid gland (derived from the third pharyngeal pouch). The superior parathyroid glands (P-IV) are located close to the upper pole of the thyroid gland, at the level with the first tracheal ring. Traditionally, a superior parathyroid gland is said to be found in an area 2 cm in diameter centred 1 cm above the intersection of the

Table 5.1 Familial conditions in which parathyroid hyperplasia or tumours develop

Syndrome	Inheritance pattern	Associated gene(s)	Parathyroid abnormality	Other abnormalities
Multiple endocrine Neoplasia type 1 (MEN-1)	Autosomal dominant	MEN1	• Multiple gland hyperplasia • Adenomas	• Pancreatic islet cell tumours • Pituitary adenomas
Multiple endocrine Neoplasia type 2 (MEN2)	Autosomal dominant	RET	• Adenomas	• Medullary carcinoma thyroid (MCT) • Pheochromocytoma
Hyperparathyroidism jaw Tumour syndrome	Autosomal dominant	HRPT2[a, b]	• Adenomas • Carcinoma (15%)	• Ossifying jaw tumours • Renal, uterine and pancreatic tumours
Familial isolated Hyperparathyroidism	Typically autosomal dominant	MEN1, RET or HRPT2	• Adenomas • Carcinoma • Hyperplasia	• Without additional syndromic features

[a](also known as *CDC73*)
[b]codes for parafibromin. Lack of parafibromin expression is now being used to assist with the histological diagnosis of parathyroid carcinoma

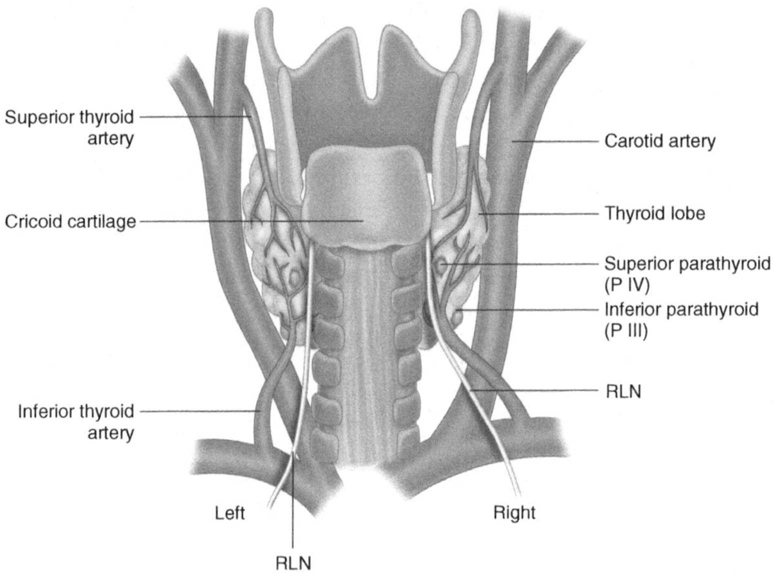

Fig. 5.2 Anatomy of parathyroid glands as viewed from posterior. Superior parathyroid glands located on posterior surface of thyroid gland near the insertion of the recurrent laryngeal nerve into the cricoid muscle. Inferior parathyroid glands are less constant but usually located on inferior and lateral surface of lower lobe of thyroid or adjacent thymus. Blood supply to parathyroid glands are from small branches of the inferior thyroid arteries

inferior thyroid artery and recurrent laryngeal nerve (RLN).

The inferior parathyroid glands have a more variable position. They are commonly visible on the anterolateral surface of the lower pole of the thyroid; however, they are often found in the thyrothymic ligament or even the thymus (Fig. 5.2).

Macroscopic Appearance of Parathyroid Glands

Normal parathyroid glands are commonly described to be the size of a grain of rice, measuring 5–8 mm in their largest dimension. The weight of a normal parathyroid gland is approximately 40 mg. They are brown-yellow in colour, a characteristic that makes it possible to distinguish them from thyroid (which is darker) and fat (which is a brighter yellow). They are very friable and can easily be "bruised" with manipulation. A fine capsule surrounds the glands and there is a single feeding artery.

Relationship of Parathyroid Glands to the Recurrent Laryngeal Nerves

If one considers a coronal plane incorporating the RLN along its trajectory from the mediastinum to the larynx, the superior parathyroid glands are posterior to that plane and the inferior parathyroid glands are in front of that plane. This relationship is important to consider when a parathyroid adenoma is approached with limited exposure of surrounding anatomical landmarks and the operating surgeon needs to anticipate if the RLN will be in front of the adenoma (as for superior glands) or posterior to the adenoma (as for inferior glands).

Blood Supply of Parathyroid Glands

Both superior and inferior glands receive branches from the inferior thyroid artery. These are often end arteries so care must be taken during dissection of the thyroid and parathyroid glands to preserve parathyroid blood supply. Venous drainage is typically is through small unnamed tributaries that join the thyroid venous branches (Fig. 5.2).

Ectopic Parathyroid Glands

Superior parathyroid glands (P-IV) have a short migration in association with the thyroid gland and as a result major ectopia of the superior parathyroid glands is rare (see also Fig. 6.1). Exceptionally, they may be "undescended" and found anywhere from the posterior pharynx or oesophagus to just above the upper pole of the thyroid. Superior parathyroid glands (P-IV) can also become included within the thyroid at the time of time of the fusion of the ultimobranchial body (carrying the calcitonin-secreting c-cells from this "fifth" pharyngeal pouch) and the median thyroid. This would lead to a truly intrathyroidal parathyroid gland. Many parathyroid glands described as intrathyroidal are simply adherent to the posterior thyroid capsule.

The inferior parathyroid glands (P-III) have a longer embryological descent in association with the thymus gland and their ectopic positions range from the angle of the mandible to the pericardium. High ectopia results from incomplete migration and is represented by glands along the carotid sheath from the angle of mandible to the lower pole of the thyroid. Low ectopias result from excessive migration and result in glands in the thymus and anterior mediastinum.

Histology

There are two main cell types found in the parathyroid gland, namely chief cells and oxyphil cells. Chief cells, or principal cells, are the more abundant cell type and are small, typical neuroendocrine cells arranged into curvilinear cords and are packed with secretory granules containing parathyroid hormone (PTH).

Oxyphil cells are larger, pale pink cells, with a smaller, darker nucleus and relatively larger amount of cytoplasm than the chief cells. The significance of the oxyphil cells is not clear. For reason difficult to explain, in parathyroid adenomas that incorporate the radioactive tracer sestamibi and can be seen visualised on nuclear medicine scans oxyphil cells make up 20% of the cell population while tumours lacking oxyphil cells do not take up the tracer.

Parathyroid Physiology

Calcium homeostasis is a phylogenetically important adaptation mechanism involving a balance between dietary intake, intestinal absorption, renal excretion, and bone deposition and breakdown. All these processes are modulated by parathyroid hormone and vitamin D. Extracellular calcium concentration is the main factor controlling the secretion of parathyroid hormone by parathyroid cells. The calcium-sensing receptor (CaSR) on the plasma membrane enables parathyroid cells them to detect and respond to minute changes in extracellular calcium. Through a classic signalling pathway involving G-protein-phospholipase C-IP_3 formation and discharge of intracellular calcium stores, high extracellular calcium is translated into high intracellular calcium levels. The high intracellular calcium inhibits PTH secretion from parathyroid cells. This inhibition of hormone secretion in response to increasing intracellular calcium is unique among endocrine cells which are usually stimulated to secrete hormones when increasing intracellular calcium promotes the docking and fusion of the secretory granules with the plasma membrane.

Abnormalities of CaSR have significant impact on parathyroid physiology. Inactivating mutations lead to the parathyroid cells not "switching off" in the presence of high extracellular calcium. In one inactivating mutation heterozygous known as Familial Hypocalciuric Hypercalcemia (FHH) or Familial Benign Hypercalcemia patients suffer from hypocalciuric hypercalcemia which is usually asymptomatic. Newborns homozygous for this inactivating CaSR mutation have Neonatal Severe Hyperparathyroidism (NSHPT) with severe hypercalcemia. Activating mutations are rare and lead to the reverse condition—hypercalciuric hypocalcaemia.

Low expression of CaSR plays a role in the secondary hyperparathyroidism associated with renal insufficiency. Pharmacological stimulation of the CaSR with a specific agonist, cinacalcet, inhibits parathyroid secretion and it is increasingly used in patients with secondary hyperparathyroidism from end-stage renal disease and in patients with parathyroid carcinoma. In the United States, the Food and Drug Administration has not approved cinacalcet for use in children.

Parathyroid Hormone

Parathyroid hormone (PTH) is an 84-aminoacid peptide with a very short half-life of only 2–5 min because of rapid degradation into an amino-terminal fragment and a carboxy-terminal fragment. Modern laboratory determinations of PTH use a double antibody immunoassay that detects only the intact molecule rather than reacting against an end fragment. The main physiological effects of PTH (Fig. 5.3) are result from PTH interaction with specific receptors located in the kidney and bone. Chondrocytes, vascular smooth muscle cells, fat cells, brain and pancreas also express PTH receptors.

In the kidney, PTH increases calcium reabsorbtion from the ascending limb on the loop on Henle and the distal tubules. Also in the kidney PTH increases the enzymatic activation of Vitamin D. The active form of Vitamin D then increases intestinal absorbtion of dietary calcium. In bone, PTH increases calcium by interacting with osteoblasts which stimulate osteoclast precursors to make more osteoclasts. Osteoclasts directly lead to bone resorption and calcium release.

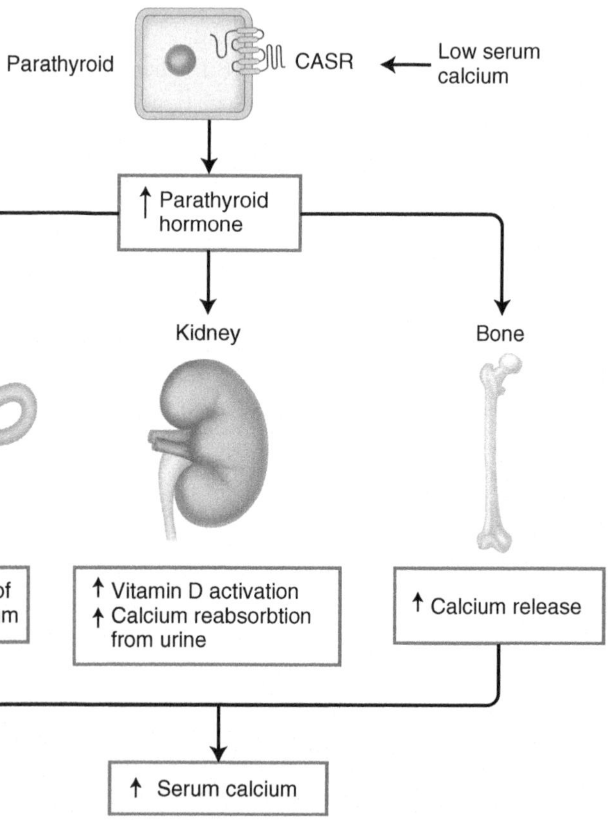

Fig. 5.3 Physiologic effects of parathyroid hormone. *CaSR* = Calcium sensing receptor

References

1. Arnault V, Beaulieu A, Lifante J-C, Serra AS, Sebag F, Mathonnet M, Hamy A, Meurisse M, Carnaille B, Kraimps J-L. Multicenter study of 19 aortopulmonary window parathyroid tumors: the challenge of embryologic origin. World J Surg. 2010;34:2211–6.
2. Leroyer-Alizon E, David L, Anast CS, Dubois PM. Immunocytological evidence for parathyroid hormone in human fetal parathyroid glands. J Clin Endocrinol Metab. 1981;52:513–6.
3. Simmonds CS, Karsenty G, Karaplis AC, Kovacs CS. Parathyroid hormone regulates fetal-placental mineral homeostasis. J Bone Miner Res. 2010;25:594–605.
4. Grigorieva IV, Mirczuk S, Gaynor Ku, Nesbit MA, Grigorieva EF, Wei Q, Ali A, Fairclough RJ, Stacey JM, Stechman MJ, Mihai R, Kurek D, Fraser WD, Hough T, Condie BG, Manley N, Grosveld F, Thakker RV. Gata3-deficient mice develop parathyroid abnormalities due to dysregulation of the parathyroid-specific transcription factor Gcm2. J Clin Invest. 2010;120(6):2144–55.
5. Chisaka O, Capecchi MR. Regionally restricted developmental defects resulting from targeted disruption of the mouse homeobox gene hox-1.5. Nature. 1991;350(6318):473–9.

6 Parathyroid Surgery in Children

Jocelyn Burke, Herbert Chen and Ankush Gosain

This chapter reviews the presentation, diagnosis, and treatment of hyperparathyroidism in children. Compared to adults, parathyroid disease is rare in children and this rarity may lead to delay in diagnosis of the parathyroid problem and delay in recognition of associated conditions. The common causes of hyperparathyroidism, such as parathyroid adenoma and hyperplasia, as well as the less common causes, such as adenocarcinoma, that require a high index of suspicion to diagnose are considered. The chapter will highlight the similarities and differences between children and adults in the diagnosis and management of parathyroid disease.

Incidence/Epidemiology

Hyperparathyroidism (HPT) is a rare disease in children, with an incidence of 2–5 per 100,000, compared to 1 per 1000 in adults [1]. Primary hyperparathyroidism (PHPT), which results from overproduction of parathyroid hormone (PTH), is the most common cause of HPT in both adults and children. A single parathyroid adenoma is the cause of 80–85% PHPT in adults, and is also the most common cause of PHPT in children. Parathyroid hyperplasia of all four glands is responsible for 10–15% of cases of PHPT in adults and is much more common in patients with hereditary conditions such as multiple endocrine neoplasia type 1 (MEN1) [2, 3].

Secondary and tertiary hyperparathyroidism are related to chronic renal failure, which results in continuous stimulation of PTH production, and are less common causes of HPT in children. In pediatric patients with chronic kidney disease (CKD) on dialysis, approximately 80% have secondary hyperparathyroidism with renal osteodystrophy, requiring medical treatment and occasionally surgery.

Parathyroid adenocarcinoma is an exceedingly rare cause of HPT, accounting for less than 1% of all cases of HPT in adults and it is probably even more uncommon in children, although no reports convincingly describe the incidence of parathyroid cancer in the pediatric population [4–9].

As in adults, HPT in children is more common in females than males, with a 3:2 ratio in a retrospective study of 52 pediatric patients [1]. In pediatric patients with sporadic (non-inherited) disease, symptomatic presentation generally occurs between age 15 and 18 years [1, 10]. Patients with MEN syndromes and other inherited forms of the HPT are often diagnosed with hyperparathyroidism earlier than patients with sporadic HPT. Children with inherited HPT might present with symptoms earlier than

J. Burke (✉) · H. Chen · A. Gosain
Department of Surgery, University of Wisconsin School of Medicine and Public Health, 600 Highland Avenue, Madison, WI 53792, USA
e-mail: jburke@uwhealth.org

H. Chen
e-mail: chen@surgery.wisc.edu

A. Gosain
e-mail: gosain@surgery.wisc.edu

D.J. Ledbetter and P.R.V. Johnson (eds.), *Endocrine Surgery in Children*,
DOI 10.1007/978-3-662-54256-9_6

adolescents with sporadic disease but the earlier diagnosis may be due to screening children who are asymptomatic but have a positive family history or other condition that heightens suspicion for HPT. Earlier detection of abnormal parathyroid glands may also occur in patients with MEN2 during their prophylactic thyroidectomy for medullary thyroid cancer.

Etiology

There are three main forms of hyperparathyroidism: primary, secondary, and tertiary. All three forms result in an overproduction of PTH. Under normal conditions, parathyroid hormone is released in response to decreased serum calcium levels. Increased PTH leads to [1] increased gastrointestinal absorption of calcium via increased renal production of 1, 25-dihydroxy vitamin D_3, [2] osteoclast activation with increased bone breakdown and release of calcium, and [3] increased renal reabsorption of calcium. All of these mechanisms increase serum calcium. Under normal circumstances calcium-sensing receptors (CaSRs) in the parathyroid glands detect the increased serum calcium and activate a negative feedback loop to decrease PTH production [3]. In primary hyperparathyroidism (PHPT), caused by parathyroid adenoma (s), hyperplasia of all four glands, or parathyroid carcinoma, the overproduction of PTH escapes this normal negative feedback loop and hypercalcemia results.

Hyperparathyroidism can manifest in newborns with neonatal severe hyperparathyroidism (NSHPT). This rare disease is associated with severe metabolic bone disease and life-threatening hypercalcemia (often >20 mg/dL) in the first week of life, and must be distinguished from transient neonatal hyperparathyroidism due to maternal hypocalcemia. NSHPT is associated with inactivating mutations in the calcium-sensing receptor genes (*CASR*), which code for the CaSR proteins. Neonates with NSHPT generally have complete or near-complete absence of functioning CaSRs in their parathyroid glands [2]. This results in parathyroid hyperplasia, increased PTH secretion and decreased renal excretion of calcium resulting in severe hypercalcemia [2]. A milder form of this condition results from a monoallelic mutation in *CASR*, which can cause an asymptomatic form of PHPT, termed familial hypocalciuric hypercalcemia (FHH). In these cases, reduced levels of functioning CaSRs result in increased secretion of PTH and modest hypercalcemia that can be managed with medical intervention alone [2].

In some cases of primary HPT, serum calcium levels are in the high-normal range, but PTH levels fail to be appropriately suppressed. This condition is sometimes referred to as "normocalcemic hyperparathyroidism" or "mild hyperparathyroidism." In the rare cases when hyperparathyroidism results from parathyroid carcinoma, patients often have extremely high levels of hypercalcemia (>14 mg/dL), arising from the overproduction of PTH from tumor cells within the parathyroid gland and metastases [4]. These patients can present in hypercalcemic crisis, which is a medical emergency described in more detail in 6.71 Preoperative Management.

Secondary hyperparathyroidism (SHPT) arises in the setting of chronic kidney failure, when vitamin D activation by the kidney declines which reduces gastrointestinal absorption of calcium. In addition, renal excretion of phosphate declines and the increasing serum phosphate binds calcium. Both processes lead to low serum calcium levels that continuously signal the parathyroid glands to produce PTH, resulting in elevated serum PTH levels and ultimately leading to four-gland hyperplasia [3].

Tertiary hyperparathyroidism (THPT) describes the condition in which a parathyroid gland subjected to prolonged stimulation from hypocalcemia, usually due to renal failure or chronic vitamin D deficiency, begins autonomous overproduction of PTH that no longer responds to negative feedback. This can result in higher levels of serum calcium than would be expected from calcium and calcitriol therapy alone [3]. THPT is most often seen after renal transplantation.

Hyperparathyroidism in children can also be a manifestation of MEN1 and MEN2 syndromes.

Parathyroid disease may be the first indicator of MEN disorders and children who present with hyperparathyroidism and have a family history of parathyroid disease or neuroendocrine tumors should undergo genetic testing for the involved genetic mutations (*MEN1* and *RET*, respectively). In MEN1, the *MEN1* gene is a putative tumor suppressor, and the development of MEN1 requires two genetic hits to result in loss of function. One mutation is inherited in the germline and is present in every cell. The second mutation is a sporadic somatic mutation in a single cell of an involved tissue that results in clonal expansion and tumor development. The MEN1 tumor syndrome includes development of parathyroid tumors, pancreatic neuroendocrine neoplasms, pituitary tumors, and bronchial carcinoids [11].

MEN2 syndrome results from an autosomal dominant inheritance of activating mutations in the *RET* proto-oncogene. *RET* (*RE*arranged during *T*ransfection) codes for a receptor tyrosine kinase involved in cellular growth. The missense mutations of the gene result in gain of function alterations in the protein, which manifest as medullary thyroid cancer (MTC) in nearly every patient, as well as varying presence of other endocrine neoplasms [11]. For more information on parathyroid disease in MEN1 and MEN2 please refer to Chaps. 30 and 31, respectively.

Pathology

In children with hyperparathyroidism, as in adults, the most common operative finding is a single adenoma and second most common operative finding is four-gland hyperplasia [1, 12]. In series of children and young adults with PHPT, 60–92% have a single adenoma and 0–40% have four-gland hyperplasia [1, 12, 13]. In a study that focused on patients under 18 years old with no family history of parathyroid or thyroid disease, 100% were found to have single adenomas [13]. Additionally, in a separate series, 10% of patients were found to have ectopic glands, including intrathymic and intrathyroidal adenomas (Fig. 6.1) [1]. On pathologic analysis, specimens show hyperplastic parathyroid tissue.

Adenocarcinoma of the parathyroid is defined by gross or histologic invasion of blood vessels, perineural tissue, thyroid gland, or other surrounding tissues and by the presence of distant metastases. Of note, fibrosis or mitotic figures can be found in adenomas without malignant potential, so these findings are not sufficient to diagnose parathyroid adenocarcinoma [3].

Clinical Presentation

History and Symptoms

Patients with hyperparathyroidism can have a wide range of symptoms, or they can be asymptomatic (Table 6.1) [1, 12]. Pediatric patients are more likely to present with symptoms than adults. While most adult series demonstrate asymptomatic rates of 30–40%, pediatric series report only 0–20% of patients as asymptomatic on presentation [1, 2, 12]. Children are also more likely to present with end organ damage, including pathologic bone fractures, osteitis fibrosa cystica, nephrolithiasis, and pancreatitis [12]. These presentations of advanced disease may be due in part to the frequent delays in diagnosis caused by a low index of suspicion and delay in appropriate confirmatory diagnostic investigations. Hyperparathyroidism is the third most frequent endocrine disease in adults (after diabetes and thyroid disease) [3] and is a commonly considered diagnosis, but in a large series of children and adolescents it took an average of 24 months to diagnose the same disease in pediatric patients [1].

In the rare patients with neonatal severe hyperparathyroidism, symptoms present in the first few days of life and include failure to thrive, hypotonia, respiratory distress, and prominent skeletal involvement. This is always combined with severe hypercalcemia that often requires urgent intervention [2].

A family history of parathyroid disease is common in pediatric patients with HPT, especially in those with genetic disorders such as

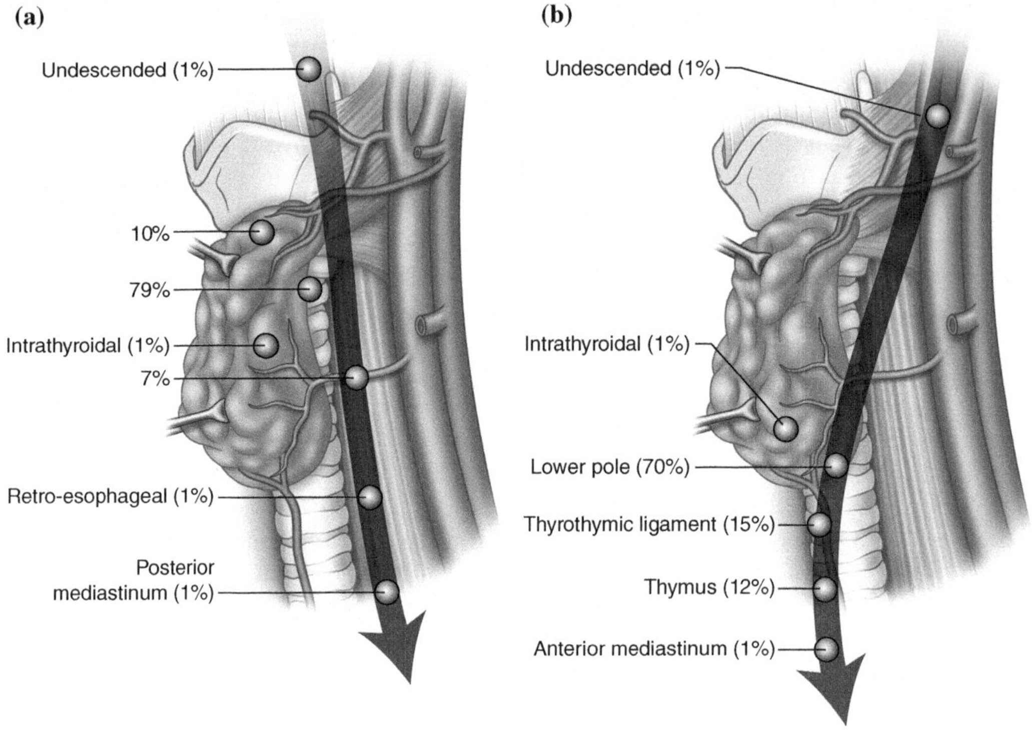

Fig. 6.1 The location and frequency of ectopic superior (**a**) and inferior (**b**) parathyroid glands. The *shaded area* indicates the embryologic of descent of the parathyroid glands

MEN1 or MEN2, or familial HPT. Patients with these inherited conditions are even more likely to present with symptoms when compared to those without a family history [1, 3, 11, 12].

Physical Examination

The physical examination in children and adolescents with HPT is usually normal. The parathyroid glands lie posterior and medial to the lateral border of the thyroid gland (see Chap. 5) and are difficult to palpate even when enlarged. When patients with HPT have palpable neck nodules, the nodules are usually not parathyroid glands [1]. Occasionally an ectopic gland may be palpated as a small (≤ 1 cm), mobile, non-tender neck nodule. Cervical lymph nodes are rarely enlarged and supraclavicular lymph nodes are even more rarely enlarged.

Blood Tests

In any child with suspected hypercalcemia and/or hyperparathyroidism, serum levels of total calcium, PTH, phosphate, and alkaline phosphatase should be checked. Serum TSH levels should be checked to rule out concomitant thyroid disease. Diagnosis of primary HPT is made with elevated PTH levels (>65 pg/mL, though the normal range varies by testing protocol) in the presence of normal or elevated serum calcium (>10.2 mg/dL, though the normal range varies by testing protocol). A PTH level that is not appropriately suppressed with a high-normal serum calcium level is also consistent with HPT. Secondary HPT, in contrast, is diagnosed when elevated PTH levels are present in the setting of hypocalcemia caused by a known separate etiology such as chronic renal failure.

Table 6.1 Clinical presentations of hyperparathyroidism

Asymptomatic
General
• Fatigue
• Weakness
• Myalgias
Neurologic/Psychiatric
• Headache
• Depression
• Cognitive impairment
Skeletal
• Bone pain
• Osteoporosis
• Pathologic fractures
• Osteitis fibrosa cystica
Gastrointestinal
• Anorexia
• Nausea
• Vomiting
• Diarrhea
• Constipation
• Pancreatitis
• Peptic ulcer disease
Renal
• Polyuria
• Polydipsia
• Kidney stones
• Hypertension

Imaging

Preoperative localization of the affected gland is important as it determines the operative approach for parathyroidectomy. If a single enlarged or hyperfunctioning gland is detected, the operation can be performed as a minimally invasive, or unilateral, parathyroidectomy (MIP). Cervical ultrasound (US) can aid both in the diagnosis of parathyroid adenomas and preoperative localization of the diseased gland. Parathyroid adenomas are recognized on ultrasound as a small, round, generally symmetrical, hypoechoic structure (Fig. 6.2). Neck ultrasound is noninvasive, relatively inexpensive, and radiation and sedation can be avoided, but the effectiveness of ultrasound is operator-dependent. Operator dependency probably explains the widely variable published accuracy rates of 48–74% [3, 14]. Ultrasound is also unable to sufficiently evaluate mediastinal glands.

One of the most common and most accurate preoperative localization studies is a dual-phase technitium-99 m sestamibi scan with single-photon emission computed tomography/computed tomography (SPECT/CT) (Fig. 6.3), with accuracy rates over 90% [3, 14, 15]. While the costs of sestamibi imaging with SPECT/CT are higher than ultrasound, this modality is less operator-dependent and is much better at detecting ectopic adenomas. However, when detection rates are based on persistent radionuclide uptake in both phase scans, the false negative rate can be as high as 40%. Recent studies including both adult and pediatric patients show that review of the early phase sestamibi scan by an experienced endocrine surgeon can result in increased preoperative localization of parathyroid adenomas, thus increasing the possibility of performing a MIP [16, 17].

Additional imaging options include CT or magnetic resonance imaging (MRI). CT images rely on the vascularity of parathyroid glands and their relative enhancement with contrast compared to the surrounding structures. CT has a sensitivity of 40–86% depending on the technique and experience of the radiologist [18]. Recently the sensitivity of CT has improved to 88% with the introduction of four-dimensional CT (4D-CT) that utilizes changes in the perfusion of contrast over time in addition to the three-dimensional images [18]. In MRI imaging, hyperfunctioning parathyroid glands show contrast enhancement on T_1-weighted images. Sensitivity for adenoma detection with this modality is 69–88% [18] and it may be preferred in pediatric patients, as there is no associated ionizing radiation and the costs are comparable with sestamibi SPECT/CT [3, 18].

Indications for Operation

The indications for operation vary based on the cause of hyperparathyroidism. In general, published indications derive from primary HPT in adult patients, as this is the most common type of HPT and the disease is uncommon in children. Any patient with elevated or inappropriately normal PTH and symptoms of hypercalcemia, including nephrolithiasis, nephrocalcinosis, renal dysfunction, osteopenia, pathologic fractures, osteitis fibrosa cystica, and altered neurologic function with obtundation, delirium, or coma, should undergo a parathyroidectomy [3, 18].

Regarding patients with asymptomatic PHPT, a National Institutes of Health (NIH) consensus conference published guidelines in 1990 that were amended in 2002 and 2008 [19] that propose surgery should be performed in the following circumstances:

- Serum calcium is more than 1 mg/dL (>0.25 mM/L) above the upper limits of normal.
- Glomerular filtration rate of <60 ml/min (per 1.73 m [2]). Below this level, elevations in serum PTH occur, and pathophysiological abnormalities associated with declining renal function may negatively influence the hyperparathyroid state.
- Reduced bone density, with a Z-score of −2.5 or less in patients younger than 50 years old, or any previous fracture or fragility.
- Age less than 50, as evidence supports a greater risk of complications from PHPT in these individuals over time [19].

Based on these recommendations, all children, adolescents, and young adults diagnosed with PHPT should undergo the appropriate operation to remove the affected gland(s).

If the patient's workup is suspicious for parathyroid carcinoma and the disease appears to be resectable, any biopsy including fine-needle aspiration should be avoided, as this can violate the capsule and increase the risk for tumor implants. The patient should proceed to operative resection, as described below [4].

The indications for operative intervention in secondary hyperparathyroidism are less clear. Medical therapy is the first-line treatment for SHPT, with the goal to increase available serum calcium and vitamin D, decrease hyperphosphatemia, and increase the sensitivity of CaSRs to serum calcium. Medical therapy with calcitriol supplementation and phosphate binders is often

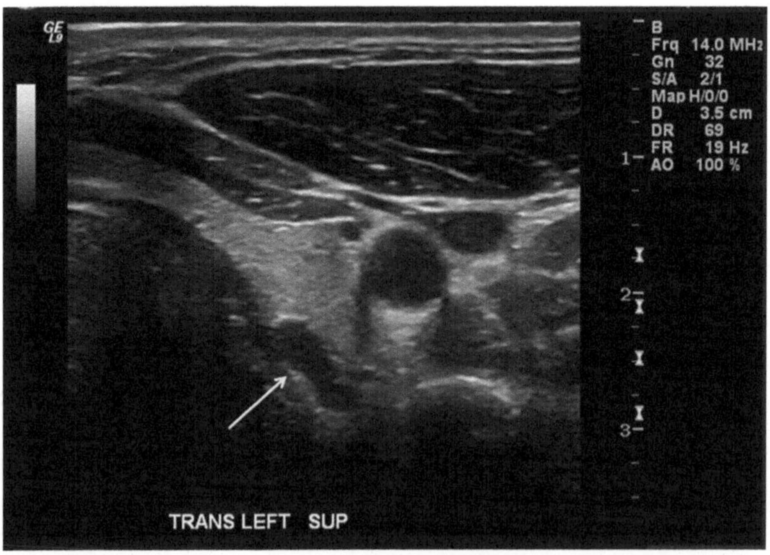

Fig. 6.2 Cervical ultrasound demonstrating a hypoechoic mass (*arrow*) consistent with a parathyroid adenoma posterolateral to the *left* thyroid lobe

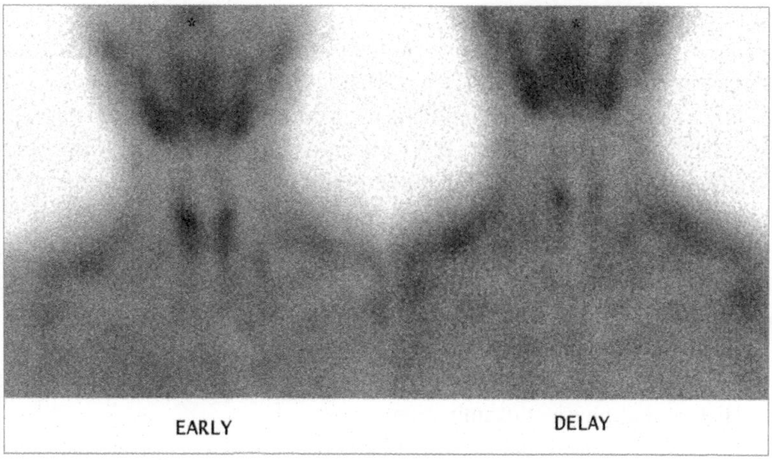

Fig. 6.3 Dual-phase technetium-99 m sestamibi scan showing increased focal uptake of the radionuclide that persists in the late phase scan, indicating a positive localization of a *right side* parathyroid adenoma

sufficient to maintain normal PTH and phosphorous levels. Pilot studies of cinacalcet, a calcimimetic that allosterically activates CaSRs, showed that a single dose predictably lowered serum PTH, calcium, and phosphorous in pediatric renal dialysis patients, which suggests this compound might have further use as medical treatment for pediatric SHPT [20]. Although in most cases calcium and PTH levels return to normal after return of normal renal function surgical treatment of SHPT should be considered in the following circumstances:

- A calcium • phosphate product >70
- Severe bone disease and pain
- Pruritus
- Extensive soft tissue calcification with tumoral calcinosis
- Calciphylaxis [21].

While the vast majority of hyperparathyroidism in the setting of CKD resolves within 6 months of renal transplantation, tertiary hyperparathyroidism (TPHT) develops in 2–3% of patients who receive a renal transplant [22]. Contrary to SHPT, the primary treatment of THPT is surgical. After receiving a kidney transplant patients with SHPT are routinely monitored for resolution of their HPT. Surgical treatment should be considered if any of the following occur after renal transplantation:

- Severe hypercalcemia (>11.5 mg/dL)
- Persistent hypercalcemia (>10.2 mg/dL more than three months after transplant)
- Severe osteopenia
- Symptomatic HPT (fatigue, pruritus, bone pain, pathologic bone fracture, peptic ulcer disease, mental status changes)
- Hypercalcemia with a history of renal calculi [23]

Management

Preoperative Management

The only curative management for PHPT is surgical removal of the diseased parathyroid gland(s). In general, no additional treatment is needed prior to parathyroidectomy. However, as described above, patients with SHPT and THPT are managed medically to control the levels of serum PTH, calcium, and phosphorous, and surgery is only performed if patients meet the indications presented above.

Hypercalcemic Crisis

Occasionally, patients present in hypercalcemic crisis with extremely high levels of serum calcium (generally above 14 mg/dL), oliguria or anuria, and changes in mental status [24]. This is more common in patients with NSHPT, in part because the syndrome is rare and the initial symptoms go unrecognized. Hypercalcemic crisis is a medical emergency, and patients need to be stabilized before they can undergo a parathyroidectomy. If this is the initial presentation of the patient for hypercalcemia (i.e., they have not previously been diagnosed with HPT), they should undergo a shortened diagnostic workup while they are being medically stabilized. This workup should include:

- History and physical examination
- X-rays of the head, thorax, vertebral column, pelvis, and long bones to look for osteolytic lesions associated with PHPT, metastases, other neoplasms
- Ultrasound examination of the abdominal organs to exclude hepatic, pancreatic, renal, or gynecologic tumors
- Laboratory studies including phosphate, potassium, creatinine, urea, alkaline phosphatase, complete blood count, and PTH [24].

While this workup is taking place, treatment for the severe hypercalcemia should begin. These patients are usually severely dehydrated, and the first step of therapy is intravenous hydration with normal saline. In addition, any medications that are associated with or adversely affected by hypercalcemia should be discontinued. Once intravascular volume is normalized then urinary excretion of calcium is encouraged by additional intravenous fluid. Loop diuretics are added to inhibit calcium reabsorption in the kidney and prevent fluid overload. Patients with renal failure may need urgent hemodialysis. Once the etiology of hypercalcemia is determined to be PHPT, the best definitive treatment is prompt surgical intervention. If surgery cannot be performed urgently, calcium can also be lowered with administration of gallium nitrate, bisphosphonates, or calcitonin, all of which act to inhibit osteoclasts and/or slow bone resorption [3]. However, due to the slow onset of therapeutic effect and long half-life of bisphosphonates, their use can lead to postoperative hypocalcemia, and in general they are not recommended when urgent surgery can be performed. If they are used, it is suggested that, due to children's highly sensitive response to bisphosphonates, only half of the normal dose should be given in the acute setting [25]. Case studies and small pilot studies indicate that cinacalcet, a calcimimetic, may be used in the pediatric population in the short term to lower calcium [20, 26]. Once patients are stabilized, they can proceed to surgery.

Operative Management

The goals of operative care are to identify and remove the diseased parathyroid gland or glands, preserve function in the remaining glands, identify and treat concomitant thyroid disease, and avoid intraoperative complications. The operative approach is determined by considering patient history and results from the preoperative imaging studies. A small series of 25 patients with PHPT demonstrated that patients younger than 18 years old with no family history of parathyroid disease uniformly had single parathyroid adenomas [13].

Parathyroidectomy is conducted either through a bilateral four-gland exploration or as a MIP (Fig. 6.4). For patients with PHPT and preoperative imaging that confirms localization of the diseased gland (as described in 6.54 Imaging), the operation of choice has been MIP. MIP has advantages over bilateral four-gland exploration including decreased operative time, lower hospital costs, shorter lengths of stay, and fewer events of postoperative hypocalcemia [27–32]. An additional benefit of MIP is the unilateral neck exploration, leaving the contralateral side relatively free of manipulation and thus scarring, making future neck operations less difficult. However, controversy around MIP has arisen due to recent large studies in adults with PHPT that indicate long-term recurrence rates may be slightly higher in patients who undergo an MIP versus bilateral exploration [33, 34]. As these findings have not been reported in children and postoperative complication rates are often higher in children than in adults [35], our center continues to perform MIPs in pediatric patients with positive preoperative localization studies. In this procedure, a small (1.5–2 cm) incision is made along an anterior neck skin fold on the side of midline identified with preoperative imaging, and unilateral exploration is completed to identify both ipsilateral parathyroid glands, taking care to identify and protect the recurrent laryngeal nerve. If an enlarged gland is encountered, it is removed and intraoperative testing modalities described below are used to confirm that the excised gland is the causative adenoma [3]. If no enlarged gland is identified, this procedure can be converted to a bilateral exploration without extension of the incision. If it is found that the patient has four-gland hyperplasia, a subtotal parathyroidectomy can be performed, with removal of 3.5 glands and an intended remnant amount of 50–75 mg. In these cases, we recommend cryopreservation of parathyroid tissue for later autotransplantation if the patient goes on to have postoperative hypoparathyroidism.

The success of MIP is enhanced with intraoperative localization adjuncts, including radioguidance and intraoperative PTH values. A radio-guided parathyroidectomy involves preoperative intravenous injection of technetium-99 m sestamibi 1–2 h prior to the operation and use of a hand-held gamma probe intraoperatively to localize hyperfunctioning parathyroid glands. Once the gland is removed, an ex vivo radionuclide count greater than 20% of background counts indicates appropriate removal of hyperfunctioning parathyroid tissue. This technique has been shown to be equally effective in children as in adults despite smaller adenomas in children [36].

Intraoperative PTH (ioPTH) monitoring is a reliable, accurate adjunct to a successful MIP [37]. After induction of anesthesia and prior to making an incision, a baseline PTH level is drawn. Once the enlarged gland is removed, a rapid PTH serum level is checked at 5, 10 and 15 min post removal. A fall in the serum PTH level to below 50% of baseline at any of these time points is indicative of cure, and the operation can be concluded. However, if the levels fail to fall by 50%, the presence of a second hyperfunctioning gland should be suspected, and cervical exploration should be continued. If a second adenoma is found and removed, this process of ioPTH measurement is repeated. In some cases, the first ioPTH shows an increase above the baseline level. This increase is attributed to manipulation of the gland during the exploration. By treating the elevated first ioPTH value as the new baseline and monitoring for a drop of later ioPTH levels by 50% below this new baseline, cure can still be accurately detected [38]. Using ioPTH decline as measurement for cure can be used effectively in children. In fact, a study of the kinetics of PTH decline in 15 pediatric patients with PHPT suggests that their serum PTH falls faster than in adults after removal of a parathyroid adenoma and 100% demonstrated cure with the 5 min ioPTH level, compared to 54% of adults by 5 min and 70% by 10 min [10]. This suggests that, in a child with PHPT, a persistently elevated ioPTH level at 5 min indicates presence of additional hyperfunctioning parathyroid tissue and operative exploration should continue in an effort to identify it.

The operative approach to SHPT assumes four-gland hyperplasia pathology, and begins with bilateral exploration. If hyperplasia indeed is present, a subtotal parathyroidectomy or total (four glands) parathyroidectomy with autotransplant is performed. A study of 105 patients undergoing parathyroidectomy for SHPT or THPT showed that ioPTH monitoring is still useful in patients as it can demonstrate cure [39]. This study gives even more striking rationale for using ioPTH monitoring in parathyroidectomy for THPT. While patients with THPT are generally assumed to have hyperplasia as well, if only one or two glands are noted to be enlarged during a bilateral exploration, these should be removed and ioPTH values should be checked. Limited resection with only one or two glands was sufficient for cure in 21% of patients with THPT [39]. Additionally, ioPTH monitoring allowed for the detection of supernumerary glands in three patients with THPT, meaning the surgical approach was altered in a total of 25% of THPT patients based on ioPTH results [39].

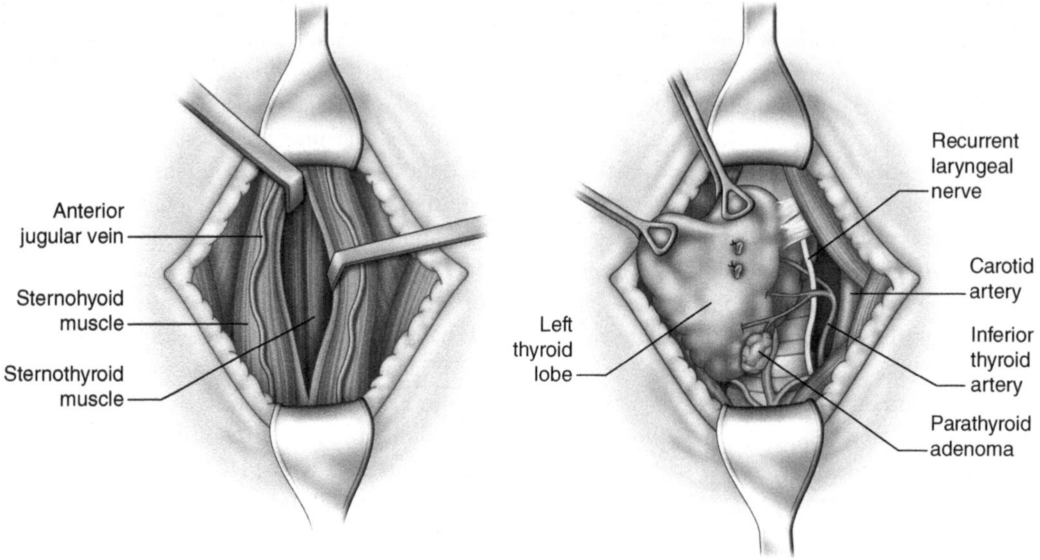

Fig. 6.4 Minimally invasive parathyroidectomy (MIP). A 1.5–2 cm transverse skin incision is made in line with the skin folds. The anterior strap muscles (sternohyoid, sternothyroid) are separated, and a unilateral exploration is undertaken to identify both ipsilateral parathyroid glands. The enlarged gland is removed, taking care to protect the recurrent laryngeal nerve

In patients with parathyroid carcinoma and no evidence of metastases, the recommended procedure is *en bloc* removal of the parathyroid cancer, with ipsilateral thyroid lobectomy, isthmectomy, tracheal skeletonization, excision of any adherent muscle, and a central lymph node dissection if deemed appropriate based on appearance and extension of the primary tumor and surrounding nodes [4]. Parathyroid carcinomas are often difficult to diagnose preoperatively, especially in children where the index of suspicion is exceedingly low. Therefore, if certain gross features, such as firm texture, thick gray or white capsule, and adherence to surrounding tissue, are encountered during the operation, the surgeon should consider carcinoma [4]. Utmost care must be taken to not violate the capsule so as to prevent spillage. Once *en bloc* resection has been performed, exploration of the remaining glands should be completed as carcinoma can coexist with multiple gland disease [4]. If the disease is metastatic, resection of the primary disease and the metastases can improve PTH and hypercalcemia [4].

Postoperative Management

In our practice, patients older than age 14 with an uneventful procedure and no comorbidities are discharged to home on the same day as their operation. Patients younger than age 10 can be admitted to the general care floor overnight with a general diet and full activity. When a patient falls between those ages, individual patient characteristics and parental comfort level are taken into account to decide whether or not to admit them to the floor postoperatively. Patients and parents are educated about the signs and symptoms of hypocalcemia, and patients are discharged with calcium carbonate (Tums), 1000–3000 mg based on age (Calcium carbonate dosing—Age 2–5 yrs: 400 mg, maximum 1200 mg daily; Age 5–11 yrs: 800 mg, maximum 2400), to be used as needed for hypocalcemia. If patients are at high risk for postoperative hypocalcemia (e.g., subtotal parathyroidectomy, redo operation), or if the patient and family would have difficulty detecting symptoms of hypocalcemia, they are discharged on 1000–3000 mg scheduled daily. Patients who undergo a total parathyroidectomy with forearm transplant of parathyroid tissue will require complete calcium and calcitriol replacement at discharge because the autograft will not become fully functional for at least 2 weeks. Patients return for a follow-up appointment one week postoperatively.

Complications

Multiple studies have indicated that high-volume endocrine surgeons have better clinical outcomes with fewer complications [35, 40, 41]. Operative complications include recurrent laryngeal nerve damage, which can cause hoarseness with unilateral injury or airway compromise if both nerves are damaged. In adults, recurrent laryngeal nerve monitors are sometimes used. These utilize a special endotracheal tube with a built-in sensor that is too large to use in most children, and thus they are not used in pediatric parathyroidectomies. Another possible complication is hematoma, though this risk is much lower than in thyroidectomy. Similarly, wound infections are possible but uncommon complications. Parathyroidectomy is considered a clean procedure and thus perioperative antibiotic prophylaxis is not recommended. If a wound infection does occur, conservative treatment with antibiotics should be attempted prior to open drainage. Due to the location of the incision on the neck, many delicate underlying structures are exposed with an open wound, and this should be prevented if possible.

Hypoparathyroidism can result from devascularization or removal of the remaining parathyroid glands and can lead to hypocalcemia. This is often transient, with symptoms resolving within the first week postoperatively. The risk of both transient and permanent hypocalcemia is higher in subtotal parathyroidectomy and in reoperative parathyroidectomy. For these reasons, it is recommended to cryopreserve some of the removed parathyroid tissue for potential autotransplantation should the patient's hypoparathyroidism persist. A study of the Healthcare Cost and Utilization Project—National Inpatient Sample demonstrated that children having parathyroidectomy have higher complication rates than adults, both general (21% vs. 12%) and endocrine-specific complications (15.2% vs. 6.2%) [35]. Age affects complication rates as well, with more complications in children age 0–6 (22%) than in those aged 7–12 (1.1%) or 13–17 (0.6%) [35]. This supports the involvement of multidisciplinary care with pediatric endocrine patients, especially in the youngest subset.

Long-Term Outcomes and Follow-up

In HPT, disease persistence is defined as elevated serum calcium within 6 months postoperatively, and disease recurrence denotes initially normal serum calcium levels that become elevated again more than 6 months postoperatively. Cure is defined based on calcium levels and not PTH levels because PTH levels can remain elevated postoperatively in 20–30% of patients. The scarce data available on cure rates and recurrence rates in pediatric patients suggest they are similar to those in adults, with 96–100% cured in reported series [1, 12, 13]. Patients should continue follow-up with their primary care provider or endocrinologist with routine monitoring for symptoms of hypercalcemia. While less than 5% will have persistent disease or develop recurrent disease, these few may require reoperative parathyroidectomy. The most common cause of persistent HPT is surgeon inexperience in locating and adequately excising the parathyroid adenomas [42].

Recurrent HPT is uncommon, but occurs more frequently in the setting of familial disease. When recurrent or persistent disease is suspected, a full workup must be completed to confirm the diagnosis. When the diagnosis is confirmed, vocal cord assessment should be performed to evaluate for occult dysfunction [42, 43]. Surgeons considering reoperative parathyroid surgery should have a higher threshold for operation than initial surgery due to the increased difficulty of reoperation. These include markedly elevated serum calcium level, recurrent nephrolithiasis, or ongoing bone loss. Patients should undergo preoperative imaging, and the operative approach must be decided based on the findings with the consideration that the diseased gland has a higher chance of being in an ectopic location. The use of intraoperative localization adjuncts is especially important in reoperative parathyroidectomies [43].

References

1. Kollars J, Zarroug AE, Van Heerden J, Lteif A, Stavlo P, Suarez L, Moir C, Ishitani M, Rodeberg D. Primary hyperparathyroidism in pediatric patients. Pediatrics. 2005;115:974.
2. Roizen J, Levine MA. Primary hyperparathyroidism in children and adolescents. J Chin Med Assoc. 2012;75(9):425–34.
3. Sosa JA, Udelsman R The Parathyroid Gland. In: Sabiston (ed) Textbook of general surgery, Section VIII Endocrine, Chapter 39, pp 924–943.
4. Adam MA, Untch BR, Olson JA. Parathyroid carcinoma: current understanding and new insights into gene expression and intraoperative parathyroid hormone kinetics. Oncologist. 2010;15:61–72.
5. Hamill J, Maoate K, Beasley SW, Corbett R, Evans J. Familial parathyroid carcinoma in a child. J Paediatr Child Health. 2002;38:314–7.
6. Fiedler AG, Rossi C, Gingalewski CA. Parathyroid carcinoma in a child: an unusual case of an ectopically located malignant parathyroid gland with tumor invading the thymus. J Pediatr Surg. 2009;44:1649–52.
7. Vinodh M, Rajeshwari A. Parathyroid carcinoma presenting as genu valgum. Indian Pediatr. 2012; 49:156.
8. Meier DE, Snyder WH, Dickson BA, Margraf LR, Guzzetta PC. Parathyroid carcinoma in a child. J Pediatr Surg. 1999;34:606–8.
9. Young TO, Saltzstein EC, Boman DA. Parathyroid carcinoma in a child: unusual presentation with seizures. J Pediatr Surg. 1984;19(2):194–6.
10. Burke JF, Schneider DF, Sippel RS, Chen H. Analysis of intraoperative parathyroid hormone levels in children: does standard protocol apply? In: Presented American Association of Pediatrics October 2012, manuscript in preparation.
11. Lairmore TC, Moley JF Multiple Endocrine Neoplasia Syndromes. Textbook of General Surgery, ed. Sabiston, Section VIII Endocrine, Chapter 42, pg 995–1010.
12. Li CC, Yang C, Wang S, Zang J, Kong XR, Ouyang J. A 10-year retrospective study of primary hyperparathyroidism in children. Exp Clin Endocrinol Diabetes. 2012;120:229–33.
13. Durkin ET, Nichol PF, Lund DP, Chen H, Sippel RS. What is the optimal treatment for children with primary hyperparathyroidism? J Ped Surg. 2010;45:1142–6.
14. Patel CN, Salahudeen HM, Lansdown M, Scarsbrook AF. Clinical utility of ultrasound and 99 mTc sestamibi SPECT/CTfor preoperative localization of parathyroid adenoma in patients with primary hyperparathyroidism. Clin Radiol. 2010;65:278–87.
15. Ciappuccini R, Morera J, Pascal P, Rame J-P, Heutte N, Aide N, Babin E, Resnik Y, Bardet S. Dual-phase 99mTc sestamibi scintigraphy with neck and thorax SPECT/CT in primary hyperparathyroidism: a single-institution experience. Clin Nucl Med. 2012;37(3):223–8.
16. Zia S, Sippel RS, Chen H. Sestamibi imaging for primary hyperparathyroidism: the impact of surgeon interpretation and radiologist volume. Ann Surg Oncol. 2012;19(12):3827–31.
17. Burke JF, Naraharisetty K, Schneider DF, Sippel RS, Chen H. Early phase technetium 99m-sestamibi scintigraphy can improve preoperative localization in primary hyperparathyroidism. Am J Surg. 2013;205(3):269–73.
18. Mohebati A, Shaha AR. Imaging techniques in parathyroid surgery for primary hyperparathyroidism. Am J Otolaryngol. 2012;33(4):457–68.
19. Bilezikian JP, Khan AA, Potts JT Jr. Guidelines for the management of asymptomatic primary hyperparathyroidism: summary statement from the third international workshop. J Clin Endocrinol Metab. 2009;94:335–9.
20. Padhi D, Langman CB, Fathalla-Shaykh S, Warady BA, Salusky IB, Lee E, Wang C, Posvar E. An open-label study to evaluate a single-dose of cinacalcet in pediatric dialysis subjects. Pediatr Nephrol. 2012;27:1953–9.
21. Clark OH (2010) Chapter 16. Thyroid and parathyroid. In: Doherty GM (ed) Current diagnosis and treatment: surgery. 13th ed. McGraw-Hill, New York.
22. Nichol PF, Starling JR, Mack E, Klovning JJ, Becker BN, Chen H. Long-term follow-up of patients with tertiary hyperparathyroidism treated by resection of a single or double adenoma. Ann Surg. 2002;235(5):673–80.
23. Pitt SC, Sippel RS, Chen H. Secondary and tertiary hyperparathyroidism, state of the art surgical management. Surg Clin North Am. 2009;89(5):1227–39.
24. Ziegler R. Hypercalcemic crisis. J Am Soc Nephrol. 2001;12:53–9.
25. Sebestyen JF, Srivastava T, Alon US. Bisphosphonates use in children. Clin Pediatr. 2012;51(11): 1011–24.
26. Wilhelm-Bals A, Parvex P, Magdelaine C, Girardin E. Successful use of bisphosphonate and calcimimetic in neonatal severe primary hyperparathyroidism. Pediatrics. 2012;129:e812.

27. Udelsman R, Lin Z, Donovan P. The superiority of minimally invasive parathyroidectomy based on 1650 consecutive patients with primary hyperparathyroidism. Ann Surg. 2011;253:585–91.
28. Chen H, Sokoll LJ, Udelsman R. Outpatient minimally invasive parathyroidectomy: a combination of sestamibi-SPECT localization, cervical block anesthesia, and intraoperative parathyroid hormone assay. Surgery. 1999;126:1016–21.
29. Goldstein RE, Blevins L, Delbeke D, Martin WH. Effect of minimally invasive radioguided parathyroidectomy on efficacy, length of stay, and costs in the management of primary hyperparathyroidism. Ann Surg. 2000;231:732–42.
30. Sidhu S, Neill AK, Russell CFJ. Long-term outcome of unilateral parathyroid exploration for primary hyperparathyroidism due to presumed solitary adenoma. World J Surg. 2003;27:339–42.
31. Bergenfelz A, Lindblom P, Tibblin S, Westerdahl J. Unilateral versus bilateral neck exploration for primary hyperparathyroidism: a prospective randomized controlled trial. Ann Surg. 2002;236 (5):543–51.
32. Norman J, Chheda H, Farrell C. Minimally invasive parathyroidectomy for primary hyperparathyroidism: decreasing operative time and potential complications while improving cosmetic results. Am Surg. 1998;64(5):391–6.
33. Norman J, Lopez J, Politz D. Abandoning unilateral parathyroidectomy: why we reversed our position after 15,000 parathyroid operations. J Am Coll Surg. 2012;214:260–9.
34. Schneider DF, Mazeh H, Sippel RS, Chen H. Is minimally invasive parathyroidectomy associated with greater recurrence compared to bilateral exploration? Analysis of more than 1000 cases. Surgery. 2012;152:1008–15.
35. Sosa JA, Tuggle CT, Wang TS, Thomas DC, Boudourakis L, Rivkees S, Roman SA. Clinical and economic outcomes of thyroid and parathyroid surgery in children. J Clin Endocrinol Metab. 2008;93(8):3058–65.
36. Burke JF, Jacobson K, Gosain A, Sippel RS, Chen H. Radioguided parathyroidectomy effective in pediatric patients. J Surg Res. 2013;184(1):312–317.
37. Chen H, Mack E, Starling JR. A comprehensive evaluation of perioperative adjuncts during minimally invasive parathyroidectomy: which is most reliable? Ann Surg. 2005;242:375–83.
38. Cook MR, Pitt SC, Schaefer S, Sippel RS, Chen H. A rising ioPTH level immediately after parathyroid resection: are additional hyperfunctioning glands always present? An application of the Wisconsin criteria. Ann Surg. 2010;251:1127–30.
39. Pitt SC, Panneerselvan R, Chen H, Sippel RS. Secondary and tertiary hyperparathyroidism: the utility of ioPTH monitoring. World J Surg. 2010;34 (6):1343–9.
40. Chen H, Zeiger MA, Gordon TA, Udelsman R. Parathyroidectomy in Maryland: effects of an endocrine center. Surgery. 1996;120:948–53.
41. Wang TS, Roman SA, Sosa JA. Predictors of outcomes following pediatric thyroid and parathyroid surgery. Curr Opin Oncol. 2008;21:23–8.
42. Solorzano CC, Mendez W, Lew JI, Rodgers SE, Montano R, Carneiro-Pla DM, Irvin GL. Long-term outcome of patients with elevated parathyroid hormone levels after successful parathyroidectomy for sporadic primary hyperparathyroidism. Arch Surg. 2008;143(7):659–63.
43. Udelsman R. Approach to the patient with persistent or recurrent primary hyperparathyroidism. J Clin Endocrinol Metab. 2011;96:2950–8.

Part III

Adrenal

Adrenal Gland Embryology, Anatomy, and Physiology

7

Sanjeev Vasudevan and Mary L. Brandt

Surgical intervention may be required for definitive treatment of adrenal gland disorders; therefore, every surgeon involved in treating children with adrenal pathology needs a thorough understanding of adrenal gland embryology, physiology, and anatomy. This chapter reviews these topics with special emphasis on how they relate to diseases of the adrenal gland and especially their surgical treatment. Adrenal gland embryology is reviewed first as it explains many unique aspects of adrenal anatomy, histology, and physiology. Adrenal physiology is then reviewed as it forms the basis to understand problems of deranged adrenal function, especially the unregulated secretion of steroids or catecholamines that are common manifestations of adrenal tumors. Finally, the anatomy of the adrenal glands and surrounding structures is considered as this explains the clinical findings of mass effects on adjacent organs of functional and nonfunctional adrenal tumors and, most importantly, forms the basis to understand the conduct of adrenal operations.

S. Vasudevan · M.L. Brandt (✉)
Department of Pediatric Surgery, Texas Children's Hospital, 6701 Fannin St # 1210, Houston, TX 77030, USA
e-mail: mary.brandt@bcm.edu; mlbrandt@texaschildrens.org

S. Vasudevan
e-mail: savasude@texaschildrens.org

Embryology

The adrenal gland is made up of two distinct types of tissue that arise from two separate origins. These two tissue types are responsible for the dual functions of the adrenal gland—steroid and catecholamine metabolism. At 5–6 weeks postconception, bilateral mesothelial proliferation occurs between the root of the dorsal mesentery and the gonadal ridges (Fig. 7.1) [1]. This tissue eventually forms the fetal cortex of the immature adrenal glands. The fetal adrenal cortex surrounds the developing adrenal medulla (Fig. 7.2), and the entire gland is encapsulated by a mesodermal layer that separates the adrenal gland from the adjacent developing gonad and kidney. The close approximation of the nascent adrenal cortex to the mesoderm destined to become the kidney and gonads explains both the normal anatomic relationship to the kidney and the occasional finding of ectopic adrenal tissue or adrenal "rests" associated with the gonadal vessels and gonads [2–4]. Up to 50% of newborns have ectopic adrenal tissue, either cortical tissue alone (if it migrated before invasion of the medullary cells) or a combination of cortical and medullary tissue. This ectopic adrenal tissue atrophies in most children so that adrenal rests are found in only 1% of adults [1].

At 9 weeks gestation the fetal adrenal cortex differentiates into histologically distinct zones—the definitive zone and the fetal zone [5]. During gestation, the fetal cortex primarily produces androgens, which along with hormones produced

D.J. Ledbetter and P.R.V. Johnson (eds.), *Endocrine Surgery in Children*,
DOI 10.1007/978-3-662-54256-9_7

by the developing gonads influence sexual differentiation of the fetus [6, 7]. In the third trimester, a third layer called the transitional zone forms between the definitive zone and fetal zone. By 6 months of life the definitive and transitional zones give rise to the zona glomerulosa, the outermost layer of the adrenal cortex which produces mineralocorticoids, and the zona fasciculata, which produces glucocorticoids. Over the first year of life, the fetal cortex involutes and the zona reticularis which produces androgens begins to develop as the inner most layer of the adrenal cortex [8]. The zona reticularis becomes a distinct layer by 3–4 years of age (Fig. 7.2).

Chromaffin cells are the functional cells of the adrenal medulla and are derived from the neural crest (Fig. 7.1). Along with chromaffin cells the neural crest also supplies the chief cells of the paraganglia and the parafollicular C cells of the thyroid to the developing endocrine system by the neural crest [9]. Chromaffin cells in the adrenal produce catecholamines, and are the cells of origin of pheochromocytomas and neuroblastomas. Chief cells, found in the varied anatomic locations of the paraganglia, are the cells of origin of extra-adrenal pheochromocytomas and neuroblastomas [9, 10].

The merging of the primitive medullary and cortical cells to create the adrenal gland is accomplished by migration of medullary cells into the cortex which begins during the seventh week of gestation. This process continues so that by the second trimester the fetal adrenal cortex surrounds the medulla and the entire gland becomes encapsulated by a mesodermal layer separating the adrenal glands from the surrounding retroperitoneal structures (Fig. 7.2) [1, 11]. Interestingly, while in mammals the medullary and cortical tissues merge into a single organ, in pre-vertebrates, they develop as two separate organs [10].

Adrenal Cortex Histology and Physiology

The fully mature adrenal cortex is made up of three layers with distinct hormonal functions (Fig. 7.3). The outer layer is the zona glomerulosa, which makes up about 10% of the adrenal cortex and consists of columnar epithelium arranged in cord-like structures [12, 13]. The cells of the zona glomerulosa have sparse cytoplasm, rounded nuclei, and a characteristic

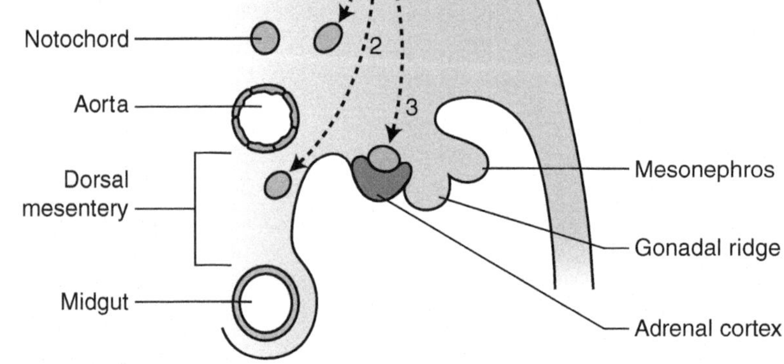

Fig. 7.1 Adrenal embryology—origins of the cortex and medulla left half of a cross section of the embryo. Adrenal cortex originates as a mesothelial proliferation between the root of the dorsal mesentery and the gonadal ridge. Adrenal medulla originates from the neural crest and migrates into the developing adrenal cortex

Age	Cross section adrenal	Inner ← Layers → Outer			
7 weeks gestation	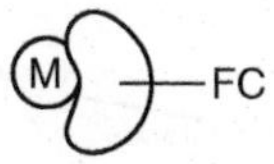 M, FC	Medulla (M)	Fetal cortex (FC)		
9 weeks gestation	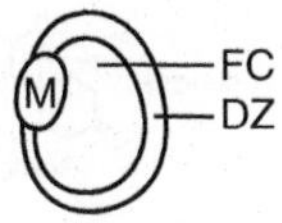 M, FC, DZ	Medulla (M)	Fetal cortex (FC)	Definitive zone (DZ)	
3rd trimester gestation	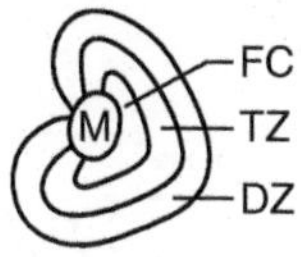 M, FC, TZ, DZ	Medulla (M)	Fetal cortex (FC)	Transitional zone (TZ)	Definitive zone (DZ)
6 months	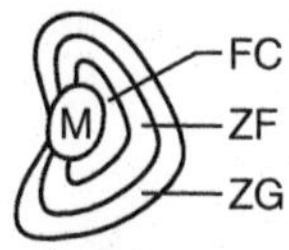 M, FC, ZF, ZG	Medulla (M)	Fetal cortex (FC)	Zona fasciculata (ZF)	Zona granulosa (ZG)
3-4 years	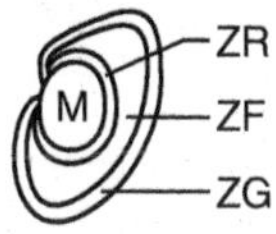 M, ZR, ZF, ZG	Medulla (M)	Zona reticularis (ZR)	Zona fasciculata (ZF)	Zona granulosa (ZG)

Fig. 7.2 Adrenal embryology—development of the mature adrenal gland. Adrenal medullary cells migrate to and begin merging with the developing adrenal cortex during the 7th week of gestation. By the second trimester the cortex surrounds the medulla and the entire gland is encapsulated by a mesodermal layer separating the adrenal glands from surrounding retroperitoneal structures. At 9 weeks gestation the cortex begins to differentiate into histologically and physiologically distinct zones and this process continues until the first few years after birth

transverse infolding of the mitochondrial cristae [13].

Activation of the renin-angiotensin axis stimulates the zona glomerulosa layer to produce and secrete aldosterone. The juxtaglomerular cells of the kidney are stimulated to secrete renin when the intrarenal blood pressure is low, when the macula densa cells in the distal renal tubule sense a decreased concentration of sodium chloride or when renal sympathetics are activated. Circulating renin then converts angiotensinogen, a serum globulin produced in the liver, to an oligopeptide, angiotensin I. Angiotensin I is converted by angiotensin-converting enzyme (ACE) to angiotensin II. Angiotensin II is a vasoconstrictor and also directly stimulates zona glomerulosa cells to synthesize and secrete aldosterone. Aldosterone causes the kidney to save sodium and lose potassium [8]. ACE inhibitor drugs decrease angiotensin II and aldosterone and are a mainstay in the treatment of hypertension.

The middle layer of the adrenal cortex is the zona fasciculata which makes up about 80% of the mature adrenal cortex. This layer has large, lipid-rich, polyhedral cells that store large amounts of cholesterol which is a precursor of cortisol [13, 14]. Zona fasciculata cells, unlike the cells in the zona glomerulosa, possess the enzymes 17α-hydroxylase and 11β-hydroxylase, which promote the conversion of progesterone to cortisol [15]. During stress cholesterol is converted to cortisol and the zona fasciculata decreases in size [14]. The adrenal cortex respond to the hypothalamic-pituitary axis (HPA) via corticotropic releasing factor (CRF) from the hypothalamus which causes the pituitary to secrete adrenocorticotropic hormone (ACTH)

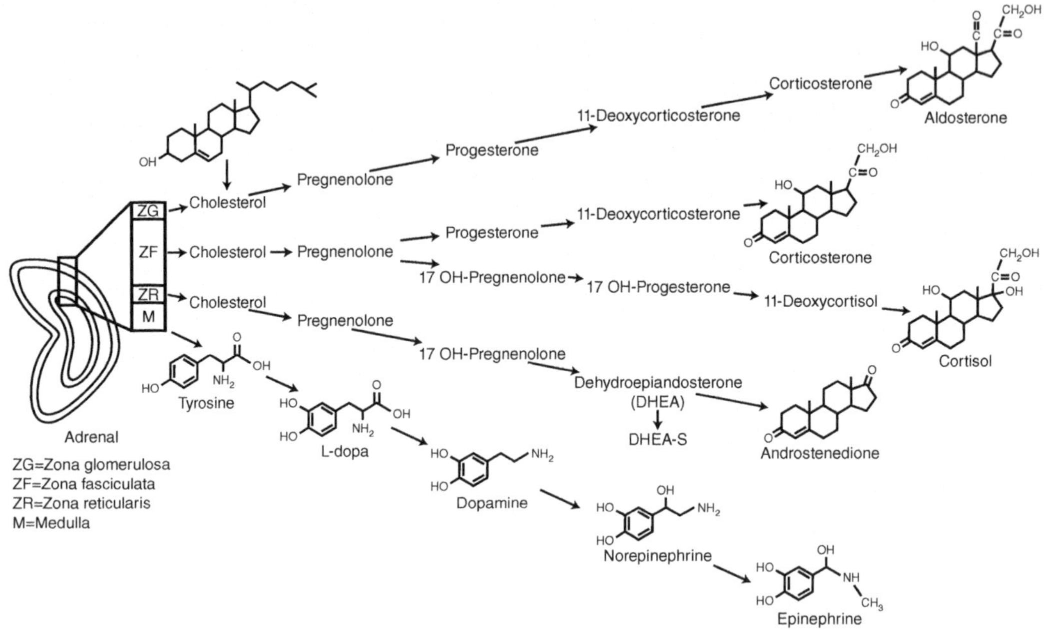

Fig. 7.3 Adrenal gland physiology. The three layers of the mature adrenal cortex produce a distinct pattern of corticosteroids from cholesterol. The adrenal medulla produces catecholamines by a stepwise enzymatic alterations of tyrosine

which acts on the zona fasciculata cells to produce cortisol. Cortisol secretion from the zona fasciculata is controlled by circadian secretion of ACTH, the stress-induced stimulation of the HPA, and the negative feedback regulation of the HPA by cortisol [8]. During stress, the adrenal medulla and zona fasciculata of the cortex can interact directly. The sympathetic nervous system can directly stimulate cortisol secretion from cells of the zona fasciculata and cortisol stimulates the chromaffin cells of the medulla to increase synthesis of catecholamines.

The innermost layer of the adrenal cortex adjacent to the medulla is the zona reticularis which makes up about 10% of the entire adrenal cortex and has a darker color than the other layers due to the pigment lipofuscin [14]. It is made up of small eosinophilic cells arranged in a cord-like fashion [16]. The zona reticularis is the site of production and secretion of dihydroepiandrosterone (DHEA) and DHEA-sulfate. Production of these androgens is also regulated by ACTH [15].

Adrenal Medulla Histology and Physiology

The adrenal medulla produces catecholamines and is regulated by the sympathetic nervous system. The central nervous system activates the sympathetic nervous system via preganglionic fibers from the spinal cord. These preganglionic fibers synapse with postganglionic fibers within the sympathetic ganglion and the postganglionic fibers carry the stimulus to end organs [17]. The adrenal medulla is unique in that it is supplied by preganglionic fibers that directly synapse to chromaffin cells which produce catecholamines. There are no postganglionic nerve fibers [17, 18]. Chromaffin cells are arranged in a reticular pattern around multiple venous channels which allows secreted catecholamines to rapidly enter the bloodstream [17].

Some medullary chromaffin cells secrete epinephrine and others secrete norepinephrine [15]. The primary substrate for catecholamine production is tyrosine. Tyrosine comes directly from dietary sources or is synthesized in the liver from dietary phenylalanine. Through stepwise enzymatic alterations, tyrosine is converted to dopamine via tyrosine hydroxylase and aromatic-L-amino acid decarboxylase (see Fig. 7.3). Dopamine can be converted to norepinephrine by dopamine-β-hydroxylase. The conversion of norepinephrine to epinephrine requires Phenylethanolamine N-methyltransferase (PNMT), an enzyme that is present in chromaffin tissue (Fig. 7.4). Cortisol from the adrenal cortex increases PNMT which, in turn, increases epinephrine production [8, 19].

Adrenal Anatomy

At birth the adrenal glands together weigh about 8 g and are nearly the size of adult adrenal glands [20]. Therefore, by weight, newborn adrenal glands are 10–20 times proportionally larger than adult adrenal glands [1, 21]. The relatively large size of the adrenal gland is obvious on newborn imaging studies where the adrenal gland may be up to one-third the size of the adjacent kidney [1]. After one year of age, the fetal cortex involutes and the adrenal gland approaches normal adult dimensions (approximately 5 × 3 × 0.6 cm) and weight (4–6 g each) [10]. The right

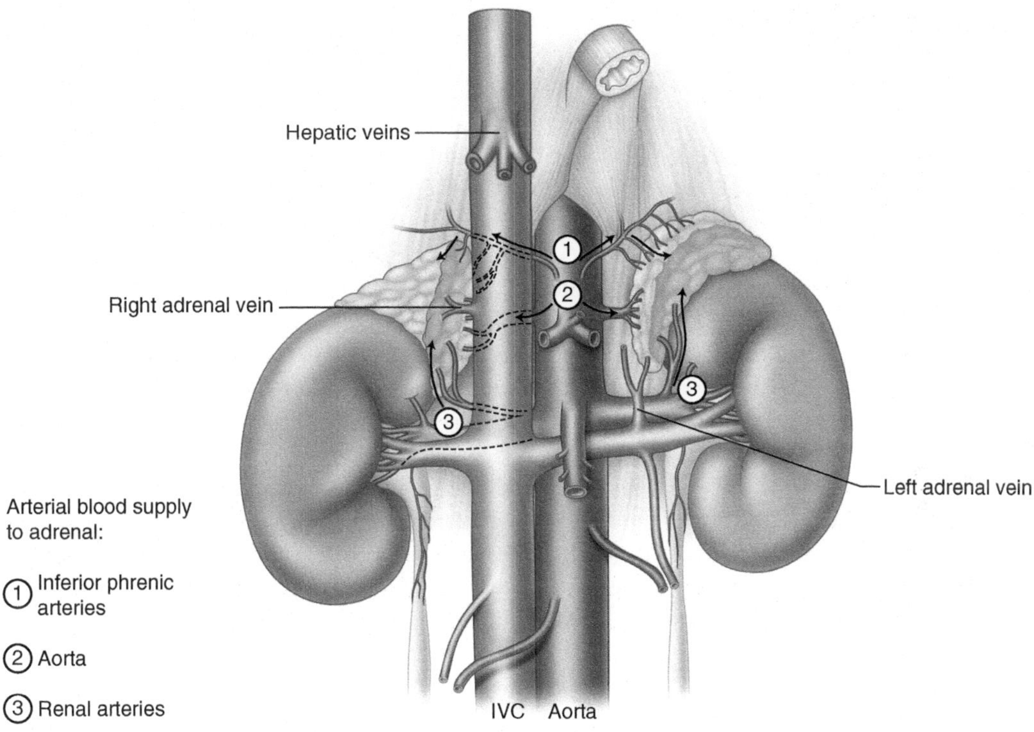

Fig. 7.4 Adrenal anatomy. Both adrenal glands are within Gerota's fascia at the superior-medial pole of the kidneys lateral to the vertebral column, in front of the 12th rib *on the right* and in front of the 11th and 12th rib *on the left*. The *right* adrenal is located against the bare area of the liver and is partially covered by the vena cava anteriorly. The *left* adrenal is behind the tail of the pancreas and is anterior to the diaphragm. The *right* adrenal vein drains directly into the inferior vena cava and is usually less than a centimeter in length. The *right* renal vein is short and drains directly into the inferior vena cava. The *left* adrenal vein is longer than the *right* adrenal vein and merges with the left inferior phrenic vein prior to draining into the *left* renal vein. The arterial blood supply to the adrenal is variable and consists of multiple small branches from the inferior phrenic arteries superiorly, the abdominal aorta medially, and the renal arteries inferiorly

adrenal gland tends to be a more triangular shape than the larger, more crescent shaped left adrenal gland [19]. The surface of the adrenal has a characteristic bright yellow-orange color which is distinct from the surrounding retroperitoneal fat. The distinctive color of the adrenal gland is more noticeable in infants and young children than in adults due to the paucity of retroperitoneal fat in younger children. This distinct color is often present in adrenal tumors and their metastases and is a helpful guide when performing gross total resections of adrenocortical carcinomas, neuroblastomas, and involved lymph nodes.

Relationship to Retroperitoneal Structures

The adrenal glands are located in the retroperitoneum, superior and slightly anterior and medial to the kidney. They are lateral to the vertebral column, in front of the 12th rib on the right and in front of the 11th and 12th rib on the left (see Fig. 7.4) [10]. On the right, the adrenal is located against the bare area of the liver and is partially covered by the vena cava anteriorly [11]. On the left, the adrenal lies behind the tail of the pancreas and is anterior to the diaphragm [11]. Both adrenal glands lie within the pararenal fat at the superior-medial pole of the kidneys within Gerota's fascia [10]. There is a fusion of the anterior and posterior Gerota's fascia between the adrenal gland and the superior pole of the kidney [10]. This connective tissue plane separates the adrenal gland and kidney and facilitates dissection of the adrenal away from the superior pole of the kidney during adrenalectomy. The renal fascia envelops the adrenal and extends cranially, where it attaches to the diaphragm and fixes the adrenal glands to the posterior abdominal wall [10]. The lateral attachments are to the superior pole of the kidney and pararenal fat. In distinction to the posterolateral anatomy, which is essentially the same for the two glands, the anterior and medial relationships are different on the right and left sides (Fig. 7.4).

Venous Anatomy

Adrenal capillaries drain into a central vein which exits the cortex at the inferomedial aspect of the gland. Each gland has a dominant vein, although smaller accessory veins are often found adjacent to the adrenal arteries [10]. Anatomic variants have been reported to occur in up to 50% of patients, although most variants are minor [22]. Significant variations probably occur in 3–5% of patients [22, 23]. Multiple adrenal veins draining via their usual pathway into the inferior vena cava IVC on the right and the left renal vein on the left are the most common anomalies [11]. Other anomalies include accessory venous drainage to the inferior phrenic vein and venous connections to the azygous vein and/or posterior gastric veins. These connections could act as shunts around an obstructed IVC or portal vein [10]. During resection of large adrenal tumors the superior pole arteries to the kidney can easily be mistaken for the adrenal vein and care must be taken to avoid inadvertent ligation of these arteries [11].

The right adrenal vein drains directly into the inferior vena cava and is usually less than a centimeter in length [10]. The short length of the right adrenal vein can make its ligation difficult during right adrenalectomy. In addition, large, right adrenal masses can significantly displace the adrenal vein and occasionally requiring circumferential mobilization of the inferior vena cava for adequate exposure and control. Anomalous drainage, such as a right adrenal vein draining into the retrohepatic vena cava at the confluence of the hepatic veins has been reported.11 [23]. The left adrenal vein is longer than the right adrenal vein and merges with the left inferior phrenic vein prior to draining into the left renal vein [10]. When dissecting large left-sided adrenal tumors, one often finds the adrenal vein flattened against the mass and stretched to a length significantly longer than normal. Once the left adrenal vein has been identified, early ligation is preferable prior to full dissection of the mass due to the risk of avulsing the attenuated vein from the left renal vein. In general, anatomic variants in venous drainage on the left are associated with an anomaly in the left renal vein. Drainage of the left adrenal vein directly into the IVC in a patient with retroaortic left renal vein has been reported [24].

Arterial Anatomy

Unlike the venous system, the arterial branches to the adrenal glands are not as distinct. These branches arise from three sources—the inferior phrenic arteries superiorly, the abdominal aorta medially, and the renal arteries inferiorly (Fig. 7.4) [10, 12, 19]. The anatomy of the arterial system is unpredictable and variable and adrenal arteries can also arise from the intercostal or gonadal arteries [11].

The arteries enter on the medial side of the glands and give rise to a dense network of vessels that supply the three layers of the adrenal cortex and the medulla. In infants and children, adrenal arteries are usually small and can be are ligated with cautery, harmonic scalpel, or fine ties. Larger arterial branches are seen when with mass lesions within the adrenal gland cause neovascularization and engorgement of the vessels. In these cases, meticulous dissection and ligation of vessels is necessary to avoid bleeding.

Lymphatic Anatomy

On the right, adrenal lymphatics drain to paracrural, paraaortic, and paracaval lymph nodes. On the left, adrenal lymphatics initially drain into paraaortic and left renal hilar lymph nodes. Adrenal lymphatics also may drain directly to the thoracic duct and posterior mediastinal nodes [10, 12]. Extension of lymphatic spread to adjacent retroperitoneal lymph node groups is common so a thorough knowledge of the adrenal lymphatic drainage patterns is critical for appropriate surgical therapy of advanced stage adrenocortical carcinoma, neuroblastoma, or malignant pheochromocytoma when gross total lymphadenectomy is often indicated.

Anatomic Basis of Surgical Approaches to the Adrenal

Operations on the adrenal glands can be done using open or minimally invasive techniques from either an anterior or posterior approach. Because the posterolateral anatomy is basically the same for both adrenal glands, the surgical approach through the flank is the same for both glands. The glands are fixed to the posterior abdominal wall by the renal fascia, allowing direct access to the glands. The posterior approach is begun with an incision made along the 12th rib, which is usually removed to facilitate exposure. The latissimus dorsi muscle is divided and the peritoneum is reflected away. To improve exposure the diaphragm can be divided to, after bluntly mobilizing the pleura. Once this is accomplished, the transversalis muscle is divided and the kidney is retracted inferiorly to expose the adrenal [10]. The posterior minimally invasive or retroperitoneoscopic approach is not commonly used in children, unless there has been extensive previous abdominal surgery or the child is obese [21]. The retroperitoneoscopic approach begins with a small incision at the tip of the 12th rib. With blunt finger dissection, a space is created to insert the first trocar. The space is opened using a balloon trocar and high (20–24 mmHg) insufflation pressures prior to placing additional trocars [25].

The anterior approach to the right and left glands is different because of the asymmetric anatomy of the glands. Open anterior adrenal procedures are most commonly performed through a subcostal incision. For bilateral lesions a chevron or midline incision can be used. The most common approach used for laparoscopic adrenal surgery is an anterior approach with the patient in a lateral position, although the procedure can be performed in the supine position as well [26]. Although single incision (SILS) laparoscopic adrenal surgery has been described, most surgeons continue to prefer a standard laparoscopic approach for adrenal procedures [27]. Whether an open or minimally invasive technique is used, the steps of the procedure are the same. On the right side, the posterior attachments of the liver to the diaphragm are divided [11]. The liver can them be retracted superiorly to expose the fascia covering the adrenal gland. If additional exposure is needed, the small veins draining the caudate lobe into the vena cava can be divided [11]. If necessary, the duodenum can mobilized medially with a Kocher maneuver to further expose the vena cava and the kidney [10, 11]. On the left side, the omentum is divided off the colon and the lesser sac entered. The inferior, avascular border of the pancreas can be dissected free and elevated to reveal the adrenal [11]. For small tumors, this direct approach through the lesser sac usually provides adequate exposure, however for large tumors visceral rotation may be required to adequately expose the adrenal gland and aorta. In this maneuver, the splenic flexure of the colon, spleen, and tail of the pancreas are mobilized and retracted medially [10]. Once the gland is adequately exposed, identification and ligation of the adrenal vein is usually carried out first. As previously noted, the right adrenal vein empties directly into the vena cava; the left vein joins the inferior phrenic vein to empty into the left renal vein. Once the vein is divided, medial and superior dissection to identify the arteries supplying the gland can be carried out.

References

1. Barwick TD, Malhotra A, Webb JA, Savage MO, Reznek RH. Embryology of the adrenal glands and its relevance to diagnostic imaging. Clin Radiol. 2005;60(9):953–9.
2. Savas C, Candir O, Bezir M, Cakmak M. Ectopic adrenocortical nodules along the spermatic cord of children. Int Urol Nephrol. 2001;32(4):681–5.
3. Iyengar V, Pittman DM. Ectopic adrenal gland tissue in inguinal hernia sac. Ann Diagn Pathol. 2007;11 (4):291–2.
4. Ketata S, Ketata H, Sahnoun A, FakhFakh H, Bahloul A, Mhiri MN. Ectopic adrenal cortex tissue: an incidental finding during inguinoscrotal operations in pediatric patients. Urol Int. 2008;81(3):316–9.
5. Moore K, Persaud T. The developing human. 8th ed. New York: WB Saunders; 2008.
6. Kempna P, Fluck CE. Adrenal gland development and defects. Best Pract Res Clin Endocrinol Metab. 2008;22(1):77–93.
7. Hanley N, Arit W. The human fetal adrenal cortex and the window of sexual differentiation. Trends Endocrinol Metab. 2006;17:391–7.
8. Cohen M, Brunt L. The endocrine system. In: O'Leary J, Capote L, editors. The physiologic basis of surgery. 4th ed. Philadelphia: Lippincott Williams & Wilkins; 2008. p. 362–404.
9. Adams MS, Bronner-Fraser M. Review: the role of neural crest cells in the endocrine system. Endocr Pathol. 2009;20(2):92–100.
10. Avisse C, Marcus C, Patey M, Ladam-Marcus V, Delattre JF, Flament JB. Surgical anatomy and embryology of the adrenal glands. Surg Clin North Am. 2000;80(1):403–15.
11. Brunt L, Cohen M. Adrenalectomy—open and minimally invasive. In: Fisher J, Bland K, editors. Mastery of surgery. 5th ed. Philadelphia: Lippincott Williams & Wilkins; 2007.
12. Clark O, Duh Q, Kebehew E. Textbook of endocrine surgery. 2nd ed. Philadelphia: WB Saunders; 2005.
13. Bravo EL. Physiology of the adrenal cortex. Urol Clin North Am. 1989;16:433–7.
14. Silverman M, Lee A. Anatomy and pathology of the adrenal glands. Urol Clin North Am. 1989;16: 417–32.
15. Molina P. Endocrine physiology. 3rd ed. New York: McGraw Hill; 2010.
16. Conram R, Cheng E, Dehmer L, Sharmada H. The Pineal, Pituitary, Parathyroid, Thyroid and Adrenal Glands. In: Stocker J, Dehner L, Husain A, editors. Stocker & Dehner's Pediatric Pathology. Philadelphia: Lippincott, Williams & Wilkins; 2011.
17. Tsapatsaris N, Breslin D. Physiology of the adrenal medulla. Urol Clin North Am. 1989;16:439–45.
18. Dimitrios L, Heerden Jv. Adrenal glands: diagnostic aspects and surgical therapy. New York: Springer; 2004.
19. Linos D, Heerden JV. Adrenal glands: diagnostic aspects and surgical therapy. New York: Springer; 2004.
20. Langlois D, Li JY, Saez JM. Development and function of the human fetal adrenal cortex. J Pediatr Endocrinol Metab. 2002;15(Suppl 5):1311–22.
21. Misseri R. Adrenal surgery in the pediatric population. Curr Urol Reports. 2007;8:89–94.
22. Parnaby CN, Galbraith N, O'Dwyer PJ. Experience in identifying the venous drainage of the adrenal gland during laparoscopic adrenalectomy. Clin Anat. 2008;21(7):660–5.
23. Sebe P, Peyromaure M, Raynaud A, Delmas V. Anatomical variations in the drainage of the principal adrenal veins: the results of 88 venograms. Surg Radiol Anat. 2002;24(3–4):222–5.

24. Stack S, Rosch J, Cook D, Sheppard B, Keller F. Anomalous left adrenal venous drainage directly into the inferior vena cava. Jl Vasc Interven Radiol. 2001;12:385–7.
25. Dickson P, Jiminez C, Chisholm G, Kannamer D, Ng C, Grubbs E, et al. Posterior retroperitoneoscopic adrenalectomy: a contemporary american experience. J Am Coll Surg. 2001;212:659–65.
26. Brunt L. Minimal access adrenal surgery. Surg Endosc. 2006;20:351–61.
27. Ishida M, Miyajima A, Takeda T, Hasegawa M, Kikuchi E, Oya M. Technical difficulties of transumbilical laparoendoscopic single-site adrenalectomy: comparison with conventional laparoscopic adrenalectomy. World J Urol. 2013;31(1):199–201.

8 Pheochromocytoma

Michael J. Stechman and Gregory P. Sadler

Tumours arising from neuroectodermal chromaffin-staining cells of the adrenal medulla are known as pheochromocytomas (PHEO). Tumours arising from neuroectodermal chromaffin-staining cells located in extra-adrenal sympathetic and parasympathetic ganglia are known as paragangliomas (PGL). Both tumours are extremely rare in children with a reported incidence of less than 0.3 cases per million [1]. Most of PHEO and sympathetic PGL secrete catecholamines including adrenaline, noradrenaline and dopamine, but 95% of head and neck PGL are derived from parasympathetic ganglia and are usually non-functioning [2, 3]. PHEO and PGL are rare compared to the usual retroperitoneal tumours of childhood such as neuroblastoma and Wilms' tumour and while neuroblastoma and Wilms' tumour usually occur in infants and toddlers, PHEO and PGL can occur at any age through to adulthood [4]. Much of the data about the natural history and management of PHEO are derived from the extensive literature of the adult disease. However, there are some important differences in the aetiology, presentation, surgical management and follow-up of children with PHEO and PGL.

Epidemiology

PHEO and PGL may occur at any age during childhood but most often arise during the early teens and with an approximately equal male to female incidence [5–8]. Between 80 and 90% of PHEO and PGL occur in adults with the remaining 10–20% occur in children. The tumours are either sporadic or familial. The majority of tumours in adults are sporadic but with advanced testing up to 30% of adult tumours initially thought to be sporadic are found to have detectable germ-line mutations [6, 9]. The incidence of detectable gene abnormalities rises to 56% in adolescents below 18 years of age and to 70% in children under 10 years of age. Mutations of several genes including *RET*, *VHL*, *SDHx*, *NF1* and *TMEM127* are associated with inherited endocrine tumour syndromes that include the development of PHEO or PGL (see Table 8.1) [10–15]. These disorders result in tumours that are more likely to be bilateral, multi-focal and extra-adrenal [7, 8, 16–19].

Aetiology and Molecular Genetics

The molecular basis of sporadic catecholamine-secreting tumours is poorly understood and few somatic mutations have been identified in tumour specimens. However, our understanding of the

M.J. Stechman
Department of Endocrine Surgery, University Hospital of Wales, Heath Park, Cardiff CF14 4XW, UK
e-mail: mstechman@doctors.org.uk

G.P. Sadler (✉)
Department of Endocrine Surgery, John Radcliffe Hospital, Headley Way, Oxford OX3 9DU, UK
e-mail: greg.sadler@ouh.nhs.uk

D.J. Ledbetter and P.R.V. Johnson (eds.), *Endocrine Surgery in Children*,
DOI 10.1007/978-3-662-54256-9_8

Table 8.1 Familial disorders with known genetic defects that are associated with the development of pheochromocytoma and/or paraganglioma

Syndrome	Gene (chromosome)[a]	Clinical manifestations	% with PHEO	% PHEO bilateral	References
von Hippel Lindau[b]	*VHL* (3p25-p26)	PHEO, cerebellar hemangioblastoma, retinal angiomas, renal cell carcinoma, pancreatic cysts, pancreatic NETs in 5–10%	10–20%	40–80	[11]
Multiple endocrine neoplasia type 2A[c] Multiple endocrine neoplasia type 2B	*RET* (10q11.2)	PHEO, MTC, hyperparathyroidism PHEO, MTC, mucosal neuromas, colonic ganglioneuromatosis, Marfanoid facies, skeletal abnormalities	50%	50–80	[10]
von Recklinghausen's disease	*NF1* (17q11.2)	Neurofibromata, >6 café au lait spots, axillary freckling, skeletal abnormalities and PHEO	5–10%	10	[15]
PGL-1	*SDHD* (11q23)	Parasympathetic head and neck PGL ± PHEO	Uncommon	–	[14]
PGL-2	*SDHAF2* (11q13.1)	Parasympathetic head and neck PGL (non-functioning)	Not described	–	[38]
PGL-3	*SDHC* (1q21)	Parasympathetic head and neck PGL, PHEO rare	Rare	–	[12]
PGL-4	*SDHB* (1p35-p36)	Sympathetic abdominal PGL and PHEO—50% malignant	PGL or PHEO in 70%		[13]
Familial pheochromocytoma	*TMEM127* (2q11)	PHEO	?	43	[40]
Familial neural crest-derived tumours	*KIF1B* (1p36.2)	PHEO or neuroblastoma	?	?	[102]

RET Rearranged during transfection; *SDH* Succinate dehydrogenase; *SDHAF2* Succinate dehydrogenase complex assembly factor 2; *TMEM127* Transmembrane 127; *NF1* Neurofibromatosis type 1; *KIF1B* Kinesin family member 1B (microtubule motor)

[a]Homozygous mutations of *SDHA* cause Leigh syndrome which is not associated with PHEO or PGL

[b]Four types of VHL disease are recognised (1, 2A, 2B and 2C)—type 1 is not associated with PHEO

[c]Medullary thyroid cancer (MTC) is usually the initial presentation. MEN2A is associated with Hirschsprung's disease in 5%

molecular basis of tumorigenesis in familial pheochromocytoma continues to develop. Experimental evidence suggests that alterations in the genes responsible for these familial pheochromocytoma (*VHL*, *RET*, *NF1* and *SDHx*) impair *c-Jun* dependent neuronal apoptosis during normal development. This unifying explanation is known as the 'developmental culling hypothesis' [20, 21]. The individual genetic disorders giving rise to PHEO and PGL are discussed below.

Von Hippel–Lindau Disease (VHL)

This autosomal-dominant disease is a significant cause of PHEO presenting in children with an incidence of 1 per 36,000 live births [22]. VHL is characterised by an increased risk of hemangioblastoma of the CNS and retina, renal cell cancer (RCC), neuroendocrine tumours of the pancreas, endolymphatic sac tumours and PHEO. 10–20% of affected patients develop PHEO and the tumours are often bilateral. Multiple cysts of the pancreas, kidney and epididymis are also common [23].

There are four subtypes of VHL: Types 1, 2A, 2B and 2C. All subtypes are due to germ-line abnormalities of the *VHL* gene on chromosome 3p25 [24]. There is a strong genotype–phenotype correlation. Type 1 disease is due to truncating *VHL* mutations that are inactivating and lead to *loss of function*. Type 1 disease is not associated with PHEO. Each of the Type 2 diseases is due to specific missense activating mutations and leads to *gain of function* of the VHL protein. Each variant has a specific tumour-risk pattern. Type 2A has an increased risk of retinal and CNS hemangioblastoma and PHEO but not RCC, Type 2B has an increased risk of RCC, hemangioblastoma and PHEO; and Type 2C has an increased risk of PHEO only [24, 25].

Nearly, all VHL families harbour specific germ-line mutations, but up to 20% of cases of VHL disease occur de novo [26]. Although malignant PHEO is reported in less than 5% of patients with VHL, those patients with subtypes that lead to RCC and hemangioblastoma have a reduced life expectancy and should be screened from 5 years of age onward with MRI of the brain and spinal cord, kidneys and adrenal glands [27]. Patients with VHL who are undergoing a surgical procedure should have preoperative evaluation of urine or plasma metanephrines to exclude occult PHEO.

Multiple Endocrine Neoplasia Type 2A and 2B (MEN 2A and 2B)

MEN 2 is an autosomal dominantly inherited endocrine tumour syndrome that affects 2–3 per 100,000 of the population. It is due to activating germ-line mutations of the gene on chromosome 10q11 that encodes the RET tyrosine kinase receptor [10]. Two main clinical subtypes are recognised, MEN 2A and MEN 2B.

MEN 2A is characterised by medullary thyroid cancer (MTC) in all patients, hyperparathyroidism in 30% and PHEO in 50%. MEN 2B is much less common accounting for only 10–15% of patients with MEN. The clinical features of MEN 2B include Marfanoid facies, skeletal deformities, mucosal neuromas of the tongue and lips, ganglioneuromatosis of the intestine, MTC and PHEO. A third disorder, familial MTC (FMTC), is also due to *RET* mutations but not associated with PHEO. Although MTC is almost always the initial presenting disorder in MEN2, as many as one-third of patients may present with MTC and PHEO simultaneously and so the latter should always be excluded prior to surgery for MTC [28].

The clinical features of the disease (phenotype), age of onset and aggressiveness of MTC are dependent upon the specific codon mutation inherited by the patient (genotype) [27, 29]. Patients with MEN 2A have mutations that affect the extracellular ligand-binding domain of the receptor (exons 10 and 11 of the RET gene) and 85% of patients have codon 634 RET mutations. The remaining 10–15% have mutations of codons 609, 611, 618 and 620 [30]. In contrast, those with MEN 2B have mutations affecting the intra-cellular, tyrosine kinase domain (exons 15 and 16) and 95% of patients have the codon 918 mutations, or more rarely codon 883 mutation [30]. Patients with FMTC have mutations affecting codons 768, 790, 791, 804 and 844 (exons 13 and 14) although mutations are described in exons 10 and 11, denoting an overlap between FMTC and MEN 2A [10]. Interestingly, although PHEO is observed in 50% of individuals with codon 634 and 918 mutations, it occurs rarely in those with mutations in exon 10 (codons 609, 611, 618 and 620) or exon 15 (codon 791 and 804) [31, 32].

Neurofibromatosis Type 1 (Von Recklinghausen Disease)

Neurofibromatosis type 1 (NF-1) is an autosomal-dominant condition that occurs in 1 in 3000 live births and is due to mutations in the *NF1* gene on chromosome 17q. Half represent de novo changes [24]. PHEO develops in 5% of those affected, usually in adulthood [33]. Diagnosis of NF-1 is usually straightforward because of the presence of cutaneous neurofibromata, café au lait spots and axillary and inguinal freckling. Genetic testing is problematic because the gene contains 60 exons with numerous pseudogenes [34]; however, it is rarely necessary due to the obvious clinical signs. Screening for PHEO should be performed in individuals with the disorder who develop hypertension.

Hereditary Paraganglioma and Pheochromocytoma Syndromes

Four inherited syndromes, PGL-1, PGL-2, PGL-3 and PGL-4 syndromes, have varying predisposition to development of PHEO, extra-adrenal sympathetic PGL and parasympathetic head and neck PGL. These syndromes are caused by germ-line mutations of genes encoding subunits of the mitochondrial complex II enzyme, succinate dehydrogenase (SDH), which is involved in the tricarboxylic acid cycle. PGL-1 syndrome is caused by *SDHD* mutations, PGL-3 syndrome is caused by *SDHC* mutations and PGL-4 syndrome is caused by *SDHB* mutations. *SDHD* mutations are also found in up to 11% of sporadic PHEO [35] and in up to 50% of sporadic head and neck PGL tumours [36]. These *SDHD* mutations have an unusual paternal origin of inheritance [37]. PGL-2 syndrome is due to mutations of the *SDHAF2* gene which encodes a protein required for flavination of the SDHA subunit [38].

PGL-1 syndrome is associated with parasympathetic head and neck PGL (chemodectoma or glomus tumour) in middle-aged patients and occasionally PHEO [14, 36]. PGL-2 is the least common syndrome and is associated with parasympathetic head and neck PGL. PGL-3 syndrome is rare with only 10 families in the literature. The disorder is associated with development of parasympathetic head and neck PGL only [36]. PGL-4 causes predominantly abdominal sympathetic PGLs and occasionally PHEO [13], but almost half are malignant [39]. Tumours may develop from the first decade of life. Diagnosis of initial tumour is at a median age of 32 years and there is an estimated penetrance of 45% by age 40 [36].

Other Genetic Disorders

Germ-line inactivating mutations of the transmembrane-encoding gene *TMEM127* on chromosome 2q11 have been shown to be associated with the development of PHEO [40]. Like *RET*, *TMEM127* acts as a tumour suppressor gene. Large-scale mutational analysis of 990 patients with sporadic PHEO revealed *TMEM127* mutations in just under 2%, with bilateral tumours in over a third of these individuals [41].

The Carney triad of gastro-intestinal stromal tumours (GISTs), pulmonary chondroma and PHEO/PGL occurs predominantly in women and is most commonly associated with deletions of chromosome 1pcen13-q21 which contains the SDHC gene although the exact genetic defect is unknown [42]. However, a separate condition, the Carney-Stratakis syndrome of GIST and PHEO/PGL, has been demonstrated to be due to *SDHB*, *SDHC* and *SDHD* mutations in a proportion of patients [36].

Genetic testing should be performed in all children and adolescents that present with PHEO or PGL. The precise order of genetic testing is dependent upon the clinical presentation. Thus, patients presenting with PHEO and MTC should undergo screening of *RET*, whereas those with isolated PHEO should undergo *VHL* and if negative, *SDHB*, *SDHD* and *SDHC* testing. Individuals with extra-adrenal tumours in the abdomen and chest should undergo *VHL*, *SDHB*, *SDHD* and *SDHC* screening, whereas those with head and neck PGL are most likely to harbour mutations in *SDHD, SDHB, SDHC, SDHAF2* and occasionally the *VHL* gene. Counselling and testing of first-degree relatives should follow the detection of index cases.

Pathology

Grossly pheochromocytomas are soft vascular tumours that when sliced are a pink/tan colour. Tumours are usually less than 5 cm in maximal diameter but can be much larger. Microscopically, tumours have a regular nested (Zellballen) pattern of polyhedral cells which stain yellow with chromic acid [43] (hence the term 'chromaffin positive') and contain large nuclei with numerous secretory granules. A layer of sustentacular cells surrounds the nests of chromaffin-positive cells. These cells are more prominent in benign tumours [44, 45] and stain positive for the immunohistochemical marker S-100. Tumours also demonstrate immunoreactivity for chromogranin A and synaptophysin [46–48].

The incidence of malignant PHEO is around 12% in children [5], but is higher in extra-adrenal sympathetic tumours, particularly those due to *SDHB* mutations. Only distant metastases and local invasion are definitive markers of malignant tumours. However, a number of surrogates suggest an increased risk of malignancy: tumour diameter >5 cm (75% prevalence of malignancy) [5]; presence of lymphovascular or capsular invasion; presence of confluent tumour necrosis; increased Ki-67 proliferation index and absent S-100 staining of sustentacular cells [45, 49–51]. Scoring systems to predict malignancy have been developed (PHEO of the Adrenal Gland Scaled Score or PASS) [52] using some of the above criteria and other histological appearances including the presence of high cellularity, tumour cell spindling, cellular monotony, increased mitotic figures, atypical mitotic figures, nuclear pleomorphism and cellular hyperchromasia. However, significant inter- and intra-observer variability of PASS component scoring highlights the limitations of current scoring systems in diagnosing malignancy [53].

Malignant tumours have increased tumour expression of some biological markers [telomerase catalytic subunit hTERT, heat shock protein (HSP) 90, cyclo-oxygenase, *N*-cadherin, vascular endothelial growth factor (VEGF)] and decreased expression of others (neuropeptide Y (NPY) and EM66) [54]. The use of these indicators to predict malignant behaviour is not routine in clinical practice.

Finally, SDHB protein expression by tumour immunohistochemistry is absent in all PHEO/PGL presenting in patients affected by SDHB, C and D mutations, but present in all those presenting as part of MEN2, VHL and NF1 and in almost 90% of those with no germ-line mutation [55]. SDHB immunohistochemistry could be a useful to guide genetic testing and, in the case of SDHB-related PHEO/PGL, assist in identifying tumours with high malignant potential.

Clinical Presentation

Sustained hypertension is the most common presenting finding in children (Table 8.2) in contrast to adults who often have the classic triad

Table 8.2 Clinical presentation of pheochromocytoma and functioning paraganglioma in children compared with adults

	Children with PHEO/PGL	Adults with PHEO/PGL[a]
Age	11 years	
Male: Female	1.6:1	1:1
Presenting symptom		
Sustained hypertension	90–100	68
Headache	81–95	90
Palpitations	35–63	72
Sweating	69–90	92
Mass effect	30–38	?

[a]Sustained hypertension is the most consistent finding in children diagnosed with chromaffin tumour, whereas adults generally present with the classic triad of headache, palpitations and sweating with episodic hypertension

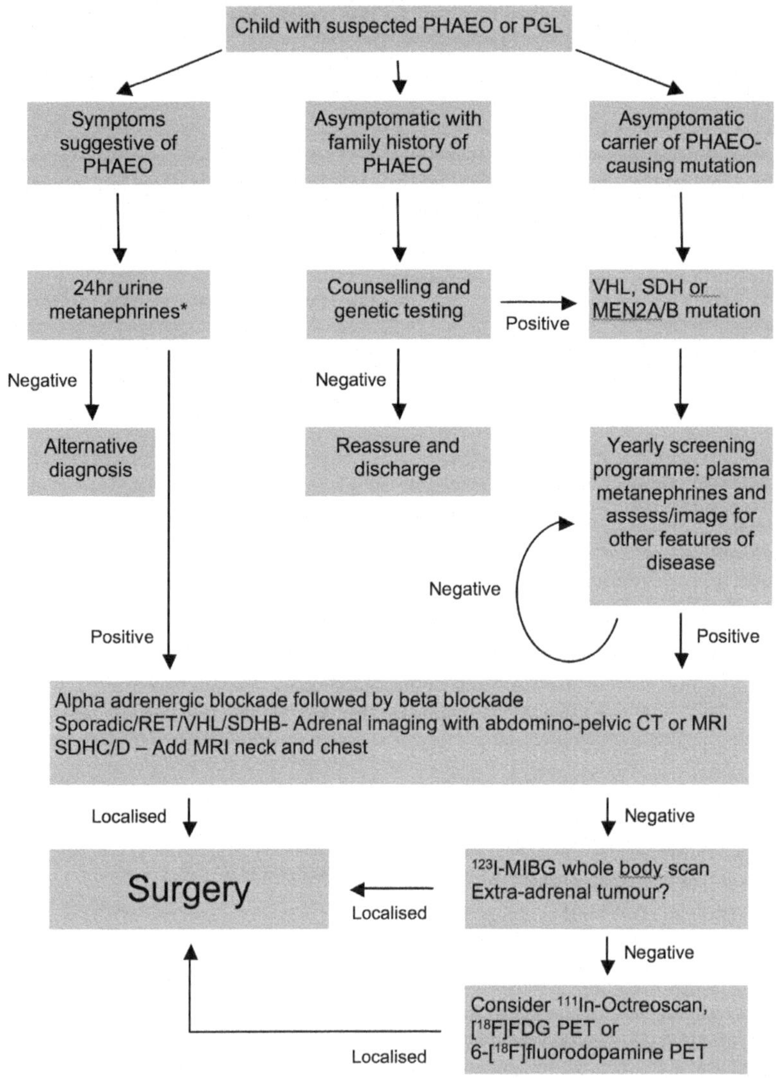

Fig. 8.1 Suggested algorithm for the investigation of a child with suspected pheochromocytoma or paraganglioma (*PHEO* pheochromocytoma, *PGL* paraganglioma, see text for other abbreviations)

of episodic sweating, palpitations and headache [19, 56]. In addition to signs and symptoms of excess catecholamines, tumours may present with local mass effects (abdominal pain with or without abdominal distension), or as an incidental finding on imaging studies, or during biochemical screening tests. A feature sometimes noted in tumours related to VHL and MEN 2 syndromes is the lack of symptoms. This may be that this is due to ascertainment bias (e.g. tumours detected on screening do not reach a size where they become symptomatic) rather than a feature of genetic tumours per se [57].

Evaluation

The approach to diagnosis in children is summarised in Fig. 8.1 with additional explanations in the following sections.

History

On presentation, the child and parents should be questioned about the presence and duration of symptoms relating to catecholamine excess such as headache, palpitations, panic attacks, sweating and about neurological symptoms such as blurred vision and weakness. In addition, specific questioning should investigate the possibility of other associated conditions such as thyroid nodules, hypercalcaemia, megacolon and renal tumours. Family history of PHEO, PGL and any related endocrine tumour (see Table 8.1) should be noted along with a pedigree of affected and unaffected family members. Finally, a full past medical history of medical problems and surgical procedures that might impact anaesthesia or operation should be documented.

Physical Examination

The most common abnormality on physical examination is hypertension but the physical examination is often normal. However, physical exam is diagnostic in patients with NF-1 (multiple cutaneous neurofibromata, café au lait spots and axillary/inguinal freckling) and in patients with MEN 2B (Marfanoid appearance, lingual neuromas, signs of Hirschsprung's megacolon, neck scar from previous thyroid surgery). Adrenal and extra-adrenal tumours are not usually palpable unless they are very large, although tumours in the neck and at the abdominal aortic bifurcation may be palpable.

Investigations

The presence of catecholamine-secreting tumours is confirmed by the biochemical testing of plasma or urine for fractionated catecholamines (adrenaline, noradrenaline and dopamine) or metanephrines (metadrenaline, normetadrenaline and 3-methoxytyramine). When catecholamine excess is determined then imaging is done to localise the tumour.

The majority of children with PHEO, particularly if symptomatic, will have increased levels of urinary catecholamines and metanephrines. Metanephrines result the enzyme catecholamine-*O*-methyltransferase (COMT) within the tumour metabolises catecholamines. Plasma and urinary metanephrines are more sensitive (99 and 97% respectively) than plasma and urinary catecholamine (86 and 84% respectively) because catecholamine secretion may be intermittent [58, 59]. Therefore, the most appropriate tests in children are urinary metanephrines or if urine collection is not feasible then plasma metanephrines. The increased sensitivity of plasma metanephrines is also valuable to detect early disease when there is a known genetic mutation that puts a patient at risk for PHEO. Elevation of metanephrines greater than 4× the upper limit of the reference range is 100% diagnostic for a chromaffin tumour [60]. Metanephrine estimations may be affected by certain drugs (e.g. monoamine oxidase inhibitors, paracetamol, tricyclic antidepressants, sympathomimetics such as ephedrine and phenylephrine, amphetamines and levodopa) so these drugs should be discontinued prior to testing [61].

Tumours may have characteristic biochemical secretions and are classified as either noradrenergic or adrenergic. For example, PGLs and PHEOs arising in association with VHL disease are noradrenergic and predominantly secrete noradrenaline and normetadrenaline [62]. This is likely due to VHL tumours having reduced expression of the enzyme phenylethanolamine-*N*-methyltransferase (PNMT), which converts noradrenaline to adrenaline [63]. Adrenergic PHEOs secrete a mixture of adrenaline/metadrenaline and noradrenaline/normetadrenaline. They may be sporadic or due to *RET* and *NF1* mutations. Dopamine and its metabolite 3-methoxytyramine are occasionally the predominant secretions, usually from PGL arising due to *SDHx* mutations. Such tumours are often asymptomatic.

Differential Diagnosis

Definitive biochemical findings of elevated catecholamines denote a PHEO or a PGL. In young children, neuroblastoma is a possibility, but may be distinguished from PHEO and PGLs because neuroblastomas do not secrete physiologically active catecholamines [19]. PHEO or PGL require preoperative alpha- and beta- adrenergic receptor blockade so it is important to distinguish these tumours from neuroblastomas. Therefore, in addition to VMA and HVA, children that present with a diagnosis of neuroblastoma and symptoms of catecholamine excess should have 24-h urinary measurements of fractionated catecholamines and metanephrines.

Imaging and Localisation

Computerised Tomography (CT) and Magnetic Resonance Imaging (MRI)

Radiological investigations to localise the tumour should only be performed after a confirmed biochemical diagnosis. Abdominal and pelvic CT and MRI have a high sensitivity (90–100%) and specificity (70–80%) [64, 65] and will detect the majority of tumours, particularly if they are symptomatic. However, CT and MRI may lack the sensitivity to localise tumours <1 cm diameter that may be detected by early biochemical screening. Contrast CT is quicker and may be more readily available, but requires exposure to radiation. Ionic contrast has been reported to precipitate catecholamine release from PHEO and 'PHEO crisis', but non-ionic contrast is safe [66]. MRI (Fig. 8.2) avoids radiation and can distinguish PHEO (which appear hyperintense on T2-weighted images) from other types of adrenal mass (usually hypointense) [67] but may require general anaesthetic in children. Ultrasound may be useful for surveillance of the neck in children at risk of head and neck PGL. Extra-adrenal PGL may occur in the head and neck (5%), the bladder (10%), along the sympathetic chain in the thorax (10%), and along the sympathetic chain in abdomen (75%), either above (juxtarenal) or below (organ of Zuckerkandl), the origin of the inferior mesenteric artery [68]. Due to the increased likelihood of extra-adrenal and multi-focal disease in children, particularly those with familial disease secondary to *SDHx* mutations, extra-adrenal sites often require investigation.

Other Imaging and Investigations

If initial imaging is negative or reveals extra-adrenal disease, functional imaging with ^{123}I-MIBG (Meta-iodobenzylguanidine) or ^{111}In-octretide may identify occult or multi-focal tumours, confirm functionality of extra-adrenal lesions and detect metastatic disease. Radiolabelled MIBG is taken-up by chromaffin cells via the vesicular monoamine transporter 1 (VMAT-1) because it resembles noradrenaline. It is 80–90% sensitive and more than 95% specific [67]. Radiolabelled octreotide binds to somatostatin receptors commonly expressed by adrenergic tissue and is 50–70% sensitive. Although less sensitive than MIBG, octreotide scanning may be useful if cross-sectional imaging and MIBG scanning are negative. Routine use of functional scans in the presence of adrenal lesions seen on CT/MRI may lead to false-positive localisation of other non-catecholamine-secreting incidentalomas [69, 70], so their use is best reserved for the detection of occult or extra-adrenal disease or for post-operative investigation of residual or metastatic disease. Various forms of positron emission tomography (PET) scanning have shown promise. In one study, imaging with 6-[^{18}F] fluorodopamine was 98% sensitive and 100% specific and was superior to ^{123}I-MIBG [71]. Factors predicting MIBG negativity were young age, hereditary aetiology and lack of VMAT-1 expression in tumours. It is therefore likely that 6-[^{18}F]fluorodopamine PET will be of use in detecting PGL in young patients when conventional imaging and MIBG have failed. It should also be considered for locating metastatic disease [2]. Finally, selective adrenal vein sampling has proved misleading in PHEO and has very limited value [69].

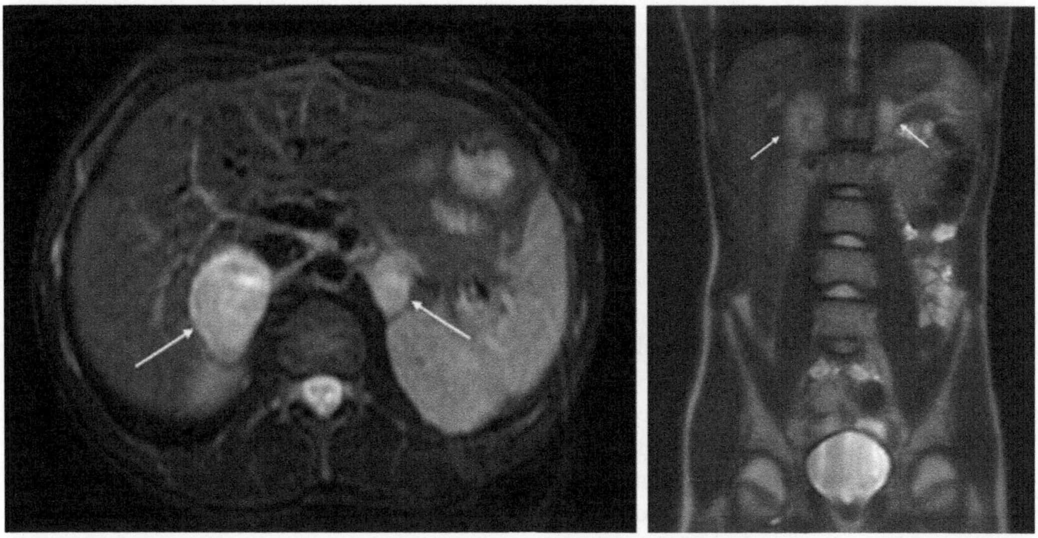

Fig. 8.2 Axial (*left*) and coronal (*right*) images from the MRI abdomen of a 13-year-old boy with VHL disease. Bilateral PHEO were diagnosed on biochemical screening. Note the hyperintense appearance of the tumours (*white arrows*) on axial T2-weighted images. He was treated with laparoscopic adrenalectomy for the 45-mm right-sided tumour and laparoscopic cortical-sparing subtotal adrenalectomy for the 20-mm left-sided tumour, performed sequentially

Management

Biochemical diagnosis and localisation of PHEO or PGL should be followed by medical preparation to control blood pressure and then prompt surgical excision.

Preoperative Management

Major operations done in the presence of undiagnosed PHEO are associated with a mortality of between 25 and 100%; therefore, preoperative preparation to protect against catecholamine excess and triggers of secretion such as induction of anaesthesia are essential for a successful outcome. Although practice varies, alpha-adrenergic blockade, with or without beta-adrenergic blockade, is the most common strategy. In the author's unit, supervised initiation of alpha blockade using oral phenoxybenzamine (0.25–1.0 mg/Kg/day in 3 divided doses) to control blood pressure is the first step. Once alpha blockade is established (usually requiring 4–7 days of therapy) then beta blockade to control tachycardia is commenced (e.g. propranolol 0.25–0.5 mg/Kg/day in 3 divided doses). This sequence of alpha blockade first and then beta blockade is important to avoid dangerous elevations in blood pressure that occur with alpha-induced vasoconstriction. Pharmacological relief of chronic vasoconstriction allows restoration of the inevitable associated depleted intravascular volume over 2–4 weeks. In the week prior to surgery, patients are admitted for supervised blood pressure monitoring and further optimisation of alpha and beta blockade to ensure a goal of a normal resting blood pressure and a postural drop in blood pressure without the normal compensatory tachycardia. At this point it is safe to proceed with an operation. Other regimens have been described, e.g. alpha blockade with doxazosin or prazosin, with and without beta blockade [72], using calcium channel blockers alone [73], and using the catecholamine synthesis blocker, metyrosine, if there are concerns about cardiac failure [74]. However, it must be stressed that preparation should be carried out by a multi-disciplinary team that is experienced in managing such patients and that the familiarity and experience of the team with the condition is probably more important than the exact regimen.

Surgery

Again, a team approach, involving personnel experienced in the surgery for PHEO/PGL, is crucial to ensure a successful outcome in children with the disease. Surgeons experienced in treating such patients will counsel children and their families about possible associated genetic disorders, surgical approach, possible steroid dependence post-operatively, and the need for long-term follow-up. PHEO and intra-abdominal PGL account for 95% of these tumours and can be dealt with by laparotomy or laparoscopic surgery.

Adrenalectomy for PHEO

Due to the rarity of PHEO in children, there are no randomised trials concerning the most appropriate method of surgical excision; however, one small, randomised study in adults reported reduced blood loss, operative time and length of hospital stay with laparoscopic resection [75]. The only disadvantage observed was an increase in intraoperative haemodynamic instability, which has been reported previously [76] but it is usually controlled without significant problems. There are several case series of adults comparing laparoscopic and open adrenalectomy for a variety of adrenal pathologies that favour the laparoscopic approach in terms of blood loss, post-operative pain, length of hospital stay, earlier return to alimentation and earlier return to normal activity [77–85]. Laparoscopic adrenalectomy has also been demonstrated to be safe in children [86] and is an accepted approach for unilateral and bilateral adrenal pathology.

Controversial issues regarding surgery for PHEO include the need of unilateral versus bilateral adrenalectomy for children with a high risk of bilateral disease when imaging has detected only one involved gland and the use of cortical-sparing resections during bilateral adrenalectomy in order to avoid long-term steroid dependence. Follow-up data suggest that unilateral laparoscopic adrenalectomy is the best approach for disease that is unilateral on imaging, followed by regular follow-up with plasma metanephrine measurements for early detection of contralateral disease [87]. Cortical-sparing surgery has been reported in retrospective studies of selected adult patients but it is probably only feasible with small tumours (e.g. <26 mm) [88]. Because a small amount of adrenal medulla is inevitably left behind with the preserved cortex there is a significant risk of recurrent disease (10–38%) [89–92]. The risk of recurrence must be carefully weighed against the substantial morbidity associated with adrenal insufficiency and Addisonian crises that 20% of children will suffer following bilateral adrenalectomy [92].

Following laparoscopic surgery, post-operative stay is <48 h for unilateral surgery but will be longer for bilateral surgery, where pain control and commencement of steroid replacement regimens tend to increase hospital length of stay.

Surgery for Thoracic and Abdominal PGL

Tumours along the sympathetic chain can be technically challenging due to their close relationship to the great vessels and visceral artery branches. For this reason, minimally invasive surgery may not be feasible, and thoracotomy and laparotomy may be the preferred options.

Surgery for Malignant PHEO

The presence of metastatic disease and local invasion is the only definite signs of malignant pheochromocytoma, but size >5 cm and history of genetic disease (*SDHB* mutations) are associated with increased risk. The choice between laparoscopic and open surgery will therefore depend upon the presence of family history combined with appearances on preoperative imaging. Large tumours with evidence of renal, vena caval, duodenal or hepatic involvement on the right side, or pancreatic, splenic, renal or colonic involvement on the left side, and/or local nodal metastases should be treated with open radical adrenalectomy and even more radical local excisions if needed. In our experience of approximately 100 adult pheochromocytomas and a small number of children, preoperative imaging signs of malignancy are rare and laparoscopic surgery is generally feasible even with larger tumours. Patients with locally advanced or metastatic disease at presentation should be treated by a combination of surgical debulking followed by adjuvant treatment to stabilise disease and treat symptoms.

Preoperative Considerations

Apart from medical preparation for surgery, preoperative preparation should include informed consent for surgery with the parents and if competent, the child. Specifically, this should include appropriate mention of steroid replacement post-operatively if bilateral tumours are present, laparoscopic and open surgical approaches and possible or serious complications. Imaging should be checked and the side of tumour marked on the patient by the operating surgeon. An anaesthetist experienced in the management of PHEO should counsel the family about the type of anaesthesia, use of regional or epidural anaesthesia and possible cardiovascular complications.

Intraoperative Considerations

Operative Technique

Laparoscopic adrenalectomy is most commonly transperitoneal, although some surgeons favour retroperitoneoscopic laparoscopy for bilateral tumours since the patient does not require repositioning during surgery [93, 94]. This section will describe transperitoneal surgery. Following general anaesthesia and arterial catheter for blood pressure monitoring, a urinary catheter and orogastric tube are inserted. The patient is then placed on the operating table with the torso in a 45° lateral decubitus position with bolsters either side of the table hinge at the level of the buttocks and shoulders. The hips are rolled slightly posterior with the arms flexed and placed at chest level with appropriate padding. The lower extremities are secured to the operating table, which is then hyper-extended or 'broken' at the level of the loin to open the space between the costal margin and iliac crest. The table is rolled away from the operating surgeon by 10°–15° so that the patient is lying firmly against the bolsters and a patient warming blanket (e.g. 'Bair Hugger', Arizant, UK) is applied. For right-sided tumours, the patient is right side up and for left-sided tumours, left side up (Fig. 8.3).

After antiseptic skin preparation, drapes are placed to expose the costal margin from the xiphoid process around to the tip of the 12th rib. Carboperitoneum, at a pressure of 10–14 mmHg, is induced by the insertion of a Veress needle approximately two-thirds of the distance along the costal margin to the mid-axillary line. Insertion of each port is preceded by infiltration of local anaesthetic at the site of incision. Safe introduction of the first 10-mm port is best achieved with an optical port (e.g. Visiport, Autosuture, UK) and further ports are inserted under direct vision of the laparoscope (Fig. 8.3).

Each adrenal gland lies on its respective diaphragmatic crus, separated from the kidney by the perinephric fat and fascia. Although right and left adrenalectomy are distinct operations, both involve dissection that is focused upon the safe identification, ligation and division of the adrenal vein as it drains into the inferior vena cava on the right and the renal vein on the left. This is followed by excision of the gland and removal using an endoscopic tissue retrieval bag.

Right Adrenalectomy

The addition of an extra 5-mm port on the right facilitates the introduction of a liver retractor into the sub-hepatic space to retract the right lobe of the liver cephalad and expose the posterior parietal peritoneum covering the inferior vena cava, perinephric fat and adrenal gland, which sit on the upper pole of the kidney (Fig. 8.3a). The peritoneum is held with an atraumatic grasper in the operator's left hand and incised with an ultrasonic dissector at the level of its reflection onto the liver, taking care to avoid contact with the vena cava. Dissection is extended along the

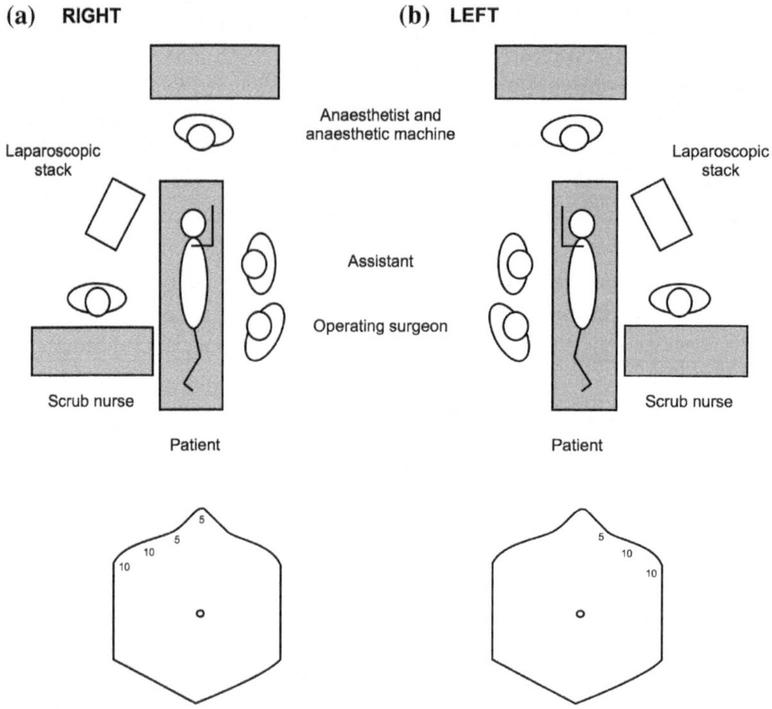

Fig. 8.3 Equipment, patient and surgeon positioning, and port sites (values are port sizes in mm) for right (**a**) and left (**b**) laparoscopic adrenalectomy

lateral border of the vena cava and the tissue plane between the vena cava and gland gently opened. In the authors' experience a 5-mm endoscopic suction device is invaluable for this part of the operation, since PHEOs are very vascular tumours and both dissection and suctioning to maintain a clear surgical field can be achieved using this instrument. The short right adrenal vein is visualised, mobilised to provide enough length to clip twice proximally and twice distally with an endoscopic clip applicator and then it is divided with endoscopic shears. Once the dominant venous drainage of a PHEO has been ligated, the patient's blood pressure will generally decrease and become less labile.

Following division of the vein the tumour can be retracted laterally and mobilised by dividing the numerous small arterial vessels arising from the aorta, inferior phrenic artery and renal artery. Larger (>5 cm) tumours may be associated with multiple fine venous and arterial collaterals that may need to be dealt with using endoscopic clips; however, most can be divided using an ultrasonic dissector. Dissection continues along the inferior and superior borders of the adrenal gland and the lateral fascial connections to the kidney are divided last to free the tumour. The adrenal bed is then irrigated with water, taking care not to brush the clips off the adrenal vein stump, and the tumour is placed in a waterproof endoscopic tissue retrieval bag (to avoid spillage of tumour cells during removal) and removed via the most lateral port. This will require the incision to be enlarged, but the tumours are usually soft and pliable and can be removed through relatively small incisions. Routine placement of drains is not necessary and the myofascial layers of the most lateral port are closed in layers with absorbable '1' or '0' braided or monofilament suture. Skin wounds are closed with subcuticular absorbable suture and adhesive skin closure strips.

Left Adrenalectomy

Tumours on the left can usually be removed using 3 ports, although a 5-mm port below the xiphoid process can be introduced to permit the use of a retractor to manoeuvre the spleen and tail of pancreas away from the renal hilum (Fig. 8.3b). First, the splenic flexure of the colon is mobilised medially, using an atraumatic grasper in the left hand and an ultrasonic dissector in the right hand to divide the splenocolic ligament and the lateral peritoneal reflection of the descending colon. The spleen and tail of pancreas are then mobilised by division of the lienorenal ligament as far posterior as possible—usually to the point when the posterior aspect of the gastric fundus is visible. Caution should be exercised in retracting the spleen and ensuring that the active blade of the dissecting device does not touch or worse still, breech the diaphragm and cause a pneumothorax.

Once the spleen and pancreas have been mobilised, they fall to the midline by rolling the patient towards the operating surgeon so that the table is horizontal. At this point the pheochromocytoma will generally be visible as a bulge through Gerota's fascia. The left adrenal gland lies medial to the kidney and the left adrenal vein, which is longer than the right, drains caudally into the left renal vein. The vein is located by incising Gerota's fascia and dissecting medially over the surface of the tumour. At the most inferior/medial point, the 5-mm suction instrument is again used for dissecting and keeping the operative field clear. The adrenal vein is identified as it drains into the left renal vein, rounded, clipped 3 times and divided. Blunt graspers are then insinuated below the tumour to lift it upward away from the renal hilum, and the caudal, cephalic and deep surfaces of the tumour are dissected. Haemostasis is achieved using an ultrasonic dissector or endoscopic clips for larger venous or arterial collaterals. Again, the lateral attachments are divided last to provide a pivot upon which to rotate the tumour away from the renal hilum. After irrigation of the adrenal bed with water to confirm haemostasis, removal of the tumour and closure of the wounds is as described for the right side.

Bilateral Laparoscopic Adrenalectomy

Bilateral tumours can be treated with sequential left and right or right and then left laparoscopic adrenalectomy or by the retroperitoneoscopic approach, starting with the larger of the tumours. If either tumour is <2.5 cm, cortical-sparing surgery is a reasonable option, provided the tumour is well circumscribed with a substantial amount of normal unaffected cortical tissue. Preoperative imaging and intraoperative laparoscopic ultrasound are helpful to determine whether sufficient unaffected cortical tissue can be preserved and gland mobilisation should be minimised to preserve the blood supply to the cortical remnant.

Open Adrenalectomy

Open adrenalectomy may be performed as a planned procedure because of concerns about tumour size and signs of malignancy on preoperative imaging, or because of conversion of an initial laparoscopic procedure due to an intraoperative suspicion of malignancy or due to a technically difficult laparoscopic procedure. Laparoscopic surgery is usually converted to open because of bleeding from the inferior vena cava on the right or the renal vein on the left. Once these issues have been dealt with (see below) the operation proceeds as already described. When malignant PHEO or PGL is suspected, the principal aim is to achieve a complete tumour resection with excision of regional para-aortic lymph nodes. If adjacent organs are involved, these should be excised *en bloc*, e.g. by nephrectomy, splenectomy and distal pancreatectomy. For right-sided tumours, adequate clearance may require partial hepatectomy with or without jugulo-caval or cardio-pulmonary bypass if reconstruction of the vena cava is required. Ex vivo techniques have also been described for dealing with tumours involving portal triad or caval structures, such that the tumour and liver are excised *en bloc*, separated on the 'back table' and the liver reimplanted [95]. Such techniques clearly require a team approach with surgeons from different specialities working in tandem.

Post-operative Care

Tumour excision is occasionally associated with post-operative hypotension due to residual alpha blockade, and this may require temporary use of pressor agents and management on an intensive care unit. However, most patients can be managed in a post-anaesthesia recovery setting for 4–6 h. Once haemodynamically stable, the arterial catheter can be removed and the patient managed in a ward setting.

Patients undergoing bilateral adrenalectomy should have intravenous glucocorticoids at induction of anaesthesia (hydrocortisone 2–3 mg/kg/day in 3 divided doses for 48–72 h). Following the institution of normal diet a maintenance dose of oral hydrocortisone is given. Fludrocortisone (0.05–0.1 mg/day), a synthetic mineralocorticoid, is required to ensure adequate salt balance and adequacy of dose is monitored by measuring supine and erect blood pressure and avoiding peripheral oedema. In the medium term, the dose can be checked by monitoring of serum sodium and potassium and if necessary, plasma renin activity, which should be at the upper limit of normal. Regimens will of course vary and joint care with a paediatric endocrinologist is essential.

Complications

Intraoperative Complications

Haemodynamic instability, myocardial ischemia, hypertensive stroke and cardiac arrest are the most serious potential complications and relate to catecholamine excess induced by anaesthesia, carboperitoneum and tumour manipulation prior to venous ligation. For the surgeon, the primary concern for right-sided tumours is safe dissection around the junction of the adrenal vein and inferior vena cava. Avulsion of the vein or dislodged endoscopic clips will result in brisk venous bleeding that should be controlled with a blunt grasper by the first assistant, while the operating surgeon performs a subcostal open incision. The area should then be packed to control bleeding and allow repair with a 5/0 polypropylene vascular suture. On the left side, colonic thermal and grasper injury are rare but potential complications, as is splenic capsular tear and thermal injury to the splenic artery, leading to haemorrhage. However, it is rare that splenic injuries necessitate splenectomy. Failure to control the left adrenal vein will result in brisk bleeding but tamponade with an endoscopic swab for 5 min should slow this enough to control haemorrhage with endoscopic clips. If this is not possible, conversion to open adrenalectomy is appropriate, to allow repair with a vascular suture.

Early Post-operative Complications

The advent of laparoscopic surgery has led to a reduction in respiratory and wound complications that were common following open unilateral and bilateral adrenalectomy and the incidence of post-operative pneumonia is now around 10–15%. Port-site hernia may occur and present as small bowel obstruction following surgery. Therefore, port sites that are enlarged for tumour removal should be formally closed. Steroid dependence is expected after bilateral and cortex-sparing surgery and should be managed administration of intravenous hydrocortisone starting at the induction of anaesthesia. Residual adrenal function after subtotal adrenalectomy should be investigated by ACTH stimulation test once the patient has fully recovered from surgery. Ileus and gastric stasis are uncommon with laparoscopic surgery and nearly all patients can drink fluids in the immediate post-operative period and resume a diet over the next 24 h if fluids are tolerated.

Late Complications

Addisonian crisis occurs in 20% of patients after bilateral adrenalectomy who are steroid-dependent. Addisonian crisis may be precipitated by an acute illness or poor medication compliance [92]. It may also occur following cortex-sparing surgery due to relative steroid deficiency. Crises are characterised by dizziness, collapse, hypotension and hyponatremia and are treated supportively with intravenous fluids, intravenous hydrocortisone and treatment of any precipitating factor. When oral intake can be tolerated then oral steroids are reintroduced. Patient and family education is important to encourage medication compliance to prevent further episodes.

Follow-Up and Prognosis

Rigorous follow-up to evaluate for recurrent and metastatic disease is mandatory for children with sporadic and familial PHEO and PGL, because of the unpredictable nature of some seemingly benign lesions. Lifelong, regular biochemical screening is necessary, with appropriate imaging for non-functioning head and neck tumours in patients with *SDHx* mutations. However, the majority of tumours will be benign and if completely excised, will result in a near-normal life expectancy for the patient.

Prognosis following surgery for malignant PHEO depends upon the presence and site of metastatic disease and completeness of surgical resection. Unfortunately, surgery for advanced disease is seldom curative. For patients with lung and liver metastases survival is generally less than 5 years, whereas those with bony metastases have a better prognosis. Overall, the 5- and 10-year survival for children with malignant PHEO is 78 and 30%, respectively. Established treatment for advanced malignant disease is either surgery with curative intent or cytoreductive surgery since this will generally improve the response to adjuvant therapies.

Other Treatment for Malignant Disease

Radioactive ^{131}I-MIBG

Positive uptake (>1% uptake of injected dose) on diagnostic ^{123}I-MIBG scanning is seen in 60% of metastases from PHEO. Patients who have positive uptake or positive expression of VMAT 1 and VMAT 2 on tumour immunohistochemistry are candidates for treatment with radioactive ^{131}I-MIBG. Review of 166 patients treated with ^{131}I-MIBG demonstrated tumour response in 30%, disease stabilisation in 40–50% and hormone response in 15–45% [54]. Response was greatest in those with limited disease. Progression occurred in 13%. Bone marrow toxicity is the principal complication and is dose related. In children, there is a risk in the long term of second malignancy [96]. The use of radiolabelled MIBG as an adjuvant treatment following potentially curative surgery remains to be validated.

Radioactive Somatostatin Analogues

The radiolabelled somatostatin analogues include ^{111}In-pentetreotide and ^{111}In-DOTA-octreotide, ^{90}Y-DOTA-octreotide and ^{177}Lu-DOTA-octreotate and radiolabelled lanreotide. Patient selection is based upon scintigraphy uptake, usually with ^{111}In-pentetreotide. Therapy is less effective than radiolabelled MIBG with disease stabilisation in only 25%. The side-effect profile is similar. Since some patients may have co-existing MIBG-positive and MIBG-negative metastases that exhibit radiolabelled somatostatin analogue uptake, combined treatment may be effective [97].

Chemotherapy, Radiotherapy and Novel Treatments

Combination chemotherapy with cyclophosphamide, vincristine and dacarbazine (CVD) improves symptoms in around 50% of those with inoperable disease but the response is short-lived and CVD does not prolong survival [98, 99]. Radiotherapy is most helpful for palliative treatment of bony metastases, and soft-tissue lesions can be treated with radiofrequency ablation, cryotherapy and arterial embolization. Experience with newer treatments including the mTOR inhibitor everolimus [100] and the combination of temozolomide and thalidomide have been [101] disappointing. The tyrosine kinase inhibitor sunitinib remains unproven but partial response to treatment has been observed in a small number of patients [54].

References

1. Goodman MT, Gurnet JG, Smith MA, Olshan AF. Sympathetic nervous system tumours. In: Ries LAG, Smith MA, Gurney JG, Linet M, Tamra T, Young JL, Bunin GR, editors. Cancer incidence and survival among children and adolescents: United States SEER Program 1975–1995. NIH Pub. No.99-4649: Bethesda, MD: National Cancer Institute; 1999. pp. 65–72.
2. Armstrong R, Sridhar M, Greenhalgh KL, Howell L, Jones C, Landes C, McPartland JL, Moores C, Losty PD, Didi M. Pheochromocytoma in children. Arch Dis Child. 2008;93(10):899–904.
3. Timmers HJ, Pacak K, Huynh TT, Abu-Asab M, Tsokos M, Merino MJ, Baysal BE, Adams KT, Eisenhofer G. Biochemically silent abdominal paragangliomas in patients with mutations in the succinate dehydrogenase subunit B gene. J Clin Endocrinol Metab. 2008;93(12):4826–32.
4. Ross JH. Pheochromocytoma. Special considerations in children. Urol Clin North Am. 2000;27 (3):393–402.
5. Barontini M, Levin G, Sanso G. Characteristics of pheochromocytoma in a 4- to 20-year-old population. Ann N Y Acad Sci. 2006;1073:30–7.
6. Neumann HP, Bausch B, McWhinney SR, Bender BU, Gimm O, Franke G, Schipper J, Klisch J, Altehoefer C, Zerres K, Januszewicz A, Eng C, Smith WM, Munk R, Manz T, Glaesker S, Apel TW, Treier M, Reineke M, Walz MK, Hoang-Vu C, Brauckhoff M, Klein-Franke A, Klose P, Schmidt H, Maier-Woelfle M, Peczkowska M, Szmigielski C, Eng C. Germ-line mutations in nonsyndromic pheochromocytoma. N Engl J Med. 2002;346(19):1459–66.
7. Beltsevich DG, Kuznetsov NS, Kazaryan AM, Lysenko MA. Pheochromocytoma surgery: epidemiologic peculiarities in children. World J Surg. 2004;28(6):592–6.
8. Ciftci AO, Tanyel FC, Senocak ME, Buyukpamukcu N. Pheochromocytoma in children. J Pediatr Surg. 2001;36(3):447–52.
9. Erlic Z, Neumann HP. When should genetic testing be obtained in a patient with pheochromocytoma or paraganglioma? Clin Endocrinol (Oxf). 2009;70 (3):354–7.
10. Mulligan LM, Kwok JB, Healey CS, Elsdon MJ, Eng C, Gardner E, Love DR, Mole SE, Moore JK, Papi L, et al. Germ-line mutations of the RET proto-oncogene in multiple endocrine neoplasia type 2A. Nature. 1993;363(6428):458–60.
11. Latif F, Tory K, Gnarra J, Yao M, Duh FM, Orcutt ML, Stackhouse T, Kuzmin I, Modi W, Geil L, et al. Identification of the von Hippel-Lindau disease tumor suppressor gene. Science. 1993;260(5112):1317–20.
12. Niemann S, Muller U. Mutations in SDHC cause autosomal dominant paraganglioma, type 3. Nat Genet. 2000;26(3):268–70.
13. Astuti D, Latif F, Dallol A, Dahia PL, Douglas F, George E, Skoldberg F, Husebye ES, Eng C, Maher ER. Gene mutations in the succinate dehydrogenase subunit SDHB cause susceptibility to familial pheochromocytoma and to familial paraganglioma. Am J Hum Genet. 2001;69(1):49–54.
14. Baysal BE, Ferrell RE, Willett-Brozick JE, Lawrence EC, Myssiorek D, Bosch A, van der Mey A, Taschner PE, Rubinstein WS, Myers EN, Richard CW 3rd, Cornelisse CJ, Devilee P, Devlin B. Mutations in SDHD, a mitochondrial complex II gene, in hereditary paraganglioma. Science. 2000;287(5454):848–51.
15. Xu W, Mulligan LM, Ponder MA, Liu L, Smith BA, Mathew CG, Ponder BA. Loss of NF1 alleles in pheochromocytomas from patients with type I neurofibromatosis. Genes Chromosom Cancer. 1992;4(4):337–42.
16. Freier DT, Tank ES, Harrison TS. Pediatric and adult pheochromocytomas. A biochemical and clinical comparison. Arch Surg. 1973;107(2):252–5.
17. Ein SH, Shandling B, Wesson D, Filler R. Recurrent pheochromocytomas in children. J Pediatr Surg. 1990;25(10):1063–5.
18. Caty MG, Coran AG, Geagen M, Thompson NW. Current diagnosis and treatment of pheochromocytoma in children. Experience with 22 consecutive tumors in 14 patients. Arch Surg. 1990;125(8):978–81.
19. Pham TH, Moir C, Thompson GB, Zarroug AE, Hamner CE, Farley D, van Heerden J, Lteif AN, Young WF Jr. Pheochromocytoma and paraganglioma in children: a review of medical and surgical management at a tertiary care center. Pediatrics. 2006;118(3):1109–17.
20. Lee S, Nakamura E, Yang H, Wei W, Linggi MS, Sajan MP, Farese RV, Freeman RS, Carter BD, Kaelin WG Jr, Schlisio S. Neuronal apoptosis linked to EglN3 prolyl hydroxylase and familial pheochromocytoma genes: developmental culling and cancer. Cancer Cell. 2005;8(2):155–67.
21. Maxwell PH. A common pathway for genetic events leading to pheochromocytoma. Cancer Cell. 2005;8(2):91–3.
22. Maher ER, Iselius L, Yates JR, Littler M, Benjamin C, Harris R, Sampson J, Williams A, Ferguson-Smith MA, Morton N. Von Hippel-Lindau disease: a genetic study. J Med Genet. 1991;28(7):443–7.

23. Maher ER, Yates JR, Harries R, Benjamin C, Harris R, Moore AT, Ferguson-Smith MA. Clinical features and natural history of von Hippel-Lindau disease. Q J Med. 1990;77(283):1151–63.
24. Maher ER. Genetics of pheochromocytoma. Br Med Bull. 2006;79–80:141–51.
25. Hes FJ, Hoppener JW, Lips CJ. Clinical review 155: pheochromocytoma in Von Hippel-Lindau disease. J Clin Endocrinol Metab. 2003;88 (3):969–74.
26. Hes FJ, van der Luijt RB, Janssen AL, Zewald RA, de Jong GJ, Lenders JW, Links TP, Luyten GP, Sijmons RH, Eussen HJ, Halley DJ, Lips CJ, Pearson PL, van den Ouweland AM, Majoor-Krakauer DF. Frequency of Von Hippel-Lindau germline mutations in classic and non-classic Von Hippel-Lindau disease identified by DNA sequencing, southern blot analysis and multiplex ligation-dependent probe amplification. Clin Genet. 2007;72(2):122–9.
27. Mulligan LM, Eng C, Healey CS, Clayton D, Kwok JB, Gardner E, Ponder MA, Frilling A, Jackson CE, Lehnert H, et al. Specific mutations of the RET proto-oncogene are related to disease phenotype in MEN 2A and FMTC. Nat Genet. 1994;6(1):70–4.
28. Petri BJ, van Eijck CH, de Herder WW, Wagner A, de Krijger RR. Pheochromocytomas and sympathetic paragangliomas. Br J Surg. 2009;96 (12):1381–92.
29. Kouvaraki MA, Shapiro SE, Perrier ND, Cote GJ, Gagel RF, Hoff AO, Sherman SI, Lee JE, Evans DB. RET proto-oncogene: a review and update of genotype-phenotype correlations in hereditary medullary thyroid cancer and associated endocrine tumors. Thyroid. 2005;15(6):531–44.
30. Raue F, Frank-Raue K. Genotype-phenotype relationship in multiple endocrine neoplasia type 2. Implications for clinical management. Hormones (Athens). 2009;8(1):23–8.
31. Machens A, Brauckhoff M, Holzhausen HJ, Thanh PN, Lehnert H, Dralle H. Codon-specific development of pheochromocytoma in multiple endocrine neoplasia type 2. J Clin Endocrinol Metab. 2005;90(7):3999–4003.
32. Quayle FJ, Fialkowski EA, Benveniste R, Moley JF. Pheochromocytoma penetrance varies by RET mutation in MEN 2A. Surgery. 2007; 142 (6):800–05. discussion 805 e801.
33. Walther MM, Herring J, Enquist E, Keiser HR, Linehan WM. von Recklinghausen's disease and pheochromocytomas. J Urol. 1999;162(5):1582–6.
34. Bausch B, Koschker AC, Fassnacht M, Stoevesandt J, Hoffmann MM, Eng C, Allolio B, Neumann HP. Comprehensive mutation scanning of NF1 in apparently sporadic cases of pheochromocytoma. J Clin Endocrinol Metab. 2006;91(9):3478–81.
35. Gimm O, Armanios M, Dziema H, Neumann HP, Eng C. Somatic and occult germ-line mutations in SDHD, a mitochondrial complex II gene, in nonfamilial pheochromocytoma. Cancer Res. 2000;60(24):6822–5.
36. Pasini B, Stratakis CA. SDH mutations in tumorigenesis and inherited endocrine tumours: lesson from the pheochromocytoma-paraganglioma syndromes. J Intern Med. 2009;266(1):19–42.
37. Heutink P, van der Mey AG, Sandkuijl LA, van Gils AP, Bardoel A, Breedveld GJ, van Vliet M, van Ommen GJ, Cornelisse CJ, Oostra BA, et al. A gene subject to genomic imprinting and responsible for hereditary paragangliomas maps to chromosome 11q23-qter. Hum Mol Genet. 1992;1(1):7–10.
38. Hao HX, Khalimonchuk O, Schraders M, Dephoure N, Bayley JP, Kunst H, Devilee P, Cremers CW, Schiffman JD, Bentz BG, Gygi SP, Winge DR, Kremer H, Rutter J. SDH5, a gene required for flavination of succinate dehydrogenase, is mutated in paraganglioma. Science. 2009;325 (5944):1139–42.
39. Gimenez-Roqueplo AP, Favier J, Rustin P, Rieubland C, Crespin M, Nau V, Khau Van Kien P, Corvol P, Plouin PF, Jeunemaitre X. Mutations in the SDHB gene are associated with extra-adrenal and/or malignant pheochromocytomas. Cancer Res. 2003; 63(17):5615–21.
40. Qin Y, Yao L, King EE, Buddavarapu K, Lenci RE, Chocron ES, Lechleiter JD, Sass M, Aronin N, Schiavi F, Boaretto F, Opocher G, Toledo RA, Toledo SP, Stiles C, Aguiar RC, Dahia PL. Germline mutations in TMEM127 confer susceptibility to pheochromocytoma. Nat Genet. 2010;42(3):229–33.
41. Yao L, Schiavi F, Cascon A, Qin Y, Inglada-Perez L, King EE, Toledo RA, Ercolino T, Rapizzi E, Ricketts CJ, Mori L, Giacche M, Mendola A, Taschin E, Boaretto F, Loli P, Iacobone M, Rossi GP, Biondi B, Lima-Junior JV, Kater CE, Bex M, Vikkula M, Grossman AB, Gruber SB, Barontini M, Persu A, Castellano M, Toledo SP, Maher ER, Mannelli M, Opocher G, Robledo M, Dahia PL. Spectrum and prevalence of FP/TMEM127 gene mutations in pheochromocytomas and paragangliomas. JAMA. 2011;304 (23):2611–9.
42. Stratakis CA, Carney JA. The triad of paragangliomas, gastric stromal tumours and pulmonary chondromas (Carney triad), and the dyad of paragangliomas and gastric stromal sarcomas (Carney-Stratakis syndrome): molecular genetics and clinical implications. J Intern Med. 2009;266 (1):43–52.
43. Kennedy JS, Symington T, Woodger BA. Chemical and histochemical observations in benign and malignant pheochromocytoma. J Pathol Bacteriol. 1961;81:409–18.
44. Lloyd RV, Blaivas M, Wilson BS. Distribution of chromogranin and S100 protein in normal and abnormal adrenal medullary tissues. Arch Pathol Lab Med. 1985;109(7):633–5.

45. Unger P, Hoffman K, Pertsemlidis D, Thung S, Wolfe D, Kaneko M. S100 protein-positive sustentacular cells in malignant and locally aggressive adrenal pheochromocytomas. Arch Pathol Lab Med. 1991;115(5):484–7.
46. Lloyd RV, Jin L, Kulig E, Fields K. Molecular approaches for the analysis of chromogranins and secretogranins. Diagn Mol Pathol. 1992;1(1):2–15.
47. Schober M, Fischer-Colbrie R, Schmid KW, Bussolati G, O'Connor DT, Winkler H. Comparison of chromogranins A, B, and secretogranin II in human adrenal medulla and pheochromocytoma. Lab Invest. 1987;57(4):385–91.
48. Wilson BS, Lloyd RV. Detection of chromogranin in neuroendocrine cells with a monoclonal antibody. Am J Pathol. 1984;115(3):458–68.
49. Linnoila RI, Keiser HR, Steinberg SM, Lack EE. Histopathology of benign versus malignant sympathoadrenal paragangliomas: clinicopathologic study of 120 cases including unusual histologic features. Hum Pathol. 1990;21(11):1168–80.
50. Brown HM, Komorowski RA, Wilson SD, Demeure MJ, Zhu YR. Predicting metastasis of pheochromocytomas using DNA flow cytometry and immunohistochemical markers of cell proliferation: a positive correlation between MIB-1 staining and malignant tumor behavior. Cancer. 1999;86 (8):1583–9.
51. Clarke MR, Weyant RJ, Watson CG, Carty SE. Prognostic markers in pheochromocytoma. Hum Pathol. 1998;29(5):522–6.
52. Thompson LD. Pheochromocytoma of the Adrenal gland Scaled Score (PASS) to separate benign from malignant neoplasms: a clinicopathologic and immunophenotypic study of 100 cases. Am J Surg Pathol. 2002;26(5):551–66.
53. Wu D, Tischler AS, Lloyd RV, DeLellis RA, de Krijger R, van Nederveen F, Nose V. Observer variation in the application of the Pheochromocytoma of the Adrenal Gland Scaled Score. Am J Surg Pathol. 2009;33(4):599–608.
54. Chrisoulidou A, Kaltsas G, Ilias I, Grossman AB. The diagnosis and management of malignant pheochromocytoma and paraganglioma. Endocr Relat Cancer. 2007;14(3):569–85.
55. van Nederveen FH, Gaal J, Favier J, Korpershoek E, Oldenburg RA, de Bruyn EM, Sleddens HF, Derkx P, Riviere J, Dannenberg H, Petri BJ, Komminoth P, Pacak K, Hop WC, Pollard PJ, Mannelli M, Bayley JP, Perren A, Niemann S, Verhofstad AA, de Bruine AP, Maher ER, Tissier F, Meatchi T, Badoual C, Bertherat J, Amar L, Alataki D, Van Marck E, Ferrau F, Francois J, de Herder WW, Peeters MP, van Linge A, Lenders JW, Gimenez-Roqueplo AP, de Krijger RR, Dinjens WN. An immunohistochemical procedure to detect patients with paraganglioma and pheochromocytoma with germline SDHB, SDHC, or SDHD gene mutations: a retrospective and prospective analysis. Lancet Oncol. 2009;10(8):764–71.
56. Stackpole RH, Melicow MM, Uson AC. Pheochromocytoma in children. Report of 9 case and review of the first 100 published cases with follow-up studies. J Pediatr. 1963;63:314–30.
57. Walther MM, Reiter R, Keiser HR, Choyke PL, Venzon D, Hurley K, Gnarra JR, Reynolds JC, Glenn GM, Zbar B, Linehan WM. Clinical and genetic characterization of pheochromocytoma in von Hippel-Lindau families: comparison with sporadic pheochromocytoma gives insight into natural history of pheochromocytoma. J Urol. 1999;162(3 Pt 1):659–64.
58. Lenders JW, Pacak K, Walther MM, Linehan WM, Mannelli M, Friberg P, Keiser HR, Goldstein DS, Eisenhofer G. Biochemical diagnosis of pheochromocytoma: which test is best? JAMA. 2002;287 (11):1427–34.
59. Ilias I, Pacak K. Diagnosis and management of tumors of the adrenal medulla. Horm Metab Res. 2005;37(12):717–21.
60. Eisenhofer G, Goldstein DS, Walther MM, Friberg P, Lenders JW, Keiser HR, Pacak K. Biochemical diagnosis of pheochromocytoma: how to distinguish true- from false-positive test results. J Clin Endocrinol Metab. 2003;88(6):2656–66.
61. Eisenhofer G, Lenders JW, Pacak K. Biochemical diagnosis of pheochromocytoma. Front Horm Res. 2004;31:76–106.
62. Eisenhofer G, Lenders JW, Linehan WM, Walther MM, Goldstein DS, Keiser HR. Plasma normetanephrine and metanephrine for detecting pheochromocytoma in von Hippel-Lindau disease and multiple endocrine neoplasia type 2. N Engl J Med. 1999;340(24):1872–9.
63. Eisenhofer G, Walther MM, Huynh TT, Li ST, Bornstein SR, Vortmeyer A, Mannelli M, Goldstein DS, Linehan WM, Lenders JW, Pacak K. Pheochromocytomas in von Hippel-Lindau syndrome and multiple endocrine neoplasia type 2 display distinct biochemical and clinical phenotypes. J Clin Endocrinol Metab. 2001;86(5):1999–2008.
64. Ilias I, Sahdev A, Reznek RH, Grossman AB, Pacak K. The optimal imaging of adrenal tumours: a comparison of different methods. Endocr Relat Cancer. 2007;14(3):587–99.
65. Pacak K, Eisenhofer G, Ahlman H, Bornstein SR, Gimenez-Roqueplo AP, Grossman AB, Kimura N, Mannelli M, McNicol AM, Tischler AS. Pheochromocytoma: recommendations for clinical practice from the first international symposium. October 2005. Nat Clin Pract Endocrinol Metab. 2007;3 (2):92–102.
66. Bessell-Browne R, O'Malley ME. CT of pheochromocytoma and paraganglioma: risk of adverse events

with i.v. administration of nonionic contrast material. AJR Am J Roentgenol. 2007; 188(4):970–4.
67. Bravo EL. Evolving concepts in the pathophysiology, diagnosis, and treatment of pheochromocytoma. Endocr Rev. 1994;15(3):356–68.
68. Whalen RK, Althausen AF, Daniels GH. Extra-adrenal pheochromocytoma. J Urol. 1992;147(1):1–10.
69. Turner MC, DeQuattro V, Falk R, Ansari A, Lieberman E. Childhood familial pheochromocytoma. Conflicting results of localization techniques. Hypertension. 1986;8(10):851–8.
70. Taieb D, Sebag F, Hubbard JG, Mundler O, Henry JF, Conte-Devolx B. Does iodine-131 meta-iodobenzylguanidine (MIBG) scintigraphy have an impact on the management of sporadic and familial pheochromocytoma? Clin Endocrinol (Oxf). 2004;61(1):102–8.
71. Fottner C, Helisch A, Anlauf M, Rossmann H, Musholt TJ, Kreft A, Schadmand-Fischer S, Bartenstein P, Lackner KJ, Kloppel G, Schreckenberger M, Weber MM. 6-18F-fluoro-L-dihydroxyphenylalanine positron emission tomography is superior to 123I-metaiodobenzyl-guanidine scintigraphy in the detection of extraadrenal and hereditary pheochromocytomas and paragangliomas: correlation with vesicular monoamine transporter expression. J Clin Endocrinol Metab. 95(6):2800–2810.
72. Weingarten TN, Cata JP, O'Hara JF, Prybilla DJ, Pike TL, Thompson GB, Grant CS, Warner DO, Bravo E, Sprung J. Comparison of two preoperative medical management strategies for laparoscopic resection of pheochromocytoma. Urology. 2010; 76 (2): 508 e506–11.
73. Lebuffe G, Dosseh ED, Tek G, Tytgat H, Moreno S, Tavernier B, Vallet B, Proye CA. The effect of calcium channel blockers on outcome following the surgical treatment of pheochromocytomas and paragangliomas. Anaesthesia. 2005;60(5):439–44.
74. Steinsapir J, Carr AA, Prisant LM, Bransome ED Jr. Metyrosine and pheochromocytoma. Arch Intern Med. 1997;157(8):901–6.
75. Tiberio GA, Baiocchi GL, Arru L, Agabiti Rosei C, De Ponti S, Matheis A, Rizzoni D, Giulini SM. Prospective randomized comparison of laparoscopic versus open adrenalectomy for sporadic pheochromocytoma. Surg Endosc. 2008; 22(6):1435–39.
76. Inabnet WB, Pitre J, Bernard D, Chapuis Y. Comparison of the hemodynamic parameters of open and laparoscopic adrenalectomy for pheochromocytoma. World J Surg. 2000;24(5):574–8.
77. Gagner M, Lacroix A, Bolte E. Laparoscopic adrenalectomy in cushing's syndrome and pheochromocytoma. N Engl J Med. 1992;327 (14):1033.
78. Naito S, Uozumi J, Ichimiya H, Tanaka M, Kimoto K, Takahashi K, Ohta J, Tanaka M, Kumazawa J. Laparoscopic adrenalectomy: comparison with open adrenalectomy. Eur Urol. 1994;26(3):253–7.
79. Prinz RA. A comparison of laparoscopic and open adrenalectomies. Arch Surg. 1995; 130(5):489–92. discussion 492-484.
80. MacGillivray DC, Shichman SJ, Ferrer FA, Malchoff CD. A comparison of open vs laparoscopic adrenalectomy. Surg Endosc. 1996;10(10):987–90.
81. Duh QY, Siperstein AE, Clark OH, Schecter WP, Horn JK, Harrison MR, Hunt TK, Way LW. Laparoscopic adrenalectomy. Comparison of the lateral and posterior approaches. Arch Surg. 1996; 131(8):870–5. discussion 875-876.
82. Gagner M, Pomp A, Heniford BT, Pharand D, Lacroix A. Laparoscopic adrenalectomy: lessons learned from 100 consecutive procedures. Ann Surg. 1997; 226(3):238–46. discussion 246-237.
83. Winfield HN, Hamilton BD, Bravo EL, Novick AC. Laparoscopic adrenalectomy: the preferred choice? a comparison to open adrenalectomy. J Urol. 1998;160(2):325–9.
84. Ramachandran MS, Reid JA, Dolan SJ, Farling PA, Russell CF. Laparoscopic adrenalectomy versus open adrenalectomy: results from a retrospective comparative study. Ulster Med J. 2006;75(2):126–8.
85. Wang HS, Li CC, Chou YH, Wang CJ, Wu WJ, Huang CH. Comparison of laparoscopic adrenalectomy with open surgery for adrenal tumors. Kaohsiung J Med Sci. 2009;25(8):438–44.
86. Miller KA, Albanese C, Harrison M, Farmer D, Ostlie DJ, Gittes G, Holcomb GW. Experience with laparoscopic adrenalectomy in pediatric patients. J Pediatr Surg. 2002; 37(7):979–82. discussion 979-982.
87. Albanese CT, Wiener ES. Routine total bilateral adrenalectomy is not warranted in childhood familial pheochromocytoma. J Pediatr Surg. 1993; 28 (10):1248–51. discussion 1251-1242.
88. Kaye DR, Storey BB, Pacak K, Pinto PA, Linehan WM, Bratslavsky G. Partial adrenalectomy: underused first line therapy for small adrenal tumors. J Urol. 2010;184(1):18–25.
89. Lee JE, Curley SA, Gagel RF, Evans DB, Hickey RC. Cortical-sparing adrenalectomy for patients with bilateral pheochromocytoma. Surgery. 1996; 120(6):1064–70. discussion 1070-1061.
90. Neumann HP, Reincke M, Bender BU, Elsner R, Janetschek G. Preserved adrenocortical function after laparoscopic bilateral adrenal sparing surgery for hereditary pheochromocytoma. J Clin Endocrinol Metab. 1999;84(8):2608–10.
91. Walther MM, Keiser HR, Choyke PL, Rayford W, Lyne JC, Linehan WM. Management of hereditary pheochromocytoma in von Hippel-Lindau kindreds with partial adrenalectomy. J Urol. 1999;161 (2):395–8.
92. Asari R, Scheuba C, Kaczirek K, Niederle B. Estimated risk of pheochromocytoma recurrence after adrenal-sparing surgery in patients with multiple endocrine neoplasia type 2A. Arch Surg. 2006; 141(12):1199–205. discussion 1205.

93. Walz MK, Alesina PF, Wenger FA, Koch JA, Neumann HP, Petersenn S, Schmid KW, Mann K. Laparoscopic and retroperitoneoscopic treatment of pheochromocytomas and retroperitoneal paragangliomas: results of 161 tumors in 126 patients. World J Surg. 2006;30(5):899–908.
94. Callender GG, Kennamer DL, Grubbs EG, Lee JE, Evans DB, Perrier ND. Posterior retroperitoneoscopic adrenalectomy. Adv Surg. 2009;43:147–57.
95. Fusai G, Steinberg R, Prachalias A, Heaton ND, Spitz L, Rela M. Ex vivo liver surgery for extraadrenal pheochromocytoma. Pediatr Surg Int. 2006;22(3):282–5.
96. Garaventa A, Gambini C, Villavecchia G, Di Cataldo A, Bertolazzi L, Pizzitola MR, De Bernardi B, Haupt R. Second malignancies in children with neuroblastoma after combined treatment with 131I-metaiodobenzylguanidine. Cancer. 2003;97(5):1332–8.
97. Ahlman H. Malignant pheochromocytoma: state of the field with future projections. Ann N Y Acad Sci. 2006;1073:449–64.
98. Averbuch SD, Steakley CS, Young RC, Gelmann EP, Goldstein DS, Stull R, Keiser HR. Malignant pheochromocytoma: effective treatment with a combination of cyclophosphamide, vincristine, and dacarbazine. Ann Intern Med. 1988;109(4):267–73.
99. Huang H, Abraham J, Hung E, Averbuch S, Merino M, Steinberg SM, Pacak K, Fojo T. Treatment of malignant pheochromocytoma/paraganglioma with cyclophosphamide, vincristine, and dacarbazine: recommendation from a 22-year follow-up of 18 patients. Cancer. 2008;113(8):2020–8.
100. Druce MR, Kaltsas GA, Fraenkel M, Gross DJ, Grossman AB. Novel and evolving therapies in the treatment of malignant pheochromocytoma: experience with the mTOR inhibitor everolimus (RAD001). Horm Metab Res. 2009;41(9):697–702.
101. Kulke MH, Stuart K, Enzinger PC, Ryan DP, Clark JW, Muzikansky A, Vincitore M, Michelini A, Fuchs CS. Phase II study of temozolomide and thalidomide in patients with metastatic neuroendocrine tumors. J Clin Oncol. 2006;24(3):401–6.
102. Schlisio S, Kenchappa RS, Vredeveld LC, George RE, Stewart R, Greulich H, Shahriari K, Nguyen NV, Pigny P, Dahia PL, Pomeroy SL, Maris JM, Look AT, Meyerson M, Peeper DS, Carter BD, Kaelin WG Jr. The kinesin KIF1Bbeta acts downstream from EglN3 to induce apoptosis and is a potential 1p36 tumor suppressor. Genes Dev. 2008;22(7):884–93.

9 Neuroblastoma

Keith Holmes

Neuroblastoma represents 10% of childhood solid tumours, with an incidence of 6–8 per million. The tumours develop in cells derived from the neural crest and may arise in any structure with the crest as its origin. There is an extra-ordinary variation in the presentation and outcome of the disease with some patients dying from extensive metastases in spite of intensive multimodal therapy and others experiencing disappearance of the tumour with no treatment.

History

"Sarcomas" of the suprarenal gland were recorded in the late nineteenth century by Virchow (1864) and Morgan (1879) [1]. "Congenital sarcomas of the suprarenal gland" were reported [2], almost certainly describing the special category of disease which occurs in the first few weeks of life. The term "Neuroblastoma" was first used in 1910 [3] in recognition of the similarity of the cells to embryonic sympathetic ganglia and the adrenal medulla.

Clinical Features

Neuroblastoma may present as incidental finding on clinical examination or imaging (Figs. 9.1a, b and 9.2) in an otherwise well child or more alarmingly as a profoundly ill child with wasting, anaemia, hypertension and a large abdominal mass with evidence of metastases. This latter situation is all too frequently preceded by symptoms and signs shared by many common childhood ailments leading to distressing delays in diagnosis and treatment.

The abdomen accounts for 60% of the primary tumours half of these arise in the suprarenal gland. A further 15% arise in the thorax; 10% in the pelvis and the remainder in other sites.

Horner syndrome may arise when a tumour develops in the cervical sympathetic chain and is usually permanent. Paralysis from spinal cord compression is a risk with intra spinal disease and is a therapeutic emergency. Paraneoplastic syndromes such as watery diarrhoea and hypertension are manifestations of tumour endocrine secretion while the explanation for the disabling Opsoclonus Myoclonus or dancing eye syndrome is not known.

Investigation

The first step is an appropriate suspicion. Listen to the parents, examine the child and if no obvious cause for illness is found then consider a

K. Holmes (✉)
Department of Paediatric Surgery, St. George's Hospital, London SW17 0QT, UK
e-mail: kholmes@doctors.org.uk

D.J. Ledbetter and P.R.V. Johnson (eds.), *Endocrine Surgery in Children*,
DOI 10.1007/978-3-662-54256-9_9

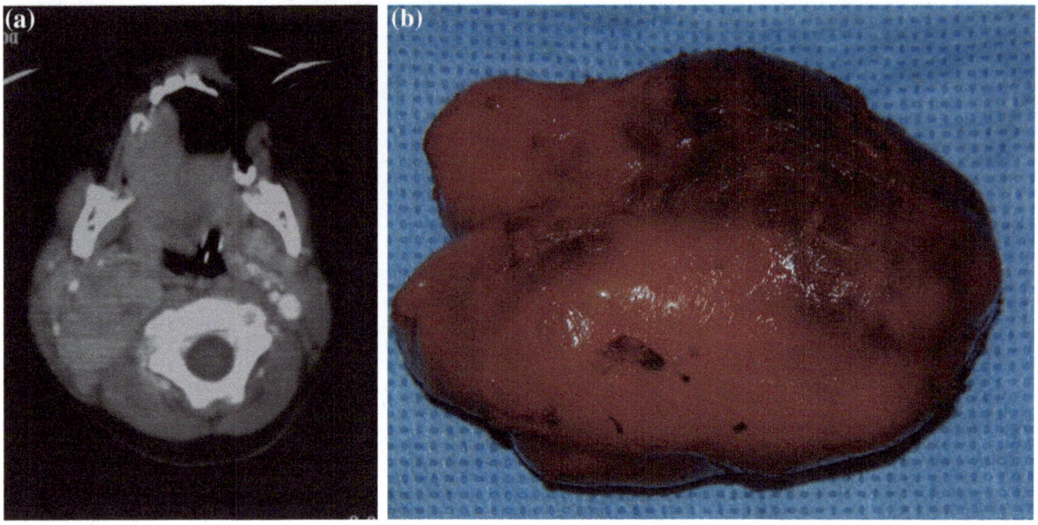

Fig. 9.1 Symptomless neck mass

readily available and non-invasive ultrasound scan.

If suspicion is confirmed, the minimum diagnostic set includes urine catecholamine assay, cross-sectional imaging and biopsy of tumour and bone marrow. The aim is to obtain a tissue diagnosis and detect metastatic disease. Ultrasound scan (US) is often the first investigation but Computed Tomography (CT) (Fig. 9.3) or Magnetic Resonance imaging (MR) are mandatory. Tissue diagnosis will require US or CT guided needle core biopsies of the primary tumour, sometimes aided by endoscopy. Multiple cores are necessary [4–9] to allow biological as well as histopathological analysis. Discrete tumours may be excised at presentation if this is deemed safe on imaging. Either way the tissue must be sent fresh to the attending pathologist and without added preservative. The majority of tumours will take up meta-iodo-benzyl guanidine (MIBG) (Fig. 9.4), a radio-labelled precursor of noradrenaline. Most

Fig. 9.2 Incidental finding on chest X-ray

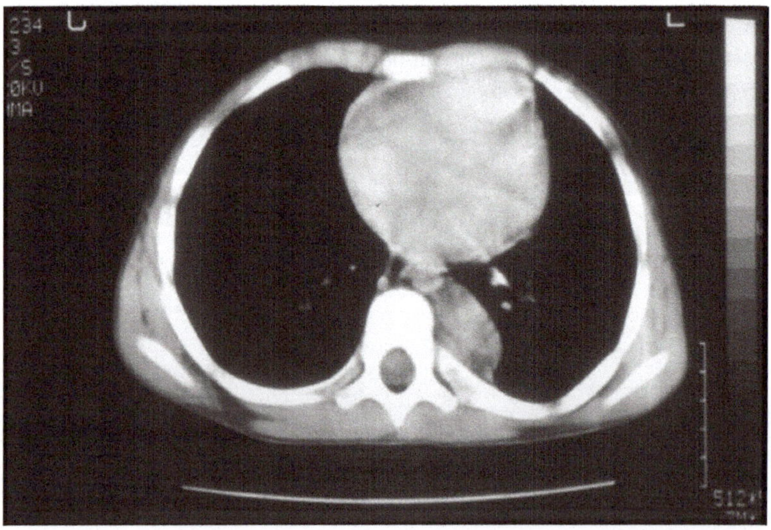

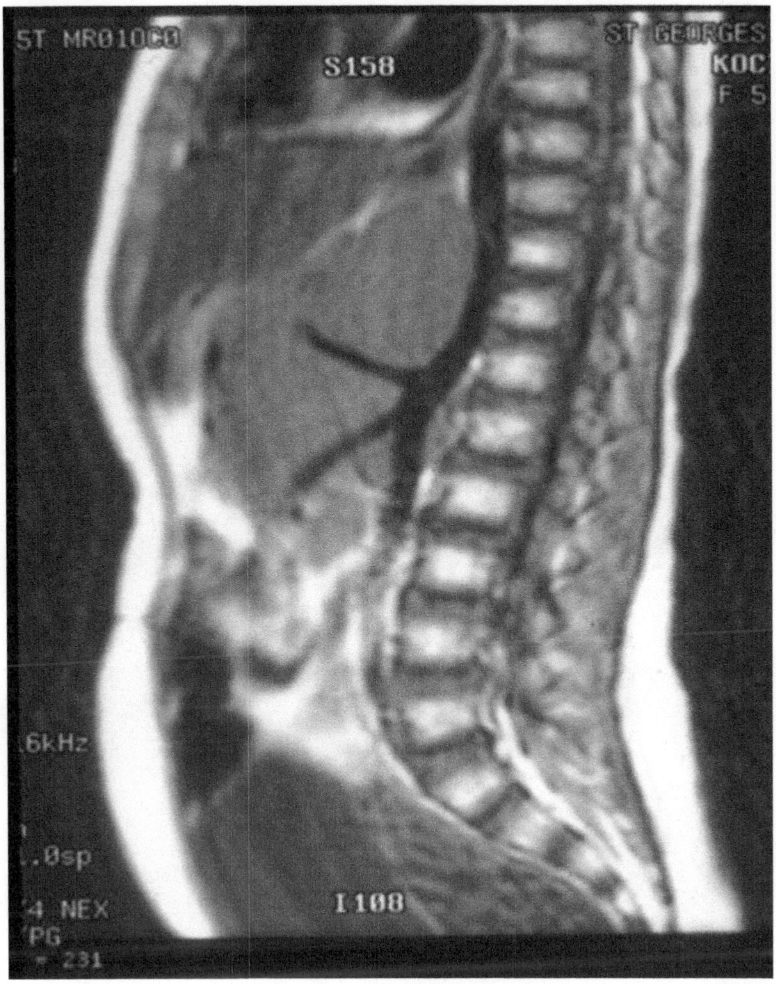

Fig. 9.3 Tendency to surround major vessels

treatment protocols now include MIBG gamma scanning to detect metastatic disease.

Treatment History

Unsurprisingly early treatment was surgical. The first recorded operation for neuroblastoma was by Bartlett in 1916 [4, 10]. The operation was a success and the patient still alive 15 years later Subsequent reports were very pessimistic with no survivors in a 1934 report [5] Prior to 1937, there were only 2 of 20 survivors without operation [6].

The addition of radiation therapy improved survival: with 21 survivors out of 24 patients in 1959, most of whom received radiation therapy after tumour excision [7]. In a similar study, the addition of radiation therapy improved survival from one of nine to six of seven following incomplete excision [8]. Radiation therapy alone resulted in five survivors [9] but all were infants, now known to have a good prognosis by virtue of their age.

Chemotherapy, now the mainstay of treatment for advanced disease was slow to gain acceptance. The Subcommittee on Childhood Solid Tumors of the National Cancer Institute USA in 1970 found no significant difference in survival when a cohort of patients treated in 1956 were compared with a similar cohort treated in 1962. These eras were before and after the use of

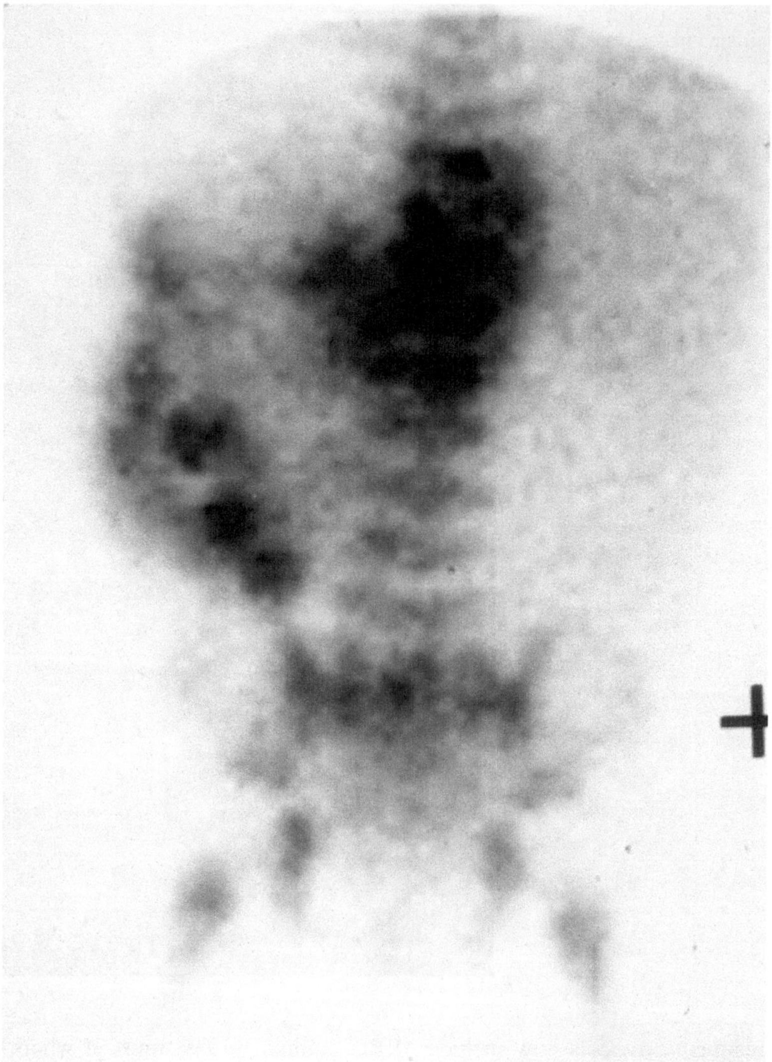

Fig. 9.4 MIBG of neuroblastoma

actinomycin D, cyclophosphamide and vincristine [11].

The St Jude Children's Research Hospital USA [12] and The Children's Cancer Study Group A (CCSGA) USA [13, 14] demonstrated a modest improvement in survival with the use of cyclophosphamide and vincristine.

Staging

Audrey Evans and others realised that there were patient and tumour characteristics which would predict survival independent of therapy. A disease staging system was proposed by the CCSGA [15] (Table 9.1) which led the way to disease risk stratification. The prognostic significance of patient age and disease stage was confirmed by analysis of the outcome of patients from CCSG and Children's Hospital of Philadelphia [16]. The staging principles were developed further by a larger group and published as the International Neuroblastoma Staging System (INSS) [17, 18] (Table 9.2). The distribution of INSS stages is shown in (Fig. 9.5).

The latest and arguably the most thoroughly researched staging system was developed by The International Neuroblastoma Risk Group (INRG)

Table 9.1 CCSG staging

Stage I	Tumour confined to the organ or structure of origin
Stage II	Tumour extending in continuity beyond the organ or structure of origin but not crossing the midline. Regional lymph nodes on the ipsilateral side may be involved
Stage III	Tumour extending in continuity beyond the midline. Regional lymph nodes may be involved bilaterally
Stage IV	Remote disease involving the skeleton, organs, soft tissue and distant lymph node groups
Stage IV-S	(Special category). Patients who would otherwise be Stage I or II but who have remote disease confined to liver, skin or bone marrow and who have no radiographic evidence of bone metastases on complete skeletal survey

From [15], with permission

Table 9.2 International staging system for neuroblastoma

Stage 1	Localised tumour confined to the area of origin; complete gross excision, with or without microscopic residual disease; identifiable ipsilateral and contralateral lymph nodes negative macroscopically
Stage 2a	Unilateral tumour with incomplete gross excision; identifiable ipsilateral and contralateral lymph nodes negative microscopically
Stage 2b	Unilateral tumour with complete or incomplete gross excision; with positive ipsilateral regional lymph nodes; contralateral lymph nodes negative microscopically
Stage 3	Tumour infiltrating across the midline with or without regional lymph node involvement; or, unilateral tumour with contralateral regional lymph node involvement; or, midline tumour with bilateral regional lymph node involvement
Stage 4	Dissemination of tumour to distal lymph nodes, bone, bone marrow, liver and/or other organs (except as defined in Stage 4S)
Stage 4S	Localised primary tumours defined for Stage 1 or 2 with dissemination limited to liver, skin and/or bone marrow

From [17], with permission

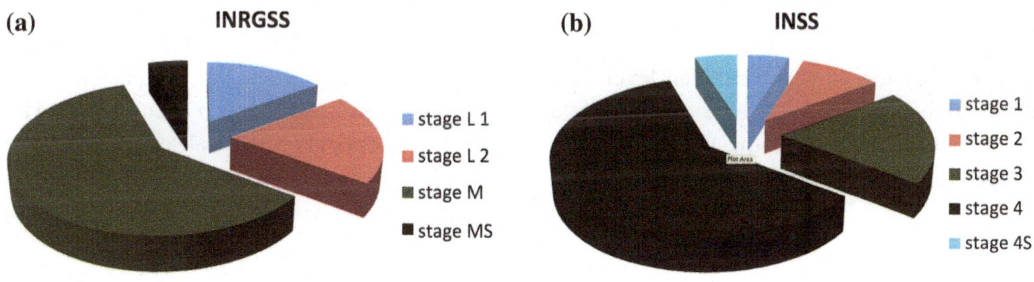

Fig. 9.5 **a** and **b** Stage distribution INRGSS with INSS

[19] and based on data from almost 9000 patients. The INRG Staging System (INRGSS) [20] was derived from an earlier study which demonstrated the importance of Surgical Risk Factors (SRF) in the prediction of the risk and effectiveness of operations to excise the tumour [21]. In essence a SRF is present when a vital structure, typically a large blood vessel, is encased by tumour [22]. The INRGSS, as it has its basis on pre-operative imaging overcomes some of the subjectivity of INSS which in part was based on operative outcome. A comparison of the distribution of stages in INSS and INRGSS is shown in (Fig. 9.5a, b). For consistency INRGSS, is used in this text except when citing a reference in which case the contemporary staging system is respected.

Pathology

The heterogeneity in behaviour of neuroblastic tumours is reflected by a wide spectrum in their microscopic morphology. The spectrum ranges from tumours with well differentiated cells which closely resemble mature neural elements to those comprised of undifferentiated small round blue cells, morphologically indistinguishable from other malignant childhood tumours and resembling undifferentiated embryonic blast cells (Fig. 9.6a, b).

The histological appearance has a profound influence on tumour behaviour [23–25]. Key variables are the degree of differentiation of the neuroblasts and the predominance of mature Schwann cells or stroma.

The International Neuroblastoma Pathology Committee (INPC) formed in 1994 with the aim of standardising histopathological definitions and tumour morphology. The Committee refined the classification as more information became available [26–28]. In ascending order of malignancy and from differentiated to undifferentiated, there are three tumour types: *ganglioneuroma*; *ganglioneuroblastoma*; *and neuroblastoma.*

Molecular Pathology

Extensive studies at a sub-cellular level have added further precision to the prediction of tumour behaviour. One of the first variables to emerge was DNA ploidy: tumours with diploid DNA have a worse prognosis than those with hyperdiploid [29]. One of the first genetic predictors of tumour behaviour to be identified was amplification of the *MYCN* oncogene [30] (Fig. 9.7a, b), which was associated with an unfavourable prognosis. Chromosomal aberrations associated with unfavourable prognosis, include 1p deletion [31]; loss of chromosome 11q [32]; gain of chromosome arm 17q [33]. Oncogenic mutations of ALK (anaplastic lymphoma kinase) are also associated with poor prognosis [34]. An elegant multivariate analysis of the impact of all these genetic variables on patient survival by Wendy London may be found in the INRG task force report [19].

Risk-Based Therapy

As overall survival improved from around 20% in 1970 to around 50% in 1990 [35, 36] it became clear that the risk of disease could be estimated by clinical and biological factors including: patient age, tumour stage, histology and MYCN status [37–39]. This information allowed the many effective therapies to be matched with the needs of the patient and the trend was for less therapy rather than more.

Patients with metastatic disease had the worst outcome and required intensive multimodal therapy while the prognosis for patients with localised disease was much better [40, 41]. Indeed some patients with localised disease, were cured by operation alone [42–44], with the

(a) (b)

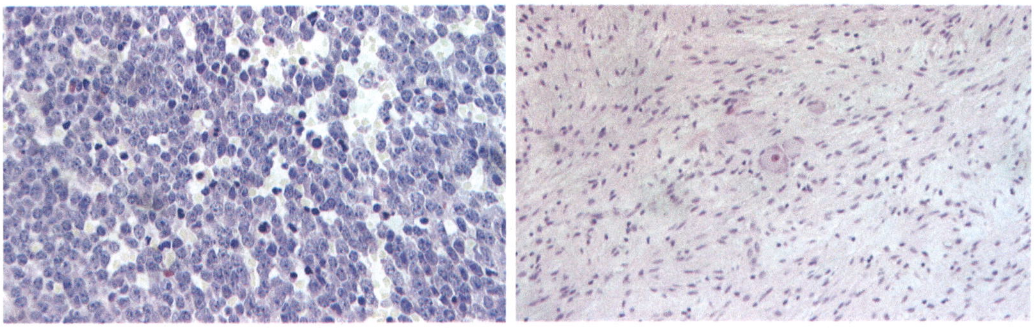

Fig. 9.6 **a** Undifferentiated cells. **b** Differentiated cells

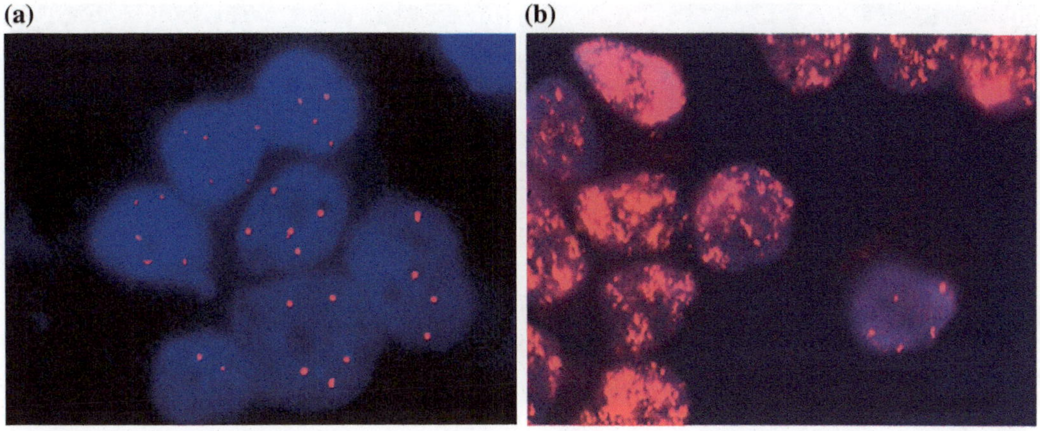

Fig. 9.7 **a** and **b** *MYCN* amplification

implication that operation was the least toxic therapy for patients with localised disease.

The trend towards less intervention was extended by the German study group (GPOH) who observed spontaneous regression in 44 of 93 infants who did not receive any treatment for their localised disease [45].

Predicting the Risk of Operation

The trend towards operation as the sole treatment for localised disease demanded that the risk of surgery be predicted with as much accuracy as possible. This was emphasised by reports of serious surgical complications and even post-operative deaths in this generally good prognosis group of patients [46, 47].

In 1995, the European Neuroblastoma Study Group opened a study to examine the risk of operation based on imaging before surgery (LNESG1). Data were collected from 107 institutions in 10 European countries. Cross-sectional imaging studies from each patient were evaluated to detect features which would predict the probability of complete tumour resection and the risk of operation complication. Surgical Risk Factors (SRF) were defined for each tumour site based on the risk of damage to neighbouring structures [21]. These risks arose as a result of the tendency for Neuroblastoma to encase vital structures, in particular major blood vessels (Fig. 9.8a and b).

The presence of SRF was associated with a complete excision rate of 46%, compared with 75% when SRF were not present. The operative complication rate was 17% if SRF were present compared with 5% in the absence of SRF.

This study was the first to estimate the variability in the complexity of operation and predict its risk and efficacy. The implication from this study was that patients with tumours which exhibit SRF should have neo-adjuvant therapy before operation in anticipation of a reduction in tumour volume and vascularity and thus a safer operation.

The tumour in patients with advanced disease INRGSS L2 and M almost invariably exhibits vascular encasement with SRF/IDRF. In spite of very effective chemotherapy, these risk factors rarely disappear completely and the surgeon is faced with technical hazards which would normally discourage operation. In spite of this, most contemporary treatment protocols include a determined attempt to remove the entire tumour at operation following more or less intensive chemotherapy.

Even in these patients with advanced disease, who may be regarded as the most challenging for the surgeon, the often lengthy operation may be accomplished with low morbidity and mortality

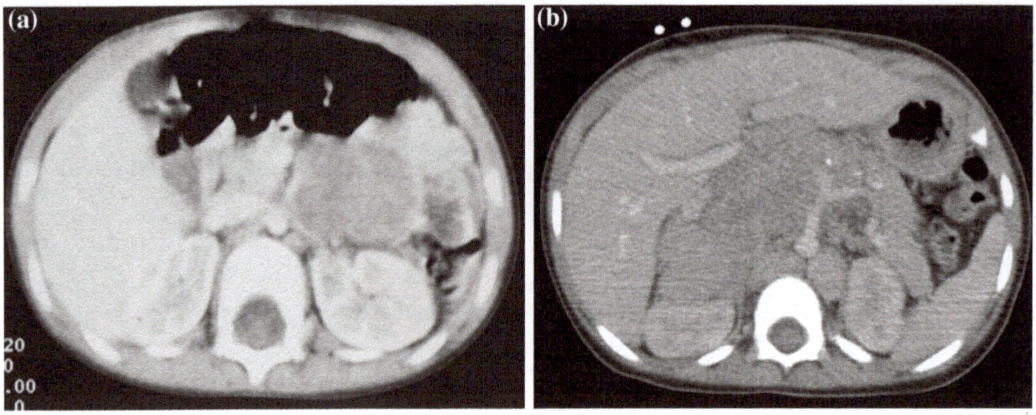

Fig. 9.8 **a** Cross-sectional imaging showing absence of risk factors (SRF/IDRF). **b** Cross-sectional imaging showing presence of risk factors

(Fig. 9.9). The death rate as a result of operation is less than 1% and the complication rate less than 10% [48–50]. The operative techniques were elegantly described by Kiely. For abdominal tumours, the overlying viscera must be dissected and reflected to expose the posterior abdominal wall. Dissection then proceeds along the major vessels starting at a section free from tumour and dissecting the latter from the vessels. Only in this way may branches and tributaries be identified and preserved.

The scope of minimally invasive surgery (MIS) for Neuroblastoma is currently under review. Smaller and localised tumours are already safely and effectively excised by MIS. It is likely that MIS will prove effective with more

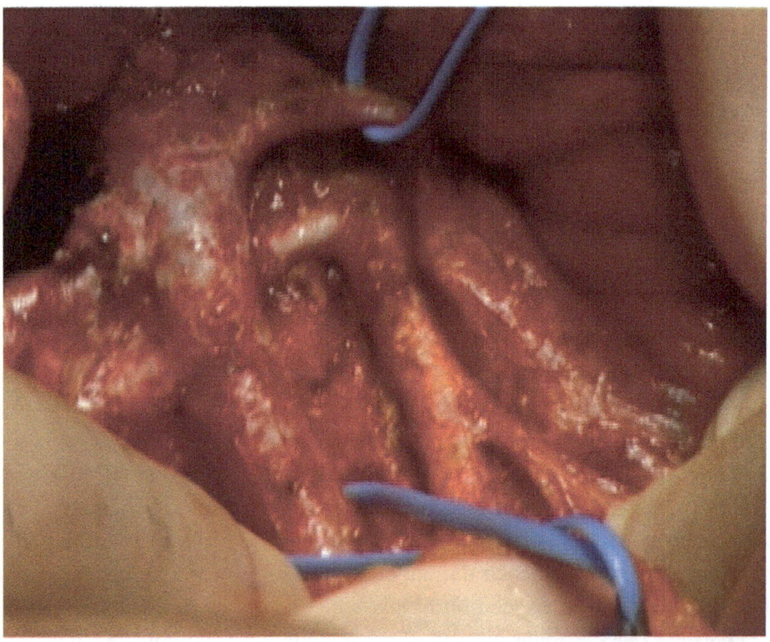

Fig. 9.9 Operation showing clearance of advanced neuroblastoma from major abdominal vessels

extensive tumours in future always with the proviso that oncological principles are respected.

Predicting the Risk of Disease

The variability in behaviour of neuroblastoma and its relation to clinical and biological variables became increasingly apparent [40, 41]. The International Neuroblastoma Risk Group (INRG) sought to develop a consensus for risk stratification before treatment [19]. In a large part, this was driven by the need for a system which would gain world-wide acceptance and thus facilitate accurate comparison of risk-based outcome studies from any national or international study group.

Data were collected from 8800 comparable patients and 13 variables analysed for prognostic significance. The most important and discriminatory factors were tumour stage, patient age, histology grade, MYCN and 11q status and DNA ploidy. Four risk groups emerged with 5 year event free survival (EFS) of: $\geq$85; $\geq$75; $\geq$50 and <50%. The INRG also introduced a novel staging system (INRGSS) again based on patient and tumour characteristics before treatment [20]. In summary, the patient stages were defined by Image Defined Risk Factors (IDRF), equivalent to SRF and based on pre-operative cross-sectional imaging. The stages were L1, a localised tumour with no IDRF; L2, a localised tumour with IDRF; M, a tumour with distant metastases and MS, a small primary tumour with metastases confined to skin and liver and in a patient less than 18 months of age. Emphasis was placed on staging before operation. In this way, the outcome of operation as a staging factor was eliminated. This cornerstone of INSS was considered an imprecise variable as it was dependent on the persistence and or skill of the surgeon and the outcome of operation.

Treatment Strategies

Neuroblastoma cells are susceptible to many therapeutic agents and sometimes undergo apoptosis. There are now strong data which allow the risk of the disease to be predicted with accuracy. For many years, a main driver of clinical research has been matching the risk of treatment with the risk of disease. For these reasons, treatment strategies will be presented in relation to the category of disease.

Localised Disease—No Image Defined Risk Factors (INSS Stage 1 and 2—INRG Stage L1)

Operative excision has proved very effective as the sole treatment for patients with localised disease [42–44]. Most relapses occur in patients with unfavourable biological features and may be salvaged with adjuvant therapy.

This strategy eliminates the acute and long-term side effects of adjuvant therapies and the safety of operation may be predicted with accuracy by careful evaluation of the pre-operative imaging [21]. For this group of patients, the relapse free survival (RFS) is 94% and overall survival (OS) is 99% [51].

Localised Disease with Risk Factors (INSS Stage 3 INRG Stage L2)

The presence of surgical or image defined risk factors (SRF or IDRF) is a contra-indication to operative excision as a first procedure. Operation in this situation is associated with a higher complication rate (17 v 5%) and a lower rate of complete excision (46 v 75%) [21]. Treatment strategies therefore employ pre-operative chemotherapy to reduce tumour volume and decrease vascularity. The European protocol for ‘unresectable localised’ Neuroblastoma involved alternating cycles of carboplatin and etoposide with cyclophosphamide, vincristine and doxorubicin (CADO). Four cycles were given before operation and two thereafter. The 5-year EFS and OS were 76 and 88% [52].

Early studies demonstrated a survival advantage of complete surgical excision [53, 54]. When the influence of biological factors was included, the benefit of operation excision was not uniform. Gross surgical resection was of benefit to patients with unfavourable biology but did not for improve outcome in patients with favourable biology [38].

Biological variation was used to stratify therapy in Memorial Sloan Kettering (MSK). A good outcome was reported following operation as the sole therapy for patients with good biology tumours [55]. The overriding importance of good biology was emphasised by the finding of spontaneous regression in 44 of 93 infants with tumours which were not resected [56].

At the other end of the biology spectrum, MSK [55] and COG [57] demonstrated a good outcome for bad biology stage 3 patients when treatment intensity was escalated and included myeloablation in addition to surgical excision. The overall survival for this group of patients was better than 85%.

Metastatic Disease in Patient Over 18 Months of Age (INSS Stage 4 INRG Stage M)

Strategies for this most dangerous end of the Neuroblastoma spectrum involve: induction chemotherapy, surgical excision and then consolidation therapy to deal with any residual disease. Although protocols vary in detail throughout the world, the principles are similar. In Europe induction is by a rapid schedule of cisplatin, vincristine, carboplatin, etoposide, and cyclophosphamide (COJEC) [58]. Treatment is given in cycles every 10 days for 70 days and then peripheral blood stem cells are harvested for bone marrow rescue. Surgical excision is then undertaken with the goal of complete resection. This is followed by high dose therapy with bone marrow ablation and stem cell rescue. Consolidation therapy, after tumour excision, comprises retinoic acid, a maturational agent and anti GD2, a monoclonal antibody.

The prognosis for patients with stage 4 disease has, until recently been uniformly dismal with overall survival rates less than 50% [35, 36]. Contemporary consolidation therapy after induction, surgical excision and bone marrow ablation shows more promising results. This therapy includes monoclonal antibody, immunomodulation and maturational therapy with retinoic acid derivatives and has resulted in very encouraging results with EFS of 66% and OS of 86% at 2 years [59].

The role of operation is impossible to estimate. "Aggressive surgery" [60] and surgical excision [61] was promoted for these patients, typically after intensive induction chemotherapy to eradicate metastatic disease and reduce tumour volume at the primary site [59, 62].

In spite of very effective chemotherapy and a very effective operation, it is difficult to estimate a benefit from complete surgical resection of the primary tumour. Complete resection was promoted by some [49, 63] but not by others [64, 65], who felt that tumour biology and intensive chemotherapy were more important.

Previous evidence of an independent benefit of complete surgical excision by the German Paediatric Oncology Group (GPOH) [66] has not been confirmed by subsequent studies [67]. There is some evidence that surgical excision of the primary tumour of benefits survival in patients over one year of age with stage 4 tumours exhibiting amplification of *MYCN* [68] and that gross total resection reduces the rate of local relapse [69].

In a recent GPOH report [70], 54.7% of 278 patients underwent complete resection after induction chemotherapy with 5 year EFS of 33.9% and OS of 43.8%. They found no correlation between the extent of surgical excision and survival.

The most recent and largest study of the impact of operation on survival in patients with high risk Neuroblastoma was from the European Study Group (SIOPEN) [50]. Five year EFS was 38% and OS 44%, the treatment strategies were broadly similar to those in the GPOH study. The SIOPEN study complete excision rate was 77% of 1462 patients with a significant increase in EFS following complete macroscopic excision: 41%; compared with incomplete excision 28% and inoperable 14%. The contrasting conclusions of these two broadly comparable studies may be due to under powering with the smaller sample size in the GPOH study and their lower complete excision rate. Another explanation is the different strategy for local control in the two studies. The SIOPEN study advised irradiation of the primary tumour site with 21 Gy in all patients independent of excision completeness. The GPOH study reserved irradiation for patients with residual disease. These different approaches may confound the different benefits of complete excision reported in the two studies.

Metastatic 'Special' in a Patient Under 18 Months of Age (INSS Stage 4S, INRG Stage MS)

This group of patients represents the most dramatic potential for Neuroblastoma to involute, often without any treatment. The prognosis for patients with 4S disease is very good with overall survival better than 90% [71]. The primary tumour is small and metastatic disease is confined to skin, liver and bone marrow. The risk to life arises from exponential growth of the hepatic metastases (Fig. 9.10) with a lethal effect on a number of organ systems: liver, lung, kidney, gut and vena cava. The risk to life and need for treatment was estimated by Evans and her team in Philadelphia [72] who developed a scoring system dependent on the degree of abnormality in each system.

Chemotherapy with carboplatin and etoposide is the first line of therapy, a single course is often effective. More intensive chemotherapy may be required if symptoms persist with external beam radiation if this is ineffective. Surgical treatment by creation of an abdominal silo and or ligation of the hepatic artery, have been used in an emergency.

Radiation Therapy

There is a long history of radiation treatment, and the Neuroblastoma cell is very radiosensitive. The long-term effects on growth mean that use is restricted to patients over one year of age.

There is no benefit to patients with INSS Stage 1 and 2 disease [38]. Patients with bad biology stage 3 disease [57] and all patients with stage 4 [73, 74] do benefit from external beam radiation to the primary tumour site.

Targeted radiation therapy may be delivered with MIBG containing an isotope of iodine, typically I^{131}. MIBG has not yet found favour as first line therapy but is frequently used for recurrent disease. Although disease remission

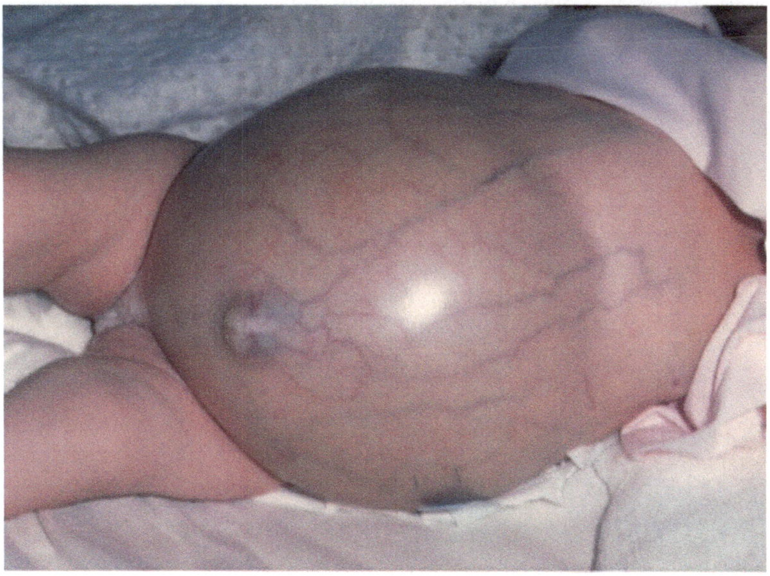

Fig. 9.10 Stage 4S

can be induced and life prolonged there are few long-term survivors [75].

Screening

Almost all neuroblastoma cells secrete catecholamines or derivatives thereof which are readily detected in random urine samples [76]. This phenomenon is important in diagnosis and has been used to screen for the disease in the hope of allowing earlier and more effective treatment. Japanese workers accumulated the largest series following the introduction of nationwide screening in 1985. Initial enthusiasm and a survival rate of 97% [77] did not stand up to long-term examination as there was no decrease in the incidence of poor prognosis tumours and no decrease in the death rate from Neuroblastoma [78]. Although there was a considerable increase in the number of cases diagnosed, the implication from long-term analysis was that screening detected good biology low stage tumours which were not a risk to life. Consistent with the benign nature of some neuroblastoma tumours and their innate tendency to apoptosis, the assumption is that many of the tumours detected by screening would have undergone natural involution. Similar conclusions followed evaluation of screening programmes in Quebec and Germany. The Japanese screening programme was stopped in 2004.

References

1. Willis RA. Pathology of tumours. 4th ed. London: Butterworth& Co; 1967. pp. 857–60.
2. Pepper W. A study of congenital sarcoma of the liver and suprarenal. Am J Med Sci. 1901;121:287–99.
3. Wright JH. Neurocytoma or neuroblastoma, a kind of tumour not generally recognised. J Exp Med. 1910;12:556–61.
4. Lehman EP. Adrenal neuroblastoma in infancy—15 year survival. Ann Surg. 1932;95:473.
5. Blacklock JWS. Neurogenic tumours of the sympathetic system in children. J Pathol Bacteriol. 1934;39:27–48.
6. Wittenborg MH. Roentgen therapy in neuroblastoma. A review of 73 cases. 1950; 54:679–88.
7. Gross RE, Farber S, Martin LW. Neuroblastoma sympatheticum: a study and report of 217 cases. Pediatrics. 1959;23:1179–91.
8. Koop CE, Johnson DG. Neuroblastoma: an assessment of therapy in reference to staging. J Ped Surg. 1971;6:595–600.
9. Swank RL II, Fetterman GH, Sieber WK, Kiesewetter WB. Prognostic factors in neuroblastoma. Ann Surg. 1971;174:428–35.
10. Lehman EP. Neuroblastoma. With report of a case. J Med Res. 1917; 36:309–26.
11. Sutow WW, Gehan EA, Heyn RM, et al. Comparison of survival curves, 1956 versus 1962, in children with Wilms' tumour and neuroblastoma. Pediatrics. 1970;45:800–11.
12. Pinkel D, Pratt C, Holton C, et al. Survival of children with neuroblastoma treated with combination chemotherapy. J Pediatr. 1968;73:928–31.
13. Leikin S, Evans A, Heyn R, Newton W. The impact of chemotherapy on advanced neuroblastoma: survival of patients diagnosed in 1956, 1962 and 1966–68 in Children's Cancer Study Group A. J Pediatr. 1974;84:131–4.
14. Sieber WK, Dibbins AW, Wiener ES. In paediatric surgery. 3d ed. In: Ravitch MM, Welch KJ, Benson CD, Aberdeen E, Randolph JG, editors. Yearbook Medical Publishers Inc; 1979. Ch. 99, p. 1095.
15. Evans AE, D'Angio GJ, Randolph J. A proposed staging system for children with neuroblastoma. Cancer. 1971;27:374–8.
16. Breslow N, McCann B. Statistical estimation of prognosis for children with neuroblastoma. Cancer Res. 1971;31:2098–103.
17. Brodeur GM, Seeger RC, Barrett A, et al. International criteria for diagnosis, staging and response to treatment in patients with neuroblastoma. J Clin Oncol. 1988;6:1874–81.
18. Brodeur GM, Pritchard J, Berthold F, et al. Revisions of the international criteria for neuroblastoma diagnosis, staging, and response to treatment. J Clin Oncol. 1993;11(8):1466–77.
19. Cohn SL, Pearson ADJ, London WB, et al. The International Neuroblastoma Risk Group classification system: an INRG task force report. J Clin Onc. 2009;27:289–97.
20. Monclair T, Brodeur GM, Ambros PF, et al. The international Neuroblastoma Risk Group (INRG) staging system: an INRG task force report. J Clin Oncol. 2009;27:298–303.
21. Cecchetto G, Mosseri V, Bernardi B, et al. Surgical risk factors in primary surgery for localised neuroblastoma: the LNESG1 study of the European International Society of Pediatric Oncology Neuroblastoma Group. J Clin Onc. 2005;23:8483–9.
22. Brisse HJ, McCarville MB, Granata C, Krug KB, Wootton-Gorges SL, Kanegawa K, … Monclair T. Guidelines for imaging and staging of neuroblastic tumors: consensus report from the International Neuroblastoma Risk Group Project. Radiology. 2011; 261:243–57.

23. Beckwith JB, Martin RF. Observations on the histopathology of neuroblastomas. J Ped Surg. 1968;3:106–10.
24. Shimada H, Chatten J, Newton WA, et al. Histopathologic prognostic factors in neuroblastic tumours: definitions of subtypes of ganglioneuroblastomaand an age linked classification of neuroblastomas. J NatCancer Inst. 1984;73:405–16.
25. Joshi VV, Cantor Altshuler G, et al. Age linked prognostic categorization based on a new histologic grading system of neuroblastomas. A clinicopathologic study of 211 cases from the Pediatric Oncology Group. Cancer. 1992;69:2197–211.
26. Shimada H, Ambros IM, Dehner LP, et al. Terminology and morphologic criteria of neuroblastic tumours: recommendations by the International Neuroblastoma Pathology Committee. Cancer. 1999;86:349–63.
27. Peuchmar M, d'Amore ES, Joshi VV, et al. Revision of the international neuroblastoma pathology classification: confirmation of the favourable and unfavourable diagnostic subsets in ganglioneuroblastoma, nodular. Cancer. 2003;98:2274–81.
28. Sano H, Bonadio J, Gerbing RB, et al. International neuroblastoma pathology classification adds independent prognostic information beyond the prognostic contribution of age. Eur J Cancer. 2006;42:1113–9.
29. Look AT, Hayes FA, Nitschke R, McWilliams NB, Green AA. Cellular DNA content as a predictor of response to chemotherapy in infants with unresectable neuroblastoma. N Eng J Med. 1984;311:231–5.
30. Brodeur GM, Seeger RC, Schwab M, Varmus HE, Bishop JM. Amplification of N-myc in untreated human neuroblastomas correlates with advanced disease stage. Science. 1984;224(4653):1121–4.
31. Brodeur GM, Sekhon G, Goldstein MN. Chromosomal aberrations in human neuroblastomas. Cancer. 1977;40:2256–63.
32. Spitz R, Hero B, Simon T, Berthold F. Loss in chromosome 11q identifies tumours with increased risk for metastatic relapses in localised and 4S neuroblastoma. Clin Cancer Res. 2006;12:3368–73.
33. Bown N, Cotteril S, Lastowska M, et al. Gain of chromosome arm 17q and adverse outcome in patients with neuroblastoma. N Eng J Med. 1999; 340:1954–61.
34. Chen Y, Takita J, Choi YL, et al. Oncogenic mutations of ALK kinase in neuroblastoma. Nature. 2008;455(7215):971–4.
35. Stiller CA. Trends in neuroblastoma in Great Britain: incidence and mortality 1971–1990. Eur J Cancer. 1993;29A:1008–12.
36. Gutierrez JC, Fischer AC, Sola JE, Perez CA, Koniaris LG. Markedly improving survival of neuroblastoma: a 30 year analysis of 1646 patients. Ped Surg Int. 2007;23:637–46.
37. Shimada H, Chatten J, Newton WA Jr, et al. Histopathologic prognostic factors in neuroblastic tumours: definition of subtypes of ganglioneuroblastoma and an age-linked classification of neuroblastomas. J Nat Cancer Inst. 1984;73:405–16.
38. Matthay KK, Perez C, Seeger RC, et al. Successful treatment of stage 3 neuroblastoma based on prospective biologic staging: a Children's Cancer Group Study. J Clin Onc. 1998;16:1256–64.
39. Perez CA, Matthay KK, Atkinson JB, et al. Biologic variables in the outcome of stages I and II Neuroblastoma treated with surgery as primary therapy: a Children's Cancer Group Study. J Clin Onc. 2000;18:18–26.
40. Brodeur GM. Neuroblastoma: biological insights into a clinical enigma. Nat Rev Cancer. 2003;3:203–16.
41. Maris JM, Hogarty MD, Bagatell R, et al. Neuroblastoma. Lancet. 2007; 369:2016–20.
42. O'Neill JA, Littman P, Blitzer P, Soper K, Chatten J, Shimada H. The role of surgery in localised neuroblastoma. J Ped Surg. 1985;20:708–12.
43. Matthay KK, Sather HN, Seeger RC, Haase GM, Hammond GD. Excellent outcome of stage II neuroblastoma is independent of residual disease and radiation therapy. J Clin Onc. 1989;7:236–44.
44. Evans AE, Silber JH, Shpilski A, D'Angio GJ. Successful management of low-stage Neuroblastoma without adjuvant therapies: a comparison of two decades, 1972 through 1981 and 1982 through 1992, in a single institution. J Clin Onc. 1996;14:2504–10.
45. Hero B, et al. Localised infant neuroblastomas often show spontaneous regression: results of the prospective trial NB95-S and NB97. J Clin Onc. 2008;26:1504–10.
46. Rubie H, Hartman O, Michon J, et al. N-Myc gene amplification is a major prognostic factor in localised neuroblastoma: results of the French neuroblastoma 90 study. J Clin Onc. 1997;15:1171–82.
47. Shamberger RC, Smith EI, Joshi W, et al. The risk of nephrectomy during local control in abdominal neuroblastoma. J Ped Surg. 1998;33:161–4.
48. Kiely E. A technique for excision of abdominal neuroblastoma. Ann RCS Eng. 2007;89:342–8.
49. LaQuaglia MP, Kushner BH, Heller G, Bonilla MA, Lindsley KL, Cheung N-KV. Stage 4 neuroblastoma diagnosed at more than 1 year of age: gross total resection and clinical outcome. J Ped Surg. 1994;29:1162–6.
50. Holmes K, et al. Advances in neuroblastoma research. Cologne: Plenary 12; 2014.
51. De Bernardi B, Mosseri V, Rubie H, et al. Treatment of localised resectable neuroblastoma. Results of the LNESG1 study by the SIOP Europe Neuroblastoma Group. Br J Cancer. 2008;99:1027–33.
52. Kohler JA, Rubie H, Castel V, et al. Treatment of children over the age of one year with unresectable

localised neuroblastoma without MYCN amplification: results of the SIOPEN study. Eur J Cancer. 2013;49(17):3671–9.
53. Haase GM, Wong KY, de Lorimer AA, Sather HN, Hammond GD. Improvement in survival after excision of primary tumor in stage III neuroblastoma. J Ped Surg. 1989;24:194–200.
54. Powis M, Imeson J, Holmes SJK. The effect of complete excision on stage III neuroblastoma: a report of the European Neuroblastoma Study Group. J Ped Surg. 1996;31:516–9.
55. Modak S, Kushner, LaQuaglia MP, Kramer K, Cheung NK. Management and outcome of stage 3 neuroblastoma. Eur J Cancer. 2009; 45:90–8.
56. Hero B, et al. Localised infant neuroblastomas often show spontaneous regression: results of the prospective trial NB95-S and NB97. J Clin Onc. 2008; 26 (9):1504–10.
57. Park JR, Villablanca JG, London WB, et al. Outcome of high risk stage 3 neuroblastoma with myeloablative therapy and 13-cis-retinoic acid: A report from the Children's Oncology Group. Ped Blood and Cancer. 2009;52:44–50.
58. Ladenstein R, Valteau-Couanet D, Brock P, et al. Randomized trial of prophylactic granulocyte colony-stimulating factor during rapid COJEC induction in pediatric patients with high-risk neuroblastoma: the European HR-NBL1/SIOPEN study. J Clin Onc. 2010; 28:3516–24.
59. Yu AL, Gilman, Ozkaynak MF, et al. Anti-GD2 antibody with GM-CSF, interleukin-2 and isotretinoin for neuroblastoma. NEng J Med. 2010; 363:1324–34.
60. Haase GM, O'Leary MC, Ramsay NK, et al. Aggressive surgery combined with intensive chemotherapy improves survival in poor risk neuroblastoma. J Ped Surg. 1991; 26:1119–23.
61. Tsuchida Y, Yokoyam J, Kaneko M, et al. Therapeutic significance of surgery in advanced neuroblastoma: a report from the Study Group of Japan. J Ped Surg. 1992; 27:616–22.
62. Rich BS, McEvoy MP, LaQuaglia MP, Wolden SL. Local control, survival and operative morbidity and mortality after re-resection and intra-operative radiation therapy for recurrent or persistent primary high-risk neuroblastoma. J Ped Surg. 2011;46: 97–102.
63. Adkins ES, Sawin R, Gerbing RB, London WB, Matthay KK, Haase GM. Efficacy of complete resection for high-risk neuroblastoma: a Children's Cancer Group Study. J Ped Surg. 2004;39:931–6.
64. Kaneko M, Ohakawa H, Iwakawa M. Is extensive surgery required for treatment of advanced neuroblastoma? J Ped Surg. 1997;32:1616–9.
65. Castel V, Tovar J, Costa J, et al. The role of surgery in stage IV neuroblastoma. J Ped Surg. 2002;37:1574–8.
66. Berthold F, Trechow R, Utsch S, Zieschang J. Prognostic factors in metastatic neuroblastoma. A multivariate analysis of 182 cases. Am J Ped Hemat Onc. 1992; 14:207–15.
67. Berthold F, Hero B, Kremens B, et al. Long-term results and risk profiles of patients in five consecutive trials (1979–1997) with stage 4 neuroblastoma over 1 year of age. Cancer Lett. 2003; 197:11–17.
68. Von Schweinitz D, Hero B, Berthold F. The impact of surgical radicality on outcome in childhood neuroblastoma. Eur J Surg. 2002;12:402–9.
69. La Quaglia MP, Kushner BH, Su W, et al. The impact of gross total resection on local control and survival in high risk neuroblastoma. J Ped Surg. 2004; 39:412–7.
70. SimonT, Haberle B, Hero B, et al. Role of surgery in the treatment of patients with stage 4 neuroblastoma age 18 months or older at diagnosis. J Clin Oncol. 2013; 31:752–8.
71. Schleiermacher G, Rubie H, Hartmann O, Bergeron C, Chastagner P, Medinaud F, Michon J. Treatment of stage 4s neuroblastoma—report of 10 years experience of French Society of Paediatric Oncology (SFOP). B J Cancer. 2003;89:470–6.
72. Hsu LL, Evans AE, D'Angio GJ. Hepatomegaly in neuroblastoma stage 4S: criteria for treatment of the vulnerable neonate. Med Ped Onc. 1996; 27:521–8.
73. Simon T, Hero B, Bongartz R, Schmidt M, Muller RP, Berthold F. Intensified external-beam radiation therapy improves the outcome of stage 4 neuroblastoma in children >1 year with residual local disease. Strahlenther Onkol. 2006;182:389–94.
74. Haas-Kogan DA, Swift PS, Selch M, et al. Impact of radiotherapy for high risk neuroblastoma: a Children's Cancer Group study. Int J Radiat Oncol Biol Phys. 2003;56:28–39.
75. Voute PA, Hoefnagel CA, De KJ, Valdes OR, Bakker DJ, van de Kleij AJ. Results of treatment with 131 I-meta-iodobenzylguanidine (131I MIBG) in patients with neuroblastoma. Future prospects of zetotherapy. Prog Clin Biol Res. 1991; 366:439–45.
76. Tuchman M, Morris CL, Ramnaraine ML, Bowers LD, Krivit W. Value of random urinary homovanillic and vanillylmandelic acid levels in the management of patients with neuroblastoma: comparison with 24 h urine collections. Pediatrics. 1985;75:234–8.
77. Sawada T. Past and future of neuroblastoma screening in Japan. Am J Pediatr Hematol Oncol. 1992;14:320–6.
78. Ajiki W, Tsukuma H, Oshima A, Kawa K. Effects of mass screening for neuroblastoma on incidence, mortality and survival rates in Osaka, Japan. Cancer Causes Control. 1998;9:631–6.

The Evaluation and Management of Adrenal Masses and Adrenocortical Tumors (Act)

10

Kenneth W. Gow

This chapter discusses the etiology, epidemiology, pathology, clinical presentation, treatment, and outcomes of adrenocortical tumors and in this context consider the general principles of evaluating adrenal masses. Before examining these topics in detail a brief review of adrenal anatomy, physiology, and masses follows.

Physiology of Adrenocortical Tumors

The adrenal glands are yellow-colored organs located within Gerota's fascia above the upper poles of the kidneys. The left gland is shaped like a crescent while the right gland is more pyramid-shaped. The arterial supply to each adrenal gland comes from three sources with branches from the inferior phrenic artery, the renal artery, and the aorta. The venous drainage of the left adrenal gland is into the left renal vein and the right adrenal gland is directly into the inferior vena cava. The lymphatic drainage is through channels towards the aortic nodes.

The adrenal gland has two distinct parts, the medulla and the cortex, with the medulla surrounded by the cortex. The cortex in turn consists of three layers, each with separate functions. From the exterior to the interior, the layers are the zona glomerulosa, zona fasciculata, and the zona reticularis.

The adrenal medulla is primarily responsible for the production of epinephrine and norepinephrine. These catecholamines are secreted into the bloodstream when the medulla is stimulated by acetylcholine release from sympathetic nerves. The adrenal cortex secretes several hormones including mineralocorticoids (e.g., aldosterone) from the zona glomerulosa, glucocorticoids (e.g., cortisol) from the zona fasciculate, and adrenal androgens [e.g., dehydroepiandrosterone (DHEA)] from the zona reticularis and fasciculata.

Adrenal masses arise from either the medulla or the cortex. Adrenal medullary lesions in children include relatively common neuroblastomas and rare pheochromocytomas. Tumors of the adrenal cortex include adenomas and carcinomas. It is difficult to distinguish a benign adrenocortical adenoma from a malignant adrenocortical carcinoma in the absence of metastatic disease, therefore in this chapter the two lesions will be grouped together under the label adrenocortical tumors (ACT). ACTs are also rare in children and their clinical characteristics and biologic behavior differs substantially from ACTs in adults and from adrenal medullary tumors.

Etiology of Adrenocortical Tumors

Most ACTs occur in children with no predisposing condition, however, there are some known molecular risk factors for developing

K.W. Gow (✉)
Department of General and Thoracic Surgery, Seattle Children's Hospital and the University of Washington, 4800 Sand Point Way NE, Seattle, WA 98105, USA
e-mail: Kenneth.gow@seattlechildrens.org

D.J. Ledbetter and P.R.V. Johnson (eds.), *Endocrine Surgery in Children*,
DOI 10.1007/978-3-662-54256-9_10

ACT including abnormalities of the p53 tumor suppressor and insulin-like growth factor 2 (IGF-2). In addition, there are less well-defined associations of ACT with other chromosomal abnormalities, tumors, birth defects, and environmental exposures.

The p53 tumor suppressor protein is important in cell cycle regulation and induces cell cycle arrest or cell death in response to DNA-damaging agents [1–4]. Mutations or deletions of the p53 gene occur in many human cancers. Li-Fraumeni syndrome (LFS), also referred to as SBLA (**S**arcoma; **B**reast and **B**rain tumors; **L**eukemia, **L**aryngeal carcinoma, and **L**ung cancer; and **A**CT) syndrome, is associated with alterations of the tumor suppressor gene p53 on the short arm of chromosome 17, band 13 [5–8]. LFS is a rare autosomal dominant condition with incomplete penetrance in which affected members develop the aforementioned tumors. In LFS patients, ACT occurs 100 times more frequently than in the general population.

The insulin-like growth factor (IGF) signaling pathway has many important roles in normal cell growth and development. All components of the IGF system are expressed by human fetal adrenal gland [9]. The IGF-2 gene maps to chromosome 11p15. Overexpression of IGF-2 is thought to contribute to tumor genesis in **Beckwith-Wiedemann Syndrome (BWS)**, which is associated with an alteration in the 11p15 region. Children with BWS, sometimes referred to as EMG (**E**xomphalos-**M**acroglossia-**G**igantism) syndrome, have an increased risk of benign and malignant tumors of multiple organs at a young age. The most common neoplasm associated with this syndrome is nephroblastoma (Wilms tumor), followed by ACT (Figs. 10.1 and 10.2) and hepatoblastoma [10]. BWS is also commonly accompanied by nonneoplastic enlargement of the adrenal glands caused by cortical hyperplasia [10]. Other possible syndromes including multiple endocrine neoplasia (MEN1), familial adenomatous polyposis coli (FAP), Lynch Syndrome, and neurofibromatosis type 1 (NF1) have been suggested but have not been universally accepted as being associated with ACTs [11, 12].

ACTs have a high frequency of chromosomal gains and amplifications, and several chromosomal subregions containing candidate proto-oncogenes have been identified [13, 14]. The most consistent findings in ACTs have been the presence of copy number gains in chromosome region 9q34 [15]. However, there is no consistent difference in chromosomal gains or losses between the adrenal adenomas and carcinomas [15].

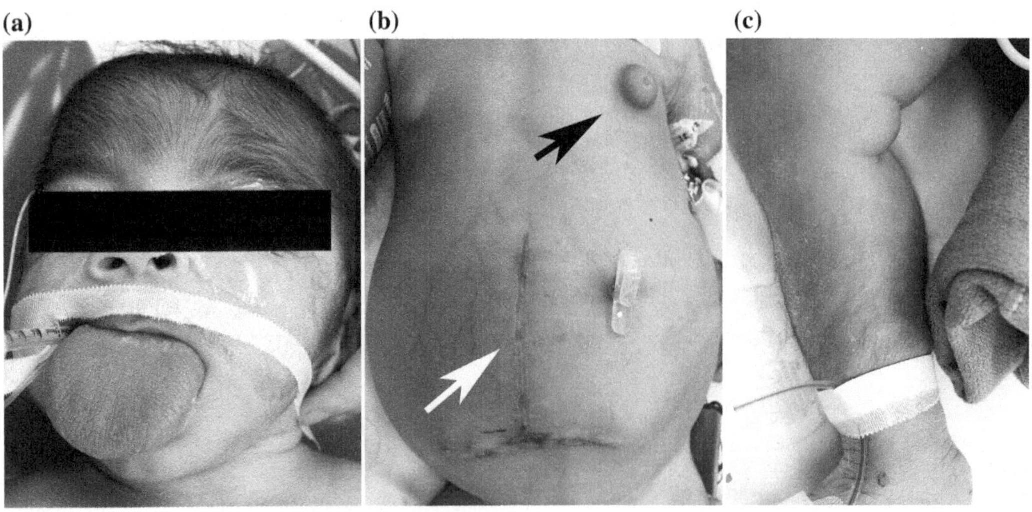

Fig. 10.1 A 3-month old with Beckwith–Wiedemann Syndrome who was born with hyperinsulinism and an omphalocele who later presented with a left adrenal mass. **a** Macroglossia and hirsutism (*forehead*). **b** Gynecomastia (*black arrow*) and a repaired omphalocele (*white arrow*). **c** Hirsutism of the leg

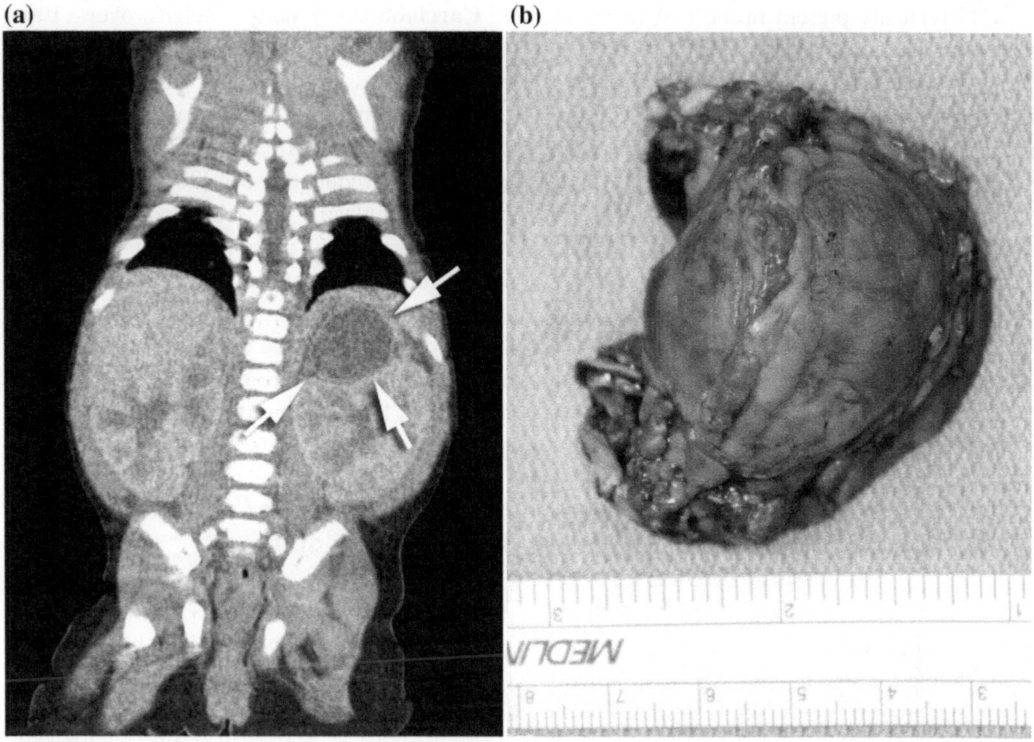

Fig. 10.2 **a** CT Scan demonstrated a left adrenal mass consistent with an ACT (*white arrows*). **b** An open left adrenalectomy was performed which confirmed an ACT with no lymphatic or vascular invasion and all nodes negative of disease

In rare cases, ACTs have been reported in association with congenital urinary tract abnormalities such as duplication of the collecting system, with tumors such as ganglioneuroma and ganglioneuroblastoma, and with congenital adrenal hyperplasia [16–20]. Environmental exposures to several agents have been postulated to be important in the development of ACTs, but these have typically been case reports with unclear mechanisms [21, 22].

Epidemiology of Adrenocortical Tumors in Children

Of the adrenal tumors of childhood, ACTs are less common than neuroblastomas but are more common than pheochromocytomas [23]. Neuroblastomas and pheochromocytomas derive from the adrenal medulla while ACTs are the most common tumor of the adrenal cortex in childhood [24, 25]. Even so, ACTs are rare in American children. It is estimated that there will be about 19 new cases of adrenocortical carcinomas in children per year in the US [26]. However, some cases of adrenocortical carcinoma may be initially misclassified as adrenocortical adenoma, so a better estimate is probably 25–30 cases per year [27]. A recent Surveillance, Epidemiology, and End Results (SEER) program study review of pediatric adrenocortical carcinoma calculated an incidence for patients under 20 years of age at 0.21 per million [28].

Interestingly, there are geographic differences in the incidence of ACT. In a region of southern Brazil, ACTs are much more common. The markedly increased incidence of ACTs in this area is probably due to the increased incidence of a p53 mutation in the population although other genetic factors and environmental exposures have been suggested.

ACTs typically present in the first five years of life with a median age of presentation between 3 and 4 years of age. However, there is a biphasic age distribution with a larger peak during infancy and a second smaller peak in adolescence [29–32]. Girls outnumber boys in all reports, with a female to male ratio of 1.5:1. This female predominance increases after adolescence to 6:1 [29, 31, 32].

Pathology of Adrenocortical Tumors in Children

Unlike similar tumors in adults, adrenocortical adenomas in children have no histopathologic features that allow them to be reliably distinguished from adrenocortical carcinomas. Also, the biologic behavior of pediatric adrenocortical neoplasms may be difficult to predict on the basis of morphologic criteria. Thus, the term adrenocortical neoplasm [or adrenocortical tumor (ACT)] is currently used to designate both benign and malignant tumors of the adrenal cortex in children [10].

Gross Features of Adrenocortical Tumors in Children

The median tumor weight of an ACT is 126 g but may range from 2 g to 6 kg. There is no tumor laterality predominance, and bilateral tumors occur in about 1% of cases [33, 34]. There are descriptions of ectopic sites within the spinal canal [35], thoracic cavity [36] and in the abdomen away from the adrenal gland. Ectopic occurrence is not surprising in view of the adrenal's close proximity to the celiac plexus, kidney, genitalia, broad ligament, epididymis, and spermatic cord during development.

Adenomas are usually spherical, unilateral, solitary, and well demarcated, but often not truly encapsulated. They typically weigh less than 50 g. Adenomas range in color from yellow to red-brown, but may appear black if the tumor contains a large amount of the pigment lipofuscin [37, 38].

Carcinomas usually weigh over 100 g although smaller malignant tumors have been reported. Grossly, they have coarse trabeculations, a multinodular contour, and are yellow to brown in color. Areas of hemorrhage and necrosis are frequently seen [38, 39]. In adrenocortical neoplasms of childhood, malignant behavior is usually associated with lesions that weigh more than 500 g, whereas most tumors that weigh less than 500 g are benign [40]. Cystic changes may be seen in both adenomas and carcinomas, but are more common in carcinomas and larger adenomas [10].

Microscopic Features of Adrenocortical Tumors in Children

Adrenal adenoma comprises a heterogeneous group of benign neoplasms that histologically resemble the appearance of the normal zona fasciculata, the zona glomerulosa, or most often, a combination of both [10]. Cells are typically arranged in nests separated by a delicate fibrovascular stroma. Cytological features vary from large, pale vacuolated cells with vesicular nuclei characteristic of the zona fasciculata to smaller cells with eosinophilic cytoplasm and condensed chromatin similar to those in the zona glomerulosa and zona reticularis [10]. In general, adrenocortical adenomas are histologically bland, with low nuclear-to-cytoplasmic ratio, very little necrosis or hemorrhage, and they rarely have mitoses or bizarre nuclear forms. In children, however, benign adrenocortical tumors are more likely to display marked nuclear atypia, polymorphism, necrosis, and mitotic activity than do similar tumors in adults. Occasionally, central degenerative changes (necrosis, hemorrhage, cystic alterations, and vascular proliferation) may be seen in adenomas. Despite some association of cell types with secretory products, it is not possible to reliably predict the endocrine function of a tumor on the basis of histologic characteristics [10].

Adrenocortical carcinoma shows a wide range of differentiation on histologic examination, not only between different tumors but also within the same tumor [10]. Morphology ranges from normal-appearing adrenal cells to completely undifferentiated cells. Broad fibrous bands often separate the tumor into multiple nodules. Most cells are lipid-poor and eosinophilic, and they may be arranged in nests, trabeculae, or sheets. Hyperchromatic nuclei, pleomorphism with bizarre giant cells and multinucleated forms, necrosis (especially confluent areas of necrosis), mitotic activity (including atypical mitoses), and vascular or capsular invasion may be seen. However, none of these histologic features is necessarily diagnostic of malignancy in ACTs in children [6, 26].

Adrenocortical Adenoma or Carcinoma?

There have been several attempts to distinguish between adrenocortical adenomas and carcinomas using clinical and pathologic features of the tumors. These studies have analyzed many different parameters with varying degrees of success. In children, clinical findings, tumor size, tumor weight, and histologic features may suggest malignant potential, but no single parameter (except the detection of metastases) allows benign tumors to be discriminated from malignant ones [10, 41]. Classification of carcinomas into low grade and high grade based on mitotic rate has also been proposed [42, 43]. However, ACTs in children cannot be reliably classified as benign or malignant using these systems [42, 44].

Special studies are often of limited value in the pathologic diagnosis of ACTs. Adrenocortical carcinomas are usually vimentin-positive and often negative for cytokeratin, epithelial membrane antigen, and carcinoembryonic antigen [10]. However the main value of immunohistochemistry of an adrenal mass is to diagnose neoplasms that metastasize to the adrenal gland rather than distinguishing between benign and malignant ACTs [45].

The **electron microscopic** appearance of adenomas resembles that of cells of the normal adrenal cortex, with steroid-producing cells showing tubulovesicular or tubular lamellar mitochondria, and an abundant, smooth endoplasmic reticulum. Adrenocortical, carcinomas may show abnormal numbers and morphology of mitochondria, and dissolution of the basement membrane surrounding alveolar groups of cells but these findings are not diagnostic [26].

Chromosomal analyses of ACTs has shown that aneuploidy tends to point toward malignancy, although this characteristic is also found in benign tumors, especially larger ones [46, 47]. Cytogenetic studies of carcinomas have shown **loss of heterozygosity** of several gene loci in some cases [47, 48]. **Mitotic rate** has been consistently reported as the most important determinant of aggressive behavior [43, 49–51]. Other histopathologic variables are also important, and it is possible to stratify the risk of recurrence based on a score that includes a combination of different histopathologic characteristics, such as venous, capsular, or adjacent organ invasion, tumor necrosis, mitotic rate, and the presence of atypical mitoses [51].

An unanswered question is how to categorize an ACT with a few "malignant" pathologic features. One approach proposed by Bugg [42] is to differentiate between those adrenocortical carcinomas with low-grade pathologic features and those with high-grade pathologic features. Another approach advocated by Dehner is to acknowledge the uncertainty by using terms such as "atypical adrenocortical neoplasm" or "adrenocortical neoplasm of uncertain or indeterminate malignant potential" for the completely resected tumor and recommend close follow-up with appropriate hormonal monitoring [52].

Evaluation of Adrenal Masses

The combination of history, physical examination, laboratory tests, and diagnostic imaging can usually distinguish adrenal cortical tumors from adrenal medullary tumors and other adrenal problems. Modern cross-sectional imaging in particular is critical in the evaluation of children with clinical features of adrenocortical hyperfunction. Finding an adrenal mass in this setting is diagnostic of an adrenocortical neoplasm.

Symptoms and Signs of Adrenal Masses

Adrenal tumors usually present with mass effects or with systemic manifestations of excessive hormone secretion. A neuroblastoma can grow quite large and present as a palpable abdominal mass or with symptoms of compression of surrounding structures, such as when the tumor extends into the spinal canal and causes paralysis. Neuroblastoma may also present with signs of metastases such as periorbital lesions causing bulging eyes or dark circles around the eyes ("black eyes" or "raccoon's eyes"), bone metastases causing bone pain, liver metastases leading to hepatomegaly and respiratory embarrassment, and subcutaneous deposits resulting in bluish lesions under the skin ("blueberry muffin"). Finally, both neuroblastoma and more commonly pheochromocytoma can present with systemic effects of catecholamine secretion such as hypertension, palpitations, sweatiness, shakiness, anxiety, and diarrhea.

In contrast to adult ACTs, most pediatric ACTs secrete hormones that lead to their presentation, usually at 5–8 months of age [29, 32, 53]. Children will present with various manifestations depending on the specific **adrenocortical hormones** secreted by the tumor. The most common presentations are virilization, feminization, Cushing's syndrome, and Conn's syndrome. Although the clinical manifestations of one endocrine syndrome may predominate, ACTs usually secretes several hormones and thus signs and symptoms of multiple syndromes may be seen.

Precocious puberty refers to secondary sex characteristics that appear in girls younger than 8 years, and in boys younger than age 9. Precocious puberty may be gonadotropin-dependent (**true precocious puberty**) or gonadotropin-independent (**pseudoprecocious puberty**). Furthermore, precocious puberty may be characterized as **isosexual** when the premature secondary sex characteristics are appropriate for the patient's gender, or **heterosexual** when the premature secondary sex characteristics are inappropriate for the patient's gender. Heterosexual precocious puberty manifests as virilization in girls and feminization in boys. Because functioning adrenocortical neoplasms represent a gonadotropin-independent source of endogenous androgens and cortisol, they usually produce pseudoprecocious puberty, Cushing's syndrome, or a mixture of the two [10].

Virilizing syndrome is the most common presentation, with about 80% due to the secretion of androgens, which cause deepening of the voice, acne, hirsutism, increased muscle mass, and secretion and proliferation of the sebaceous glands. Specifically, in girls, there is clitoral enlargement, facial and pubic hair, amenorrhea, advanced bone age, and occasionally male pattern hair changes [10]. In boys, there is early development of acne, pubic hair, penile enlargement, and precocious isosexual pseudopuberty [10].

Cushing's syndrome results from the production of autogenous corticosteroids and occurs in about one third of patients with ACTs. Children with Cushing's syndrome present with moon facies, weight gain, centripetal distribution of fat, plethora, hypertension, and striae. In addition, most patients who present with Cushing's syndrome will also have signs and symptoms of virilization.

Conn's syndrome is also known as primary aldosteronism and may be caused by adrenal cortical carcinoma, adrenal adenoma, or bilateral cortical hyperplasia. Aldosterone-producing adenoma is rare in children [54]. Symptoms associated with Conn's syndrome include headache, weakness of proximal muscle groups, polyuria, tachycardia, hypocalcemia, and hypertension. As with Cushing's syndrome, a patient's presentation may be complicated by manifestations of other hormones secreted by the ACT.

Laboratory Investigation of Adrenal Masses

The laboratory investigation of adrenal masses includes measuring the abnormal hormone secretions of medulla (catecholamines) or cortex (mineralocorticoids, glucocorticoids, androgens) and evaluating systemic effects of the tumor or its abnormal hormonal production. When medullary tumors are suspected urine or blood may be collected for substances secreted by the tumor including homovanillic acid (HMA), vanillylmandelic acid (VMA), dopamine, and norepinephrine.

Laboratory testing for ACTs includes evaluation of androgen and glucocorticoid levels and their breakdown products. Measurements of urinary 17-ketosteroids (17-KS) are the most important marker for ACT. 17-KS levels are elevated in the majority of patients with ACTs regardless of whether the tumor is associated with Cushing's syndrome or virilization [31]. Plasma dehydroepiandrosterone sulfate (DHEA-S) levels are abnormal in about 90% of patients with ACTs, making this the second most sensitive tumor marker. Abnormal urinary DHEA is less sensitive, with only two thirds of cases with detectable elevation. Urinary 17-hydroxycorticosteroid (17-OH) levels are elevated in patients with clinical signs of excessive glucocorticoids. Therefore, evaluation of patients suspected of having an ACT includes determination of urinary 17-KS and 17-OH, urinary or plasma cortisol (either baseline or suppressed), plasma DHEA-S, testosterone, androstenedione, 17-hydroxyprogesterone, aldosterone, renin activity, 11-deoxycorticosterone (DOC) and other 17-deoxysteroid precursors. The hormone activity will not help differentiate benign from malignant lesions since both will have a significant elevation in these markers [55]. Additional useful tests include serum electrolytes, especially potassium, which would be low with increased aldosterone, and serum glucose, which can be elevated with, increased corticosteroids.

Imaging Evaluation of Adrenal Masses

By the time that most children present with an adrenal mass, the mass is visible with diagnostic imaging; however, small lesions with hormonal activity may be radiologically occult. With current imaging technology, the scenario of delayed diagnosis of a functional adrenal tumor that was common in the past has largely been eliminated [23, 25].

Plain radiography has limited value but can reveal a mass effect of the tumor on surrounding organs or calcifications, which suggest neuroblastoma or previous adrenal hemorrhage. In the past excretory urography and nephrotomograms were often performed, which would show the mass effect of an adrenal lesion on the kidney and urinary collecting system however, these tests have been replaced by ultrasound and cross-sectional imaging.

Ultrasonography (US) is often the first imaging procedure performed in children with abdominal masses since it can be performed easily and without sedation. US can determine the location of a mass and its relationship to surrounding vessels and organs, determine if the mass is cystic or solid, assess the vascularity of the mass, and identify associated liver metastases. US serves as a good initial study to define the next step of management (Fig. 10.3a). However, US is most useful for large masses and the majority of lesions of the adrenal cortex tend to be small and are often difficult to visualize. Doppler US is a valuable tool to evaluate for associated tumor extension into the renal vein, inferior vena cava, and right atrium (Fig. 10.3b). Hamper et al described the sonographic features of ACTs including a wide range in size (range 3–22 cm), a round or ovoid circumscribed shape commonly displaying a lobulated border, and in a quarter of the cases, a thin echogenic capsule-like rim. The adrenocortical carcinomas less than 6 cm were homogenous solid masses and were nearly isoechoic to renal cortex. Larger lesions tended to be heterogeneous and to contain central or diffuse hypoechoic regions that corresponded to necrotic areas in the surgical pathology specimens. The term "scar sign" refers to radiating linear echoes that suggest adrenocortical carcinoma [56].

Computerized Axial Tomography (CT) is the imaging procedure of choice for evaluating adrenal lesions. CT provides accurate definition of the adrenal size, location, and appearance (Fig. 10.4a). Furthermore, it assesses local and vascular invasion, enlargement of lymph nodes,

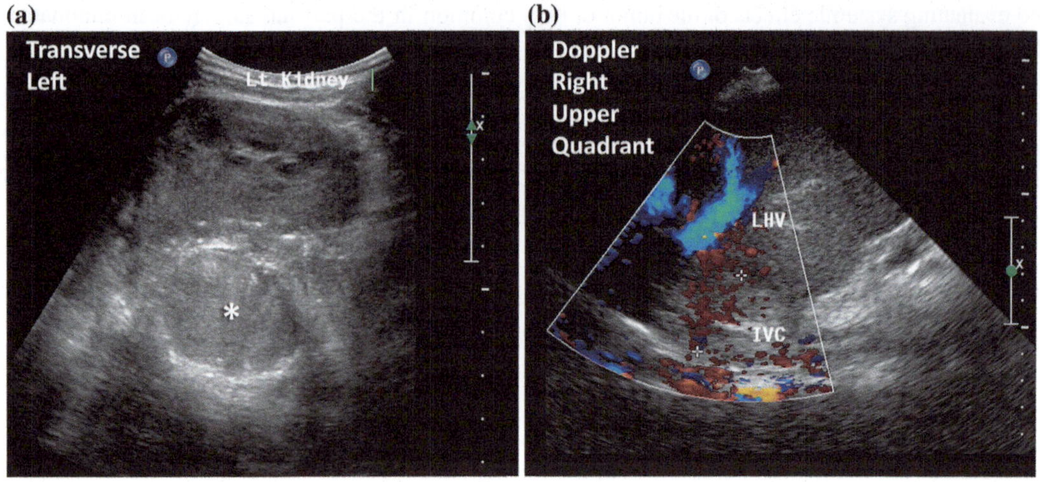

Fig. 10.3 An 11-year-old female presented with a large left sided abdominal mass. A CT scan and MRI were performed which demonstrated a left adrenal primary tumor with tumor extension through the adrenal veins into bilateral renal veins, hepatic veins, IVC, and into the right atrium. Her treatments consisted of biopsy, neoadjuvant chemotherapy, resection of primary and thrombus under cardiopulmonary bypass, and Mitotane therapy. **a** Transverse ultrasound of the left upper quadrant demonstrating the left kidney displaced inferiorly and a large mass in the left suprarenal space (*). **b** Doppler ultrasound of the right upper quadrant demonstrating a partial occluding tumor thrombus (+) in the inferior vena cava (IVC)

and the presence of metastases within in the abdomen or distant sites (Fig. 10.4b). On CT, ACTs are typically circumscribed, appear variably heterogeneous due to hemorrhage and necrosis, and may display a thin capsule-like rim [10]. Larger lesions tend to enhance heterogeneously with IV contrast.

Magnetic resonance imaging (MRI) may also define the extent of the adrenal lesion including its relationship to surrounding organs and vessels (Fig. 10.5). It may provide some advantages over CT, as it involves no radiation, displays different planes, and may better characterize tumor thrombus (Fig. 10.5). ACTs have intermediate signal intensity on T1-weighted MR images, and high signal intensity relative to liver on T2-weighted images [10]. Also, MR may help differentiate benign from malignant lesions based on the enhancement with gadolinium [57].

Nuclear scans may also be helpful in the evaluation of adrenal masses in some specific situations. **Metaiodobenzylguanidine (MIBG)** scans may be used to detect adrenal medullary tumors, pheochromocytomas, and neuroblastomas due to MIBG affinity for medullary tissue. MIBG scans may be particularly useful in localizing such tumors in extra-adrenal sites. Iodocholesterol-labeled analogs may be used to detect primary adrenocortical tumors or metastases. Dexamethasone administered before the scan may make the test more sensitive by suppressing autologous ACTH-responsive adrenal tissue.

More recently, **positron emission technology (PET) scanning** has been used to study recurrent or metastatic adrenal tumors. However, its role has yet to be fully elucidated.

Differential Diagnosis of Adrenal Masses

The differential diagnosis of an ACT includes a variety of benign and malignant conditions and some of the more common considerations are discussed below.

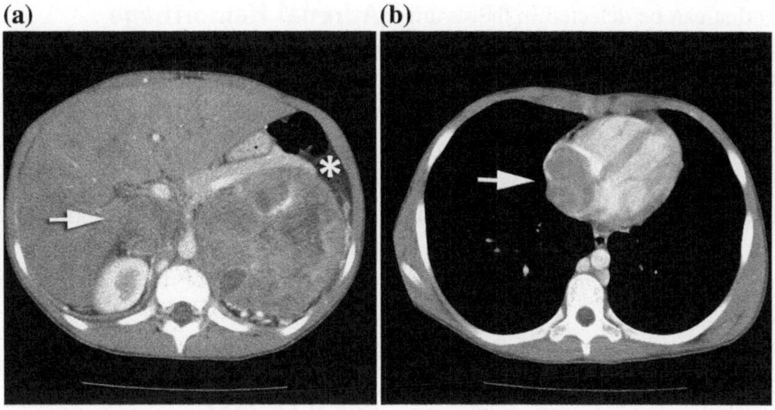

Fig. 10.4 An 11-year-old female presented with a large left sided abdominal mass. **a** Axial CT scan with a 10.1 X 10.2 cm heterogeneous left adrenocortical carcinoma (*) displacing the pancreatic tail superiorly and the left kidney inferiorly with left renal vein and IVC tumor thrombus (*white arrow*). **b** Axial CT scan with more cranial views demonstrating right atrial tumor thrombus (*white arrow*)

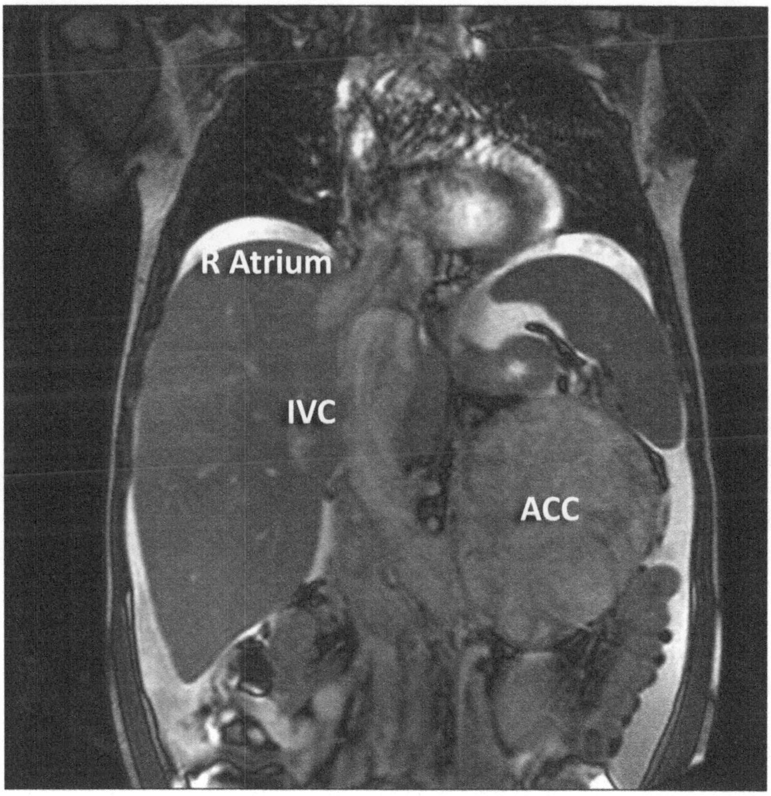

Fig. 10.5 An 11-year-old female presented with a large left sided abdominal mass. Coronal MRI demonstrating left adrenocortical carcinoma (ACC) with left renal vein and IVC tumor thrombus (IVC) and extending into the right atrium (R Atrium)

Neuroblastoma

Neuroblastoma is a neoplasm of the adrenal medulla or extra-adrenal sympathetic tissue that typically affects young children. The age at diagnosis and some clinical manifestations may overlap with the presentation of ACTs, however, neuroblastomas usually produce excessive catecholamines that can be detected in the serum and urine. Also, children with neuroblastoma are much more likely to present with metastases compared to children with ACTs. Furthermore, neuroblastomas may be associated with paraneoplastic syndromes of myoclonic encephalopathy and tumor elaboration of vasoactive intestinal peptide.

On imaging the typical neuroblastoma is a large, irregular, retroperitoneal mass that frequently encases vascular structures, often contains characteristic punctate calcifications, and may extend through neural foramina into the extradural spinal canal. However, neuroblastoma may also appear as a circumscribed suprarenal mass that is indistinguishable from an ACT. One imaging study that may be helpful in distinguishing an ACT from a neuroblastoma is the MIBG scan, which will be positive in patients with neuroblastoma.

Pheochromocytoma

Pheochromocytoma is a neoplasm derived from neural crest tissue. Similar to neuroblastoma, a pheochromocytoma secretes catecholamines and concentrates MIBG, however, pheochromocytomas usually occur in older children (6–14 years) compared to neuroblastomas and ACTs that usually occur in infants and toddlers. Children with pheochromocytomas typically present with constant or paroxysmal hypertension with resulting headaches [58, 59]. Pheochromocytomas may occur in patients with neurofibromatosis, von Hippel-Lindau disease, Sturge-Weber syndrome, and multiple endocrine neoplasia types IIA and IIB. Less than 10% of pheochromocytomas in children are malignant [10]. On imaging, they tend to be rounded, circumscribed masses. On T1-weighted MR, a pheochromocytoma has lower signal intensity than that of the liver and on T2-weighted images a higher signal intensity than ACTs [59].

Adrenal Hemorrhage

Adrenal hemorrhage typically occurs in neonates, which would be an unusual age of presentation for adrenocortical tumors. Adrenal hemorrhage can be distinguished from a neoplastic adrenal mass by serial sonograms that demonstrate a temporal evolution of the mass through stages of liquefaction, clot retraction, and eventual shrinkage.

Renal Lesions

Large adrenocortical neoplasms may appear on imaging to invade or arise from the upper pole of the kidney. **Solid renal neoplasms** of childhood include Wilms tumor (nephroblastoma), mesoblastic nephroma, renal cell carcinoma, clear cell sarcoma, and rhabdoid tumor of the kidney. None of the renal tumors produces the clinical findings of hormonally active ACTs. However, rhabdoid tumor and mesoblastic nephroma may be associated with hypercalcemia.

ACTH-Independent Macronodular Adrenal Hyperplasia (AIMAH)

AIMAH, also known as massive macronodular adrenocortical disease (MMAD) [60–62], is a benign proliferative disorder of the adrenal cortex that presents with ACTH-independent Cushing's syndrome. Steroid hormone secretion is ACTH independent and associated with both undetectable plasma levels of ACTH and the inability to suppress cortisol secretion with high dose dexamethasone [63]. Histologically, it is composed of nodules with two cell types, lipid rich cells with clear cytoplasm and lipid-poor cells with a compact cytoplasm [60]. Although corticosteroid secretion is independent of ACTH the cells express the ACTH receptor and patients will respond to exogenous ACTH [61, 64]. The increased steroid hormone synthesis in AIMAH is thought to be due to an overall increase in adrenocortical mass rather than augmented synthesis within each cell [64]. AIMAH may be associated with McCune-Albright syndrome, an autosomal dominant disorder characterized by polyostotic fibrous dysplasia, café-au-lait spots, precocious puberty, and hyperfunctioning endocrine glands [65]. McCune-Albright syndrome is caused by an activating mutation in the GNAS1 gene.

Primary Pigmented Nodular Adrenocortical Disease (PPNAD)

PPNAD is similar to AIMAH but it does not respond to ACTH [61, 66]. Both AIMAH and PPNAD are benign proliferative disorders. PPNAD is characterized by nodules usually less than 4–6 mm in diameter with a brown or black color. The color is a result of large cells containing a granular, pigment-containing cytoplasm. The internodular adrenal cortex is atrophic and disorganized, and the adrenal glands are usually normal weight and size [67, 68]. PPNAD can be seen isolation, but it is usually associated with the Carney complex, an autosomal dominant syndrome that includes perioral, ocular, or genital schwannomas, and endocrine gland hyperactivity. Affected patients often have tumors of two endocrine glands. The most common tumor in the Carney complex is PPNAD and other tumors include prolactin or growth hormone secreting pituitary tumors, thyroid adenomas or carcinomas, testicular large-cell calcifying Sertoli cell tumors, and ovarian cysts [69–71]. Clinically evident PPNAD is seen in 25–30% of patients with Carney complex and it usually presents in childhood, late adolescence, or early adulthood [67, 71, 72]. Such patients have been treated successfully with bilateral adrenalectomies [68].

Surgery for Adrenocortical Tumors

Surgery is the single most important aspect of treatment of an ACT. Surgery requires careful perioperative planning. All patients with a functioning tumor should be treated with the assumption that there will be suppression of the contralateral adrenal gland and therefore requires "stress" steroid supplementation for the perioperative period. Also, special attention to electrolyte balance, blood pressure, wound care, and infection prevention is paramount.

The use of open procedures such as laparotomy or a thoracoabdominal approach in general will allows the surgeon the best chance to completely excise the tumor. A curative, complete resection may be attempted in the 70–75% of patients who present without distant metastases. Total excision should be attempted even if it requires removal of adjacent structures, such as ipsilateral nephrectomy [55], since total resection is essential for cure. Many series have noted that patients with incomplete resection or distant metastases died, whereas those with localized or regional disease that was totally resected survived [53]. Extreme care must be exercised during surgery as the tumor tends to be friable, and tumor spillage occurs in about 20% of initial operations, and in 43% of operations done for tumor recurrence [29, 31]. Since tumor spillage worsens prognosis [29] any maneuver that reduces the risk of tumor spill is advocated. Also, infiltration of the vena cava with tumor thrombus may occur in up to 20% of the patients and may make complete resection challenging [29, 50]. In patients with extensive vascular infiltration, cardiopulmonary bypass may be necessary to achieve the vascular control needed for thrombectomy and vascular reconstruction [73]. When ACTs are completely resected, then no further therapy recommended. However, close follow-up with imaging and endocrine studies is needed to detect possible tumor recurrence. Even in patients with metastatic disease, complete resection is warranted if it is feasible [55]. However, when lesions are not resectable, then tumor ablation by injection with ethanol may be the only option for local control.

Retroperitoneal Lymph Node Dissection (RPLND)

The lymph node drainage of the adrenal gland is complex. There is an extensive subserosal network of lymphatic channels around the gland, crossing several levels in different directions inside the fascia and connective tissue involving the adrenal gland. The incidence of lymph node involvement with ACTs is not known, although some studies report it to be close to 40% in adults [74, 75]. The low frequency with which lymph nodes are resected reflects the standard surgical practice in which lymph node sampling is not routinely performed, except if there is obvious lymph node enlargement. A current Children's Oncology Group (COG) study, ARAR0332 has as one of its hypotheses that residual tumor in lymph nodes may contribute to relapse, so it specifies that patients with large tumors (Stage II) should have an ipsilateral retroperitoneal lymph nodes dissection.

Minimally Invasive Surgery for Adrenocortical Tumors in Children

While a laparotomy is still the most common approach for adrenalectomy in children, there has been an increase in laparoscopic adrenalectomy with the aim to improve operative visualization and to minimize postoperative pain [76–80]. The International Pediatric Endosurgery Group (IPEG) has released guidelines for the surgical treatment of adrenal masses in children [81]. The recommendations primarily address the use of laparoscopy in children with adrenal neuroblastoma, as this is the condition for which there is the most evidence. Nonetheless, IPEG mentions that there is no absolute contraindication to the laparoscopic approach for ACT, but notes that principles of cancer surgery must be adhered to. They conclude that the recommendation for the laparoscopic resection of adrenal tumors is supported by class 3 evidence (descriptive case series and opinions of expert panels). In general, the use of open procedure is recommended for adrenocortical carcinoma, and a laparoscopic approach for benign lesions [55, 78, 82]. Unfortunately, preoperative diagnosis of malignancy may be difficult so it is suggested that a laparoscopic approach be limited to children with small, localized lesions [55].

Staging of Adrenocortical Tumors

Staging of adrenocortical tumors is based on preoperative imaging and operative findings. Preoperative imaging defines the primary mass and is essential for surgical planning. Specifically, imaging will define the local extent of the tumor and distant metastases. Direct extension of tumor thrombus from the adrenal veins into the inferior vena cava (IVC) represents an important mechanism of nonhematogenous malignant spread and may occur in up to a third of patients. The lung is the most common site of distant metastases of adrenocortical carcinoma, followed by the liver [10]. Other metastatic sites include the peritoneum (29% of cases), pleura or diaphragm (24%), abdominal lymph nodes (24%), and kidney (18%) [26].

The staging system as modified from Sandrini et al is based on disease stage and tumor size [29, 31] (Table 10.1).

Adjuvant Therapy

The role of chemotherapy in the management of childhood ACT has not been well established. However, for patients with advanced disease or with a high risk of recurrence, the use of systemic therapy with mitotane or chemotherapy should be considered even though its impact on the overall outcome is minimal.

Table 10.1 Staging of Adrenocortical Tumors

Stage	Description
I	Tumor totally excised with negative margins. The tumor weight is ≤ 200 g, there is no evidence of metastasis and the abnormal hormone levels return to normal after surgery
II	Tumor totally excised with negative margins. The tumor weight is >200 g, or there is persistence of abnormal hormone levels after surgery Gross tumor excision with microscopic residual tumor
III	Gross residual tumor or inoperable tumors
IV	Distant metastasis

Mitotane

Mitotane is an insecticide derivative that produces adrenocortical necrosis and it has been used extensively in adults with ACT. Mitotane inhibits corticoid biosynthesis and destroys adrenocortical cells. Mitotane acts on the adrenocortical mitochondria and inhibits the 11-β-hydroxylase and the cholesterol side-chain cleavage enzymes. At higher doscs it also destroys mitochondria, resulting in necrosis of the adrenal cortex. At low plasma concentrations, mitotane suppresses the secretion of adrenal steroids, providing symptomatic improvement and regression of some of the endocrine dysfunction in patients with functioning tumors. However, higher levels are required for an adrenolytic effect [83, 84]. In patients with advanced disease, objective responses may be obtained in 20–30% of the cases using mitotane alone [83–86]. However, these responses are usually transient and the effect on prolongation of survival is uncertain [83–85]. In children, the use of mitotane for advanced ACT has not been evaluated systematically. There have been several reports of complete responses in children with advanced or metastatic ACT, but these appear to be rare events [87, 88]. In the Brazilian experience, there have been three patients who had locally unresectable tumors who received mitotane for a total of 8 months and were alive without evidence of disease after more than five years follow-up. Nonetheless, there appears to be growing movement away from Mitotane in view of the lack of demonstrable beneficial effects [89].

Chemotherapy

A variety of antineoplastic agents including cisplatin (or cisplatinum), carboplatinum, etoposide, 5-fluorouracil with leucovorin, and ifosfamide have been used in patients with ACTs but the small numbers of patients treated make definitive conclusions problematic. Cisplatin as a single agent may induce responses in approximatcly 25% of patients with advanced disease [90], and several authors have evaluated cisplatin-based regimens. Combinations of cisplatin with doxorubicin and either cyclophosphamide [91] or 5-fluorouracil [92] have resulted in responses of 20–40% of patients. Cisplatin has also been investigated in combination with etoposide (VP-16), with similar results [84, 93]. The combination of mitotane with cisplatin, etoposide, and doxorubicin has been extensively used in children with ACT by investigators of the International Pediatric Adrenocortical Tumor Registry (IPACTR) [29]. The current COG protocol, ARAR0332, will study a regimen that incorporates mitotane, cisplatin, etoposide, and doxorubicin, which has been used before and has been well tolerated [29].

Radiotherapy

Adjuvant radiation therapy has not been thoroughly evaluated in childhood ACT. Generally, it is accepted that ACT is radioresistant [84]. Also, because many children with ACT carry cancer-predisposing germline p53 mutations that could potentiate genomic instability, there is a concern that radiation may increase the incidence of secondary tumors. Driver et al reported that among 5 long-term survivors of pediatric ACT, 3 died because of secondary sarcoma arising within the radiation fields [94].

Future Therapeutic Options

There are a several novel therapies that are being developed [95–97]:

(i) Radionuclide therapy—Radiolabeled metomidate, a tracer that binds to adrenal 11B-hydroxylase (P450C11) has shown some promise in distinguishing neoplasms of adrenocortical origin from other lesions. Iodine-labeled metomedate may, in the future hold therapeutic potential as a specific adrenocortical radionuclide.

(ii) Epidermal Growth Factor Receptor inhibitors—The overexpression of the epidermal growth factor receptor (EGFR) protein in ACT's has provided the rationale for the use of EGFR inhibitors. However results to date in adults have been disappointing.

(iii) Angiogenesis inhibitors—angiogenesis and neovascularization are critical for tumor growth. Vascular endothelial growth factor (VEGF) is a proangiogenic growth factor that binds to the tyrosine kinase VEGF receptor, resulting in the activation of several intracellular signaling pathways. VEGF has been shown to be upregulated in ACT tissue. Therefore there has been interest in the targeting of VEGF signaling. However, early results in adults have not been encouraging.

(iv) IGF receptor antagonists—due to the importance of the IGF receptors in activating PI2K/Akt and MAPK pathways in cellular proliferation, differentiation, and survival, some have looked at receptor antagonists as a therapeutic option. Overexpression of IGF-II and/or IGF-1R is possibly the most frequent genetic alteration in ACT. While a possible option in the future for adults, its role in childhood may be less helpful in children.

(v) B-catenin antagonists–The B-catenin gene is an important element of signal transduction in Wnt signaling. There is some early work on antagonists of this pathway as a potential target however to date, there have only been animal models of this an no applications in patients.

(vi) Steroidogenic factor 1 (SF-1) inverse agonists–Steroidogenic factor-1 is a nuclear receptor transcription factor that has been identified to act in the regulation of promoter activity of cytochrome P450 steroid hydroxylase genes in steroidogenic cell lines. If is known that SF-1 plays a decisive role in the regulation of adrenal development. SF-1 amplification and overexpression has been described in pediatric ACT. There has only been early work towards using SF-1 inverse agonists in vivo models of ACT.

(vii) mTOR antagonists—Phosphatidylinositol 3-kinase (PI3K)/akt/mammalian target of rapamycin inhibitor (mTOR) deregulation is commonly associated to human cancer pathogenesis. Several new drugs have been developed to inhibit this pathway. Recently IGF-IR/mTOR signaling was demonstrated to be activated in childhood ACT at multiple levels. Use of mTOR inhibitors has effect in vitro in mice and may have potential in patients with ACT.

(viii) Gene therapy—the use of gene therapy is an evolving approach for cancer treatment with its aim being reactivation of oncosuppressor genes and/or inhibit oncogenes, who expression is deregulated during tumor progression. However, early results have been poor thus far.

(ix) Immunotherapy—Immunotherapy is a therapeutic approach based on the stimulation of the immune response against cancer cells. Currently being studied is the use of dendritic cells to induce antiturmor immune responses in ACTs. Early work is encouraging but has more work is needed.

Outcomes

Due to the heterogeneity and rarity of ACT, prognostic factors have not been well defined and outcomes are hard to predict. In addition, the difficulty in distinguishing malignant from benign tumors complicates any analysis.

In the older literature, a relatively poor prognosis had been predicted for children with ACTs [26]. In a report up to 1962, only 23 of 222 patients survived 2 or more years after treatment [98]. However, more recent studies suggest a better outcome for children with ACT with overall survival at 5 years of 54–74% [31, 32, 42]. In a large series of 54 patients with known outcomes, 24 (44%) died and 30 (56%) have been disease-free for periods of 1–214 months from diagnosis [31]. Improved survival rates in more recent times may reflect the benefits of earlier detection due to improved imaging, and refinements in surgical technique and postoperative care [10].

The prognosis of adrenocortical carcinoma in children is more favorable than the prognosis of adults, whose overall survival is 10–30% at 5 years [51, 52]. The improved outcome of younger patients with malignant ACTs is especially apparent in children less than 5 years who have a significantly better survival than older children and adolescents, whose tumors behave more like adrenocortical carcinoma in adults [51, 52]. A recent **Surveillance, Epidemiology, and End Results** (SEER) program study review of patients demonstrated that younger patients (≤ 4 years) were noted to have more favorable features than older patients (5–19 years) including more local disease, more likely to be <10 cm, and better 5 year survival. After adjustment the most significant predictors of cancer-specific death were age 5–19 years, and distant metastatic disease. After accounting for tumor size, only age maintained statistical significance [28].

The prognostic importance of histology has been controversial [42, 43, 99] but in general, lesions that are classified as an adenoma or benign histology are associated with good prognosis, although the rarity of ACTs in the pediatric age group tempers this expectation. Another factor complicating the ascertainment of outcomes is a tendency to over-diagnose lesions as carcinomas [26, 40]. Unless metastases are present, this difficulty in distinguishing adenoma from carcinoma is compounded by the absence of universally accepted histologic prognostic factors.

There have been attempts to predict outcome based on tumor characteristics. In one study tumor size larger than 10.5 cm, tumor weight >400 g, invasion into the surrounding soft tissue, and extension into the IVC were significant markers for a poor prognosis on univariant analysis. However, in a multivariate analysis only local invasion and extension into the IVC were independent predictors of an unfavorable outcome. These authors stressed the importance of an accurate diagnosis of ACT and they defined 9 pathologic features of malignancy and correlated the number of these features in a particular neoplasm and clinical outcome [32]. Three or fewer unfavorable pathologic features appears to be the threshold between the clinically benign and malignant ACT.

Most deaths caused by adrenocortical carcinoma occur within 1–2 years after diagnosis [26]. Sites of metastases include liver, lungs, and regional lymph nodes. The median time to tumor recurrence was 6 months (range 1–48 months with a median time to recurrence of 6 months. Only 2 of 15 patients relapsed more than 1 year from the initial surgery (1.8 and 4.0 years, respectively). Recurrences in this series were rapidly fatal in nearly all cases with a median time from relapse to death of 5 months (range, 2–11 months).

In the IPACTR, the revised staging system appears to be highly predictive of outcome in children with Stage I and Stage IV disease, with long-term survival of >90% of patients with Stage I disease and only 10% of those with Stage IV disease. Predicting outcome for patients with intermediate stages of disease is much more difficult. For example, despite presumed complete tumor resection, local recurrence will occur in 30–50% of patients with Stage II disease. In general, patients with Stage III disease will have a poor outcome similar to those with Stage IV disease.

Future Considerations

Advances in basic science, surgical techniques, and national and international collaboration have set the stage for further investigations of ACTs in children. Since surgical resection seems to be an important part of successful treatment, the Children's Oncology Group (COG) is evaluating the effect of the extent of surgical resection of the primary tumor and regional lymph nodes. As mitotane has not been found to be of significant benefit, it will not be used in patients who have a complete resection. Children who recur locally will have further attempts at complete resection of disease and are candidates for systemic chemotherapy. Also, the observations that Southern Brazilian children with ACT carry a specific germline p53 mutation [27, 57] has led to investigations looking for the molecular lesion responsible for tumor development in other patients and may ultimately allow further characterization of pathogenesis. Finally, an international registry has been established which may provide more insight into this rare tumor of childhood.

References

1. Harris CC, Hollstein M. Clinical implications of the p53 tumor-suppressor gene. The New England journal of medicine. 1993;329(18):1318–27.
2. Hollstein M, Sidransky D, Vogelstein B, Harris CC. p53 mutations in human cancers. Science. 1991;253 (5015):49–53.
3. Kern SE, Kinzler KW, Bruskin A, et al. Identification of p53 as a sequence-specific DNA-binding protein. Science. 1991;252(5013):1708–11.
4. Levine AJ. The p53 tumor-suppressor gene. The New England journal of medicine. 1992;326 (20):1350–2.
5. Fraumeni JF Jr, Li FP. Hodgkin's disease in childhood: an epidemiologic study. J Natl Cancer Inst. 1969;42(4):681–91.
6. Grayson GH, Moore S, Schneider BG, Saldivar V, Hensel CH. Novel germline mutation of the p53 tumor suppressor gene in a child with incidentally discovered adrenal cortical carcinoma. The American journal of pediatric hematology/oncology. 1994;16 (4):341–7.
7. Li FP, Fraumeni JF Jr, Mulvihill JJ, et al. A cancer family syndrome in twenty-four kindreds. Cancer Res. 1988;48(18):5358–62.
8. Malkin D, Li FP, Strong LC, et al. Germ line p53 mutations in a familial syndrome of breast cancer, sarcomas, and other neoplasms. Science. 1990;250 (4985):1233–8.
9. Ilvesmaki V, Blum WF, Voutilainen R. Insulin-like growth factor binding proteins in the human adrenal gland. Mol Cell Endocrinol. 1993;97(1–2):71–9.
10. Agrons GA, Lonergan GJ, Dickey GE, Perez-Monte JE. Adrenocortical neoplasms in children: radiologic-pathologic correlation. Radiographics: a review publication of the Radiological Society of North America, Inc. 1999;19(4):989–1008.
11. Else T. Association of adrenocortical carcinoma with familial cancer susceptibility syndromes. Mol Cell Endocrinol. 2012;351(1):66–70.
12. Raymond VM, Everett JN, Furtado LV, et al. Adrenocortical carcinoma is a lynch syndrome-associated cancer. Journal of clinical oncology: official journal of the American Society of Clinical Oncology. 2013;31(24):3012–8.
13. Dohna M, Reincke M, Mincheva A, Allolio B, Solinas-Toldo S, Lichter P. Adrenocortical carcinoma is characterized by a high frequency of chromosomal gains and high-level amplifications. Genes Chromosom Cancer. 2000;28(2):145–52.
14. Figueiredo BC, Stratakis CA, Sandrini R, et al. Comparative genomic hybridization analysis of adrenocortical tumors of childhood. The Journal of clinical endocrinology and metabolism. 1999;84 (3):1116–21.
15. Figueiredo BC, Ribeiro RC, Zambetti G, et al. Amplification of 9q34 in childhood adrenocortical tumors: a specific feature unrelated to ethnic origin or living conditions. *Brazilian journal of medical and biological research = Revista brasileira de pesquisas medicas e biologicas/ Sociedade Brasileira de Biofisica... [et al.].* Oct 2000;33(10):1217–1224.
16. Bauman A, Bauman CG. Virilizing adrenocortical carcinoma. Development in a patient with salt-losing congenital adrenal hyperplasia. JAMA, J Am Med Assoc. 1982;248(23):3140–1.
17. Daeschner GL. Adrenal Cortical Adenoma Arising in a Girl with Congenital Adrenogenital Syndrome. Pediatrics. 1965;36:141–2.
18. Dahms WT, Gray G, Vrana M, New MI. Adrenocortical adenoma and ganglioneuroblastoma in a child. A case presenting as Cushing syndrome with virilization. Am J Dis Child. 1973;125(4):608–11.
19. Gershanik JJ, Elmore M, Levkoff AH. Congenital concurrence of adrenal cortical tumor, ganglioneuroma, and toxoplasmosis. Pediatrics. 1973;51 (4):705–9.
20. Pang S, Becker D, Cotelingam J, Foley TP Jr, Drash AL. Adrenocortical tumor in a patient with

congenital adrenal hyperplasia due to 21-hydroxylase deficiency. Pediatrics. 1981;68(2):242–6.
21. Hornstein L, Crowe C, Gruppo R. Adrenal carcinoma in child with history of fetal alcohol syndrome. Lancet. 1977;2(8051):1292–3.
22. Mann JR, Cameron AH, Gornall P, Rayner PH, Shah KJ. Transplacental carcinogenesis (adrenocortical carcinoma) associated with hydroxyprogesterone hexanoate. *Lancet.* Sep 3 1983;2(8349):580.
23. Stewart DR, Jones PH, Jolleys A. Carcinoma of the adrenal gland in children. J Pediatr Surg. 1974;9 (1):59–67.
24. Daneman A, Chan HS, Martin J. Adrenal carcinoma and adenoma in children: a review of 17 patients. Pediatr Radiol. 1983;13(1):11–8.
25. Zaitoon MM, Mackie GG. Adrenal cortical tumors in children. Urology. 1978;12(6):645–9.
26. Lack EE, Mulvihill JJ, Travis WD, Kozakewich HP. Adrenal cortical neoplasms in the pediatric and adolescent age group. Clinicopathologic study of 30 cases with emphasis on epidemiological and prognostic factors. *Pathology annual.* 1992;(27) Pt 1:1–53.
27. Ribeiro RC, Michalkiewicz EL, Figueiredo BC, et al. Adrenocortical tumors in children. *Brazilian journal of medical and biological research = Revista brasileira de pesquisas medicas e biologicas / Sociedade Brasileira de Biofisica ... [et al.].* Oct 2000;33(10):1225–1234.
28. McAteer JP, Huaco JA, Gow KW. Predictors of survival in pediatric adrenocortical carcinoma: a Surveillance, Epidemiology, and End Results (SEER) program study. J Pediatr Surg. 2013;48 (5):1025–31.
29. Michalkiewicz E, Sandrini R, Figueiredo B, et al. Clinical and outcome characteristics of children with adrenocortical tumors: a report from the International Pediatric Adrenocortical Tumor Registry. Journal of clinical oncology: official journal of the American Society of Clinical Oncology. 2004;22(5):838–45.
30. Ribeiro RC, Sandrini Neto RS, Schell MJ, Lacerda L, Sambaio GA, Cat I. Adrenocortical carcinoma in children: a study of 40 cases. *Journal of clinical oncology: official journal of the American Society of Clinical Oncology.* Jan 1990;8(1):67–74.
31. Sandrini R, Ribeiro RC, DeLacerda L. Childhood adrenocortical tumors. The Journal of clinical endocrinology and metabolism. 1997;82(7):2027–31.
32. Wieneke JA, Thompson LD, Heffess CS. Adrenal cortical neoplasms in the pediatric population: a clinicopathologic and immunophenotypic analysis of 83 patients. Am J Surg Pathol. 2003;27(7):867–81.
33. Hauffa BP, Roll C, Muhlenberg R, Havers W. Growth in children with adrenocortical tumors. Klinische Padiatrie. Mar-Apr. 1991;203(2):83–7.
34. Loridan L, Senior B. Cushing's syndrome in infancy. The Journal of pediatrics. 1969;75(3):349–59.
35. Kepes JJ, O'Boynick P, Jones S, Baum D, McMillan J, Adams ME. Adrenal cortical adenoma in the spinal canal of an 8-year-old girl. Am J Surg Pathol. 1990;14(5):481–4.
36. Medeiros LJ, Anasti J, Gardner KL, Pass HI, Nieman LK. Virilizing adrenal cortical neoplasm arising ectopically in the thorax. The Journal of clinical endocrinology and metabolism. 1992;75(6):1522–5.
37. Kay S. Hyperplasia and neoplasia of the adrenal gland. Pathol Annu. 1976;11:103–39.
38. Tang CK, Gray GF. Adrenocortical neoplasms. Prognosis and morphology. *Urology.* May 1975;5 (5):691–695.
39. Gandour MJ, Grizzle WE. A small adrenocortical carcinoma with aggressive behavior. An evaluation of criteria for malignancy. *Archives of pathology & laboratory medicine.* Nov 1986;110(11):1076–1079.
40. Cagle PT, Hough AJ, Pysher TJ, et al. Comparison of adrenal cortical tumors in children and adults. Cancer. 1986;57(11):2235–7.
41. Hough AJ, Hollifield JW, Page DL, Hartmann WH. Prognostic factors in adrenal cortical tumors. A mathematical analysis of clinical and morphologic data. Am J Clin Pathol. 1979;72(3):390–9.
42. Bugg MF, Ribeiro RC, Roberson PK, et al. Correlation of pathologic features with clinical outcome in pediatric adrenocortical neoplasia. A study of a Brazilian population. Brazilian Group for Treatment of Childhood Adrenocortical Tumors. Am J Clin Pathol. 1994;101(5):625–9.
43. Weiss LM, Medeiros LJ, Vickery AL Jr. Pathologic features of prognostic significance in adrenocortical carcinoma. Am J Surg Pathol. 1989;13(3):202–6.
44. Dehner LP. Neoplasms of the adrenal cortex. Preoccupation bordering on obsession. Am J Clin Pathol. 1994;101(5):557–8.
45. Cote RJ, Cordon-Cardo C, Reuter VE, Rosen PP. Immunopathology of adrenal and renal cortical tumors. Coordinated change in antigen expression is associated with neoplastic conversion in the adrenal cortex. *The American journal of pathology.* May 1990;136(5):1077–1084.
46. Cibas ES, Medeiros LJ, Weinberg DS, Gelb AB, Weiss LM. Cellular DNA profiles of benign and malignant adrenocortical tumors. Am J Surg Pathol. 1990;14(10):948–55.
47. Medeiros LJ, Weiss LM. New developments in the pathologic diagnosis of adrenal cortical neoplasms. A review. Am J Clin Pathol. 1992;97(1):73–83.
48. Fogt F, Vargas MP, Zhuang Z, Merino MJ. Utilization of molecular genetics in the differentiation between adrenal cortical adenomas and carcinomas. Hum Pathol. 1998;29(5):518–21.
49. Harrison LE, Gaudin PB, Brennan MF. Pathologic features of prognostic significance for adrenocortical carcinoma after curative resection. Arch Surg. 1999;134(2):181–5.
50. Kendrick ML, Lloyd R, Erickson L, et al. Adrenocortical carcinoma: surgical progress or status quo? Arch Surg. 2001;136(5):543–9.

51. Stojadinovic A, Ghossein RA, Hoos A, et al. Adrenocortical carcinoma: clinical, morphologic, and molecular characterization. Journal of clinical oncology: official journal of the American Society of Clinical Oncology. 2002;20(4):941–50.
52. Dehner LP. Pediatric adrenocortical neoplasms: on the road to some clarity. Am J Surg Pathol. 2003;27 (7):1005–7.
53. Ciftci AO, Senocak ME, Tanyel FC, Buyukpamukcu N. Adrenocortical tumors in children. J Pediatr Surg. 2001;36(4):549–54.
54. Streeten DH, Tomycz N, Anderson GH. Reliability of screening methods for the diagnosis of primary aldosteronism. The American journal of medicine. 1979;67(3):403–13.
55. Rescorla FJ. Malignant adrenal tumors. Semin Pediatr Surg. 2006;15(1):48–56.
56. Prando A, Wallace S, Marins JL, Pereira RM, de Oliveira ER, Alvarenga M. Sonographic features of benign intraperitoneal lipomatous tumors in children–report of 4 cases. Pediatr Radiol. 1990;20 (8):571–4.
57. Ribeiro J, Ribeiro RC, Fletcher BD. Imaging findings in pediatric adrenocortical carcinoma. Pediatr Radiol. 2000;30(1):45–51.
58. Abramson SJ. Adrenal neoplasms in children. Radiol Clin North Am. 1997;35(6):1415–53.
59. Velchik MG, Alavi A, Kressel HY, Engelman K. Localization of pheochromocytoma: MIBG [correction of MIGB], CT, and MRI correlation. Journal of nuclear medicine: official publication, Society of Nuclear Medicine. 1989;30(3):328–36.
60. Aiba M, Hirayama A, Iri H, et al. Adrenocorticotropic hormone-independent bilateral adrenocortical macronodular hyperplasia as a distinct subtype of Cushing's syndrome. Enzyme histochemical and ultrastructural study of four cases with a review of the literature. Am J Clin Pathol. 1991;96(3):334–40.
61. Bourdeau I, Stratakis CA. Cyclic AMP-dependent signaling aberrations in macronodular adrenal disease. Ann N Y Acad Sci. 2002;968:240–55.
62. Orth DN. Cushing's syndrome. The New England journal of medicine. 1995;332(12):791–803.
63. Cheitlin RA, Westphal M, Cabrera CM, Fujii DK, Snyder J, Fitzgerald PA. Cushing's syndrome due to bilateral adrenal macronodular hyperplasia with undetectable ACTH: cell culture of adenoma cells on extracellular matrix. Horm Res. 1988;29(4):162–7.
64. Morioka M, Ohashi Y, Watanabe H, et al. ACTH-independent macronodular adrenocortical hyperplasia (AIMAH): report of two cases and the analysis of steroidogenic activity in adrenal nodules. Endocr J. 1997;44(1):65–72.
65. Sutter JA, Grimberg A. Adrenocortical tumors and hyperplasias in childhood–etiology, genetics, clinical presentation and therapy. Pediatric endocrinology reviews: PER. 2006;4(1):32–9.
66. Lamberts SW, Zuiderwijk J, Uitterlinden P, Blijd JJ, Bruining HA, de Jong FH. Characterization of adrenal autonomy in Cushing's syndrome: a comparison between in vivo and in vitro responsiveness of the adrenal gland. The Journal of clinical endocrinology and metabolism. 1990;70 (1):192–9.
67. Koch CA, Pacak K, Chrousos GP. The molecular pathogenesis of hereditary and sporadic adrenocortical and adrenomedullary tumors. The Journal of clinical endocrinology and metabolism. 2002;87 (12):5367–84.
68. Storr HL, Mitchell H, Swords FM, et al. Clinical features, diagnosis, treatment and molecular studies in paediatric Cushing's syndrome due to primary nodular adrenocortical hyperplasia. Clin Endocrinol. 2004;61(5):553–9.
69. Agarwal SK, Kennedy PA, Scacheri PC, et al. Menin molecular interactions: insights into normal functions and tumorigenesis. *Hormone and metabolic research = Hormon- und Stoffwechselforschung = Hormones et metabolisme.* June 2005;37(6):369–374.
70. Kirschner LS, Carney JA, Pack SD, et al. Mutations of the gene encoding the protein kinase A type I-alpha regulatory subunit in patients with the Carney complex. Nat Genet. 2000;26(1):89–92.
71. Stratakis CA, Kirschner LS, Carney JA. Clinical and molecular features of the Carney complex: diagnostic criteria and recommendations for patient evaluation. The Journal of clinical endocrinology and metabolism. 2001;86(9):4041–6.
72. Libe R, Bertherat J. Molecular genetics of adrenocortical tumours, from familial to sporadic diseases. European journal of endocrinology/ European Federation of Endocrine Societies. 2005;153(4):477–87.
73. Godine LB, Berdon WE, Brasch RC, Leonidas JC. Adrenocortical carcinoma with extension into inferior vena cava and right atrium: report of 3 cases in children. *Pediatric radiology.* 1990;20(3):166–168; discussion 169.
74. Crucitti F, Bellantone R, Ferrante A, Boscherini M, Crucitti P. The Italian Registry for Adrenal Cortical Carcinoma: analysis of a multiinstitutional series of 129 patients. The ACC Italian Registry Study Group. Surgery. 1996;119(2):161–70.
75. Lee JE, Berger DH, el-Naggar AK, et al. Surgical management, DNA content, and patient survival in adrenal cortical carcinoma. *Surgery.* Dec 1995;118 (6):1090–1098.
76. Hallfeldt KK, Mussack T, Trupka A, Hohenbleicher F, Schmidbauer S. Laparoscopic lateral adrenalectomy versus open posterior adrenalectomy for the treatment of benign adrenal tumors. Surg Endosc. 2003;17(2):264–7.
77. Imai T, Kikumori T, Ohiwa M, Mase T, Funahashi H. A case-controlled study of laparoscopic compared with open lateral adrenalectomy. *American journal of surgery.* Jul 1999;178(1):50–53; discussion 54.

78. Pillinger SH, Bambach CP, Sidhu S. Laparoscopic adrenalectomy: a 6-year experience of 59 cases. ANZ journal of surgery. 2002;72(7):467–70.
79. Prinz RA. A comparison of laparoscopic and open adrenalectomies. *Archives of surgery.* May 1995;130 (5):489–492; discussion 492–484.
80. Thompson GB, Grant CS, van Heerden JA, et al. Laparoscopic versus open posterior adrenalectomy: a case-control study of 100 patients. Surgery. 1997;122 (6):1132–6.
81. International Pediatric Endosurgery G. IPEG guidelines for the surgical treatment of adrenal masses in children. *Journal of laparoendoscopic & advanced surgical techniques. Part A.* Mar 2010;20(2):vii-ix.
82. Smith CD, Weber CJ, Amerson JR. Laparoscopic adrenalectomy: new gold standard. World J Surg. 1999;23(4):389–96.
83. Vassilopoulou-Sellin R, Schultz PN. Adrenocortical carcinoma. Clinical outcome at the end of the 20th century. Cancer. 2001;92(5):1113–21.
84. Wajchenberg BL, Albergaria Pereira MA, Medonca BB, et al. Adrenocortical carcinoma: clinical and laboratory observations. Cancer. 2000;88(4):711–36.
85. Luton JP, Cerdas S, Billaud L, et al. Clinical features of adrenocortical carcinoma, prognostic factors, and the effect of mitotane therapy. The New England journal of medicine. 1990;322(17):1195–201.
86. van Slooten H, Moolenaar AJ, van Seters AP, Smeenk D. The treatment of adrenocortical carcinoma with o, p'-DDD: prognostic implications of serum level monitoring. European journal of cancer & clinical oncology. 1984;20(1):47–53.
87. Netto AD, Wajchenberg BL, Ravaglia C, et al. Treatment of Adrenocortical Cancer with O,P'-Ddd. *Annals of internal medicine.* Jul 1963;59:74–78.
88. Ostuni JA, Roginsky MS. Metastatic adrenal cortical carcinoma. Documented cure with combined chemotherapy. Arch Intern Med. 1975;135 (9):1257–8.
89. Bapat AA, Demeure MJ, Bussey KJ. A fly in the ointment: reassessing mitotane's role in the treatment of adrenocortical carcinoma. Pharmacogenomics. 2012;13(11):1207–9.
90. Michalkiewicz EL, Sandrini R, Bugg MF, et al. Clinical characteristics of small functioning adrenocortical tumors in children. Med Pediatr Oncol. 1997;28(3):175–8.
91. van Slooten H, van Oosterom AT. CAP (cyclophosphamide, doxorubicin, and cisplatin) regimen in adrenal cortical carcinoma. Cancer Treat Rep. 1983;67(4):377–9.
92. Schlumberger M, Brugieres L, Gicquel C, Travagli JP, Droz JP, Parmentier C. 5-Fluorouracil, doxorubicin, and cisplatin as treatment for adrenal cortical carcinoma. Cancer. 1991;67(12):2997–3000.
93. Williamson SK, Lew D, Miller GJ, Balcerzak SP, Baker LH, Crawford ED. Phase II evaluation of cisplatin and etoposide followed by mitotane at disease progression in patients with locally advanced or metastatic adrenocortical carcinoma: a Southwest Oncology Group Study. Cancer. 2000;88(5):1159–65.
94. Driver CP, Birch J, Gough DC, Bruce J. Adrenal cortical tumors in childhood. Pediatric hematology and oncology. Nov-Dec. 1998;15(6):527–32.
95. Maluf DF, de Oliveira BH, Lalli E. Therapy of adrenocortical cancer: present and future. American journal of cancer research. 2011;1(2):222–32.
96. Stigliano A, Cerquetti L, Sampaoli C, Bucci B, Toscano V. Current and emerging therapeutic options in adrenocortical cancer treatment. Journal of oncology. 2012;2012:408131.
97. Tacon LJ, Prichard RS, Soon PS, Robinson BG, Clifton-Bligh RJ, Sidhu SB. Current and emerging therapies for advanced adrenocortical carcinoma. Oncologist. 2011;16(1):36–48.
98. Hayles AB, Hahn HB Jr, Sprague RG, Bahn RC, Priestley JT. Hormone-secreting tumors of the adrenal cortex in children. Pediatrics. 1966;37 (1):19–25.
99. Weiss LM. Comparative histologic study of 43 metastasizing and nonmetastasizing adrenocortical tumors. Am J Surg Pathol. 1984;8(3):163–9.

Part IV

Pancreas

Pancreas Embryology, Anatomy, and Physiology

11

Joseph Fusco, Yousef EL-Gohary and George K. Gittes

The term 'pancreas' is derived from the Greek word meaning 'all flesh' [1]. It is endodermally derived, consisting of two morphologically distinct tissues, the exocrine and endocrine pancreas, which are derived from a single epithelium (endoderm) (Fig. 11.1). The pancreas has two major functions, the production of digestive enzymes by the exocrine tissue, and the production of metabolically active hormones by the endocrine tissue. These two tissues exist together within the pancreas despite their disparate morphology and function. The endocrine pancreas, which compromises only 2% of the adult pancreatic mass, is organized into islets of Langerhans consisting of five cell subtypes, α, β, δ, ε, and PP cells secreting glucagon, insulin, somatostatin, ghrelin, and pancreatic polypeptide hormones, respectively. The exocrine tissue on the other hand, which forms nearly 98% of the adult pancreatic mass, is composed of acinar and ductal epithelial cells [1]. We will be reviewing in this chapter the basic anatomical and embryological development of the pancreas.

J. Fusco · Y. EL-Gohary · G.K. Gittes (✉)
Department of Pediatric Surgery, Children's Hospital of Pittsburgh, 4401 Penn Ave, Pittsburgh, PA 15224, USA
e-mail: george.gittes@chp.edu

J. Fusco
e-mail: Joseph.Fusco@chp.edu

Basic Anatomy

The human pancreas is a long tapered glandular organ, which lies in the retroperitoneum. It is divided into four anatomical regions, the head, neck, body and tail, along with one accessory lobe or 'uncinate process', with the head lying within the curve of the second part of the duodenum. It extends transversely towards the hilum of the spleen, measuring between 12 and 15 cm long in adults. The digestive enzymes and bicarbonates are secreted by the exocrine acinar tissue. The acini (the name stems from the Greek word 'acinus' meaning grape) are an accumulation of acinar cells at the termination of ducts, and then drain into a centrally located acinar spaces connected to tiny pancreatic tubular ductal networks. These networks eventually join to form the larger pancreatic ducts namely the main pancreatic duct of Wirsung, and the accessory duct of Santorini. The main duct drains into the duodenum via the major duodenal papilla (Ampulla of Vater), while the main pancreatic duct may have a separate accessory pancreatic duct (derived from proximal duct of Santorini), which drains the uncinate process and lower part of the head of the pancreas into the duodenum via the minor duodenal papilla. Incomplete stet of the dorsal and ventral pancreatic ducts results in pancreas divisum, which is the most common congenital pancreatic ductal anatomic variant, but many anatomical variations of the pancreatic ductal drainage system do exist (Fig. 11.2). Blockage of the main pancreatic duct can lead to

D.J. Ledbetter and P.R.V. Johnson (eds.), *Endocrine Surgery in Children*,
DOI 10.1007/978-3-662-54256-9_11

stasis of the digestive enzymes, which can then become activated and begin an auto-digestion process within the pancreas, resulting in pancreatitis. The endocrine hormones are produced in the islets of Langerhans, which are scattered throughout the pancreas, drained by a network of

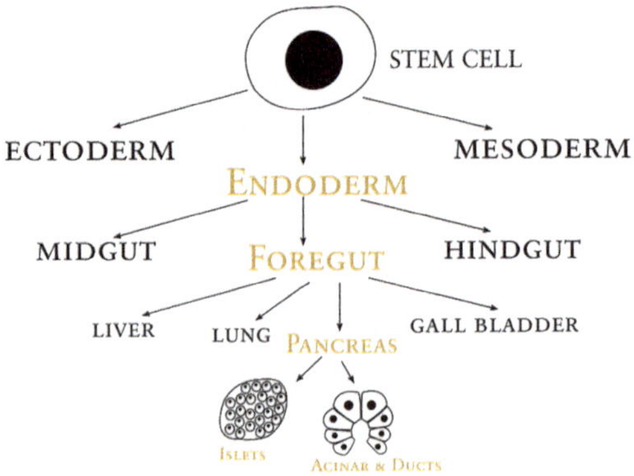

Fig. 11.1 Cell lineage schematic for pancreatic development from a multipotent progenitor stem cell

capillaries that invade the islet, and are thus delivered into the main bloodstream [2]. The distribution of endocrine cells within the islet is species-dependent. In rodents, the core of the islet is occupied by the β-cells surrounded in the periphery by a ring of α-cells, whereas in humans and monkeys all the endocrine cell types are intermingled with each other [3]. Non-endocrine cells also exist in the islet, including endothelial cells, neurons, dendritic cells, macrophages, and fibroblasts (Fig. 11.3).

A sound knowledge of the anatomical relationship of the pancreas to other surrounding structures is important when performing pancreatic surgery. The pancreatic head lies in front of the inferior vena cava, right renal artery, both renal veins and the superior mesenteric vessels, whereas the uncinate process lies posterior to the superior mesenteric vessels. The neck of the pancreas lies directly over the portal vein and vertebral bodies L1 and L2; this region is where the splenic vein unites with the superior mesenteric vein to form

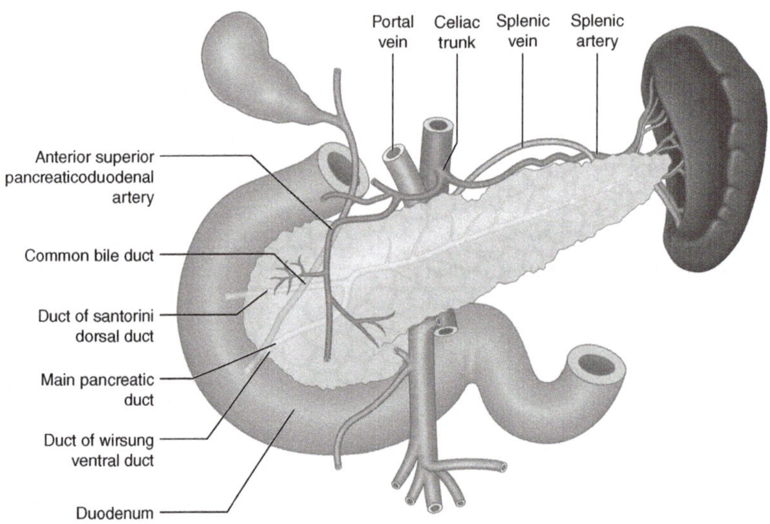

Fig. 11.2 Schematic illustration of the anatomical relationship of the pancreas in relation to other anatomical structures. The pancreatic head lies in front of the IVC and SMV, whereas the uncinate process lies posterior to the SMV. The stomach lies anterior to the pancreas, whereas the aorta, left adrenal gland and left kidney lie posterior to the body of the pancreas. The tail lies in the hilum of the spleen with the splenic artery running along the superior border of the pancreas. Major blood supply for the pancreas arises from the celiac trunk and superior mesenteric arteries, with the superior pancreaticoduodenal artery running anterior to head of pancreas. Innervation of the pancreas is derived from the vagal and splanchinic nerves. The pancreas is drained by multiple lymph node groups. The body and tail drain mostly into pancreatico-splenic nodes, whereas the head and neck drain more widely into nodes along the superior mesenteric, hepatic and pancreaticoduodenal arteries

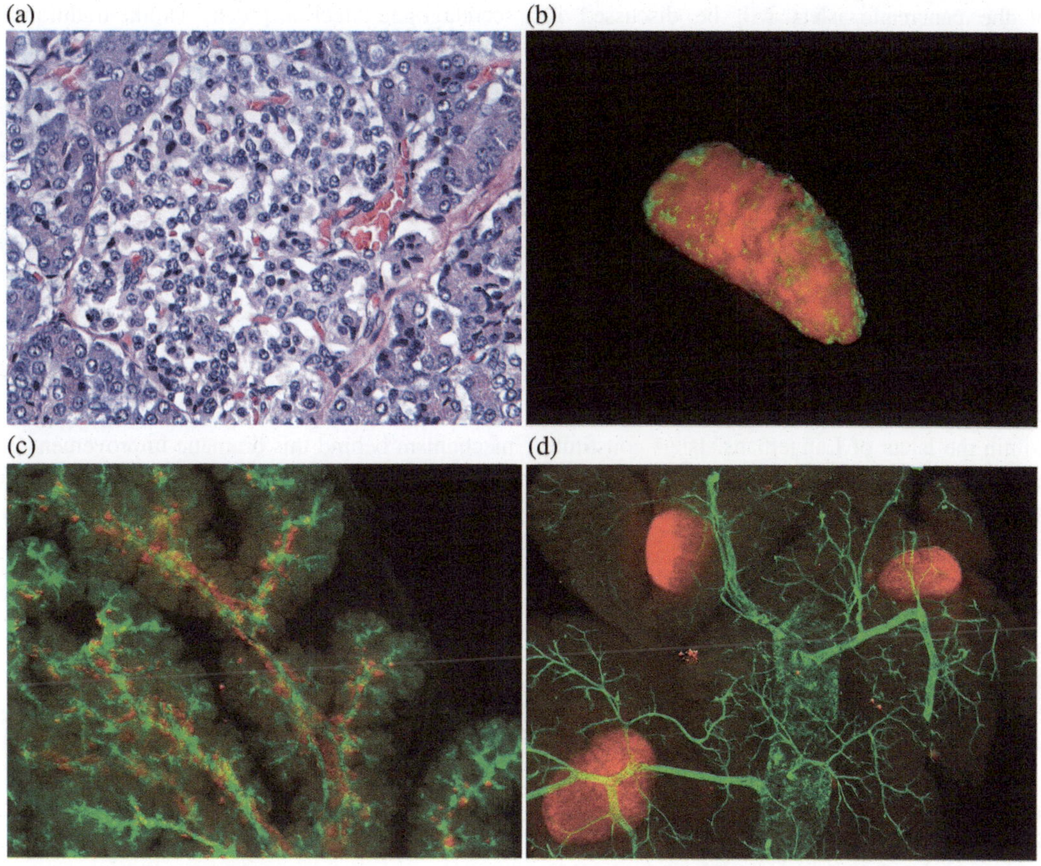

Fig. 11.3 Standard histological section of a human pancreas specimen, **a** illustrating a small, relatively pale-staining cell known as the islet of Langerhans, which is embedded in darker-stained exocrine tissue. **b** Adult mouse pancreas wholemount image showing an isolated islet stained with insulin, with glucagon in the periphery. **c** Wholemount image of embryonic day (E) 16.5 pancreas illustrating close relationship between insulin cells and pancreatic ducts. **d** Wholemount image of an adult mouse pancreas stained with insulin and DBA for pancreatic ducts

the portal vein. The splenic vein receives the inferior mesenteric vein near the tail of the pancreas. Anterior–posterior blunt trauma can thus lead to pancreatic tissue damage as well as ductal injury. The common bile duct passes in a deep groove on the posterior aspect of the pancreatic head until it joins the main pancreatic duct at the ampulla of Vater in the pancreatic parenchyma. The stomach lies anterior to the body and tail of the pancreas, whereas the aorta, left adrenal gland and left kidney lie posterior to the body of the pancreas. The tail lies in the hilum of the spleen with the splenic artery, which is often tortuous, running along the superior border of the pancreas (Fig. 11.2).

The major blood supply to the pancreas arises from multiple branches of the celiac trunk and superior mesenteric arteries, which form arterial arcades within the body and tail of the pancreas. The splenic and common hepatic arteries arise from the celiac trunk. The dorsal and greater pancreatic arteries branch from the splenic artery, whereas the gastroduodenal artery branches from the common hepatic artery, then dividing around the head of the pancreas into anterior and posterior superior pancreaticoduodenal branches that anastomose with the anterior and posterior branches of the inferior pancreaticoduodenal artery, which are branches of the superior mesenteric artery (Fig. 11.2). The vascularization of the pancreatic islets will be discussed in greater detail later in the chapter. Venous drainage of the pancreas mainly flows into the portal system, with the head and neck draining primarily through the superior and inferior pancreaticoduodenal veins, whereas the body and tail drain into the splenic vein.

Physiology

The pancreas is responsible for regulating the body's glycemia through the endocrine cells within the islets of Langerhans. Islets constitute nearly 2% of the total pancreatic tissue. This regulation is delicately balanced through the actions of the hormones insulin and glucagon. Insulin is the hormone of energy storage, and induces an increase in amino acid uptake as well as glucose uptake, increasing protein synthesis, decreasing lipolysis and glycogenolysis, especially post-prandially or in a hyperglycemic state. Whereas glucagon is viewed as the hormone of energy release, stimulating higher blood glucose levels by the stimulation of gluconeogenesis, glycogenolysis and lipolysis in the setting of hypoglycemia.

β-cells secrete insulin based on blood glucose levels as well as neural and humoral factors. The stimulus for insulin release into the bloodstream is far greater when glucose is ingested enterally compared to the parenteral route, indicating that a 'feed-forward' mechanism in the digestive tract is activated, anticipating the rise in blood glucose. This anticipation is mediated by *incretins*. There are two main incretin hormones, glucose-dependent insulinotropic peptide; also known as gastric inhibitory peptide (GIP) and glucagon-like peptide-1 (GLP-1). Both are secreted by endocrine cells located in the small intestinal epithelium when the luminal concentration of glucose increases in the digestive tract, and subsequently they stimulate the β-cells to secrete 'more' insulin. Hence, the great interest in the pharmaceutical industry to develop incretin-based therapies to treat diabetes, particularly type 2, because of its potent secretagogue effect on β-cells. Unlike traditional medications that stimulate β-cells to secrete insulin regardless of blood glucose level, incretins augment the β-cell response to blood glucose levels in a glucose-dependent manner, in addition to GLP-1's inhibitory effect on glucagon secretion and the ability to increase food transit time in the stomach [4, 5]. A peculiar phenomenon observed is type 2 diabetic patients undergoing Roux-en-Y (RYGBP) surgery is that they experience a dramatic amelioration of blood glucose homeostasis and insulin sensitivity even before weight loss. The underlying mechanism behind this dramatic improvement is not fully understood. The dumping of nutrients into the distal small intestine stimulates an exaggerated GLP-1 peptide release from intestinal endocrine L-cells into the portal vein, stimulating insulin release. Humoral inhibitors for insulin release include somatostatin, amylin, leptin and pancreastatin. Vagus nerve generally stimulates insulin release, whereas the sympathetic nervous system inhibits it, mediated by various peptidergic molecules secreted from nerve fibers such as substance P, VIP, and neurotensin.

The exocrine pancreas on the other hand consists of two morphologically distinct structures. Acinar cells, the functional unit of the exocrine pancreas which secrete digestive enzymes, and duct cells that mainly secrete bicarbonate-rich fluid. The total external secretion of the pancreas consists of clear, colorless, bicarbonate-rich alkaline solution of about 2.5 L per day. Exocrine secretion is stimulated by the hormones secretin and cholecystokinin (CCK), and by parasympathetic vagal discharge. Serum amylase is usually measured to diagnose pancreatitis, which is usually 2.5× normal within 6 h after the onset of an acute episode, and then returns to normal within 3–7 days. However, the major limitation with the use of serum amylase measurement to diagnose pancreatitis is the lack of specificity as several clinical conditions can result in an elevated amylase. In addition, a normal serum amylase certainly does not exclude pancreatitis. The amylase-to-creatinine ratio

(ACR) may help in differentiating acute pancreatitis from other conditions using the following equation:

$$\left(\text{Urine}_{\text{amy}}\text{U/L} \times \text{Serum}_{\text{Cr}}\text{mg/dL}\right)/\left(\text{Serum}_{\text{amy}}\text{U/L} \times \text{Urine}_{\text{Cr}}\text{mg/dL}\right) \times 100$$

An ACR greater than 5% suggests acute pancreatitis, and ratios less than 1% suggest macroamylasemia. Serum lipase levels, on the other hand, are thought to be more specific in diagnosing pancreatic tissue damage because it is only produced in the pancreas. Lipase tends to be higher in alcoholic pancreatitis and the amylase level higher in gallstone pancreatitis, hence the lipase-to-amylase ratio has been suggested as means to distinguish between the two.

Imaging

There are several imaging modalities that are useful for investigating pancreatic disease overall. Each modality has its advantages and drawbacks. Often a combination of methods is required for the accurate diagnosis of conditions of the endocrine pancreas.

Plain Abdominal Radiographs

Although not useful for directly imaging the pancreas, plain abdominal radiographs may indirectly reveal an inflamed pancreas, demonstrating a 'sentinel loop', which is an isolated bowel segment (jejunum, transverse colon or duodenum) that is dilated next to the inflamed pancreas. Plain radiographs may also reveal the 'colon cutoff sign'. This sign represents the abrupt termination of gas within the proximal colon at the level of the radiographic splenic flexure which is caused by colonic spasm secondary to pancreatic inflammation. It must be noted however, that both signs are nonspecific for pancreatitis. In the setting of endocrine insufficiency in chronic pancreatitis, calcification may be visualized. Patients may also develop pleural effusions which can be seen on chest X-rays. Structural abnormalities such as annular pancreas may be associated with duodenal obstruction/atresia resulting in the classic 'double-bubble' sign on an abdominal X-ray.

Abdominal Ultrasonography (US)

US is a helpful imaging modality to examine the pancreas in pediatric patients, although overlying bowel gas can make imaging variable. It can be used as a simple, noninvasive test for diagnosing a mass within the pancreas, and can demonstrate a peri-pancreatic fluid collection and edema.

Abdominal Computed Tomography (CT) Scans

CT scans offer much better resolution of the pancreas than US in terms of assessing the size and location of an endocrine tumor within the pancreas or a tumor within the gastrinoma triangle. It is the imaging of choice for assessing complications of pancreatitis but it should be noted that inflammatory changes are not usually radiographically present during the first 72 h of pancreatic inflammation [6].

Endoscopic Retrograde Cholangiopancreatography (ERCP)

ERCP is increasingly being used in children with pancreaticobiliary disease, both as a diagnostic procedure and therapeutic tool, with complication rates similar to that seen in adults [7]. As a result, ERCP is now considered a safe and useful tool for use in children in the hands of a well-trained endoscopist.

Magnetic Resonance Cholangiopancreatography (MRCP)

MRCP is a noninvasive and safer test compared with ERCP in diagnosing choledocholithiasis in the setting of pancreatitis, especially if there is real concern that ERCP may worsen pancreatitis. Although it is not as sensitive as ERCP, with sensitivity reported as low as 38%. However, the use of secretin has shown very promising results with sensitivity and specificity approaching 98% up to 100% in assessing patients with pancreatic divisum or common bile duct obstruction, respectively [7]. It is now the initial imaging of choice in evaluating pancreatic ductal anatomy in children with unexplained or recurrent pancreatitis [8].

Other Imaging Modalities for the Endocrine Pancreas

Many researchers are looking into developing simple, noninvasive methods to image the β-cells in vivo in order to measure their mass, function, severity of disease and inflammation. With recent advances in imaging technology such as magnetic resonance imaging (MRI), positron emission tomography (PET), ultrasound backscatter microscopy, and fluorescence spectroscopy, this is starting to be a reality. Type 1 diabetics have a decrease in β-cell mass due to autoimmune destruction whereas type 2 patients have initially an increase in β-cell mass due to insulin resistance, but the increase can no longer compensate for the increase in insulin demand. Currently, the only true marker of β-cell mass in vivo that can be realistically used is insulin (or the pro-insulin by-product C-peptide). However, more than 90% of β-cells must be lost in order to detect inappropriate decreases in insulin and C-peptide levels relative to glucose levels. So essentially, no useful in vivo islet imaging modality currently exists, which is also due to other logistical problems such as the fact that islets make up only 2% of the whole pancreas, which lies in a retroperitoneal position.

Presently, researchers are looking at certain surface markers on β-cells, which could logically serve as a guide to measuring β-cell mass, such as glucose transporter-2 and glucagon-like peptide-1 receptor which are significantly downregulated during hyperglycemia. In addition, unique β-cell metabolism may provide a target for PET scans to target lymphocytes which infiltrate islets in type 1 diabetic patients. These lymphocytes may be tagged with an imaging contrast agent to monitor inflammation, and antibody-guided targeting of ultrasound-detectable micro-bubbles aggregating in the islet microcirculation to allow for sufficient β-cell mass imaging to name but a few. The ultimate aim is to develop a simple and reliable bedside method for monitoring disease progress and measuring the clinical response to therapy in diabetic patients.

Basic Pancreatic Embryology

The embryonic pancreas is known to pass through three stages of development [9]. The first is the undifferentiated stage where the endoderm evaginates to initiate pancreatic morphogenesis, with only insulin and glucagon genes being expressed at this stage [10]. The second phase involves epithelial branching morphogenesis with simultaneous formation of primitive ducts. This stage involves the separation of islet progenitors beginning to differentiate and losing their attachments to the basement membrane [11]. The third and final stage begins with the formation of acinar cells at the apices of the ductal structures, with the development of zymogen granules containing enzymes. Acinar cells usually commence enzyme secretion shortly after birth [9, 12].

Organogenesis of the pancreas is initiated with the regional specification of the undifferentiated primitive foregut tube by transcription factors pancreatic and duodenal homeobox 1 (Pdx1), which marks the pre-pancreatic endoderm and by pancreas transcription factor (PTF1a), where both are expressed in multipotent pancreatic progenitor cells [13]. The first appearance of the pancreas appears morphologically as a mesenchymal condensation at the level of the duodenal anlagen, distal to the stomach on the dorsal aspect of the foregut tube at embryonic day (E) 9.0 in mice. All cells expressing Pdx1 and PTF1a in the endoderm will eventually give rise to all of the epithelial cells in the adult pancreas, which includes endocrine, acinar, and

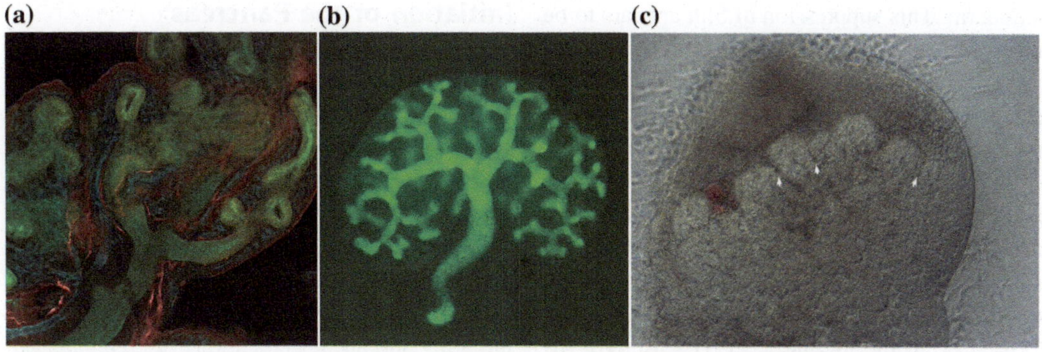

Fig. 11.4 Pancreatic branching morphogenesis is different than other organ systems such as lung and kidney. **a** Wholemount of E12.5 lung stained for Ecad, PGP9.5 (a neuronal marker) and CD31. **b** E11.5 kidney cultured for 3 days and stained with the epithelial marker Calbindin-D28 k, both demonstrating 90° branching pattern. **c** E11 whole pancreas from CD-1 cultured for five days revealing acute branching pattern mesenchymal exclusion zones (*arrow-head*). Mesenchyme contains factors that regulate pancreatic growth and differentiation

duct cells [1]. At around E9.5 gestation in mice and the twenty-sixth day of gestation in humans, the dorsal bud begins to evaginate into the overlying mesenchyme while retaining luminal continuity with the gut tube [14]. Approximately 12 h later in mice, and six days after dorsal bud evagination in humans, the ventral bud begins to arise. Gut rotation will bring the ventral lobe dorsally, ultimately fusing with the dorsal pancreatic bud (this event corresponds to around the sixth to seventh week of gestation in humans or E12-E13 in mice) contributing to the formation of the uncinate process and inferior part of the head of the pancreas, while the rest of the pancreas arises from the dorsal pancreatic bud. The entire ventral pancreatic duct and the distal part of the dorsal pancreatic duct fuse together to form the main pancreatic duct of Wirsung. The remaining proximal part of the dorsal pancreatic duct is either obliterated or persists as a small accessory pancreatic duct of Santorini [15]. This fusion of the two buds is followed by elongation of the pancreatic bud stalk region (precursor to the main pancreatic duct) and branching morphogenesis of the apical region of the bud. Unlike the usual branching morphogenesis growth patterns seen in the developing kidney, lung, and salivary gland, in which the branching morphogenesis occurs at 90° angles, the pancreas grows in an acute-angled branching pattern, which leads to the exclusion or 'squeezing out' of mesenchyme from between the closely apposed branches of epithelium (Fig. 11.4). This exclusion of mesenchyme may influence epithelial–mesenchymal interactions and lineage selection. The pancreas then undergoes major amplification of the endocrine cell population through two distinct waves of differentiation within the pancreatic epithelium during embryogenesis, an early primary wave (pre E13.5 in mice), followed by the secondary wave of differentiation (E13.5-E16.5 in mice) [1]. Over a similar gestational window the exocrine pancreatic precursors undergo an exponential increase in branching morphogenesis and acinar cell differentiation.

Dorsal and Ventral Pancreatic Bud Development

It is important to note that while the morphological development of the ventral and dorsal pancreatic buds may be similar, they differ markedly at the molecular level, with various lines of evidence suggesting that there are differences in the specification between both pancreatic rudiments, with the notochord playing a key role. Sonic hedgehog (Shh), which is a potent intercellular patterning molecule, is expressed along the entire foregut, is noticeably suppressed in the prospective pancreatic endoderm. This suppression of Shh appears to be necessary for dorsal pancreatic development, permitting the expression of pancreas specific genes including pdx1 and insulin. Deletion of the notochord in chick embryo cultures leads to ectopic Shh being seen in the pancreatic region of the foregut endoderm, with subsequent failure of the pancreas to develop [16]. Furthermore, the pancreatic anlage normally remains in contact with the notochord in mice until the paired dorsal aortae fuse in the midline (~E8.0). Activin-βB (a member of the transforming growth factor-β family) and FGF2 (fibroblast growth factor) both mimic notochord activity in inducing pancreatic genes [16]. In stark contrast to the dorsal bud, developmental gene expression in the ventral pancreatic anlage is not affected when the notochord is removed [17]. It appears that ventral pancreatic bud development is under the control of signals from the overlying cardiogenic mesenchyme, which also produces pro-hepatic signals (FGFs) to induce liver formation. Lack of pro-hepatic FGF signaling in regions of the cardiogenic mesenchyme will lead to the endoderm by 'default' differentiating into ventral pancreas [18]. When ventral foregut endoderm is cultured in the absence of cardiac mesoderm or FGF, it fails to activate liver specific genes, with instead pdx1 being expressed. Cardiac mesoderm, through FGF, induces liver formation from the ventral endoderm, and simultaneously inhibits pancreatic development [18]. Further differences between ventral and dorsal pancreas are demonstrated in Hlxb9 mutant mice. The homeobox gene Hlxb9, which is transiently expressed in the endoderm in the region of the dorsal and ventral pancreatic anlage, when inactivated in mice, only dorsal pancreatic development is blocked [19]. Hex is an early marker of the anterior endoderm [20] and is expressed at E7.0 in the cells that will subsequently gives rise to the ventral pancreas and liver. Hex null mutant embryos have specific failure of ventral pancreatic bud development, with the dorsal bud developing normally [21]. These examples underscore the significantly different molecular controls governing dorsal and ventral pancreatic bud development.

Initiation of the Pancreas with Endodermal Patterning

The signaling molecules that govern the specification of the primitive gut tube into different specialized domains remains yet to be fully elucidated [22]. The pancreas and other endoderm-derived organs develop through 'cross-talk' between the endoderm and the surrounding mesenchyme, which is a critical step in initiating organ specification or '*endodermal patterning*' along the anterior–posterior axis of the foregut endoderm. Endodermal patterning is manifested by the regional expression of transcription factors in the primitive gut tube; for example, Hex1 (Hematopoietically expressed homeobox1, an early marker of anterior endoderm) and Nkx2.1 (also known as Thyroid transcription factor 1) are expressed at E8.5 in defined foregut domains along the anterior–posterior axis of the primitive gut tube, giving rise to liver and lung/thyroid respectively. Pdx1 and PTF1a are co-expressed in the foregut–midgut endoderm boundary, defining the pancreas and duodenum, whereas Cdx1, and Cdx4 (early markers of posterior endoderm) are expressed in the posterior midgut and hindgut domains that will give rise to the small and large intestines. Thus, various domains of the primitive gut tube are specified [23, 24].

Mesenchyme-induced endodermal patterning is necessary before the initiation of organogenesis. When the pancreatic mesenchyme is removed from the pancreatic epithelium in explant cultures, it results in disrupted pancreatic cell differentiation, with the endocrine lineage being favored over exocrine [9].

The primitive gut tube is divided into three domains, foregut, midgut, and hindgut regions, each of which will give rise to specialized structures [13]. This subdivision into presumptive gut tube domains is governed by different molecular markers in the gastrula stage endoderm (E7.5) [13, 25, 26]. The endoderm toward the anterior side of the embryo generates the ventral foregut, which will later give rise to the liver, lung, thyroid, and the ventral pancreas. The dorsal region of the definitive endoderm, on the other hand, contributes to the formation of the esophagus, stomach, dorsal pancreas, duodenum, and intestines. The pancreas has been found to form as a result of the actions of some key specific transcription factors and signaling pathways. Fore example, FGF4 and Wnt signaling from the posterior mesoderm are specifically inhibited in the anterior endoderm to allow foregut development. FGF signaling is required to initially determine, and then to maintain gut tube domains, as demonstrated with cultured mouse endoderm and by in vivo studies in chick embryos. FGF4 is normally expressed in the mesoderm and ectoderm adjacent to the developing midgut–hindgut endoderm, and when isolated mouse endoderm is cultured in the presence of high concentrations of FGF4, a posterior (intestinal) endoderm was induced. On the other hand, lower concentrations of FGF4 induced a more anterior (pancreas–duodenal) cell fate. Similarly in chick embryos in vivo, when treated with FGF4, Hex1 (anterior endodermal marker) expression domain was reduced, whereas CdxB (posterior endodermal marker) expression expanded anteriorly, inhibiting the development of the foregut [23, 27]. Therefore, FGF4 plays a critical role in endodermal patterning by repressing anterior (foregut) fate and promoting posterior (intestinal) endoderm fate. Another molecular pathway that has linked endodermal patterning to the initiation of pancreatic development is Wnt/β-catenin signaling, as demonstrated in frog (*Xenopus*) studies [28]. β-catenin repression in the anterior endoderm is specifically necessary to initiate liver and pancreas development, and to maintaining foregut identity. Conversely, forcing high β-catenin activity in the posterior endoderm promotes intestinal development and inhibits foregut development. McLin et al. [28] demonstrated that forced β-catenin expression in the anterior endoderm (where β-catenin is usually repressed) led to downregulation of Hhex, as well as other foregut markers for liver (*for1*), pancreas (*pdx1*), lung/thyroid (*nkx2.1*), and intestine (*endocut*) [25], resulting in inhibition of foregut fate, namely liver and pancreas formation. Repressing β-catenin in the posterior endoderm (future hindgut that normally expresses β-catenin) induced ectopic liver and pancreas markers (hhex,pdx1, elastase, and amylase) with subsequent ectopic liver bud initiation and pancreas development [28]. The homeobox-containing gene Hhex, is a direct target of β-catenin and is one of the earliest foregut markers [20] and is essential for normal liver and ventral pancreas development in mice [21, 29]. *Hex* expression was noted to have an important role in the specification and differentiation of the ventral pancreas, where $Hex^{-/-}$ null mutant mouse embryos lacked a ventral pancreas, and lacked liver, thyroid, and parts of the forebrain [21, 30].

Retinoic acid (RA) signaling has been implicated as an important molecule for endodermal patterning in zebrafish. RA-signaling is necessary for specification and differentiation of both liver and pancreas [31]. As with RA, BMP signaling has also been shown to have a role in endodermal patterning and in the normal development of the pancreas in zebrafish, but neither RA nor BMP affect the induction of endodermal precursors [32]. Targeted disruption of the Pdx1 gene in mice also prevented pancreatic development [33]. A critical role for Pdx1 in pancreatic initiation and patterning of foregut endoderm in mice was further demonstrated by humans with Pdx1 mutations being apancreatic [34]. Unfortunately, despite our knowledge of many molecular signals mediating cross-talk between the pancreatic mesenchyme and the epithelium, most pathways remain poorly understood.

Pancreatic Mesenchyme

Following regional specification of the foregut tube, the pancreatic epithelium becomes enveloped by the pancreatic mesenchyme. Mesenchymal factors then promote growth and differentiation of the developing pancreas, specifically inducing growth of the endocrine cell population and rapid branching morphogenesis [1]. The early stages of pancreatic development involve a lineage selection by the pancreatic epithelium between endocrine and exocrine lineages [9], which is regulated by stimuli from the pancreatic mesenchyme [1]. This interaction between pancreatic mesenchyme and epithelium is a vital process for pancreatic development. Pure pancreatic epithelium (E11) without its mesenchyme failed to develop at all, however, the epithelium grew into a fully differentiated pancreas (acinar, ductal, and endocrine structures), when cultured with its mesenchyme [9]. The pancreatic mesenchyme has a pro-exocrine effect on the epithelium through cell–cell contact, and then also a pro-endocrine effect, mediated by diffusible factors secreted from the mesenchyme [35]. Mesenchymal contact with the epithelium both enhances notch signaling (Hes1), which favors the acinar lineage, and also inhibits neurogenin 3 expression (Ngn3) leading to the suppression of endocrine differentiation [36]. The 'default' differentiation of the pancreatic epithelium in the absence of mesenchyme is endocrine [9]. Interestingly, culturing pure pancreatic epithelium in a basement membrane rich gel, without its mesenchyme, led to the predominant formation of ductal structures. These results suggest that the basement membrane has factors or components which are conducive to ductal development [9]. To further illustrate the importance of the mesenchyme and mesenchymal signaling in embryonic and organ development, when the normal embryonic separation that occurs between the spleen and the pancreas-associated mesenchyme does not occur in Bapx1 null mutant embryos, the dorsal pancreatic bud gets intestinalized [37]. Activin A, which is expressed in the splenic mesenchyme, is a possible mediator for this transdifferentiation since exposing pancreatic buds to activin A in an in vitro culture system, leads to intestinalization [38].

Some signaling pathways have been implicated in mediating this epithelial–mesenchymal interaction, such as the FGF's. Specifically, FGF's 1, 7, and 10, which are expressed in the pancreatic mesenchyme, mediate their effects through FGF receptor 2B (FGFR2B), which is expressed in the pancreatic epithelium. Mesenchymal FGF signaling has been shown to induce epithelial proliferation favoring exocrine differentiation [39]. Similarly, null mutation of the receptor FGFR2B or the ligand FGF10 lead to blunting of early branching pancreatic morphogenesis, with inhibition of proliferation of endocrine progenitor cells and premature endocrine differentiation, indicating that FGF10 normally induces proliferation of epithelial cells, and prevents endocrine differentiation [40, 41]. Despite the positive role that FGF plays in dorsal pancreatic development, it seems to play a different role in ventral pancreatic bud development. FGF's secreted from the cardiogenic mesenchyme inhibit ventral pancreatic bud formation and favor liver development [18]. BMP ligands in pancreatic mesenchyme induce epithelial branching and inhibit endocrine differentiation [42].

Key Signaling Molecules

TGF-β Signaling

Transforming growth factor-beta (TGF-β) superfamily signaling has been implicated in many developmental processes, including pancreatic development. The superfamily consists of three main subfamilies, TGF-β isoforms (numbered 1–3 in mammals), BMP's, and activins. TGF-β isoform receptors during the early stages of pancreatic development are distributed throughout the pancreatic epithelium and mesenchyme, but then gradually become restricted to the pancreatic islets and ducts [43]. TGF-β ligands (TGF-β1, -β 2, and -β3) on the other hand are specifically localized to the pancreatic embryonic epithelium as early as E12.5, and then progressively become focused to the acinar cells, where they mediate their actions through TGF-β receptor type II [43]. Blocking TGF-β signaling in the embryonic pancreas, either with the in vivo overexpression of dominant-negative TGF-β type II receptor, or with the in vitro TGF-β-specific pan-neutralizing antibody, leads to a profound increase in the number of proliferating endocrine cells. This expansion of endocrine cells occurred in the periductal area [85]. Thus overall, TGF-β isoform signaling suppresses the transition of endocrine cells from the ducts in the embryonic pancreas, and TGF-β isoform inhibition allows pancreatic ductal epithelial cells to proliferate and differentiate into endocrine cells [43].

Once TGF-β ligands bind to their receptor, intracellular signaling is mediated by Smads. Interestingly smad4 mutations were specifically mutated in 50% of pancreatic cancers [44]. However, a key role for smad4 has not been identified yet in pancreatic development [45]. Smad7 on the other hand, which acts as a general TGF signaling inhibitor, when expressed under the pdx1 promoter, resulted in a 90% decrease in β-cells at birth, which were replaced by glucagon cells [46].

Notch Signaling

Notch signaling has been identified as an important regulator of the decision between endocrine and exocrine pancreatic lineages [47]. Activation of the Notch receptor leads to the activation of HES1 (Hairy-Enhancer of Split 1) and repression of genes such as Ngn3 (neurogenin3, a prerequisite marker for pancreatic endocrine lineage development) [47]. Notch also serves to maintain cells in an undifferentiated progenitor-like state. Impairing Notch signaling leads to premature differentiation of pancreatic progenitor cells into endocrine cells. However, the exact mechanism for Notch signaling in pancreatic lineage selection remains elusive, and ambiguity still surrounds the exact role of Notch signaling in pancreatic development.

Hedgehog Signaling

The mammalian hedgehog family consists of sonic hedgehog (Shh), desert hedgehog (Dhh), and Indian hedgehog (Ihh). *Shh* signaling is essential for foregut differentiation towards a gastrointestinal fate [48] and its suppression in the prospective pancreatic endoderm is a prerequisite for pancreas formation. However, targeted deletion of *Shh* in the foregut of mice does not lead to an expanded pancreatic field as would be expected [49, 50]. Null mutant mice for Indian hedgehog (Ihh) develop a small pancreas, indicating a pro-pancreatic role for Ihh [51]. Furthermore, combining a *Shh* null mutation with a heterozygous mutation for *Ihh* results in an annular pancreas.

There appears to be a link between aberrant Hh signaling and pancreatic exocrine neoplasia, with the upregulation of *Shh* ligand being observed in noninvasive lesions preceding pancreatic adenocarcinoma [52]. In addition, it has been demonstrated that *Shh* ligand secreted by pancreatic cancer epithelium binds to stromal cells in a paracrine fashion, causing proliferation and 'desmoplasia' [53–55]. Clinical trials are in place to neutralize and target Hh molecules in patients with pancreatic adenocarcinoma [56]. Shh was not thought to be expressed in the normal pancreas [16] until recently when Strobel et al. [57] identified expression in a specialized compartment within the proximal ductal system, known as the pancreatic duct glands (PDGs), which are blind-ending outpouches, that specifically produce Shh ligand. When exposed to chronic injury, PDGs grow, associated with an upregulation of Shh expression (along with gastric mucins and other progenitor markers such as pdx1 and hes1). This process leads to a Shh-mediated mucinous gastrointestinal metaplasia with features of a pancreatic intraepithelial neoplasia (PanIN). PanIN's are pancreatic cancer precursor lesions of unclear origin that are known to aberrantly express Shh and gastrointestinal mucins. They are thought to arise from ducts, and thus PDG may be the missing link between Shh, mucinous metaplasia, and neoplasia [48].

Wnt's

Wnt signaling plays a role in early endodermal specification of pancreas since β-catenin repression in the anterior endoderm is necessary to initiate liver and pancreas development (see earlier section). However, beyond endodermal patterning Wnt signaling has multiple pancreatic roles which depend on the time and place of Wnt signaling. Transgenic expression of Wnt1 or Wnt5a in the pancreatic epithelium leads to pancreatic agenesis or severe hypoplasia, respectively, confirming that early Wnt signaling is detrimental to pancreatic development. Others found a role for Wnt signaling in promoting post-natal pancreatic growth [58], illustrating the complex and multiple roles that Wnt's play in pancreatic development.

Endothelial Cells and Oxygen Tension

It has been shown that cells exposed to low oxygen tensions go through adaptive changes such anaerobic metabolism, increased angiogenesis, and erythropoeisis [59]. In pancreatic development, beta cell differentiation seems to be influenced by oxygen tension. A key mediator for this adaptive response by cells is hypoxia-inducible factor (HIF) [60]. HIF1α is expressed strongly in the rat pancreatic epithelium and mesenchyme at E11.5, then gradually decreases and is virtually undetectable by birth. Hypoxia leads to the stabilization of HIF1α, resulting in absent Ngn3 expression and thus arresting beta cell differentiation. Increasing oxygen tension leads to upregulation of beta cell differentiation with degradation of HIF1α, and restoration of Ngn3. Similarly, inhibiting the degradation of HIF1α resulted in the repression of Ngn3 and arrest of beta cell differentiation, even in normoxia [60].

Endothelial Cells

Islet transplantation entails an enzymatic digestion process that also removes some intraislet endothelial cells [61, 62]. This endothelial removal may take away an important vascular niche for the β-cells. Pancreatic islets are highly vascularized, embedded in a capillary network that is five to ten times denser than that of the exocrine pancreas, and allows efficient secretion of islet hormones into the bloodstream [63]

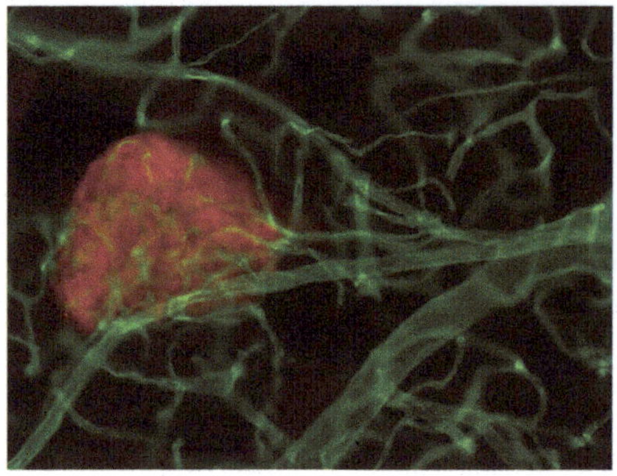

Fig. 11.5 Wholemount adult mouse pancreas, stained with CD31 and insulin demonstrating the complex microcapillary network within the islet

(Fig. 11.5). During development, β-cells aggregate to form islets, and express high levels of vascular endothelial growth factors (VEGF) to attract endothelial cells [64]. β-cells deficient in VEGF-A form islets with less capillaries, and experimental overexpression of VEGF-A has improved islet graft vascularization [64, 65]. Thus, there is an intimate relationship between blood vessels and the pancreatic cells during embryonic development. As the embryonic pancreas progresses through the different developmental stages, it receives signals from different adjacent structures, including notochord, cardiac mesoderm, and the doral aortae. Removal of the dorsal aorta from Xenopus embryos led to the absence of pancreatic endocrine development [66]. In addition, aortic endothelial cells can induce dorsal pancreatic bud and β-cell formation in vitro from endoderm. Interestingly, ventral pancreas development seems not to be dependent on the endothelium, despite its close proximity to the vitelline veins [67]. This difference was corroborated in a human with aortic coarctation. The patient lacked the pancreatic body and tail, but not the head of the pancreas, with the latter arising from the ventral bud and develops independently of the aortae [68]. Here, the prospective pancreatic endoderm presumably lost the inducing signal from the 'narrowed' aorta, leading to dorsal pancreatic agenesis.

Extracellular Matrix

The pancreatic epithelium is contained within a continuous sheath of basement membrane, which constitutes the epithelial–mesenchymal interface, and plays an important role in guiding pancreatic development [69]. Basement membrane has also been shown to play an important role in regulating branching morphogenesis in many other organs, with laminin and collagen IV the major protein components of all basement membranes [70]. Laminin-1 was found to induce duct formation in isolated E11 mouse pancreatic epithelium [26], and to mediate the pro-exocrine inductive effect of the mesenchyme, as well as the pro-β-cell role later in gestation [35, 71]. β-cells are unable to form their own basement membrane but depend on the endothelial cells to produce a vascular basement membrane. Endothelial cells also produce collagen IV, which interacts with α1β1 integrin to increase insulin secretion [72]. Cadherins (**Ca**lcium-dependent **ad**hesion molecules), which are critical for cell–cell adhesion, play an essential role in migration and differentiation of pancreatic endocrine progenitor cells. E-cadherin and R-cadherin are initially localized to the ducts, and then become downregulated in endocrine progenitor cells as they move out of the ducts to form islets [73, 74]. N-CAM is a cell adhesion molecule that is expressed in mature α- and PP cells [75] and is necessary for aggregation of endocrine cells within the islet [76].

Glucagon

The first detectable endocrine cells during pancreatic development are the glucagon-containing cells at around E9 in the mouse, and recent studies have shown that glucagon signaling is necessary for early differentiation of insulin expressing cells, which appear at E10-E13 [14, 77]. Glucagon is generated from pro-glucagon by the action of pro-hormone convertase 2 (PC2). When PC2 or the glucagon receptor is knocked out, mutant mice lack glucagon and have delayed islet cell differentiation and maturation, but still show the large amplification of insulin-positive cells ('secondary wave') later in gestation [78]. These studies strongly support the role of glucagon signaling, through its receptor, in initiating early insulin differentiation. Recently it has been demonstrated that α-cells can be reprogrammed to form new β-cells during regeneration after ablating nearly 99% of the existing β-cells [79].

Transcription Factors

Transcription factors are key elements to orchestrating the formation of all endocrine and exocrine cell lineages, and their roles have been extensively studied in pancreatic development. The most heavily studied transcription factor is pdx1, one of the earliest markers for pancreatic progenitors that later is expressed only in β-cells. It is expressed in the pre-pancreatic region of the primitive foregut tube at E8.5 then expands to be expressed in distal stomach, common bile duct, and duodenum by E10.5-11.5 [1]. Pdx1 is initially expressed throughout the epithelium, however, its expression becomes suppressed in cells as they commit to the endocrine lineage or ducts. It then reappears as cells differentiate to the insulin-positive-β-cell lineage. Pdx1 null mutant mice and humans that lack pdx1 gene have pancreatic agenesis [34]. Delayed pdx1 inhibition using a tetracycline regulatable transgenic knock-in system demonstrated severe blunting of pancreatic development with complete absence of acini and β-cells [80], indicating that pdx1 continues to have a role in pancreas development beyond early regional specification during endodermal patterning.

PTf1a

Pancreas specific transcription factor 1a (PTF1a) is an early marker of pancreatic progenitor cells, expressed slightly later than pdx1 at around E9.5, and then becomes localized to the acini by E18.5 [81]. PTF1a null mutant mice develop severe pancreatic hypoplasia and absent acini and ducts, however endocrine cells still develop and, interestingly, the endocrine cells migrate out through the pancreatic mesenchyme to form islets in the spleen [82].

Ngn3

The transcription factor Ngn3 is required for endocrine lineage development. It is first expressed at E9.0, and then peaks at around E15.5, and is thought to be antagonized by Notch signaling through Hes1 in cells with an acinar fate [83]. Ngn3 cells proliferate, giving rise to post-mitotic endocrine progenitor cells expressing transcription factors neuroD, nkx6.1, and pax6. Ngn3 shuts off at around E17.5 [83, 84]. When Ngn3 is deleted from cells, it leads to the absence of the four endocrine cell types (α, β, δ, and PP) that produce glucagon, insulin, somatostatin, and pancreatic polypeptide, respectively [85]. Thus, Ngn3 appears to be a critical and essential factor for pancreatic endocrine differentiation acting as a pro-endocrine gene.

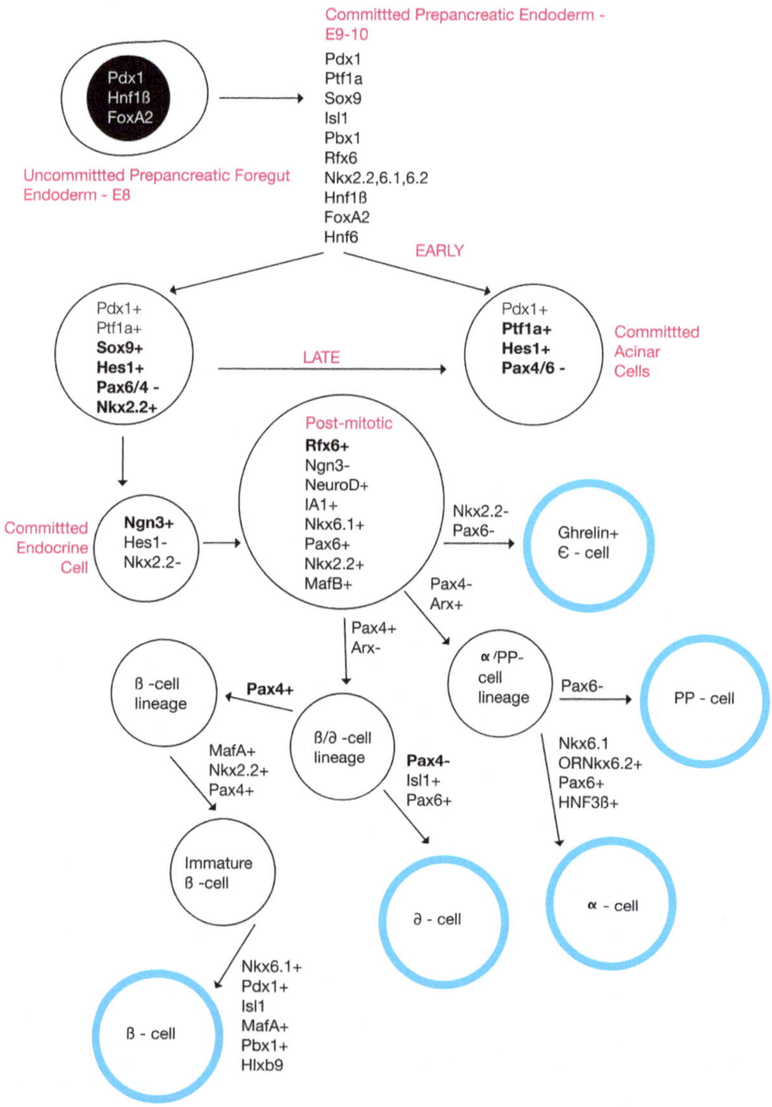

Fig. 11.6 Overview of the pancreatic endocrine and exocrine cell lineage

Rfx6

Rfx6 is a transcription factor downstream of Ngn3 that has been identified as a key pro-endocrine regulator that directs islet cell differentiation. Mice that are null-mutant for Rfx6 fail to generate all islet cell types except pancreatic polypeptide cells (insulin, glucagon, somatostatin, and ghrelin). A human syndrome of neonatal diabetes (patients lack pancreatic endocrine cells) with bowel atresia was show to have mutations in the Rfx6 gene [86].

Nkx2.2

Nkx2.2 is expressed as early as E9.5, is co-expressed with pdx1 as a marker of multipotent pancreatic progenitor cells, and eventually becomes restricted to Ngn3-positive cells, persisting in all endocrine lineages except for δ-cells [87]. Nkx2.2 null mutant mice develop with no β-cells, reduced PP cells, 80% reduction in α-cells, but no effect on δ-cells. Interestingly, a large number of ghrelin-positive ε-cells with no glucagon co-expression were seen, indicating that Nkx2.2 normally induces insulin-positive differentiation and represses ε-cell formation [87].

MafA/B

There are two distinct waves of amplification of the endocrine cell population, primary (pre E13.5) and secondary (E13.5-E16.5) transition periods. MafB is expressed in endocrine cells during both waves. As insulin-positive cells form into mature β-cells, MafB turns off and the cells then express MafA [88]. MafA is first expressed only in the secondary wave β-cells and in adult β-cells. MafA is a critical regulator of the insulin gene, and is viewed as the only transcription factor specific to β-cells. However, it is not absolutely necessary for β-cell formation since mafA null mutant mice have a normal proportion of insulin-positive cells at birth [89].

Sox9

Sox9 is a marker for those pancreatic progenitor cells that can give rise to all pancreatic cell types, and is necessary for maintaining those cells in a progenitor state [90]. Postnatally, sox9 expression becomes restricted to the ductal and centroacinar cell compartment [91]. Sox9 mutants display pancreatic hypoplasia as a result of depletion of the pancreatic progenitor pool [91] (Fig. 11.6).

References

1. Gittes GK. Developmental biology of the pancreas: a comprehensive review. Dev Biol. 2009;326:4–35.
2. Gray S. Russo K Gray's anatomy, Ill. Woodstock: Dramatic Publishing; 2008.
3. Kim A, Miller K, Jo J, et al. Islet architecture: a comparative study. Islets. 2009;1:129–36.
4. Baggio LL, Drucker DJ. Biology of incretins: GLP-1 and GIP. Gastroenterology. 2007;132:2131–57.
5. Scheen AJ. Radermecker RP Addition of incretin therapy to metformin in type 2 diabetes. Lancet. 2010;375:1410–2.
6. Imamura Y, Hirota M, Ida S, et al. Significance of renal rim grade on computed tomography in severity evaluation of acute pancreatitis. Pancreas. 2010;39:41–6.
7. Paris C, Bejjani J, Beaunoyer M, et al. Endoscopic retrograde cholangiopancreatography is useful and safe in children. J Pediatr Surg. 2010;45:938–42.
8. Neblett WW 3rd, O'Neill JA Jr. Surgical management of recurrent pancreatitis in children with pancreas divisum. Ann Surg. 2000;231:899–908.
9. Gittes GK, Galante PE, Hanahan D, et al. Lineage-specific morphogenesis in the developing pancreas: role of mesenchymal factors. Development. 1996 122:439–447 (Cambridge, England).
10. Gittes GK, Rutter WJ. Onset of cell-specific gene expression in the developing mouse pancreas. Proc Natl Acad Sci U S A. 1992;89:1128–32.
11. Argent BE, Githens S, Kalser S, et al. The pancreatic duct cell. Pancreas. 1992;7:403–19.
12. Kolacek S, Puntis JW, Lloyd DR, et al. Ontogeny of pancreatic exocrine function. Arch Dis Child. 1990;65:178–81.
13. Moore-Scott BA, Opoka R, Lin SC, et al. Identification of molecular markers that are expressed in discrete anterior-posterior domains of the endoderm from the gastrula stage to mid-gestation. Dev Dyn. 2007;236:1997–2003.

14. Pictet RL, Clark WR, Williams RH, et al. An ultrastructural analysis of the developing embryonic pancreas. Dev Biol. 1972;29:436–67.
15. Sadler TW, Langman J. Langman's medical embryology. Philadelphia: Lippincott Williams & Wilkins; 2006.
16. Hebrok M, Kim SK, Melton DA. Notochord repression of endodermal Sonic hedgehog permits pancreas development. Genes Dev. 1998;12:1705–13.
17. Kim SK, Hebrok M, Melton DA. Notochord to endoderm signaling is required for pancreas development. Development. 1997;124:4243–52 (Cambridge, England).
18. Deutsch G, Jung J, Zheng M, et al. A bipotential precursor population for pancreas and liver within the embryonic endoderm. Development 2001;128:871–81 (Cambridge, England).
19. Li H, Arber S, Jessell TM, et al. Selective agenesis of the dorsal pancreas in mice lacking homeobox gene Hlxb9. Nat Genet. 1999;23:67–70.
20. Thomas PQ, Brown A, Beddington RS. Hex: a homeobox gene revealing peri-implantation asymmetry in the mouse embryo and an early transient marker of endothelial cell precursors. Development 1998;125:85–94 (Cambridge, England).
21. Bort R, Martinez-Barbera JP, Beddington RS, et al. Hex homeobox gene-dependent tissue positioning is required for organogenesis of the ventral pancreas. Development 2004;131:797–806 (Cambridge, England).
22. Wells JM, Melton DA. Vertebrate endoderm development. Annu Rev Cell Dev Biol. 1999;15:393–410.
23. Dessimoz J, Opoka R, Kordich JJ, et al. FGF signaling is necessary for establishing gut tube domains along the anterior-posterior axis in vivo. Mech Dev. 2006;123:42–55.
24. Ehrman LA, Yutzey KE. Anterior expression of the caudal homologue cCdx-B activates a posterior genetic program in avian embryos. Dev Dyn. 2001;221:412–21.
25. Costa RM, Mason J, Lee M, et al. Novel gene expression domains reveal early patterning of the Xenopus endoderm. Gene Expr Patterns. 2003;3:509–19.
26. Grapin-Botton A. Antero-posterior patterning of the vertebrate digestive tract: 40 years after Nicole Le Douarin's PhD thesis. Int J Dev Biol 2005;49:335–47.
27. Shamim H, Mason I. Expression of Fgf4 during early development of the chick embryo. Mech Dev. 1999;85:189–92.
28. McLin VA, Rankin SA, Zorn AM. Repression of Wnt/beta-catenin signaling in the anterior endoderm is essential for liver and pancreas development. Development 2007;134:2207–17 (Cambridge, England).
29. Keng VW, Yagi H, Ikawa M, et al. Homeobox gene Hex is essential for onset of mouse embryonic liver development and differentiation of the monocyte lineage. Biochem Biophys Res Commun. 2000;276:1155–61.
30. Martinez Barbera JP, Clements M, Thomas P, et al. The homeobox gene Hex is required in definitive endodermal tissues for normal forebrain, liver and thyroid formation. Development 2000;127:2433–45 (Cambridge, England).
31. Stafford D, Hornbruch A, Mueller PR, et al. A conserved role for retinoid signaling in vertebrate pancreas development. Dev Genes Evol. 2004;214:432–41.
32. Tiso N, Filippi A, Pauls S, et al. BMP signalling regulates anteroposterior endoderm patterning in zebrafish. Mech Dev. 2002;118:29–37.
33. Ahlgren U, Jonsson J, Edlund H. The morphogenesis of the pancreatic mesenchyme is uncoupled from that of the pancreatic epithelium in IPF1/PDX1-deficient mice. Development 1996;122:1409–16 (Cambridge, England).
34. Stoffers DA, Zinkin NT, Stanojevic V, et al. Pancreatic agenesis attribu to a single nucleotide deletion in the human IPF1 gene coding sequence. Nat Genet. 1997;15:106–10.
35. Li Z, Manna P, Kobayashi H, et al. Multifaceted pancreatic mesenchymal control of epithelial lineage selection. Dev Biol. 2004;269:252–63.
36. Duvillie B, Attali M, Bounacer A, et al. The mesenchyme controls the timing of pancreatic beta-cell differentiation. Diabetes. 2006;55:582–9.
37. Asayesh A, Sharpe J, Watson RP, et al. Spleen versus pancreas: strict control of organ interrelationship revealed by analyses of Bapx1−/− mice. Genes Dev. 2006;20:2208–13.
38. van Eyll JM, Pierreux CE, Lemaigre FP, et al. Shh-dependent differentiation of intestinal tissue from embryonic pancreas by activin A. J Cell. 2004;117:2077–86.
39. Elghazi L, Cras-Meneur C, Czernichow P, et al. Role for FGFR2IIIb-mediated signals in controlling pancreatic endocrine progenitor cell proliferation. Proc Natl Acad Sci U S A. 2002;99:3884–9.
40. Bhushan A, Itoh N, Kato S, et al. Fgf10 is essential for maintaining the proliferative capacity of epithelial progenitor cells during early pancreatic organogenesis. Development 2001;128:5109–17 (Cambridge, England).
41. Pulkkinen MA, Spencer-Dene B, Dickson C, et al. The IIIb isoform of fibroblast growth factor receptor 2 is required for proper growth and branching of pancreatic ductal epithelium but not for differentiation of exocrine or endocrine cells. Mech Dev. 2003;120:167–75.
42. Ahnfelt-Ronne J, Ravassard P, Pardanaud-Glavieux C, et al. Mesenchymal bone morphogenetic protein signaling is required for normal pancreas development. Diabetes 59:1948–1956.
43. Tulachan SS, Tei E, Hembree M, et al. TGF-beta isoform signaling regulates secondary transition and mesenchymal-induced endocrine development in the

embryonic mouse pancreas. Dev Biol. 2007;305:508–21.
44. Hahn SA, Schutte M, Hoque AT, et al. DPC4, a candidate tumor suppressor gene at human chromosome 18q21.1. Science. 1996;271:350–3.
45. Bardeesy N, Cheng KH, Berger JH, et al. Smad4 is dispensable for normal pancreas development yet critical in progression and tumor biology of pancreas cancer. Genes Dev. 2006;20:3130–46.
46. Smart NG, Apelqvist AA, Gu X, et al. Conditional expression of Smad7 in pancreatic beta cells disrupts TGF-beta signaling and induces reversible diabetes mellitus. PLoS Biol. 2006;4:e39.
47. Apelqvist A, Li H, Sommer L, et al. Notch signalling controls pancreatic cell differentiation. Nature. 1999;400:877–81.
48. Maitra A. Tracking down the hedgehog's lair in the pancreas. Gastroenterology. 2010;138:823–5.
49. Litingtung Y, Lei L, Westphal H, et al. Sonic hedgehog is essential to foregut development. Nat Genet. 1998;20:58–61.
50. Ramalho-Santos M, Melton DA, McMahon AP Hedgehog signals regulate multiple aspects of gastrointestinal development. Development 2000;127:2763–72 (Cambridge, England).
51. Hebrok M, Kim SK, St Jacques B, et al. Regulation of pancreas development by hedgehog signaling. Development 2000;127:4905–13 (Cambridge, England).
52. Pasca di Magliano M, Sekine S, Ermilov A, et al. Hedgehog/Ras interactions regulate early stages of pancreatic cancer. Genes Dev. 2006;20:3161–73.
53. Bailey JM, Swanson BJ, Hamada T, et al. Sonic hedgehog promotes desmoplasia in pancreatic cancer. Clin Cancer Res. 2008;14:5995–6004.
54. Olive KP, Jacobetz MA, Davidson CJ, et al. Inhibition of Hedgehog signaling enhances delivery of chemotherapy in a mouse model of pancreatic cancer. Science. 2009;324:1457–61.
55. Yauch RL, Gould SE, Scales SJ, et al. A paracrine requirement for hedgehog signalling in cancer. Nature. 2008;455:406–10.
56. Hidalgo M, Maitra A. The hedgehog pathway and pancreatic cancer. N Engl J Med. 2009;361:2094–6.
57. Strobel O, Rosow DE, Rakhlin EY, et al. Pancreatic duct glands are distinct ductal compartments that react to chronic injury and mediate Shh-induced metaplasia. Gastroenterology. 2010;138:1166–77.
58. Heiser PW, Lau J, Taketo MM, et al. Stabilization of beta-catenin impacts pancreas growth. Development 2006;133:2023–2032 (Cambridge, England).
59. Semenza GL. Life with oxygen. Science. 2007;318:62–4.
60. Heinis M, Simon MT, Ilc K, et al. Oxygen tension regulates pancreatic beta-cell differentiation through hypoxia-inducible factor 1alpha. Diabetes. 2010;59:662–9.
61. Couzin J. Diabetes. Islet transplants face test of time. Science. 2004;306:34–7.
62. Konstantinova I, Lammert E. Microvascular development: learning from pancreatic islets. BioEssays. 2004;26:1069–75.
63. Eberhard D, Kragl M. Lammert E 'Giving and taking': endothelial and beta-cells in the islets of Langerhans. Trends Endocrinol Metab. 2010;21:457–63.
64. Lammert E, Gu G, McLaughlin M, et al. Role of VEGF-A in vascularization of pancreatic islets. Curr Biol. 2003;13:1070–4.
65. Zhang N, Richter A, Suriawinata J, et al. Elevated vascular endothelial growth factor production in islets improves islet graft vascularization. Diabetes. 2004;53:963–70.
66. Lammert E, Cleaver O, Melton D. Induction of pancreatic differentiation by signals from blood vessels. Science. 2001;294:564–7.
67. Yoshitomi H, Zaret KS. Endothelial cell interactions initiate dorsal pancreas development by selectively inducing the transcription factor Ptf1a. Development 2004;131:807–17 (Cambridge, England).
68. Kapa S, Gleeson FC, Vege SS. Dorsal pancreas agenesis and polysplenia/heterotaxy syndrome: a novel association with aortic coarctation and a review of the literature. JOP. 2007;8:433–7.
69. Hisaoka M, Haratake J, Hashimoto H. Pancreatic morphogenesis and extracellular matrix organization during rat development. Differ; Res Biol Divers. 1993;53:163–72.
70. Hallmann R, Horn N, Selg M, et al. Expression and function of laminins in the embryonic and mature vasculature. Physiol Rev. 2005;85:979–1000.
71. Jiang FX, Georges-Labouesse E, Harrison LC. Regulation of laminin 1-induced pancreatic beta-cell differentiation by alpha6 integrin and alpha-dystroglycan. Mol Med. 2001;7:107–14 (Cambridge, Mass).
72. Kaido T, Yebra M, Cirulli V, et al. Regulation of human beta-cell adhesion, motility, and insulin secretion by collagen IV and its receptor alpha1beta1. J Biol Chem. 2004;279:53762–9.
73. Dahl U, Sjodin A, Semb H. Cadherins regulate aggregation of pancreatic beta-cells in vivo. Development 1996;122:2895–902 (Cambridge, England).
74. Sjodin A, Dahl U, Semb H. Mouse R-cadherin: expression during the organogenesis of pancreas and gastrointestinal tract. Exp Cell Res. 1995;221:413–25.
75. Cirulli V, Baetens D, Rutishauser U, et al. Expression of neural cell adhesion molecule (N-CAM) in rat islets and its role in islet cell type segregation. J Cell Sci. 1994;107(Pt 6):1429–36.
76. Esni F, Taljedal IB, Perl AK, et al. Neural cell adhesion molecule (N-CAM) is required for cell type segregation and normal ultrastructure in pancreatic islets. J Cell Biol. 1999;144:325–37.
77. Prasadan K, Daume E, Preuett B, et al. Glucagon is required for early insulin-positive differentiation in the developing mouse pancreas. Diabetes. 2002;51:3229–36.

78. Vincent M, Guz Y, Rozenberg M, et al. Abrogation of protein convertase 2 activity results in delayed islet cell differentiation and maturation, increased alpha-cell proliferation, and islet neogenesis. Endocrinology. 2003;144:4061–9.
79. Thorel F, Nepote V, Avril I, et al. Conversion of adult pancreatic alpha-cells to beta-cells after extreme beta-cell loss. Nature. 2010;464:1149–54.
80. Holland AM, Hale MA, Kagami H, et al. Experimental control of pancreatic development and maintenance. Proc Natl Acad Sci U S A. 2002;99:12236–41.
81. Cras-Meneur C, Li L, Kopan R, et al. Presenilins, Notch dose control the fate of pancreatic endocrine progenitors during a narrow developmental window. Genes Dev. 2009;23:2088–101.
82. Kawaguchi Y, Cooper B, Gannon M, et al. The role of the transcriptional regulator Ptf1a in converting intestinal to pancreatic progenitors. Nat Genet. 2002;32:128–34.
83. Jensen J, Heller RS, Funder-Nielsen T, et al. Independent development of pancreatic alpha- and beta-cells from neurogenin3-expressing precursors: a role for the notch pathway in repression of premature differentiation. Diabetes. 2000;49:163–76.
84. Gu G, Dubauskaite J, Melton DA. Direct evidence for the pancreatic lineage: NGN3+ cells are islet progenitors and are distinct from duct progenitors. Development 2002;129:2447–2457 (Cambridge, England).
85. Gradwohl G, Dierich A, LeMeur M, et al. neurogenin3 is required for the development of the four endocrine cell lineages of the pancreas. Proc Natl Acad Sci U S A. 2000;97:1607–11.
86. Smith SB, Qu HQ, Taleb N, et al. Rfx6 directs islet formation and insulin production in mice and humans. Nature. 2010;463(7282):775–80.
87. Sussel L, Kalamaras J, Hartigan-O'Connor DJ, et al. Mice lacking the homeodomain transcription factor Nkx2.2 have diabetes due to arrested differentiation of pancreatic beta cells. Development 1998;125:2213–21 (Cambridge, England).
88. Artner I, Hang Y, Mazur M, et al. MafA and MafB regulate genes critical to beta cells in a unique temporal manner. Diabetes. 2010;59(10):2530–9.
89. Nishimura W, Bonner-Weir S, Sharma A. Expression of MafA in pancreatic progenitors is detrimental for pancreatic development. Dev Bio. 2009;333:108–20.
90. Akiyama H, Kim JE, Nakashima K, et al. Osteo-chondroprogenitor cells are derived from Sox9 expressing precursors. Proc Natl Acad Sci U S A. 2005;102:14665–70.
91. Seymour PA, Freude KK, Tran MN, et al. SOX9 is required for maintenance of the pancreatic progenitor cell pool. Proc Natl Acad Sci USA. 2007;104:1865–70.

12 Congenital Hyperinsulinism

Khalid Hussain, Shireen A. Nah and Agostino Pierro

Congenital hyperinsulinism (CHI) is a condition characterised by the inappropriate secretion of insulin from the pancreatic β-cell. The unregulated insulin secretion leads to severe and profound hypoglycaemia which is a major cause of mental retardation, epilepsy and cerebral palsy [1]. CHI typically presents in the newborn period with severe hypoglycaemia but can also present in the infancy and childhood periods where it tends to be milder. The incidence of CHI can vary from 1 in 40,000–50,000 in the general population to 1 in 2500 in some isolated communities with high rates of consanguinity [2]. Mutations in genes which play a role in regulating insulin secretion underlie the genetic basis of CHI.

The biochemical diagnosis of CHI involves the documentation of inappropriate insulin secretion in the presence of hypoglycaemia [2]. The key step in the management of patients with CHI is the avoidance of hypoglycaemia by providing concentrated intravenous dextrose infusions and or high calorie oral feeds. Specific pharmacological intervention is attempted with drugs, such as diazoxide, octreotide and glucagon but some patients do not respond to these medications. In those patients who show no response to medical therapy the surgical option is the only route. Histological examination of pancreatic tissue from patients who have undergone a pancreatectomy shows that there are two major histological forms of CHI, namely diffuse and focal [3]. Pre-operative differentiation of these two histological subgroups is crucial before any surgical intervention is planned, as the surgical approach will be different for diffuse and focal forms [4]. Traditionally, those patients with diffuse CHI will require a near total pancreatectomy (95–98%), whereas those patients with the focal type will only require a limited pancreatectomy which provides a cure for the patient from the hypoglycaemia point [5].

The field of CHI has exploded in the last a few years with advances in molecular genetics, novel imaging modalities and advances in laparoscopic surgery for medically unresponsive focal and diffuse forms of CHI. This chapter will provide an overview of CHI focussing on the clinical presentation, diagnosis, pathophysiology, the histological subtypes of CHI, imaging techniques used in CHI patients and discuss the role of surgery in patients with medically unresponsive forms of CHI.

K. Hussain (✉)
Department of Paediatrics, Division of Endocrinology, Sidra Medical and Research Centre, OPC, C6-337, Doha PO Box 26999, Qatar
e-mail: khussain@sidra.org

S.A. Nah
The Surgery Unit2, UCL Institute of Child Health, Great Ormond Street Hospital for Children, NHS Trust, University College London, London, UK

A. Pierro
Department of Pediatric General and Thoracic Surgery, Hospital for Sick Children, 555 University Avenue, Toronto, ON M5G 1X8, Canada

D.J. Ledbetter and P.R.V. Johnson (eds.), *Endocrine Surgery in Children*,
DOI 10.1007/978-3-662-54256-9_12

Clinical Presentation and Diagnosis

CHI most commonly presents in the newborn with severe and persistent hypoglycaemia but it can also present during infancy and childhood where it tends to be milder. The hypoglycaemia is usually refractory to oral feeds and normoglycaemia can only be maintained by giving large volumes of concentrated dextrose infusions [2]. Patients can present either with mild non-specific symptoms of hypoglycaemic (such as poor feeding, lethargy and irritability) or more severe symptoms (such as apnoea, seizures or even coma). As a result of the in utero hyperinsulinaemia newborns with CHI are typically macrosomic, however the absence of macrosomia does not exclude CHI. Fetal hyperinsulinaemia also accounts for the hypertrophic cardiomyopathy and hepatomegaly (increased storage of glucose as glycogen) that is commonly observed in patients with CHI. In most forms of CHI the hypoglycaemia typically presents during fasting but in some cases the hypoglycaemia is provoked by protein/leucine loading or even exercise [2].

CHI may also be associated with certain syndromes, with Beckwith–Wiedemann (BWS) syndrome being the most common. Patients with this syndrome have prenatal and/or postnatal overgrowth, macroglossia, anterior abdominal wall defects, organomegaly, hemihypertrophy, ear lobe creases, helical pits, and renal tract abnormalities. A small number of patients with BWS have severe CHI which requires surgical intervention in the form of a near total pancreatectomy. An insulinoma is a rare cause of hyperinsulinaemic hypoglycaemia and must be considered in older children or adolescents presenting with recurrent hypoglycaemia. Insulinomas may be a part of multiple endocrine neoplasia syndrome type 1 (MEN1) and hence a family history may provide a diagnostic clue in the familial cases.

The early diagnosis of CHI is fundamentally important for preventing hypoglycaemic brain injury. In the history, it is important to establish the duration of fasting and whether the hypoglycaemia is precipitated by meals (protein sensitivity) or by exercise. Typically, newborns with CHI have markedly reduced fasting tolerance (less than 1 h). A powerful clue to the dysregulated insulin secretion is the increased intravenous glucose infusion rate required to maintain normoglycaemia (>8 mg/kg/min with normal being 4–6 mg/kg/min). Biochemically, there is inappropriate concentration of serum insulin (and/or c-peptide) for the level of blood glucose (spontaneous or provoked). The metabolic effect of this inappropriate insulin secretion is reflected by the inappropriately low levels of serum ketone bodies and fatty acids during the hypoglycaemic episode [2]. It is this metabolic profile (hypoglycaemia associated with inappropriately low fatty acids and ketone bodies) which increases the risk of brain damage in CHI patients.

Pathophysiology of CHI

The genetic basis of CHI involves mutations in genes that play a role in regulating insulin secretion from the pancreatic ß-cell. Mutations in these genes perturb the normal physiological mechanisms that regulate glucose metabolism and insulin secretion. The pancreatic ß-cell adenosine triphosphate-sensitive potassium channels (K_{ATP} channels) play a critical role in glucose stimulated insulin secretion. These channels are heterooctameric complexes comprising of four inwardly rectifying potassium channel (Kir6.2) subunits and four of the sulphonylurea receptor 1 (SUR1) subunits. The channels link glucose metabolism to membrane electrical activity and insulin release in pancreatic ß-cells. Glucose metabolism leads to an increase in the intracellular ratio of nucleotides such as ATP/ADP within the ß-cell causing closure of the channels; this results in cell membrane depolarization, Ca^{2+} influx via voltage gated calcium channels and insulin exocytosis.

The SUR1 and Kir6.2 proteins are encoded by the *ABCC8* and *KCNJ11* genes, respectively. Loss of function mutations in these two genes are the most common cause of severe medically unresponsive CHI [6–8]. The majority of K_{ATP}

channel mutations have been thought to act recessively. However, recent reports of autosomal dominantly inherited mutations in patients with CHI suggest that they may be more common than recognized [9]. Mutations in *ABCC8* and *KCNJ11* result either in a trafficking defect with the SUR1 and Kir6.2 proteins not getting to the membrane surface or cause dysregulation in the way that SUR1 and Kir6.2 respond to changes in the nucleotide ratio [10].

Other rare forms of HI involve metabolic disturbances in enzymes regulating insulin secretion from the pancreatic ß-cells. These include dominant forms of CHI due to mutations in the *GLUD1* (encoding the enzyme glutamate dehydrogenase associated with a high serum ammonia level), *GK* (encoding the enzyme glucokinase) and *SLC16A1* (encoding the monocarboxylate transporter MCT-1) genes [11–13]. Another rare recessive form of CHI involves defects in the enzyme short-chain L-3-hydroxyacyl-CoA dehydrogenase (SCHAD) which is encoded by the *HADH* gene [14]. More recently, heterozygous loss-of-function mutations in the Hepatocyte Nuclear Factor 4A (*HNF4A*) gene resulting in transient or persistent CHI have been described [15]. Mutations in *HNF4A* not only lead to CHI but also to maturity-onset diabetes of the young (MODY). Virtually all of these types of CHI are medically responsive and will not require surgery.

Medical Management

The early diagnosis and immediate meticulous management will be important in preventing brain injury in patients with CHI. Once the diagnosis is established the priority is to maintain the normal blood glucose levels (3.5–6 mmol/L). In some patients normoglycaemia can only be maintained by giving concentrated solutions of glucose intravenously and this often require the insertion of a central venous catheter (such as a Hickman line). A combination of oral feeds with a glucose polymer (such as Maxijul or Polycal) and intravenous fluids are used to keep the patient stable until further procedures are planned.

In an emergency situation where venous access is difficult to obtain, intramuscular glucagon (0.5–1 mg) can be administered in order to temporarily stabilize blood glucose concentrations. Glucagon acts by immediately releasing hepatic stores of glycogen and also has actions on gluconeogenesis, ketogenesis and lipolysis. In the acute management of infants with CHI it can be administered alone or in combination with octreotide as an intravenous or subcutaneous infusion to stabilize blood glucose concentrations. Prolonged periods of intravenous/nasogastric or gastrostomy feeding can lead to problems with 'orality' in infants with CHI and ultimately delay in establishing full oral feeds. Gastro-oesophageal reflux and foregut dysmotility are commonly observed in CHI infants which complicates the feeding problems [2]. Early treatment of gastro-oesophageal reflux and the introduction of oral feeds with avoidance of force-feeding are thus recommended. In some cases the expertise of a skilled speech and language therapist may be required to help establish a normal feeding pattern.

The most commonly used medication for CHI infants is diazoxide- a drug that binds to the intact SUR1 component of the K_{ATP} channels [2]. It acts by keeping the K_{ATP} channels open, thereby preventing depolarisation of the ß-cell membrane and insulin secretion. In newborns it is used in conjunction with chlorothiazide, a diuretic with hyperglycaemic properties. Diazoxide is effective in virtually all forms of CHI except in diffuse CHI due to inactivating mutations in *ABCC8* and *KCNJ11* and in patients with focal CHI. Diazoxide can cause fluid retention (especially in newborns) and hence it must be used with caution especially in patients who are receiving large volumes of intravenous fluids/oral feeds. Octreotide (a somatostatin analogue) is the second line of therapy for patients with diffuse disease who show no response to oral diazoxide. Table 12.1 outlines the different drugs used for the treatment of patients with CHI.

Table 12.1 Summary of the medications used in the treatment of CHI

Drug	Dose	Route of administration	Side effects
Diazoxide	5–20 mg/kg/day divided into three doses	Oral	Fluid retention, hypertrichosis
Chlorothiazide (in conjunction with diazoxide)	7–10 mg/kg/day divided into two doses	Oral	Hyponatraemia, hypokalaemia
Glucagon	1–10 μg/kg/h 0.5–1 mg for emergency treatment of hypoglycaemia	SC/IV infusion IM/IV	Nausea, vomiting, skin rashes. Paradoxical hypoglycaemia in high doses
Octreotide	5–35 μg/kg/day	SC as a continuous infusion or 6–8 hourly injections	Common—tachyphylaxis Others—Suppression of GH, TSH, ACTH, glucagon; diarrhoea, steatorrhoea, cholelithiasis, abdominal distension, growth suppression

Diazoxide is the mainstay of therapy for patients with CHI. However, the vast majority of patients with defects in the K_{ATP} channels will not respond to diazoxide

Histological Subtypes of Phhi

Histologically, there are two major subtypes of CHI, diffuse and focal [4] (Fig. 12.1). However, patients have been described with atypical histological forms of CHI which do not fit into the classification of diffuse or focal [16, 17]. The diffuse form of CHI affects all the ß-cells within the islets of Langerhans (Fig. 12.2). The histological subtype of CHI can be a guide as to the mode of inheritance. Diffuse disease can be familial or sporadic and can result from recessively inherited or dominantly acting mutations in the genes previously described whilst focal disease is always sporadic [18]. The diffuse and focal forms of CHI are histologically unrelated to nesidioblastosis [19] (which describes the proliferation of islets cells budding off from pancreatic ducts).

Focal pancreatic lesions appear as small regions of islet adenomatosis (nodular hyperplasia of islet-like cell clusters, including ductuloinsular complexes) measuring 2–10 mm which are characterised by ß-cells with enlarged nuclei surrounded by normal tissue [18, 20] (Fig. 12.2). Focal disease results from paternal uniparental disomy (UPD) encompassing chromosome11p15.5-11p15.1 within a single pancreatic ß-cell which unmasks a paternally inherited K_{ATP} channel mutation at 11p15.1 [21, 22]. Paternal UPD at 11p15.5 causes altered expression of a number of imprinted genes, including the maternally expressed tumour suppressor genes *H19* and *CDKN1C*, and the paternally expressed growth factor *IGF2*, likely leading to clonal expansion of the single cell and dysregulated insulin secretion from the resulting focal lesion [21, 22].

Differential of Focal and Diffuse

In patients that are unresponsive to medical therapy with diazoxide it is essential to differentiate focal from diffuse disease as the surgical approaches are radically different [23]. Infants with diffuse and focal disease are clinically and biochemically undistinguishable, thus there is no biochemical marker which will help in the differentiation. The precise preoperative localisation and limited surgical removal of the focal domain "cures" the patient from the hypoglycaemia and minimizes the risk of pancreatic exocrine insufficiency. Focal lesions are typically invisible to the naked eye at the time of the operation (size can vary from 2 to 10 mm in diameter) and in most cases buried deep within the pancreas [4]. In contrast, patients with diffuse disease will require a near total pancreatectomy which will

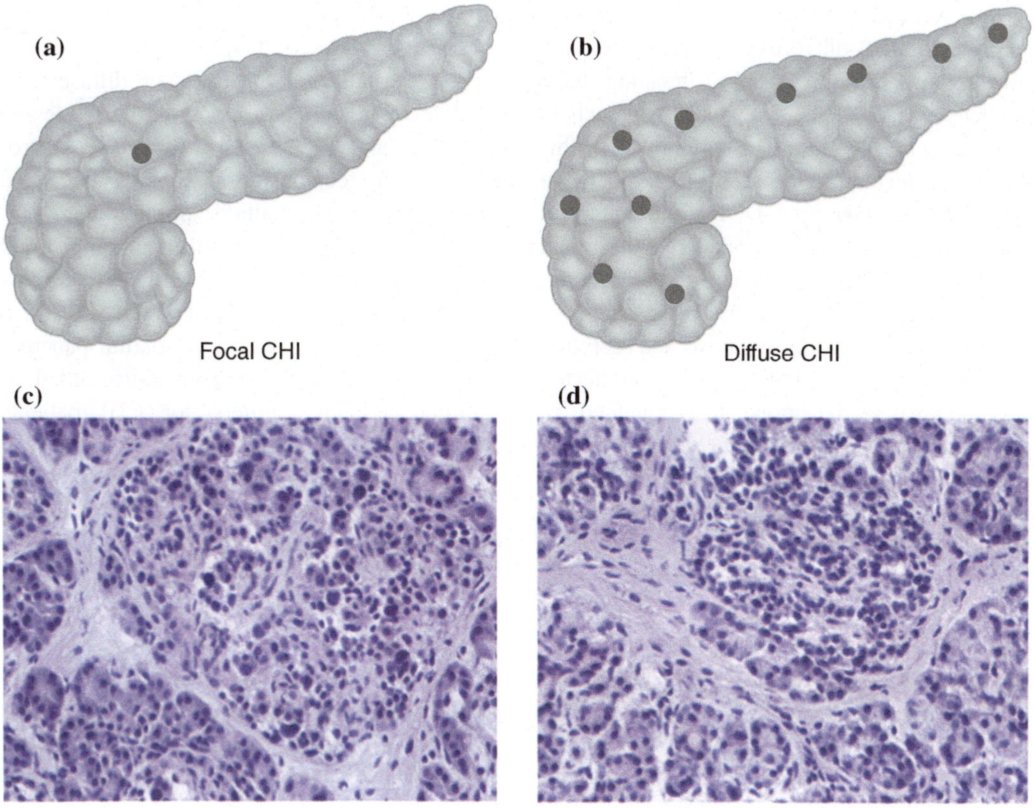

Fig. 12.1 Histological subtypes of CHI. **a** and **b** The focal form is localised to a single region of the pancreas whereas the diffuse form affects the whole pancreas. **c** and **d** On H&E staining there is marked hyperplasia of the islets in focal disease

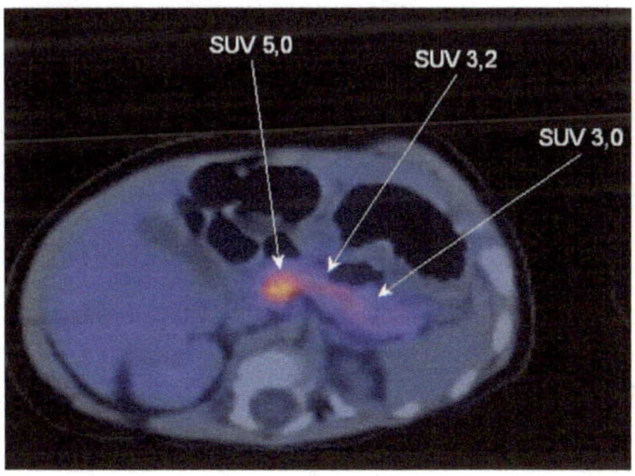

Fig. 12.2 ^{18}F-DOPA-PET/CT scan of focal lesion located in the head of the pancreas. The standard uptake value (SUV) of Fluorine-18-L-3,4-dihydroxyphenylalanine is highest in the head of the pancreas (5.0) compared to the body and tail of the pancreas. At surgery a focal lesion was found located between the superior mesenteric vein and the portal vein

have life-long implications (with a high risk of developing diabetes mellitus and pancreatic exocrine insufficiency). Patients with diffuse CHI that are medically managed also have a high risk of developing diabetes mellitus [16].

In the past methods for identifying children with a focal CHI included intrahepatic pancreatic portal venous sampling (PVS), arterial calcium stimulation/venous sampling, acute insulin response testing to intravenous glucose, calcium and tolbutamide and biopsy of the tail of the pancreas. However, these investigations are not only technically difficult and challenging but also have poor sensitivity and specificity. Focal lesions cannot be visualized with magnetic resonance imaging (MRI) or computerized tomography (CT) scans.

However, recent advances in ^{18}F-DOPA-PET (Fluorine-18-L-3,4-dihydroxyphenylalanine positron emission tomography) imaging have completely changed the diagnostic approach to these patients [24–30]. The principle of this radiological technique is based on the fact that pancreatic islets take up L–DOPA and convert it into dopamine by the aromatic amino acid decarboxylase [28]. The uptake of the positron emitting tracer ^{18}F-DOPA is increased in ß-cells with a high rate of insulin synthesis and secretion (increased metabolism) compared to unaffected areas. Dopamine receptors are expressed in pancreatic ß-cells suggesting a possible role in regulating insulin secretion. However, the precise role of dopamine in the pancreatic ß-cells is still unclear.

The detection limit of PET imaging using ^{18}F-DOPA-PET is equivalent to 10^5–10^6 cells and a diameter of approximately 1 mm [6]. The recent introduction of the integrated ^{18}F-DOPA-PET/CT technique allows more precise preoperative localization of the focal lesion [31]. The new ^{18}F-DOPA-PET/CT technique allows visualization of the splenic artery, portal vein, superior mesenteric and inferior mesenteric arteries as well as the duodenum and enables exact anatomical and functional description of the pancreatic focus [31]. Ectopic focal lesions (in the wall of the jejunum and the ileum) can also be detected by ^{18}F-DOPA-PET [32, 33]. ^{18}F-DOPA-PET/CT scan is indicated in those patients who have the genotype of a focal lesion (namely a paternally inherited mutation in *ABCC8* or *KCNJ11*) or have no mutations in the *ABCC8/KCNJ11* genes. If the patient has a homozygous or compound heterozygote mutation in *ABCC8* or *KCNJ11* then this is likely to be associated with diffuse disease and an ^{18}F-DOPA-PET/CT is not required these cases. The aim of the ^{18}F-DOPA-PET/CT is to allow pre-operative localisation of the focal domain [25, 26]. We recently reviewed our experience in the PET-CT localization of focal CHI and this suggests that in focal lesions, ^{18}F-DOPA-PET scan is useful in defining the site and dimension of the focal lesion in 2/3 of patients [34].

Surgery for CHI

Surgery is indicated for cases of diffuse CHI which are medically unresponsive (diazoxide and octreotide) and in all cases of focal disease provided that the focal lesion is accurately localised pre-operatively. A multidisciplinary team (involving the endocrinologist, histopathologist and surgeon) approach to patients with CHI can help in distinguishing focal from diffuse disease, locate focal lesions, and permit partial pancreatectomy with cure in most patients [5, 35]. It is recommended that surgery for CHI patients should be done in centers of expertise where all the facilities and resources are available. The surgeon has to work very closely with the histopathologist as intra-operative examination of pancreatic specimens will guide the surgeon on the extent of resection required [36]. Surgeons need to be aware about the limitations of ^{18}F-DOPA-PET in identifying the exact location and the dimension of the focal lesion and should always rely on the intra-operative histological confirmation of complete excision of the focal lesion [34].

Surgery for Diffuse CHI

The extent of pancreatic resection for diffuse disease is controversial, however most of the current literature recommends a near total or 95% pancreatectomy [23]. The aim of doing a near total pancreatectomy for diffuse disease ideally is to remove enough pancreatic tissue so that the child can become independent of intravenous glucose infusion and maintain normoglycaemia on bolus enteral feeds. However, there is a very delicate balance between removing too much or too little pancreatic tissue. The child will still have hyperinsulinaemic hypoglycaemia following post pancreatectomy if too little pancreatic tissue is removed (which may require another pancreatectomy) and early diabetes mellitus will develop if too much tissue is resected. There are currently no markers which can be used during the intra-operative period to direct the extent of

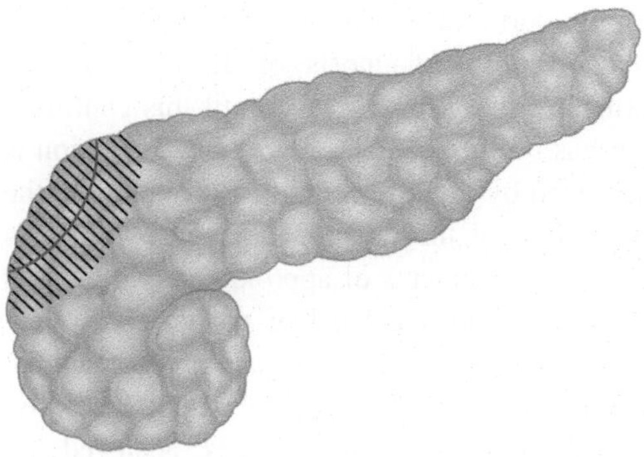

Fig. 12.3 Near-total pancreatectomy. The *shaded area* indicates the remaining pancreas after resection, leaving behind pancreatic tissue around the common bile duct and along the medial border of the duodenum

pancreatic resection. Thus not having a precise marker for the extent of pancreatic resection makes surgery complicated for diffuse disease. In near-total (95%) pancreatectomy, the tail, body, uncinate process and part of pancreatic head are resected, leaving pancreatic tissue surrounding the common bile duct and along the duodenum [37] (Fig. 12.3).

Open Near-Total Pancreatectomy

Pancreatic resection for the diffuse type of CHI has traditionally been carried out by the open approach. The abdomen is accessed via a generous transverse supraumbilical incision. The lesser sac is entered through the gastrocolic omentum; Kocherisation of the duodenum allows full exposure of the pancreas. The tail of the pancreas is sent for intraoperative frozen section histology and the diagnosis of diffuse CHI is confirmed before proceeding with pancreatectomy.

A stay suture is placed in the tail of the pancreas to allow traction of the pancreas facilitating its dissection since direct handling of the pancreas results in fracture of this friable organ. The tail of the pancreas is carefully dissected away from the hilum of the spleen, and the short pancreatic vessels are coagulated. Dissection of the pancreas is carried out in a medial direction towards the head of the pancreas. Pancreatic vessels passing from the splenic vessels into the pancreas are coagulated and divided using bipolar diathermy. Meticulous care is taken with the splenic artery and vein which are closely related to the pancreas, as the spleen should be preserved. Once dissection has arrived at the superior mesenteric vessels, the uncinate process is mobilised. A sling may be placed around the superior mesenteric vessels, retracting them away from the uncinate process.

As the head of pancreas is approached, attention is directed to identifying the course of the common bile duct. A sling is placed around the bile duct superior to the first part of the duodenum. A blunt forceps is then passed from within the C-loop of the duodenum behind the first part of the duodenum to grasp the sling, bringing it out superior to the head of pancreas. This becomes the guide to the position of the common bile duct during subsequent dissection of the pancreas. The head of the pancreas is mobilised, and the superior and inferior pancreaticoduodenal vessels are divided. The pancreatic duct is ligated with non-absorbable sutures and divided. A rim of pancreatic tissue surrounding the common bile duct and along the duodenum is left remaining after near-total (95%) pancreatectomy (Fig. 12.3). The abdomen is closed in layers using absorbable sutures. Postoperatively, the patient has both nasogastric tube and bladder catheter. Enteral feeds are restarted after the gastrointestinal function has returned.

Near-total pancreatectomy has been associated with a range of complications [23, 38, 39].

The intra-operative complications which have been reported include bleeding, splenic injury, bile duct injury and small bowel injury. The postoperative complications reported include biliary leak, delayed development of bile duct stricture, wound infections, prolonged ileus, adhesion obstruction, persisting hyperinsulinaemic hypoglycaemia (which may require another pancreatectomy) and the development of diabetes mellitus with pancreatic exocrine insufficiency. Rarely patients have died following a near total pancreatectomy [38].

There have been recent reports of laparoscopic surgery being performed in CHI patients [40–46]. The use of laparoscopy represents a new approach to the diagnosis and management of patients with CHI. Laparoscopic pancreatectomy is attractive since it should be associated with less operative trauma. The laparoscopic approach offers other theoretical advantages. This procedure is relatively quick, associated with faster recovery, decreased post-operative pain, decreased wound related complications and faster post-operative recovery times. Laparoscopic exploration for focal lesions in CHI has been used to locate and excise the focal area thus curing the patient [45]. More recently, laparoscopic surgery in combination with ^{18}F-DOPA-PET/CT has proved a very powerful technique for removing focal lesions around the tail region of the pancreas [31]. Laparoscopic near-total pancreatectomy for diffuse disease has now been devised and introduced in our centre by one of the authors (AP). It seems to be comparable to open surgery but with the added benefits as listed above. In one study [40] 12 patients with diffuse PHHI underwent laparoscopic near total pancreatectomy with no major pre or post-operative complications.

Laparoscopic Near-Total Pancreatectomy

An umbilical 10 mm Hasson port is inserted by an open technique and a 5 mm 30° camera is introduced. Three additional ports are placed: a 5 mm port in the left lower quadrant, a Nathanson retractor at the epigastrium and a further working port (3 or 5 mm) in the right flank. The gastro-colic omentum is divided and the lesser sac is entered. The Nathanson retractor is used to retract the stomach. The head of the patient is elevated. A stay suture is inserted into the tail of the pancreas which is used to retract the pancreas superiorly. Dissection of the pancreas proceeds towards the head. The short pancreatic vessels passing from the splenic vessels into the pancreas are divided using a 3 mm hook diathermy at very high coagulation settings. These vessels are the most common source of intra-operative haemorrhage, which may be controlled by applying gentle pressure using an atraumatic bowel grasper. The pancreatic tail is transected using the Harmonic Scalpel® (Ethicon Endosurgery). The pancreatic tail is removed via the umbilical 10 mm port and sent for frozen section analysis to confirm the diagnosis of diffuse CHI. No further resection takes place until this confirmation has been obtained. Subsequent dissection is facilitated by the insertion of a stay suture at the cut surface of the remaining pancreas which is resected in segments of approximately 2 cm. As dissection nears the head of the pancreas, stay sutures are placed in the uncinate process and the head of pancreas which are retracted superiorly. A near-total pancreatectomy is achieved by leaving a small rim of pancreas along the medial border of the duodenum where the common bile duct is expected (Fig. 12.3). Port sites are closed using absorbable sutures. No drains are used.

Surgery for Focal CHI

In patients with focal CHI, a localised resection of the focal lesion is curative [5]. Prior to surgery, the diagnosis of focal CHI is confirmed using a combination of genetic analysis and findings on 18F-DOPA-PET-CT scan. The site of the lesion seen on PET-CT Scan allows preoperative planning of the anticipated procedure. However, it should be noted that the accuracy of localization in PET-CT Scan is approximately 70% [34]. In proximal lesions in the head and neck of the pancreas, open resection of the lesion with a small rim of surrounding normal pancreatic tissue is carried out and pancreaticojejunostomy is performed to allow drainage of the distal pancreas. In distal lesions, a distal pancreatectomy may be done laparoscopically (Fig. 12.3).

The abdomen is accessed laparoscopically as described earlier. The pancreas is inspected and palpated for a nodular area indicating the site of the focal lesion. In focal CHI, the lesion is often deep within the parenchyma of the pancreas and may not be visually evident. An intraoperative biopsy is performed for frozen section histological examination. Histology may reveal the following: [1] the presence of the focal lesion completely resected (normal pancreas at the resection margin); [2] focal lesion not completely resected; [3] the presence of normal pancreas excluding the presence of diffuse CHI and

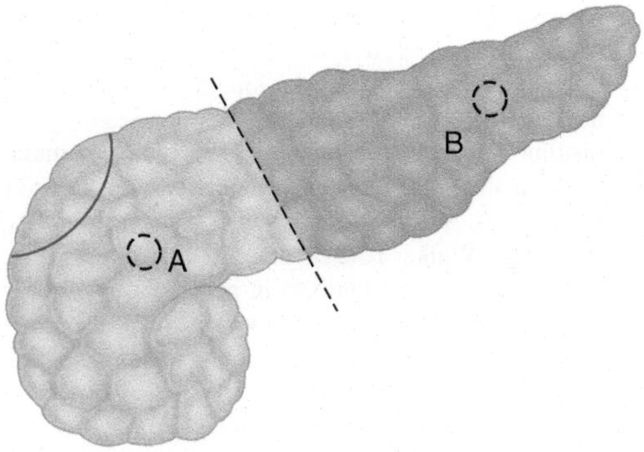

Fig. 12.4 Focal CHI. **a** Lesion in the head or neck of pancreas (*zone A*: *unshaded area*). Surgery: Open excision of focal lesion and pancreaticojejunostomy. **b** Lesion in the body or tail of pancreas (*zone B*: *shaded area*). Surgery: Laparoscopic distal pancreatectomy

indicating that the focal lesion has not yet been excised.

Focal Lesion in Head or Neck of Pancreas

When the focal lesion is deep in the head or neck of the pancreas, the procedure may be converted to open and dissection of the head of the pancreas is commenced (Fig. 12.4a). Superficial lesions may be enucleated laparoscopically. A sling may be passed behind the neck of the pancreas to facilitate traction of the pancreas away from the pancreatic bed. Short pancreatic vessels are meticulously ligated using bipolar diathermy and divided. The head of the pancreas is dissected in the direction of the duodenum, carefully avoiding the common bile duct. A pancreaticojejunostomy is then constructed to allow drainage of the distal pancreas.

Focal Lesion in Body or Tail of Pancreas

In more distal lesions, the entire procedure may be completed either laparoscopically or open (Fig. 12.4b). Once histological confirmation of focal disease is obtained, the pancreas is dissected as described previously. Dissection is performed until the resected specimen includes the lesion. The pancreas is transacted using Harmonic Scalpel® (Ethicon Endosurgery). An adequate resection margin is confirmed by further frozen section analysis. There is no need for drains.

Summary

The pre-operative histological differentiation of CHI is crucial as the surgical management of the two major subgroups is radically different. Genetic analysis and ^{18}F-DOPA-PET/CT scan allows differentiation between diffuse and focal disease. A preoperative ^{18}F-DOPA-PET/CT also assists in determining the size and location of focal lesions in approximately 70% of patients with focal disease, which can then be surgically, resected thus curing the patient. Laparoscopic distal pancreatectomy can be performed for focal lesions in the body or tail of the pancreas. For more proximal lesions, partial excision of the head of the pancreas and pancreaticojejunostomy is required. The management of the severe diffuse form of the disease, however still remains a challenge as the treatment options are unsatisfactory with lifelong implications. Near-total pancreatectomy is necessary in children who do not respond to medical treatment, which carries a risk of endocrine and exocrine insufficiency. Laparoscopic near-total pancreatectomy is an option in centers with advanced laparoscopic expertise.

References

1. Menni F, de Lonlay P, Sevin C, Touati G, Peigne C, Barbier V, Nihoul-Fékété C, Saudubray JM, Robert JJ. Neurologic outcomes of 90 neonates and infants with persistent hyperinsulinemic hypoglycemia. Pediatrics. 2001;107:476–9.
2. Aynsley-Green A, Hussain K, Hall J, Saudubray JM, Nihoul-Fékété C, De Lonlay-Debeney P, Brunelle F, Otonkoski T, Thornton P, Lindley JK. The practical management of hyperinsulinism in infancy. Arch Dis Child Fetal Neonatal Ed. 2000;82:F98–107.
3. Rahier J, Guiot Y, Sempoux C. Persistent hyperinsulinaemic hypoglycaemia of infancy: a heterogeneous syndrome unrelated to nesidioblastosis. Arch Dis Child Fetal Neonatal Ed. 2002;82(2) F108–12.
4. Rahier J, Sempoux C, Fournet JC, Poggi F, Brunelle F, Nihoul-Fekete C, Saudubray JM, Jaubert F. Partial or near-total pancreatectomy for persistent neonatal hyperinsulinaemic hypoglycaemia: the pathologist's role. Histopathology. 1998;32(1):15–9.
5. Crétolle C, Fékété CN, Jan D, Nassogne MC, Saudubray JM, Brunelle F, Rahier J. Partial elective

pancreatectomy is curative in focal form of permanent hyperinsulinemic hypoglycaemia in infancy: a report of 45 cases from 1983 to 2000. J Pediatr Surg.2002;37(2):155–8.
6. Thomas P, Ye Y, Lightner E. Mutation of the pancreatic islet inward rectifier Kir6.2 also leads to familial persistent hyperinsulinemic hypoglycemia of infancy. Hum Mol Genet. 1996;5:1813–22.
7. Thomas PM, Cote GJ, Wohllk N, Haddad B, Mathew PM, Rabl W, Aguilar-Bryan L, Gagel RF, Bryan J. Mutations in the sulfonylurea receptor gene in familial persistent hyperinsulinemic hypoglycemia of infancy. Science 1995;268(5209):426–9.
8. Dunne MJ, Kane C, Shepherd RM, Sanchez JA, James RF, Johnson PR, Aynsley-Green A, Lu S, Clement JP IV, Lindley KJ, Seino S, Aguilar-Bryan L. Familial persistent hyperinsulinemic hypoglycemia of infancy and mutations in the sulfonylurea receptor. N Engl J Med. 1997;336:703–6.
9. Huopio H, Reimann F, Ashfield R, Komulainen J, Lenko HL, Rahier J, Vauhkonen I, Kere J, Laakso M, Ashcroft F, Otonkoski T. Dominantly inherited hyperinsulinism caused by a mutation in the sulfonylurea receptor type 1. J Clin Invest. 2000;106: 897–906.
10. Kane C, Shepherd RM, Squires PE, Johnson PRV, James RFL, Milla PJ, Aynsley-Green Lindley KJ, Dunne MJ. Loss of functional K_{ATP} channels in β-cells causes persistent hyperinsulinaemic hypoglycaemia on infancy. Nat Med. 1996;2:1344–7.
11. Stanley CA, Lieu YK, Hsu BY, Burlina AB, Greenberg CR, Hopwood NJ, Perlman K, Rich BH, Zammarchi E, Poncz M. Hyperinsulinism and hyperammonemia in infants with regulatory mutations of the glutamate dehydrogenase gene. N Engl J Med. 1998;338(19):1352–7.
12. Glaser B, Kesavan P, Heyman M, Davis E, Cuesta A, Buchs A, Stanley CA, Thornton PS, Permutt MA, Matschinsky FM, Herold KC. Familial hyperinsulinism caused by activating glucokinase mutation. N Engl J Med. 1998;338(19) 226–30.
13. Otonkoski T, Jiao H, Kaminen-Ahola N, Tapia-Paez I, Ullah MS, Parton LE, Schuit F, Quintens R, Sipilä I, Mayatepek E, Meissner T, Halestrap AP, Rutter GA, Kere J. Physical exercise-induced hypoglycemia caused by failed silencing of monocarboxylate transporter 1 in pancreatic beta cells. Am J Hum Genet. 2007;81(3):467–74.
14. Clayton PT, Eaton S, Aynsley-Green A, Edginton M, Hussain K, Krywawych S, Datta V, Malingre HE, Berger R, van den Berg IE. Hyperinsulinism in short-chain L-3-hydroxyacyl-CoA dehydrogenase deficiency reveals the importance of beta-oxidation in insulin secretion. J Clin Invest. 2001;108(3): 457–65.
15. Pearson ER, Boj SF, Steele AM, Barrett T, Stals K, Shield JP, Ellard S, Ferrer J, Hattersley AT. Macrosomia and Hyperinsulinaemic Hypoglycaemia in Patients with Heterozygous Mutations in the HNF4A Gene. PLoS Med. 2007;4(4):e118.
16. Gussinyer M, Clemente M, Cebrián R, Yeste D, Albisu M, Carrascosa A. Glucose intolerance and diabetes are observed in the long-term follow-up of nonpancreatectomized patients with persistent hyperinsulinemic hypoglycemia of infancy due to mutations in the ABCC8 gene. Diabetes Care. 2008;31 (6):1257–9.
17. Jack MM, Walker RM, Thomsett MJ, Cotterill AM, Bell JR. Histologic findings in persistent hyperinsulinemic hypoglycemia of infancy: Australian experience. Pediatr Dev Pathol. 2000;3(6):532–47.
18. Sempoux C, Guiot Y, Dahan K, Moulin P, Stevens M, Lambot V, de Lonlay P, Fournet JC, Junien C, Jaubert F, Nihoul-Fekete C, Saudubray JM, Rahier J. The focal form of persistent hyperinsulinemic hypoglycemia of infancy: morphological and molecular studies show structural and functional differences with insulinoma. Diabetes. 2003;52 (3):784–94.
19. Laidlaw GF. Nesidioblastoma, the islet tumor of the pancreas. Am J Pathol. 1938;14:125–34.
20. Sempoux C, Guiot Y, Jaubert F, Rahier J. Focal and diffuse forms of congenital hyperinsulinism: the keys for differential diagnosis. Endocr Pathol. Fall. 2004;15(3):241–6.
21. De Lonlay P, Fournet JC, Rahier J, Gross-Morand MS, Poggi-Travert F, Foussier V, Bonnefont JP, Brusset MC, Brunelle F, Robert JJ, Nihoul-Fekete C, Saudubray JM, Junien C. Somatic deletion of the imprinted 11p15 region in sporadic persistent hyperinsulinemic hypoglycemia of infancy is specific of focal adenomatous hyperplasia and endorses partial pancreatectomy. J Clin Invest. 1997; 100(4):802–7.
22. Verkarre V, Fournet JC, Delonlay P. Paternal mutation of the sulphonylurea receptor (SUR 1) gene and maternal loss of the 11p15 imprinted genes lead to persistent hyperinsulinism in focal adenomatous hyperplasia. J Clin Invest. 1998;102:1286–91.
23. Fékété CN, de Lonlay P, Jaubert F, Rahier J, Brunelle F, Saudubray JM. The surgical management of congenital hyperinsulinemic hypoglycemia in infancy. J Pediatr Surg. 2004;39(3):267–9.
24. Arbizu Lostao J, Fernández-Marmiesse A, Garrastachu Zumarrán P, Martino Casado E, Azcona San Julián C, Carracedo A, Richter Echevarría JA. [18F-fluoro-L-DOPA PET-CT imaging combined with genetic analysis for optimal classification and treatment in a child with severe congenital hyperinsulinism. Pediatr (Barc). 2008;68(5):481–5.
25. Capito C, Khen-Dunlop N, Ribeiro MJ, Brunelle F, Aigrain Y, Crétolle C, Jaubert F, De Lonlay P, Nihoul-Fékété C. Value of 18F-fluoro-L-dopa PET in the preoperative localization of focal lesions in congenital hyperinsulinism. Radiology. 2009;253(1):216–22.
26. Hardy OT, Hernandez-Pampaloni M, Saffer JR, Scheuermann JS, Ernst LM, Freifelder R, Zhuang H, MacMullen C, Becker S, Adzick NS, Divgi C, Alavi A, Stanley CA. Accuracy of [18F] fluorodopa positron emission tomography for

diagnosing and localizing focal congenital hyperinsulinism. J Clin Endocrinol Metab. 2007;92(12): 4706–11.
27. Hardy OT, Hernandez-Pampaloni M, Saffer JR, Suchi M, Ruchelli E, Zhuang H, Ganguly A, Freifelder R, Adzick NS, Alavi A, Stanley CA. Diagnosis and Localization of Focal Congenital Hyperinsulinism by (18)F-Fluorodopa PET Scan. J Pediatr. 2007;150(2):140–145.
28. Mohnike K, Blankenstein O, Minn H, Mohnike W, Fuchtner F, Otonkoski T. [F]-DOPA Positron Emission Tomography for Preoperative Localization in Congenital Hyperinsulinism. Horm Res. 2008;70(2): 65–72.
29. Otonkoski T, Nanto-Salonen K, Seppanen M, Veijola R, Huopio H, Hussain K, Tapanainen P, Eskola O, Parkkola R, Ekstrom K, Guiot Y, Rahier J, Laakso M, Rintala R, Nuutila P, Minn H. Noninvasive diagnosis of focal hyperinsulinism of infancy with [18F]-DOPA positron emission tomography. Diabetes. 2006;55(1):13–8.
30. Ribeiro MJ, Boddaert N, Bellanné-Chantelot C, Bourgeois S, Valayannopoulos V, Delzescaux T, Jaubert F, Nihoul-Fékété C, Brunelle F, De Lonlay P. The added value of [(18)F]fluoro-L: -DOPA PET in the diagnosis of hyperinsulinism of infancy: a retrospective study involving 49 children. Eur J Nucl Med Mol Imaging. 2007;34(12):2120–8.
31. Barthlen W, Blankenstein O, Mau H, Koch M, Höhne C, Mohnike W, Eberhard T, Fuechtner F, Lorenz-Depiereux B, Mohnike K. Evaluation of (18F)FDOPA PET-CT for surgery in focal congenital hyperinsulinism. J Clin Endocrinol Metab. 2008;93(3): 869–75.
32. Hussain K, Seppanen M, Nanto-Salonen K, Adzick NS, Stanley C, Thornton P, Minn H. The diagnosis of ectopic focal hyperinsulinism of infancy with [18F]-DOPA positron emission tomography. J Clin Endocrinol Metab. 2006;91(8):2839–42.
33. Peranteau WH, Bathaii SM, Pawel B, Hardy O, Alavi A, Stanley CA, Adzick NS. Multiple ectopic lesions of focal islet adenomatosis identified by positron emission tomography scan in an infant with congenital hyperinsulinism. J Pediatr Surg. 2007; 42(1):188–92.
34. Zani A, Nah SA, Ron O, Totonelli G, Ismail D, Smith VV, Ashworth M, Blankenstein O, Mohnike W, De Coppi P, Eaton S, Hussain K, Pierro A. The predictive value of preoperative ^{18}Fluoro-L-DOPA-PET-CT scans in children with congenital hyperinsulinism of infancy. J Pediatr Surg 2011. 2010;46(1):204–8.
35. Adzick NS, Thornton PS, Stanley CA, Kaye RD, Ruchelli E. A multidisciplinary approach to the focal form of congenital hyperinsulinism leads to successful treatment by partial pancreatectomy. J Pediatr Surg. 2004;39(3):270–5.
36. Suchi M, Thornton PS, Adzick NS, MacMullen C, Ganguly A, Stanley CA, Ruchelli ED. Congenital hyperinsulinism: intraoperative biopsy interpretation can direct the extent of pancreatectomy. Am J Surg Pathol. 2004;28(10):1326–35.
37. Spitz L. Surgery for hyperinsulinaemic hypoglycaemia. Spitz L, Coran AG, editors. Operative pediatric surgery 6th ed, London:Hodder Arnold. 2006. p. 733–738.15.
38. Lovvorn HN 3rd, Nance ML, Ferry RJ Jr, Stolte L, Baker L, O'Neill JA Jr, Schnaufer L, Stanley CA, Adzick NS. Congenital hyperinsulinism and the surgeon: lessons learned over 35 years. J Pediatr Surg. 1999;34(5):786–92.
39. McAndrew HF, Smith V, Spitz L. Surgical complications of pancreatectomy for persistent hyperinsulinaemic hypoglycaemia of infancy. J Pediatr Surg. 2003;38(1):13–6.
40. Al-Shanafey S, Habib Z, AlNassar S. Laparoscopic pancreatectomy for persistent hyperinsulinemic hypoglycemia of infancy. J Pediatr Surg. 2009; 44(1):134–8.
41. Al-Shanafey S. Laparoscopic vs open pancreatectomy for persistent hyperinsulinemic hypoglycemia of infancy. J Pediatr Surg. 2009;44(5):957–61.
42. Bax KN, van der Zee DC. The laparoscopic approach toward hyperinsulinism in children. Semin Pediatr Surg. 2007;16(4):245–5.
43. Bax NM, van der Zee DC, de Vroede M, Jansen M, Nikkels J. Laparoscopic identification and removal of focal lesions in persistent hyperinsulinemic hypoglycemia of infancy. Surg Endosc. 2003;17(5):833.
44. Blakely ML, Lobe TE, Cohen J, Burghen GA. Laparoscopic pancreatectomy for persistent hyperinsulinemic hypoglycemia of infancy. Surg Endosc. 2001;15(8):897–8.
45. De Vroede M, Bax NM, Brusgaard K, Dunne MJ, Groenendaal F. Laparoscopic diagnosis and cure of hyperinsulinism in two cases of focal adenomatous hyperplasia in infancy. Pediatrics. 2004;114(4): e520–2.
46. Liem NT, Son TN, Hoan NT. Laparoscopic near-total pancreatectomy for persistent hyperinsulinemic hypoglycemia of infancy: report of two cases. J Laparoendosc Adv Surg Tech A. 2010; 20(1):115–7.

13 Pancreatic Neuroendocrine Tumours

Paul R.V. Johnson

Pancreatic tumours are rare in children overall [1, 2]. Of those presenting in the under 20-year-old age-group, 30% are reported to be pancreatic neuroendocrine tumours (PaNETs), although due to their frequently asymptomatic and indolent nature, PaNETs are probably under-diagnosed in children [3]. Pa NETs are the second commonest manifestation of MEN1, occurring in up to 80% of patients [4]. Although encountered infrequently, PaNETs can present significant diagnostic and treatment challenges for the paediatric endocrinologist and paediatric surgeon. This chapter aims to provide an overview of PaNETs and emphasises the importance of a multi-disciplinary approach to ensure optimal care for children with these rare endocrine tumours.

Aetiology

The exact aetiology of PaNETs is unclear. The majority is sporadic, but some are associated with specific inherited familial syndromes including part of an associated syndrome, e.g. Multiple Endocrine Neoplasia 1 (MEN 1) or Wermer Syndrome (see Chap. 30), Von Hippel–Lindau, neurofibromatosis, and tuberous sclerosis. [5, 6]. Indeed, PNETs are the second commonest manifestation of MEN1, occurring in up to 80% of patients [4]. In addition to the genetic mutations identified with the familial syndromes above, a number of novel genetic mutations have been identified in association with PaNETs [7]. One in six well-differentiated PaNETs have mutations in the mTOR pathway genes (including TSC2, PTEN, and PUK3CA [8]. In addition, about 40% of PaNETs are associated with mutations in the ATRX and DAXX genes that are part of a recently discovered cancer pathway [9]. These genetic mutations are distinct from those previously identified in pancreatic adenocarcinoma.

Pathology and Classification

PaNETs are slow growing tumours that arise from cells within the neuroendocrine system. They are an example of a 'small blue cell tumour'. As with all neuroendocrine tumours, PaNETs demonstrate positive reactions to markers of neuroendocrine tissue, including neuron-specific enolase, synaptophysin and chromogranin [10–12], but vary in other histological features due to their pancreatic location. Previously, the embryological origin of all neuroendocrine tumours was believed to be from cells migrating from the neural crest. However,

P.R.V. Johnson (✉)
Academic Pediatric Surgery Unit, Nuffield Department of Surgical Sciences, John Radcliffe Hospital, University of Oxford and Oxford Islet Transplant Programme, Headley Way, Oxford OX3 9RZ, UK
e-mail: Paul.Johnson@nds.ox.ac.uk

D.J. Ledbetter and P.R.V. Johnson (eds.), *Endocrine Surgery in Children*,
DOI 10.1007/978-3-662-54256-9_13

this is no longer believed to be the case, and it is now postulated that the origin of gut and pancreatic neuroendocrine tumours is from pluripotential progenitor cells that develop a neuroendocrine phenotype [13].

PaNETs are usually multiple and can occur throughout the head, body and tail of the pancreas. They can be benign or malignant, and can range from microadenomas, to macroadenomas, to invasive/metastatic carcinomas.

Both the 2000 and 2010 WHO 2010 classifications of neuroendocrine tumours distinguishes tumours based on their degree of differentiation [14, 15]. The 2000 WHO system included the three groups: well-differentiated neuroendocrine tumours, well-differentiated (low grade) neuroendocrine carcinomas, and poorly differentiated (high grade) neuroendocrine carcinomas [14]. The WHO 2010 Classification includes a three-tier tumour grading system that is based on the mitotic count or Ki-67 index [16] (Ki67 antigen is a nuclear protein expressed by proliferating cells). G1 is defined as a mitotic count of <2 mitoses per High Power Field (HPF) and/or Ki-67 index of $\leq 2\%$; G2 as a mitotic count of 2–20 mitoses/10 HPF and/or Ki-67 index of 3–20%; and G3 as a mitotic count of >20 mitoses/10 HPF AND/OR ki-67 index of >20% [15]. Staging is by the European Neuroendocrine Tumour Society's (ENETS's) TNM system [17, 18].

Most PaNETs secrete pancreatic peptide hormones (functioning PaNETs). Indeed, they can simultaneously produce several pancreatic hormones including gastrin, insulin, glucagon or vasoactive intestinal polypeptide (VIP). However, the clinical presentation, and hence primary nomenclature, of a PaNET reflects the predominant hormone being secreted in excess (e.g. gastrinoma or insulinoma, etc.) (see Clinical Presentation below). A proportion of PaNETs, possibly the majority in children, is labelled as non-secretory (non-functioning PaNETs) and are detected incidentally or on radiological screening in patients with the MEN1 mutation [3]. However, Kimura et al. have demonstrated that many of these so-called 'non-functioning' PaNETs still produce sub-clinical levels of hormone [19].

Clinical Presentation

Functioning PaNETs

Gastrinomas

Over 50% of PaNETs are either gastrinomas or insulinomas (Table 13.1). While insulinomas are the commonest functioning PaNET in adults, gastrinomas are the most frequently occurring PaNET overall in children if both sporadic and familial (MEN1) PaNETs are taken into account. Gastrinomas classically present with the Zollinger-Ellison syndrome comprising recurrent peptic ulceration and diarrhoea [20]. Gastrinomas are usually multiple and most commonly occur in the anatomical region termed the 'gastrinoma triangle'. This is the area defined by the cystic and common bile ducts, the junction of the second and third part of the duodenum, and the junction of the neck and body of the pancreas. Although the majority of gastrinomas are situated within the wall of the duodenum, those situated within the pancreas are reported as having greater malignant potential. Pancreatic gatsrinomas are also seen more commonly in patients with MEN1 [21]. Up to 65% of gastrinomas are malignant at presentation.

Gastrinomas are diagnosed by an increased gastric acid output with pH <2.0 in association with raised fasting serum gastrin levels [20, 21]. It is important to ensure that proton pump inhibitors have been stopped for at least 1 week prior to gastrin levels being measured, as these agents can lead to a falsely elevated gastrin level.

Diagnostic localisation of gastrinomas can be achieved through cross-sectional imaging (CT and MRI), functional positron emission tomography (PET), and octreoscan/single photon emission tomography (SPECT). Given the multiple nature of these tumours, it is important to visualise the whole gastrinoma triangle, as well as carefully evaluating the liver for potential metastatic disease.

Insulinomas

Insulinomas are insulin-secreting PaNETs arising from the beta cells of the islets of Langerhans and, as such, patients present with symptoms of

Table 13.1 The clinical features of the most common functioning pancreatic NETs are determined by the predominant hormone being secreted by the tumour

Tumour	Symptoms
Insulinoma	Confusion, sweating, weakness, unconsciousness, relief of symptoms with eating
Gastrinoma	Peptic ulceration and diarrea (Zollinger-Ellison syndrome, or diarrea alone
Glucagonoma	Weight loss, diabetes mellitus, diarrea, necrolytic migratory erythema
VIPoma	Profuse diarrea and marked hypokalaemia (Verner-Morrison syndrome)
Somatostatinoma	Weight loss, diarrea, steatorrhea, diabetes mellitus

Data from [25]

hyperinsulinism. Depending on the age of the child, symptoms include sweating, weakness, unconsciousness, and confusion. Symptoms improve with feeding. Biochemical diagnosis demonstrates fasting hypoglycaemia with inappropriately raised plasma insulin, and C-peptide levels [22]. The combination of symptoms of hypoglycaemia (especially after fasting or heavy exercise), a low plasma glucose measured during these symptoms, and relief of the symptoms once blood glucose has been normalised, is termed the Whipple's triad.

Other Functioning PNETs

Vasoactive intestinal polypeptide (VIP)-omas are rare PanNETs secrete VIP that cause the WDHA or Verner-Morrison syndrome. This comprises watery diarrhoea, hypokalaemia and achlorhydria, resulting in severe acidosis and dehydration. Unlike in adults, VIPomas in children are mainly non-pancreatic in origin.

Glucagonomas arise from the glucagon-secreting pancreatic alpha cells. Glucagonomas present with weight loss, anaemia, hyperglycaemia, and a characteristic rash known as necrolytic migratory erythema.

Somatostatinomas arise from islet delta-cells and usually present with weight loss, diarrhoea, steatorrhea and diabetes mellitus. *Pancreatic polypeptide (PP)-omas* secrete PP. However, elevated serum PP is also found in association with some 'non-functioning' PanNETs. However, PPomas and somatostatinomas are often asymptomatic [23, 24]. Sporadic glucagonomas and somatostatinomas do not seem to have been reported in children.

Other rare forms of functioning PaNETs include PaNETs that secrete adrenocorticotropic hormone (ACTH), corticotropin-releasing hormone (CRH), parathyroid hormone-related peptide (PHRP), growth hormone-releasing hormone (GHRH), gonadotropin-releasing hormone (CRH) or calcitonin (GRF).

Non-functioning PaNETs

Non-functioning PaNETs can be large and often present late. Indeed, about 50% of non-functioning PaNETs have metastasised by the time of clinical presentation [25]. Symptoms may be due to the local effects of the pancreatic mass and/or the hepatic metastases.

Diagnosis

Diagnosis is based on a combination of clinical presentation, detection of circulating NET secretions, and a range of different imaging techniques [25]. Tissue diagnosis by histopathology then confirms the diagnosis. Children with a family history of MEN1 or who are known to have a genetic predisposition to developing PNETs, should be screened for possible tumours. There is however, an ongoing debate concerning at what age screening should commence.

Biochemical Tests

Measuring the specific secretions produced by functioning PaNETS helps make the diagnosis in the first place, as well as being a useful way of monitoring tumour progression and resolution following treatment [26]. In addition, there are a number of less-specific substances that are produced by many gastro-pancreatic NETs regardless of their anatomical location and regardless of whether they are clinically functional tumours. These include pancreatic polypeptide which is produced by more than 30% of GEP-NETs, and also chromogranin A (CgA) [25, 27]. However, care has to be taken to recognise that CgA is also elevated in patients with atrophic gastritis, renal insufficiency, and who are on treatment with proton pump inhibitors [28].

Imaging

Diagnostic imaging consists of a combination of routine and specialist radiological and nuclear investigations [25, 28]. Most NETs require a multi-modality approach for accurate localisation and staging. Cross-sectional imaging (CT and MRI) plays an important role in initial localisation, as somatostatin receptor scintigraphy (SSRS). MIBG Scintigraphy can be useful in diagnosing PaNETs that do not take up somatostatin analogues. PET/CT is the imaging of choice for localising insulinoma in adults with either FDOPA or GLP-1 as the isotope. However, this is unavailable for children in most centres. Serial venous sampling therefore, still has a place as a localisation modality. Endoscopic ultrasound can be useful for detecting pancreatic GEP-NETs, and intraoperative ultrasound can help identify tumour extent and the presence of multifocal disease at the time of surgery.

Management

Due to the rare and complex nature of PaNETs in children, it is paramount that these are managed within a multi-disciplinary team. Such a team should comprise a paediatric surgeon, a paediatric endocrinologist, an adult pancreatic surgeon, experienced diagnostic and interventional radiologist, and an oncologist with experience of managing advanced and malignant PaNETs. Combining the expertise of paediatric and adult specialists ensures that children with PaNETs have the very best care possible for this rare and challenging condition.

Consensus guidelines exist for the management of many PaNETs [25]. However, most of these have been designed for adults rather than children. Modified guidelines are needed for children, although the rarity of these cases in this age-group means that these are hard to generate in an evidence-based manner.

Management of Functioning PaNETs

Surgical Management

Complete surgical resection offers the only curative treatment for neuroendocrine tumours. However, radical resection may be required, and the tendency to multifocal disease must always be taken into account in planning surgical treatment. When non-resectable or metastatic disease is present, surgery aimed at ablating or debulking the tumour burden can significantly improve length of patient survival, and it can contribute considerably to quality of life [28]. The use of novel intraoperative techniques, such as radio-frequency ablation and cryotherapy, have further aided the surgical treatment of advanced disease. Recent advances in medical treatment for advanced PaNETs has been encouraging with early evidence of prolonged survival.

The optimal surgical therapy for gastrinomas remains controversial [29]. Surgery for gastrinomas is rarely curative due to their small size and multiplicity.

Curative surgery to enucleate the tumour or a partial pancreatic resection is the aim of treatment for patients with these symptomatic functioning pancreatic tumours.

Pancreatic resection is beneficial for functioning glucagonoma and VIPoma NETs, as medical therapy is unsatisfactory.

Non-operative Management

Medical therapies for gastrinomas include proton pump inhibitors and somatostatin analogues to suppress hyperacidity. Treatment of inoperable or metastatic PNETs includes biotherapy (e.g. somatostatin analogues and interferon-α), targetted radionuclide therapy, locoregional treatments and chemotherapy [13, 27, 30, 31]. Inhibitors of tyrosine kinase receptors (TKRs) and of the mammalian target of rapamycin (mTOR) signalling pathway have recently been reported to be effective in treating PaNETs [32, 33]. Sunitinib, which inhibits TKRs, and Everolimus, which is an inhibitor of mTOR, in randomised placebo-controlled trials improved median progression-free survival when compared to patients treated with placebo (11.4 months vs. 5.5 months and 11.0 months vs. 4.6 months, respectively, $P < 0.001$) in adults with advanced or progressive well-differentiated pancreatic NETs [32, 33]. Somatostatin biotherapy has antitumour and antiproliferative effects, and the CLARINET phase III trial of depot lanreotide treatment significantly prolonged progression-free survival in patients with metastatic pancreatic NETs [34].

Periodic endoscopic surveillance of the upper gastrointestinal tract in those with hypergastrinemia is beneficial for the identification of peptic ulcer disease and gastric carcinoid tumours [35].

Management of Non-functioning PaNETs

The role of surgery for non-functioning pancreatic tumours is controversial, but should be considered for tumours that demonstrate significant growth over 6 months or are >1 cm in size [3, 29].

Outcomes and Prognosis

The outcome of PaNETs is highly dependent on the type of tumour, the degree of differentiation, the proliferative activity and the TNM stage of the tumour at the time of diagnosis. Of all gastrointestinal NETs, pancreatic tumours overall are associated with a poorer outcome [25]. The SEER registry identified 481 cases of malignant NETs (all sites) in children aged between 3 and 19 of age, and reported an overall 5-year survival rate of 78% [36]. Ninety-one percent of the children with localised tumours were alive at 5 years, compared with only 35% of those with metastatic disease. The WHO classifications have helped provide some more meaningful prognostic comparisons between different tumour grades and stages. Overall, the 5 year survival rates for grades 1, 2 and 3 tumours are 96, 73, and 28%, respectively, whereas the survival for stages I, II, III and IV GEP-NETs are 100, 90, 79, and 55%, respectively [37]. Early diagnosis is key. With this in mind, proactive screening of all children with a family history of MEN1 or who demonstrate genetic predisposition to NET tumours is important to ensure early diagnosis and curative treatment. However, there is currently no consensus on what age such screening should begin, and also how regularly imaging should be conducted in children who have been found to have small, non-functioning tumours. Although these tumours are very rare overall, paediatric-specific guidelines need to be developed to ensure optimal management for any child who develops a PaNET.

Acknowledgements The author would like to acknowledge the contribution of Gerard Walls to this chapter.

References

1. Jaksic T, Yaman M, Thorner P, Wesson DK, Filler RM, Shandling B. A 20-year review of pediatric pancreatic tumors. J Pediatr Surg. 1992;27 (10):1315–7.
2. Vane DW, Grosfeld JL, West KW, Rescorla FJ. Pancreatic disorders in infancy and childhood: experience with 92 cases. J Pediatr Surg. 1989;24(8): 771–6.
3. Newey PJ, Jeyabalan J, Walls GV, Christie PT, Gleeson FV, Gould S, et al. Asymptomatic children with multiple endocrine neoplasia type 1 mutations may harbor nonfunctioning pancreatic neuroendocrine

tumors. J Clin Endocrinol Metab. 2009;94(10):3 640–6.
4. Trump D, Farren B, Wooding C, Pang JT, Besser GM, Buchanan KD, et al. Clinical studies of multiple endocrine neoplasia type 1 (MEN1). QJM. 1996;89(9):653–69.
5. Jensen RT, Berna MJ, Bingham DB, et al. Inherited pancreatic endocrine tumour syndromes: advances in molecular pathogenesis, diagnosis, management, and controversies. Cancer. 2008;113(7 Suppl):1807–43.
6. Lodish MB, Stratakis CA. Endocrine tumours in neurofibromatosis type 1, tuberous sclerosis, and related syndromes. Best Pract Res Clin Endocrinol Metab. 2010;24(3):439–49.
7. Rindi G, Klöppel G, Alhman H, et al. All other Frascati Consensus Conference participants.; European Neuroendocrine Tumor Society (ENETS). TNM staging of foregut (neuro)endocrine tumors: a consensus proposal including a grading system. Virchows Arch 2006;449(4):395–401.
8. Sobin LH, Gospodarowicz MK, Wittekind C, editors. TNM classification of malignant tumours. Oxford: Wiley-Blackwell; 2009.
9. Jiao Y, Shi C, Edil BH, et al. DAXX/ATRX, MEN1, and mTOR pathway genes are frequently altered in pancreatic neuroendocrine tumours. Science. 2011;331(6021):1199–203.
10. Berretta M. Biomarkers in neuroendocrine tumors. Front Biosci. 2010;S2:332.
11. Ferolla P, Faggiano A, Mansueto G, et al. The biological characterization of neuroendocrine tumors: the role of neuroendocrine markers. J Endo Invest. 2008;31(3):277–86.
12. Kulke MH, Mayer RJ. Carcinoid Tumors. N Engl J Med. 1999;340:858–68.
13. Kloppel G. Classification and pathology of gastroenteropancreatic neuroendocrine neoplasms. Endocr Relat Cancer. 2011;18:S1–16.
14. Klimstra DS, Modlin IR, Coppola D, et al. The pathologic classification of neuroendocrine tumors. Pancreas. 2010;39(6):707–12.
15. Bosman FT, Carneiro F, Hruban RH, et al. WHO classification of tumours of the digestive system. Lyon: IARC; 2010.
16. Sokmensuer C, Gedikoglu G, Uzunalimoglu B. Importance of proliferation markers in gastrointestinal carcinoid tumours: a clinicopathologic study. Hepatogastroenterology. 2001;48:720–3.
17. Rindi G, Falconi M, Klersy C, et al. TNM staging of neoplasms of the endocrine pancreas: results from a large international cohort study. J Natl Cancer Inst. 2012;104(10):764–77.
18. Falconi M, Eriksson B, Kaltas G, Bartsch DK, Capdevilla J, Caplin M, Kos-Kudla B. ENETS consensus guidelines update for the management of patients with functional pancreatic neuroendocrine tumors and non-functional pancreatic neuroendocrine tumors. Neuroendocrinology. 2016;103(2):153–71.
19. Kimura W, Kurodan A, Morioka Y. Clinical pathology of endocrine tumors of the pancreas. Analysis of autopsy cases. Dig Dis Sci. 1991;36(7):933–42.
20. Zollinger RM, Ellison EH. Primary peptic ulcerations of the jejunum associated with islet cell tumors of the pancreas. 1955. CA Cancer J Clin. 1989;39(4): 231–4.
21. Pipeleers-Marichal M, Somers G, Willems G, Foulis A, Imrie C, Bishop AE, et al. Gastrinomas in the duodenums of patients with multiple endocrine neoplasia type 1 and the Zollinger-Ellison syndrome. N Engl J Med. 1990;322(11):723–7.
22. Brandi ML, Gagel RF, Angeli A, Bilezikian JP, Beck-Peccoz P, Bordi C, et al. Guidelines for diagnosis and therapy of MEN type 1 and type 2. J Clin Endocrinol Metab. 2001;86(12):5658–71.
23. Levy-Bohbot N, Merle C, Goudet P, Delemer B, Calender A, Jolly D, et al. Prevalence, characteristics and prognosis of MEN 1-associated glucagonomas, VIPomas, and somatostatinomas: study from the GTE (Groupe des Tumeurs Endocrines) registry. Gastroenterol Clin Biol. 2004;28(11):1075–81.
24. Akerström G, Hellman P. Surgical aspects of neuroendocrine tumours. Eur J Cancer. 2009;45 (Suppl 1):237–50.
25. Ramage JK, Ahmed A, Ardill J, et al. Guidelines for the management of gastroenteropancreatic neuroendocrine (including carcinoid) tumors (NETs). Gut. 2012;61:6–32.
26. Ardil JE. Circulating markers for endocrine tumours of the gastroenteropancreatic tract. Ann Clin Biochem. 2008;45:539–59.
27. Eriksson B, Annibale B, Bajetta E, Mitry E, Pavel M, Platania M, et al. ENETS consensus guidelines for the standards of care in neuroendocrine tumors: chemotherapy in patients with neuroendocrine tumors. Neuroendocrinology. 2009;90(2):214–9.
28. Maroun J, Koch W, Kvols L, et al. Guidelines for the diagnosis and management of carcinoid tumours. Part 1: the gastrointestinal tract. A statement from a Canadian national carcinoid expert group. Curr Oncol. 2006;13(2):67–76.
29. Thakker RV, Newey PJ, Walls GV, Bilezikian J, Dralle H, Ebeling PR, et al. Clinical practice guidelines for multiple endocrine neoplasia type 1 (MEN1). J Clin Endocrinol Metab. 2012;97(9): 2990–3011.
30. Oberg K, Ferone D, Kaltsas G, Knigge UP, Taal B, Plockinger U. ENETS consensus guidelines for the standards of care in neuroendocrine tumors: biotherapy. Neuroendocrinology. 2009;90(2):209–13.
31. Kwekkeboom D, Rindi G, Kloppel G, Reed N, Klanmanesh R, Jensen RT. Vienna consensus conference particpants. ENETS consensus guidelines update for the management of patients with functional pancreatic neuroendocrine tumors and non-functional pancreatic neuroendocrine tumors. Neuroendocrinology. 2016;103(2):153–71.

32. Raymond E, Dahan L, Raoul JL, Bang YJ, Borbath I, Lombard-Bohas C, et al. Sunitinib malate for the treatment of pancreatic neuroendocrine tumors. N Engl J Med. 2011;364(6):501–13.
33. Yao JC, Shah MH, Ito T, Bohas CL, Wolin EM, Van Cutsem E, et al. Everolimus for advanced pancreatic neuroendocrine tumors. N Engl J Med. 2011;364 (6):514–23.
34. Caplin ME, Pavel M, Ćwikła JB, Phan AT, Raderer M, Sedláčková E, et al. Lanreotide in metastatic enteropancreatic neuroendocrine tumors. N Engl J Med. 2014;371(3):224–33.
35. Berna MJ, Annibale B, Marignani M, Luong TV, Corleto V, Pace A, et al. A prospective study of gastric carcinoids and enterochromaffin-like cell changes in multiple endocrine neoplasia type 1 and Zollinger-Ellison syndrome: identification of risk factors. J Clin Endocrinol Metab. 2008;93(5):1582–91.
36. Allan B, David J, Perez E, et al. Malignant neuroendocrine tumors: incidence and outcomes in paediatric patients. Eur J Paed Surg. 2013;23:394–9.
37. Pape UF, Jann H, Muller-Nordhorn J, et al. Prognostic relevance of a novel TNM classification system for upper gastroenteropancreatic neuroendocrine tumors. Cancer. 2008;113:256–65.

Islet Cell Transplantation

14

Antonio Bruni, Michael McCall and A.M. James Shapiro

Diabetes mellitus currently affects more than 200 million people worldwide, with projections of it affecting 5% of the world population by 2025 [1]. Type 1 diabetes mellitus (T1DM), the most severe form of this disease, represents approximately 10% of all cases of diabetes and is characterized by a progressive autoimmune disorder resulting in the destruction of insulin-producing β-cells within the pancreatic islets of Langerhans. Due to progressive chronic micro- and macrovascular complications, T1DM is a major source of morbidity and mortality. Whilst T1DM has become a manageable condition, largely owing to the availability of exogenous insulin following the discovery of insulin by Banting, Best, Collip and McLeod [2, 3], many patients still develop a multitude of chronic complications of diabetes including nephropathy, neuropathy, retinopathy, peripheral vascular disease and coronary artery disease. Although the etiology of these complications is multifactorial, the Diabetes Control and Complications Trial (DCCT) clearly demonstrated that their development can be reduced by tight glycemic control. This was achieved in the trial by the use of intensive rather than conventional insulin therapy [4–6]. However, one of the downsides of intensive insulin was a substantial increase in life-threatening hypoglycemia [5].

Safer and innovative means to tighten glycemic control have been developed, including the use of insulin pumps, dynamic continuous glucose monitoring, and closed loop systems. These have achieved improved glycemic control, reduced hypoglycemic risk, and moderate improved protection from secondary diabetic complications. However, while these technological advances offer patients improved benefit, they continue to fall short as a definitive, robust cure for diabetes. Indeed, these treatments all involve the use of exogenous insulin and work by better 'controlling' diabetes rather than by 'reversing' it. An alternative approach is to attempt to actually restore the destroyed beta (β)-cell mass by transplanting the insulin-producing tissue, either in the form of a whole vascularized pancreas transplant, or by a cellular islet transplant.

First attempted in 1966, whole pancreas transplantation initially showed poor clinical outcomes [7]. However, following considerable advances in surgical technique, immunosuppressive strategies, and postoperative management, the results have improved drastically, with 80–85% of patients remaining insulin independent for at least a year following this procedure. However, it remains a major intra-abdominal surgical procedure, with significant morbidity

A. Bruni · M. McCall
5-040 Li Ka Shing Health Research, 112 Street and 87 Avenue, Edmonton, AB T6G 2E1, Canada
e-mail: bruni1@ualberta.ca

M. McCall
e-mail: mmccall@ualberta.ca

A.M. James Shapiro (✉)
2000 College Plaza, 8215 112 Street, Edmonton, AB T6G 2C8, Canada
e-mail: amjs@islet.ca

D.J. Ledbetter and P.R.V. Johnson (eds.), *Endocrine Surgery in Children*,
DOI 10.1007/978-3-662-54256-9_14

and a mortality rate of 4–7% in leading centers around the world. In addition, as the pancreas only comprises 2% endocrine tissue, it could be argued that patients with T1DM receiving a whole pancreas graft are receiving 98% of pancreatic tissue that they do not require! It is therefore, very unlikely that this treatment will become a routine treatment for children with T1DM.

Conversely, pancreatic islet cell transplantation is a minimally invasive procedure, involving only the implantation of the pancreatic endocrine component. In addition, as a cellular transplant, islet transplants have the real potential to be immunomodified or immunoisolated at the time of transplantation, meaning that in the future it may be possible to undertake an islet transplant without the need for immunosuppression. This, combined with the simplicity of the procedure, mean that this therapy has real potential for future use in children.

In this chapter, we provide a historical perspective of islet transplantation; outline the challenges of donor selection; provide an overview of human islet isolation; discuss the different aspects of the islet transplant procedure, including some of the challenges; a review of the current outcomes of clinical islet transplantation; and finally, discuss the potential use of islet transplantation in children.

Islet Transplantation: A Historical Perspective

The work of von Mering and Minkowski in 1889, was essential for first identifying the pivotal link between the pancreas and elevated blood glucose levels, when they showed that total pancreatectomy in dogs resulted in fatal diabetes [8]. Two decades later, Sharpey-Shafer's hypothesis provided insight into the link between diabetes and insulin, a key chemical found within pancreas. However, although the recognition of diabetes and the hypothesis about insulin were monumental, it was not until Banting, Best, Collip, and McLeod discovered and isolated insulin in 1922, that diabetes became a chronically manageable condition [2, 3]. The introduction of intensive blood glucose monitoring and the frequent daily administration of exogenous insulin improved things further, and therapeutic efforts shifted more from the acute phase of the disease to strategies to stabilize, reverse, or ideally prevent the chronic complications of the disease [9]. As highlighted above, however, focus has turned to strategies that enable true reversal of diabetes, and currently this can only be achieved by restoring β-cell mass through transplantation.

One of the most important advances that enabled clinical islet transplantation to be made possible was the ability to isolate sufficient numbers of human islets from a donor pancreas. The isolation of rodent islets was first accomplished by Lacy in the 1960s when a number of islets were isolated following the enzymatic digestion of rodent pancreases from obese animals with hypertrophic islets [10]. Further refinements by Lacy and Kostianovsky then established the technical ability to isolate hundreds of metabolically active and structurally intact islets from the pancreas of normal rats [11]. While several authors reported the correction of hyperglycemia in diabetic mice using varied islet doses and success rates via the intraperitoneal route, the work of Reckard and Barker in 1973 was the first to effectively cure diabetes in a chemically induced model of diabetes [12]. Yet despite these successes, the same methods of islet isolation and purification could not be applied to larger animals or humans, whose pancreases contain several million islets, and whose pancreatic structure differs greatly from rodents [11, 13].

Further refinements to the methods of islet isolation and purification for islet transplantation continued for decades (and still do continue), with improved success in isolating greater quantities with greater purity. Injection of collagenase into the pancreatic duct proved an effective method for successful islet isolation from large animals and humans [13, 14]. However, it was the development of the Ricordi digestion chamber in 1988, enabling a semi-automated process for human islet isolation, that was instrumental in enabling sufficient isolation and purification of islets for clinical use [13, 15]. This method of islet isolation is still considered the universal 'gold standard', and has made clinical islet transplantation a reality [13].

With regard to islet transplantation itself, outcomes have progressed significantly since clinical islet transplants were first performed. This is partly due to improved islet manufacturing processes, but has also been greatly facilitated by the availability of more effective induction and maintenance immunosuppression to protect against both auto- and alloreactivity [16]. In subjects with poor glycemic control, islet-alone transplantation has recently become an accepted practice to stabilize frequent hypoglycemia or severe glycemic lability [17]. While Lacy's work established the liver as an ideal site for islet transplantation [18], further work by Najarian et al. in 1977 reported the first successful clinical islet transplant paired with the administration of azathioprine and corticosteroids [19]. In spite of these achievements, only 9% of the 267 islet transplant recipients since 1999 were insulin independent for >1 year [20]. It was not until 2000 that the 'Edmonton Protocol' reported insulin independence in seven consecutive T1DM patients over a median follow-up of 11.9 months with sustained C-peptide [16]. Patients had received at least two different islet transplants and a mean islet mass of 13,000 IEQ/kg. Perhaps most notably, patients received a steroid-free immunosuppressive regimen of anti-interleukin (IL)-2 receptor antagonist antibody therapy, daclizumab. These monumental results were pivotal in driving forward both interest and activity in clinical islet transplantation over the subsequent decade, which resulted in the expansion of islet transplantation programs in North America and abroad through remarkable inter-center collaboration.

The success of the Edmonton Group ignited widespread enthusiasm. However, the initial waning of complete insulin independence by 3–5 years post-transplantation raised further concerns that islet transplantation could not permanently ameliorate the diabetic state in patients. Strategies to improve islet transplantation outcomes have continued over subsequent years, including but not limited to, improved donor selection, optimized techniques for organ donation and preservation and immunosuppression regimens. Undoubtedly, such refinements will enable this treatment to fulfill its potential in the coming decades and expand its therapeutic benefit to patients afflicted with this debilitating illness.

Donor Selection and Donor Availability

The number of patients that can receive an islet transplant is largely limited by the availability of donor pancreases. In addition, optimal donor selection is an important factor influencing successful islet transplant outcome. Several donor-related variables that may contribute to islet isolation outcomes have been demonstrated through single-center retrospective studies. Variables include donor age, cause of death, body mass index (BMI), cold ischemia time, length of hospitalization, use of vasopressors, and blood glucose levels [21–28]. In spite of the observation that a larger pancreas contains a larger β-cell mass, pancreas weight does not appear to correlate directly with successful islet yield [27, 29]. In a study analyzing data from 345 deceased donors, it was determined that although BMI correlates with pancreas weight, body surface area is a better predictor of pancreas weight than BMI [29]. Several other groups have indicated that BMI itself positively affects islet yield [30], leading many to consider BMI as an important donor predictor islet isolation outcome [25–27]. This view, however, has led to the misconception that an obese donor is a good candidate for successful transplantation, whereas it is important to distinguish between factors that lead to a high islet yield, and those that correlate with optimal islet physiology.

With regard to pancreas allocation, in most countries to date, 'optimal' pancreases are still prioritized for whole organ transplantation before they are offered to islets. A review by Berney and Johnson concluded that transplanted islet mass does not unequivocally correlate with islet graft function (also see below), further arguing that based on this premise, donor selection criteria for islet transplantation and hence allocation rules (pancreas for whole organ or islet transplant) may need to be redefined [31]. A joint whole pancreas and islet donor allocation system for whole pancreas and islet transplantation has now been introduced in the United Kingdom.

O'Gorman et al. developed a scoring system based on donor characteristics that can predict islet isolation outcomes and has been an instrumental tool in assessing whether a pancreas should be processed for islet isolation [32]. Though this tool has been sufficient for determining which organs are optimal for islet isolation in terms of islet yields and crude islet function, it does not predict optimal islet transplant outcome. Similarly, other published studies investigating optimal donor factors for islet isolation have not taken transplant outcome into consideration [21, 22, 24, 25, 26, 27, 28]. Lakey et al. retrospectively reviewed human islet isolation preparations and studied the effects of donor age on islet yield and function (insulin secretory capabilities) [25]. Their study suggested that older donors (51–65 years old) are more likely to produce a transplantable yield of islets when compared with their younger donor counterparts (83% compared to 37% in 19–28 year old donors). However, the secretory capabilities of these islets were significantly reduced. Other studies have confirmed these results and shown higher rates of diabetes reversal in immunodeficient diabetic mice receiving human islet grafts from younger donors [23]. While this would point to younger donors as 'ideal' for islet transplantation, one must also realize that digestion of a young pancreas is also technically more difficult and hence islet yields lower. The more 'fibrous' nature of the pancreatic matrix within young donors considerably reduces the success rate and yield of islets. More recently, groups from Minnesota and San Francisco in the US have modified islet isolation protocols for optimized success with the younger human pancreas.

Prolonged cold ischemic time for the pancreas during shipment from the donor center to the isolation center can be injurious to human islet isolation (both islet yield and function), with times exceeding 6–8 h being less optimal than locally procured donors [24]. While pancreatic transport in University of Wisconsin (UW) solution was standard previously, most transplant programs (at least in Canada and in parts of the US) have switched to histidine-tryptophan-ketoglutarate (HTK) solution, which may be less optimal for pancreas storage [33]. The two-layer oxygenated UW–perfluorodecalin method for pancreas transportation initially looked promising, but with increased use, it appeared to add little protection to the islets prior to isolation, and has therefore been abandoned by most programs at the present time [34].

Human Islet Isolation

One of the most important prerequisites of successful clinical islet transplantation is an optimized islet isolation process. Unquestionably, human islet isolation requires considerable skill and involves a significant financial cost, especially now that the regulation of human islet isolation has become so stringent around the world. Whereas in the 1990s, human islet isolation was performed in modified research laboratories, this now has to be conducted in ultraclean Good Manufacturing Practice (GMP) facilities that meet strict national governmental oversight. This has led over recent years to the development of a number of 'hub and spoke' clinical islet transplant networks, in which islet isolation is only performed in one or two 'clinical-grade' isolation facilities that provide quality islets for a network of different islet transplant centers. Successful networks include the GRAGIL Network in Switzerland and France [35], the NORDIC network in Scandinavia, and the UK Islet Transplant Consortium (UKITC) in Britain. Clinical islets have also been successfully shipped between centers in the US [36]. This approach allows resources and expertise to be centralized, making the clinical islet isolation process much more cost-effective.

The process of islet isolation starts at the time of cadaveric organ donation with the need for meticulous surgery and minimal handling of the pancreas during procurement. This is combined with rapid cooling of the lesser sac at the time of aortic cross-clamp placement and arterial flushing. Once procured, the pancreas is then placed in a cold storage solution and transported to the islet isolation facility.

The challenge of islet isolation is to produce high yields of 'in tact' islets of optimal viability, purity, and function. Human islet isolation involves three steps, namely pancreas digestion, density gradient purification, and islet culture.

Pancreas Digestion

The pancreas is digested by a combination of physical and enzymatic dissociation. This stage is intended to liberate islets from the surrounding pancreatic exocrine matrix, producing a pancreatic digest in which both islets and exocrine sit. This digestion stage is performed within a Ricordi chamber (Fig. 14.1) and uses commercially available collagenase enzyme produced from the bacteria Clostridum histolyticum. An efficient enzymatic digestion is critical for successful islet isolation, and this is achieved by a careful balance of enzyme composition and duration of

(a) (b) (c) (d)

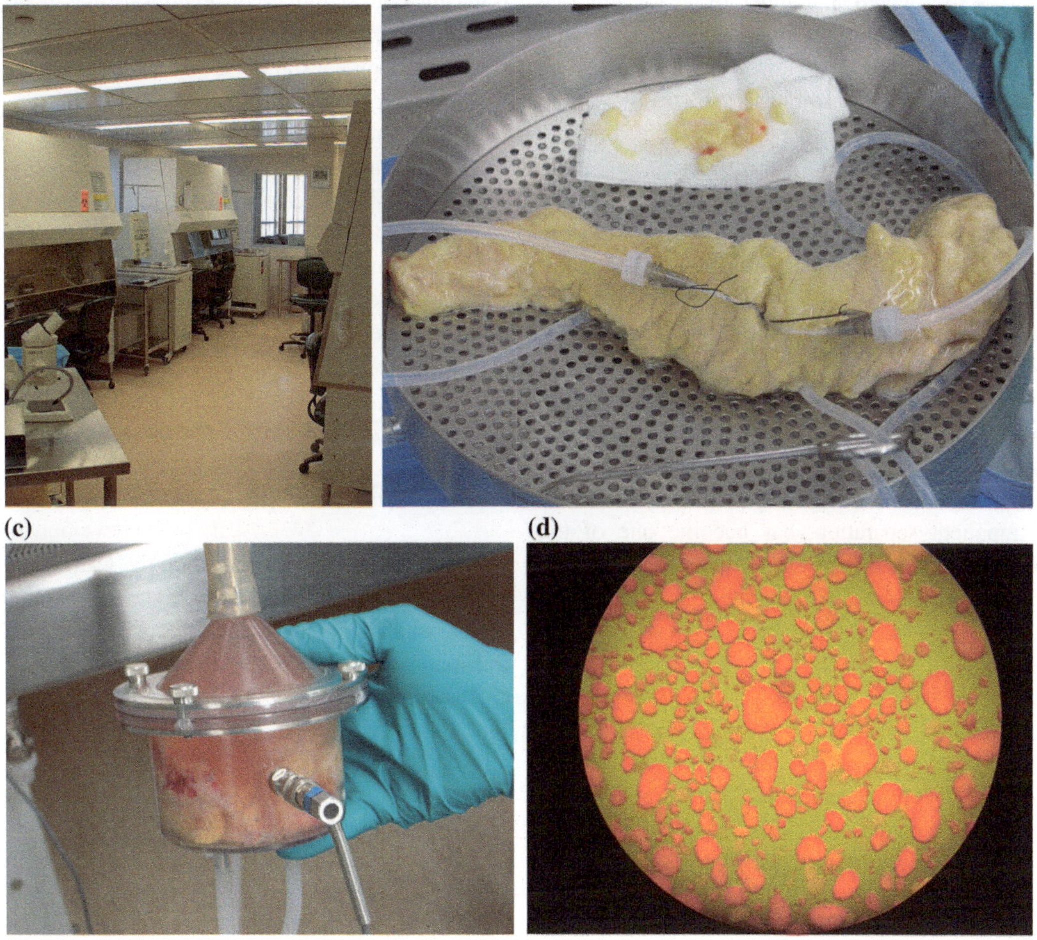

Fig. 14.1 Human islet isolation. **a** Human islet isolation occurs in a specialized laboratory. **b** The pancreatic duct is cannulated after the pancreas is trimmed. **c** The sectioned pancreas is loaded into the Ricordi chamber for digestion. **d** Isolated islets are stained with dithizone and counted

collagenase digestion [37]. Suboptimal collagenase composition, or insufficient collagenase exposure, leads to incomplete liberation of islets from the exocrine tissue resulting in low islet yields of decreased purity. However, overactive collagenase or increased duration of collagenase exposure, can lead to islet fragmentation. Thus, one of the greatest challenges for islet transplant programs has for many years been the 'batch-to-batch' variability and non-reproducibility of collagenase preparations [38, 39].

Density Gradient Purification

It was discovered a number of years ago that islets infused into the portal vein with large amounts of accompanying exocrine tissue can lead to portal vein thrombosis which can be fatal [40]. The pancreatic digest is therefore, purified by density gradient centrifugation, enabling 'pure' islets to be retrieved. Islet purification takes advantage of the fact that islets and exocrine tissue have different buoyant densities. When placed in specially developed media of known density and spun on a centrifuge, tissue will migrate to a layer corresponding to their own density, with the less dense islets settling at a higher density than exocrine tissue. The introduction of the COBE 2991 machine by the Leicester Group, originally utilized for blood component separation, has become one of the key factors in achieving sufficient numbers of purified islets for clinical use [41].

Islet Culture

While the islets used in the original Edmonton Protocol were transplanted immediately after isolation, culturing islets post-isolation is believed to be important for their recovery from isolation-induced damage and enables islets to be carefully assessed before infusion. It also enables immunomodulatory therapy to be started in the recipient and potentially reduces the immunogenicity of the graft. A culture period also greatly enhances the practicality of an islet transplant in terms of planning for the patient's admission and the availability of the radiology suite. However, this may be at the cost of impaired revascularization subsequent to transplant, due to the loss of intra-islet endothelial cells during this culture period. Therefore, essential components of the culture conditions for human islet preparations are sufficient oxygen and nutrient supply. During the culture stage, the maintenance of the tridimensional islet cluster and preventing islet mass loss should be accomplished during the culturing phase. To date, sufficient investigation of optimal culture conditions has occurred, yet in spite of this, protocols have yet to be standardized and culture conditions may vary between islet isolation centers [42]. Other considerations like media composition, seeding density, and incubation temperature play a significant role in maintaining viability and recovery [42].

During the 24–48 h of islet culture, 10–20% of the islet mass is 'lost' due to islet disaggregation and islet death. However, these 'lost' islets would probably not have survived in the recipient, and a period of islet culture enables more extensive evaluation of the graft pre-transplantation.

The Islet Transplant Procedure

Pre-transplant Preparation

Once a patient has been placed on the waiting list for islet transplantation, they await a suitable donor pancreas for islet isolation and subsequent transplantation. Once the islet yield of the matched pancreas has been confirmed to be sufficient for transplanting into that recipient (usually ≥ 5000 islet equivalents (IEQ) per kg, where an IEQ is an islet count that has been adjusted to standardize the islet diameter to 150 μm), the patient is admitted to the transplant centre to begin immunosuppressive induction therapy. Prior to the introduction of the Edmonton Protocol in the late 1990s, corticosteroids were a mainstay component of the immunosuppressive protocol. It is widely known, however, that these medications are themselves diabetogenic and are particularly damaging to newly transplanted islets. The Edmonton Protocol provided a steroid-free approach, employing sirolimus and low-dose tacrolimus maintenance therapy after the potent induction agent daclizumab, an anti-CD25 (IL-2R) monoclonal antibody [16]. Since the removal of daclizumab from the market after patent expiry, other T-cell depletional agents have been used including thymoglobulin (antithymocyte globulin), basiliximab (Il-2R antibody) and, more recently, some of the best results have been used with the anti-CD52 alemtuzumab. At some centers, sirolimus is being replaced from post-transplant immunosuppressive protocols by the better tolerated mycophenolate mofetil.

Many centers are employing adjuvant regimens to enhance outcomes. The blockade of tumor necrosis factor α (TNFα) as a means to prevent its inflammatory attack on islets post-transplantation has been used in the form of Etanercept [43, 44] and Infliximab [45]. Exenatide (a GLP-1 agonist) has found use in patients with graft dysfunction, promoting insulin secretion and improving islet function [46, 47]. In fact, the combination of Etanercept and Exenatide may enhance islet engraftment when given in combination [48]. All patients are given broad-spectrum prophylactic antibiotics shortly before the procedure.

The Transplant Procedure

Today, most clinical islet transplants are performed using percutaneous intrahepatic islet infusion via the portal vein under radiological control. However, a few centers still prefer the surgical mesenteric cannulation approach for additional safety.

Portal infusion offers a minimally invasive procedure, accomplished without need for surgery or general anaesthesia, with the ability to regulate glycemic levels through portal insulin delivery [49]. Once at the confluence of the portal vein, islets are infused aseptically under gravity while the portal venous pressure is monitored. Heparin (70 units/kg) is included in the islet preparation to minimize the chance of portal vein thrombosis. While catheter tract bleeding is a known complication, multiple approaches can be used to prevent this including D-STAT [50], coils and gelfoam or microfibrillary collagen (Avitene®) paste. However, although rare, this percutaneous approach still has some potential procedural risks, including portal thrombosis and bleeding [51].

The surgical approach to portal venous access is less commonly used, though it may be necessary if the percutaneous approach cannot be utilized (e.g., large right-sided liver hemangioma). In this instance, a mesenteric vein is cannulated, utilizing complete surgical control to prevent bleeding. However, this approach has the inherent risks of laparotomy/laparoscopy including bleeding, infection, adhesion formation, and wound breakdown/incisional hernia (especially if on sirolimus).

The liver is the currently the preferred transplant site for a number of reasons. It is easily accessible percutaneously, it has high a vascularity supplying sufficient oxygen and nutrients during the revascularization period, and it contains a sinusoidal structure that enables islets to become trapped and engrafted. Having islets placed within the liver also ensures a physiological release of insulin into the portal vein, although compared with the native pancreas, it suffers from a low oxygen content. Moreover, a significant amount of intraportal islet mass is lost immediately post-transplant due to innate immune pathways involving platelet and complement activation.

To date, numerous alternative islet transplantation sites have been proposed and tested, both experimentally and in some cases clinically. These include the kidney subcapsule, the spleen, pancreas, omentum, gastrointestinal wall, immune privileged sites such as the eye and testis/ovary, and the subcutaneous spaces. Though some alternative sites offer advantageous results in experimental models, their feasibility and translation into clinical settings have been limited. Undoubtedly, ongoing experimental and clinical investigation is required to elucidate an optimal islct transplant site with efforts aimed to improve islet engraftment, long-term insulin independence, and transplant outcomes from single donors.

Post-transplant Care

To minimize stress on the newly transplanted islets, tight glycemic control is maintained using an insulin/glucose sliding scale. It is known that islets engraft more readily if they are able to do so in a euglycemic environment [52]. However, apoptotic islets will release insulin, making the patient susceptible to hypoglycemia. To prevent portal vein thrombosis and combat IBMIR (instant blood mediated inflammatory reaction), unfractionated heparin is infused in the postoperative period. Ultrasonography is routinely performed at day one and one week post-transplant to rule out intraperitoneal hemorrhage and ensure patency of the portal vein. In addition to immunosuppressive drugs, patients are discharged home 1–2 days later on a range of post-transplant medications.

Complications

Procedure-Related Complications

Portal vein thrombosis and major hepatic bleeding account for two of the most serious complications associated with the percutaneous approach to islet transplantation [53]. Portal vein is extremely uncommon now, especially as we now transplant purer islet preparations and use heparin in the preparation and also systemically in the patient. The incidence of bleeding from the catheter tract was not uncommon in the early incidences of clinical islet transplantation [53]. Many of these events have all but been eliminated through methods to reduce the catheter tract. The clinical islet transplantation site in Edmonton currently utilizes Avitene® paste to seal and abate the catheter tract. Although segmental vein thrombosis can occur (5% in the above-mentioned series), main portal vein thrombosis is extremely rare. This risk is largely reduced through the administration of unfractionated heparin (70 units/kg) in the islet preparation, as well as through instituting systemic anticoagulation, post-procedure.

Immunosuppression-Related Complications

Corticosteroids used to form the backbone of immunosuppression regimes in early clinical islet transplantation settings and were found to be quite toxic to islets. The success of the 'Edmonton Protocol' is attributed to the immunosuppression scheme that utilized the combination of sirolimus, low-dose tacrolimus and daclizumab in an effort to prevent the deleterious effects of calcineurin inhibitors and steroids [54]. In spite of these refinements, most patients returned to modest amounts of insulin despite the elimination of recurrent hypoglycemia by 5 years post-transplant, clearly indicating room for improvement [55]. Moreover, β-cell survival and function are also compromised due to the proximity of the transplanted islets to high concentrations of these drugs in the hepatoportal circulation [56, 57].

Due to the multiple pathways known to contribute to β-cell attrition and the alloresponse to foreign antigens, it is unlikely that a monotherapy will optimize clinical islet transplantation outcomes and lead to single donor recipients [55]. The implementation of highly potent and selective biological agents for the initiation and maintenance of immunosuppression has made significant progress in reducing the frequency of acute rejection, prolonging graft survival and minimizing the complications of these therapeutic schemes [58, 59]. The University of Minnesota reported improvements to single donor success rates as a result of combining anti-inflammatory biologics to maintenance immunosuppression [43, 60]. In addition, peri-transplant insulin and heparin administration greatly increased the success rate of single donor islet transplants from 10 to 40% [61].

Furthermore, the blockade of tumor necrosis factor alpha with etanercept has also enhanced single donor islet transplant outcomes [43, 61, 62, 63, 64].

The successful establishment of an immunosuppressive regimen that promotes self-tolerance is critical for the long-term success of clinical islet transplantation. A tolerizing regimen that utilizes biologics and techniques that selectively target donor-reactive T cells while expanding populations of regulatory T cells, in an 'islet friendly' manner will undoubtedly lead to the definitive cure of T1DM.

Islet transplant recipients often have some degree of renal impairment at the time of transplantation, which can be exacerbated by calcineurin inhibitors. This is true even with the low doses used currently, which can be compounded with the use of sirolimus [65, 66]. Consequently, renal function of islet transplant recipients must be monitored diligently. In addition, islet recipients are prone to the more generalized immunosuppressive complications including leucopenia, mouth ulcers, infections, and malignancy.

Clinical Islet Transplantation Outcomes

Since the inception of the Edmonton Protocol, over 750 islet transplants have been performed in over 30 International transplant centers around the world. Unquestionably, the concept of islet transplantation has evolved in a number of countries from an experimental procedure to one that recognized standard clinical therapy.

To date, 677 allogeneic islet transplants have been reported to the Collaborative Islet Transplant Registry (CITR). Of these, 44% were insulin independent at three years post-transplant in the 'new era' of islet transplants (2007–2010), as compared to 27% of clinical islet transplant recipients in 1999–2002 [67, 68] (Fig. 14.2a). Moreover, marked improvements in clinical islet transplantation have been observed from 2007 to 2010, as evidenced by retained C-peptide levels, reduction in HbA1c levels and reduced islet reinfusion rates [68]. Shifts in immunosuppression strategies can account for these success rates, though improvements to islet engraftment and subsequent survival are paramount to achieving durable insulin independence.

In spite of marked improvements in clinical islet transplantation outcomes and substantial transplant activity in international islet transplant centers, few centers are currently active in North America. In the United States, islet transplantation is still classified as an experimental therapy, and as a result immensely lacks the available funds necessary to conduct and support large-scale clinical trials. In an effort to support the FDA biological license application mandate, two pivotal Phase III clinical trials are currently being conducted in specialized islet transplantation centers through the Clinical Islet Transplant (CIT) Consortium (CIT-06 and CIT-07, Clinical Trials.gov NCT00468117 and NCT00434811, respectively). Successful licensure will inevitably recognize islet transplantation as a clinical therapy, thus expanding its therapeutic applicability to patients with T1DM in the United States.

The University of Alberta's Clinical Islet Transplant Program remains an active site, and in 2013 alone, 66 islet transplants were conducted at the Edmonton site (Fig. 14.2b). The Edmonton Group reports that of over 200 patients transplanted with more than 400 intraportal islet preparations, 79% of recipients continue to show full or partial islet graft function [69]. Notably, the median duration of insulin independence is 34.6 and 11 months for subjects with full or partial graft function. Moreover, the duration of C-peptide is 53.3 and 70.4 months, respectively, for those same patients [70–72].

To date, the application of islet allotransplantation is only suitable for patients with unstable glycemic control that is life-threatening (e.g., hypoglycemia unawareness) and that cannot be corrected by standard conventional and intensive insulin therapies [17]. Patients who exhibit good glycemic control, as well as children, are not currently considered for islet allotransplantation, largely owing to the need for lifelong, chronic immunosuppression. In a recent trial by Ly et al.,

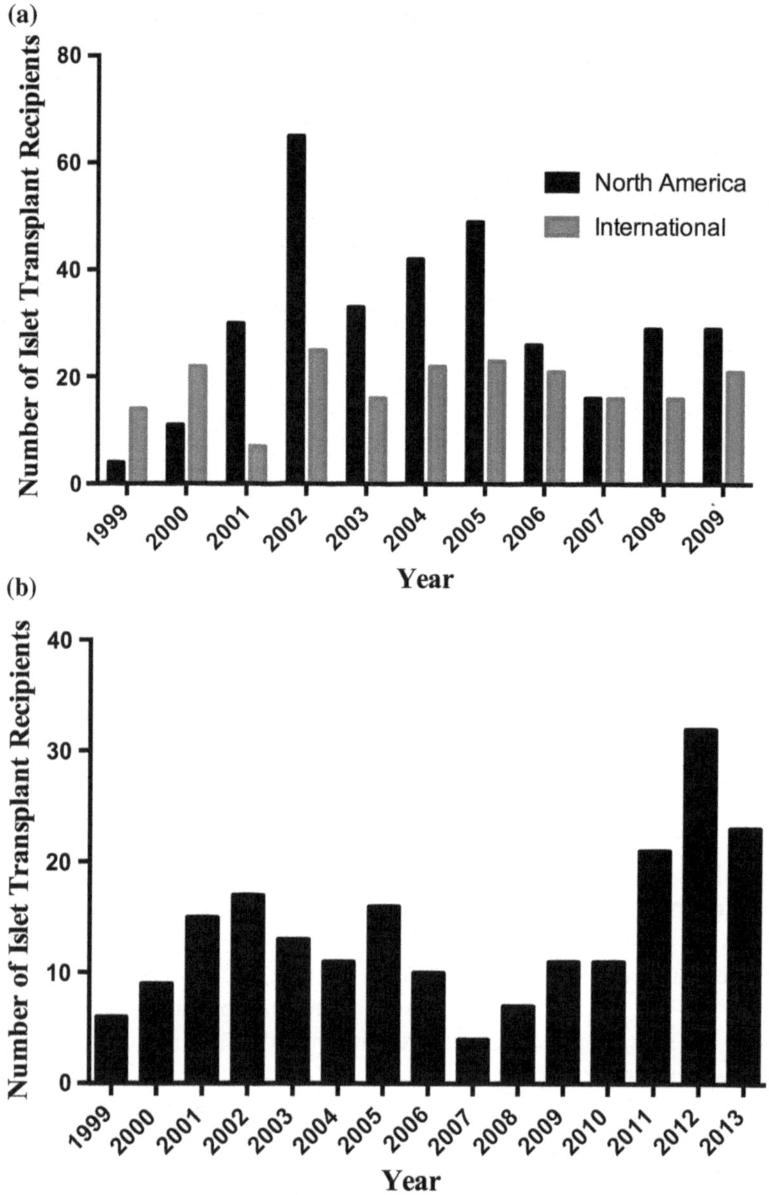

Fig. 14.2 Clinical islet transplant recipients per year. **a** Number of islet transplant recipients per year completed in North America and Internationally, registered by the CITR. **b** Number of islet transplant recipients completed by the Edmonton Clinical Islet Transplant Program

sensor-augmented pump therapy with automated insulin suspension reduced the rate of moderate and severe hypoglycemia, as well as impaired hypoglycemia awareness over a 6-month period in trial participants. Yet, when compared to the standard insulin pump control group, no change in glycosylated hemoglobin (HbA1C) was observed [72]. Conversely, in islet transplant recipients, HbA1C levels were corrected to levels that could predictably reverse the secondary consequences of diabetes [73]. Moreover, a one-way crossover study conducted by Thompson and colleagues demonstrated that clinical islet transplantation was more effective in reducing progression of diabetic retinopathy and nephropathy than intensive medical therapy [74]. In this therapeutic setting, the lifelong need for immunosuppressive therapy may be readily justified.

Indications and Patient Selection for Islet Transplantation

As noted, the current indications for islet allotransplantation do not include the pediatric population, though the potential applicability to children will be explored below (Table 14.1). Indeed, islet transplantation has been carried out in children, although most have been in the setting of total pancreatectomy and islet autotransplantation for hereditary pancreatitis. In this clinical setting the necessity for immunosuppression is not required.

Secondary to the procedure and consequences of the immunosuppressive therapies, there are a number of risks associated with islet transplantation. As such, adult patients selected for islet transplantation must have T1DM with life-threatening complications to justify these risks. Suitable patient populations include those with severe and recurrent hypoglycemic unawareness and/or those with unstable glucose control despite an optimized insulin regime (glycemic lability). The latter includes those requiring hospitalization for hypoglycemia or ketoacidosis. Those with advanced secondary complications of T1DM may also be considered.

In addition to thorough characterization of secondary complications, patient selection also involves the determination of metabolic status. Typically, patients are selected provided there is no endogenous insulin reserve, indicated by the absence of C-peptide. Patients with elevated BMI (>30 kg/m^2) or weight > 90 kg may be excluded since the transplanted islet tissue may not meet metabolic demand. The evaluation of hypoglycemia and glycemic lability is assessed through the HYPO score and Lability Index (LI), respectively, developed by Ryan et al. [75]. While the former is based on the frequency, severity and degree of unawareness of the hypoglycemia, the latter is calculated based on the change in glucose levels over time. Patients ranking in the 90th percentile for either score are given consideration for islet transplantation.

Patients selected for islet transplantation undergo a full cardiac assessment and should have no evidence of uncontrolled hypertension, absence of myocardial infarction in the preceding six months and left ventricular ejection fraction >30%. Since immunosuppressive therapy (specifically tacrolimus and sirolimus) may exacerbate renal failure, a glomerular filtration rate of >80 ml/min/1.73 m^2 and no evidence of macroscopic proteinuria is preferred. All recipients are also screened for any evidence of early neoplasias.

Pediatric Islet Allotransplantation—A Real Possibility?

In the history of solid organ transplantation, it did not take long for life-saving transplants and the need for chronic immunosuppression in adults to be translated to the pediatric population. Some of the earliest successful liver transplants were carried out in children, and today end-stage renal failure in children is optimally managed with renal transplantation and chronic immunosuppression. The risks associated with immunosuppression (increased rates of infection and

Table 14.1 Indications and exclusions for islet allotransplantation

Indications for islet transplantation	Exclusions for islet transplantation
• Type 1 diabetes for >5 years • Above 18 years old • Negative stimulated C-peptide (<0.3 ng/ml) • Despite adequate insulin therapy: – Hypoglycemic unawareness[a] – Glycemic lability[b] – Composite score >75th percentile	• Uncontrolled hypertension • Severe cardiac disease • Macroalbuminuria • Glomerular filtration rate <80 ml/min/1.73 m^2 • Potential inability to comply with imunosuppression

[a]Clark Score >4, HYPO score > 90th percentile
[b]Lability index >90th

malignancy, renal impairment and specific drug-related side effects) are well defined in the pediatric and adult populations. Whole pancreas transplantation has rarely been applied to children, largely owing to the risk associated with surgical intervention of such magnitude, as well as the life-threatening complications. Consequently, such a procedure would be difficult to justify in a child with T1DM without other life-threatening complications. It is often questioned when islet transplantation would be a suitable therapy for children. If the need for lifelong immunosuppression could be negated through the induction of tolerance, then islet transplantation in children could adequately be justified. Conversely, with today's standard of care treatment, the lifelong commitment to immunosuppression represents a challenging balance against the known, unmitigated complications associated with T1DM.

Alarmingly, the incidence of both T1DM and type 2 diabetes mellitus (obesity-related diabetes) is progressively rising in children globally. To mitigate the long-term complications associated with diabetes, tight glycemic control must be maintained, though this is not without inherent risks. Notably, in children, there are increased risks of fatal hypoglycemia, behavioral and cognitive impairment and the masking of future episodes of hypoglycemia [4, 76, 77].

There are numerous obstacles that are associated with the optimal care of this age group, including accuracy of blood glucose monitors, family commitment and the compliance of the patient as they reach adolescence [78]. Children occasionally face life-threatening, asymptomatic nocturnal hypoglycemia despite adequate exogenous insulin therapy [78]. Challenges arise in adequately identifying these risks at an appropriate time and improving insulin management while ensuring the prevention of a fatal hypoglycemic episode. Unquestionably, islet transplantation will likely become a therapeutic strategy in children with unstable and recalcitrant forms of T1DM. As inroads continue to be made in the safety of the procedure itself, as well as improvements to the side effects associated with acute and chronic immunosuppression therapies. Moreover, effective control of the autoimmune process in type 1 diabetes will be essential if these approaches are to move forward successfully.

In the adult population, islet transplantation has proven effective in preventing hypoglycemic events and enabling insulin independence. The requirement for chronic, long-term immunosuppression, paired with their potential side effects, limits its use in this population. As newer, less toxic immunosuppressive regimens and the potential for both steroid and calcinerin inhibitor-free protocols are developed, islet transplantation may be a possible therapy in very select groups of children. These include:

- Children suffering from recurrent, severe hypoglycemic events despite diet and insulin alterations.
- Children who develop secondary complications of diabetes, especially retinopathy and nephropathy, likely leading to severe deficits in adulthood.
- Those children already on immunosuppression for a previous solid organ allograft.

From a practical perspective, the first and third groups would derive the most benefit in light of the risks associated with islet transplantation and immunosuppression. However, the optimization of diet and insulin therapy would need to be considered in order for islet transplantation to be implemented. For islet transplantation to be widely implemented in children, a number of key questions will need to be answered, including [78]:

- Will the recipient outgrow the islet mass or will the islet mass expand over time as the patient develops?
- Will islets from one donor be sufficient to promote insulin independence?
- Will adolescent patients be able to comply with maintenance immunotherapy after successful islet transplantation?
- How should immunosuppressive regimens be tailored in female patients who wish to conceive in early adulthood?

Elucidating answers to these questions are critical for the application of clinical islet transplantation in children afflicted with T1DM.

Concluding Remarks

Undoubtedly, improvements in human islet isolation, the introduction of the 'Edmonton Protocol', and more recent developments in anti-inflammatory and immunosuppressive strategies have played a major role in improving the results and activity of clinical islet transplantation. Islet transplantation cannot currently be defined as a cure for T1DM, though this therapeutic treatment can offer an improved quality of life in recipients, evidenced by remarkable stability of glycemic control and correction of HbA1C. Such clinical outcomes provide an increasing number of patients with sustained periods of complete independence from insulin. Prevention of life-threatening hypoglycemia is a major advance that can often not be sustained by optimized exogenous insulin therapy. Continued, concerted efforts are still required to further establish islet transplantation as a suitable treatment modality for all patients afflicted with T1DM. The applicability of whole organ allotransplantation in children emphasizes the ongoing need to establish less toxic immunosuppression regimes aimed to improve all lives of those afflicted with T1DM. This need calls for a continued rapid drive to transition islet transplantation as a treatment for some, to a therapy for all.

References

1. King H, Aubert RE, Herman WH. Global burden of diabetes, 1995–2025: prevalence, numerical estimates, and projections. Diabetes Care. 1998;21(9): 1414–31.
2. Polonsky KS. The past 200 years in diabetes. New Engl J Med. 2012;367(14):1332–40.
3. Banting FG, Best CH, Collip JB, Campbell WR, Fletcher AA. Pancreatic extracts in the treatment of diabetes mellitus. Can Med Assoc J. 1922;12(3): 141–6.
4. The Diabetes Control and Complications Trial Research Group. The effect of intensive treatment of diabetes on the development and progression of long-term complications in insulin-dependent diabetes mellitus. New Engl J Med. 1993;329(14): 977–86.
5. Keen H. The diabetes control and complications trial (DCCT). Health Trends. 1994;26(2):41–3.
6. Nathan DM, Lachin J, Cleary P, Orchard T, Brillon DJ, Backlund JY, et al. Intensive diabetes therapy and carotid intima-media thickness in type 1 diabetes mellitus. New Engl J Med. 2003;348(23):2294–303.
7. Kelly WD, Lillehei RC, Merkel FK, Idezuki Y, Goetz FC. Allotransplantation of the pancreas and duodenum along with the kidney in diabetic nephropathy. Surgery. 1967;61(6):827–37.
8. Brogard JM, Vetter T, Blickle JF. Discovery of pancreatic diabetes in Strasbourg. Diabete Metabol. 1992;18(2):104–14.
9. Agarwal A, Brayman KL. Update on islet cell transplantation for type 1 diabetes. Semin Intervent Radiol. 2012;29(2):90–8.
10. Lacy PE, Kostianovsky M. Method for the isolation of intact islets of Langerhans from the rat pancreas. Diabetes. 1967;16(1):35–9.
11. Misler S. The isolated pancreatic islet as a micro-organ and its transplantation to cure diabetes: celebrating the legacy of Paul Lacy. Islets. 2010;2(4): 210–24.
12. Reckard CR, Ziegler MM, Barker CF. Physiological and immunological consequences of transplanting isolated pancreatic islets. Surgery. 1973;74(1):91–9.
13. Shapiro AM. A historical perspective on experimental and clinical islet transplantation. Informa Health Care. 2007;1.
14. Lakey JR, Warnock GL, Shapiro AM, Korbutt GS, Ao Z, Kneteman NM, et al. Intraductal collagenase delivery into the human pancreas using syringe loading or controlled perfusion. Cell Transplant. 1999;8(3):285–92.
15. Ricordi C, Lacy PE, Scharp DW. Automated islet isolation from human pancreas. Diabetes. 1989;38 (Suppl 1):140–2.
16. Shapiro AM, Lakey JR, Ryan EA, Korbutt GS, Toth E, Warnock GL, et al. Islet transplantation in seven patients with type 1 diabetes mellitus using a glucocorticoid-free immunosuppressive regimen. New Engl J Med. 2000;343(4):230–8.
17. Ryan EA, Bigam D, Shapiro AM. Current indications for pancreas or islet transplant. Diabetes Obes Metab. 2006;8(1):1–7.
18. Scharp DW, Kemp CB, Knight MJ, Ballinger WF, Lacy PE. The use of ficoll in the preparation of viable islets of langerhans from the rat pancreas. Transplantation. 1973;16(6):686–9.
19. Najarian JS, Sutherland DE, Matas AJ, Steffes MW, Simmons RL, Goetz FC. Human islet transplantation: a preliminary report. Transpl Proc. 1977;9(1):233–6.

20. Brendel M HB, Shulz A, Bretzel R. International islet transplant registry report. 1999.1–20.
21. Benhamou PY, Watt PC, Mullen Y, Ingles S, Watanabe Y, Nomura Y, et al. Human islet isolation in 104 consecutive cases. Factors affecting isolation success. Transplantation. 1994;57(12):1804–10.
22. Goto M, Eich TM, Felldin M, Foss A, Kallen R, Salmela K, et al. Refinement of the automated method for human islet isolation and presentation of a closed system for in vitro islet culture. Transplantation. 2004;78(9):1367–75.
23. Ihm SH, Matsumoto I, Sawada T, Nakano M, Zhang HJ, Ansite JD, et al. Effect of donor age on function of isolated human islets. Diabetes. 2006;55(5):1361–8.
24. Lakey JR, Rajotte RV, Warnock GL, Kneteman NM. Human pancreas preservation prior to islet isolation. Cold ischemic tolerance. Transplantation. 1995;59(5):689–94.
25. Lakey JR, Warnock GL, Rajotte RV, Suarez-Alamazor ME, Ao Z, Shapiro AM, et al. Variables in organ donors that affect the recovery of human islets of Langerhans. Transplantation. 1996;61(7):1047–53.
26. Matsumoto I, Sawada T, Nakano M, Sakai T, Liu B, Ansite JD, et al. Improvement in islet yield from obese donors for human islet transplants. Transplantation. 2004;78(6):880–5.
27. Nano R, Clissi B, Melzi R, Calori G, Maffi P, Antonioli B, et al. Islet isolation for allotransplantation: variables associated with successful islet yield and graft function. Diabetologia. 2005;48(5):906–12.
28. Zeng Y, Torre MA, Karrison T, Thistlethwaite JR. The correlation between donor characteristics and the success of human islet isolation. Transplantation. 1994;57(6):954–8.
29. Kin T, Murdoch TB, Shapiro AM, Lakey JR. Estimation of pancreas weight from donor variables. Cell Transplant. 2006;15(2):181–5.
30. Brandhorst H, Brandhorst D, Hering BJ, Federlin K, Bretzel RG. Body mass index of pancreatic donors: a decisive factor for human islet isolation. Exp Clin Endocrinol Diabetes. 1995;103(Suppl 2):23–6.
31. Berney T, Johnson PR. Donor pancreata: evolving approaches to organ allocation for whole pancreas versus islet transplantation. Transplantation. 2010; 90(3):238–43.
32. O'Gorman D, Kin T, Murdoch T, Richer B, McGhee-Wilson D, Ryan E, et al. The standardization of pancreatic donors for islet isolation. Transpl Proc. 2005;37(2):1309–10.
33. de Boer J, De Meester J, Smits JM, Groenewoud AF, Bok A, van der Velde O, et al. Eurotransplant randomized multicenter kidney graft preservation study comparing HTK with UW and Euro-Collins. Transpl Int. 1999;12(6):447–53.
34. Hering BJ, Matsumoto I, Sawada T, Nakano M, Sakai T, Kandaswamy R, et al. Impact of two-layer pancreas preservation on islet isolation and transplantation. Transplantation. 2002;74(12):1813–6.
35. Benhamou PY, Oberholzer J, Toso C, Kessler L, Penfornis A, Bayle F, et al. Human islet transplantation network for the treatment of Type I diabetes: first data from the Swiss-French GRAGIL consortium (1999–2000). Groupe de Recherche Rhin Rhjne Alpes Geneve pour la transplantation d'Ilots de Langerhans. Diabetologia. 2001;44(7):859–64.
36. Goss JA, Schock AP, Brunicardi FC, Goodpastor SE, Garber AJ, Soltes G, et al. Achievement of insulin independence in three consecutive type-1 diabetic patients via pancreatic islet transplantation using islets isolated at a remote islet isolation center. Transplantation. 2002;74(12):1761–6.
37. Wolters GH, Vos-Scheperkeuter GH, van Deijnen JH, van Schilfgaarde R. An analysis of the role of collagenase and protease in the enzymatic dissociation of the rat pancreas for islet isolation. Diabetologia. 1992;35(8):735–42.
38. Johnson PR, White SA, London NJ. Collagenase and human islet isolation. Cell Transplant. 1966;15(4):437–52.
39. Wang X, Meloche M, Verchere CB, Ou D, Mui A, Warnock GL. Improving islet engraftment by gene therapy. J Transplant. 2011;2011:594851.
40. Mehigan DG, Bell WR, Zuidema GD, Eggleston JC, Cameron JL. Disseminated intravascular coagulation and portal hypertension following pancreatic islet autotransplantation. Ann Surg. 1980;191(3):287–93.
41. Lake SP, Bassett PD, Larkins A, Revell J, Walczak K, Chamberlain J, et al. Large-scale purification of human islets utilizing discontinuous albumin gradient on IBM 2991 cell separator. Diabetes. 1989;38(Suppl 1):143–5.
42. Ichii HPA, Khan A, Fraker C, Ricordi C. Culture and transportation of human islets between centers. Islet transplantation and beta cell replacement therapy. New York: Informa healthcare; 2007. p. 251.
43. Hering BJ, Kandaswamy R, Ansite JD, Eckman PM, Nakano M, Sawada T, et al. Single-donor, marginal-dose islet transplantation in patients with type 1 diabetes. JAMA. 2005;293(7):830–5.
44. Gangemi A, Salehi P, Hatipoglu B, Martellotto J, Barbaro B, Kuechle JB, et al. Islet transplantation for brittle type 1 diabetes: the UIC protocol. Am J Transplant. 2008;8(6):1250–61.
45. Froud T, Ricordi C, Baidal DA, Hafiz MM, Ponte G, Cure P, et al. Islet transplantation in type 1 diabetes mellitus using cultured islets and steroid-free immunosuppression: Miami experience. Am J Transplant. 2005;5(8):2037–46.
46. Froud T, Faradji RN, Pileggi A, Messinger S, Baidal DA, Ponte GM, et al. The use of exenatide in islet transplant recipients with chronic allograft dysfunction: safety, efficacy, and metabolic effects. Transplantation. 2008;86(1):36–45.

47. Ghofaili KA, Fung M, Ao Z, Meloche M, Shapiro RJ, Warnock GL, et al. Effect of exenatide on beta cell function after islet transplantation in type 1 diabetes. Transplantation. 2007;83(1):24–8.
48. Faradji RN, Tharavanij T, Messinger S, Froud T, Pileggi A, Monroy K, et al. Long-term insulin independence and improvement in insulin secretion after supplemental islet infusion under exenatide and etanercept. Transplantation. 2008;86(12):1658–65.
49. Rajab A. Islet transplantation: alternative sites. Curr Diab Rep. 2010;10(5):332–7.
50. Froud T, Yrizarry JM, Alejandro R, Ricordi C. Use of D-STAT to prevent bleeding following percutaneous transhepatic intraportal islet transplantation. Cell Transplant. 2004;13(1):55–9.
51. Barshes NR, Lee TC, Goodpastor SE, Balkrishnan R, Schock AP, Mote A, et al. Transaminitis after pancreatic islet transplantation. J Am Coll Surg. 2005;200(3):353–61.
52. Biarnes M, Montolio M, Nacher V, Raurell M, Soler J, Montanya E. Beta-cell death and mass in syngeneically transplanted islets exposed to short- and long-term hyperglycemia. Diabetes. 2002;51(1): 66–72.
53. Owen RJ, Ryan EA, O'Kelly K, Lakey JR, McCarthy MC, Paty BW, et al. Percutaneous transhepatic pancreatic islet cell transplantation in type 1 diabetes mellitus: radiologic aspects. Radiology. 2003;229(1):165–70.
54. Ryan EA, Paty BW, Senior PA, Bigam D, Alfadhli E, Kneteman NM, et al. Five-year follow-up after clinical islet transplantation. Diabetes. 2005;54(7):2060–9.
55. Gala-Lopez B, Pepper AR, Shapiro AM. Biologic agents in islet transplantation. Curr Diab Rep. 2013;13(5):713–22.
56. Bloom SR, Polak JM. Somatostatin. Br Med J. 1987;295(6593):288–90.
57. Korsgren O, Lundgren T, Felldin M, Foss A, Isaksson B, Permert J, et al. Optimising islet engraftment is critical for successful clinical islet transplantation. Diabetologia. 2008;51(2):227–32.
58. Shapiro AM. A historical perspective on experimental and clinical islet transplantation. In: Shapiro AM, Shaw JA, editors. Islet transplantation and beta cell replacement therapy. New York, London: Informa Healthcare; 2007.
59. Gabardi S, Martin ST, Roberts KL, Grafals M. Induction immunosuppressive therapies in renal transplantation. Am J Health-System Pharm: AJHP: Official J Am Soc Health-System Pharmacists. 2011;68(3):211–8.
60. Hering BJ. Repurification: rescue rather than routine remedy. Am J Transplant. 2005;5(1):1–2.
61. Koh A, Senior P, Salam A, Kin T, Imes S, Dinyari P, et al. Insulin-heparin infusions peritransplant substantially improve single-donor clinical islet transplant success. Transplantation. 2010;89(4):465–71.
62. Matsumoto S, Takita M, Chaussabel D, Noguchi H, Shimoda M, Sugimoto K, et al. Improving efficacy of clinical islet transplantation with iodixanol based islet purification, Thymoglobulin induction and blockage of IL-1-beta and TNF-alpha. Cell Transplant. 2011;20(10):1641–7.
63. Shapiro AM, Ricordi C. Unraveling the secrets of single donor success in islet transplantation. Am J Transplant. 2004;4(3):295–8.
64. Xenos ES, Farney AC, Widmer MB, Casanova D, Stevens RB, Blazar BR, et al. Effect of tumor necrosis factor alpha and of the soluble tumor necrosis factor receptor on insulin secretion of isolated islets of Langerhans. Transpl Proc. 1992;24 (6):2863–4.
65. Senior PA, Paty BW, Cockfield SM, Ryan EA, Shapiro AM. Proteinuria developing after clinical islet transplantation resolves with sirolimus withdrawal and increased tacrolimus dosing. Am J Transplant. 2005;5(9):2318–23.
66. Kaplan B, Schold J, Srinivas T, Womer K, Foley DP, Patton P, et al. Effect of sirolimus withdrawal in patients with deteriorating renal function. Am J Transplant. 2004;4(10):1709–12.
67. The CITR Coordinating Center and Investigators. The collaborative islet transplant registry (CITR) 2011 seventh annual report. https://web.emmes.com/study/isl/reports/01062012_7thAnnualReport.pdf. Accessed 27 Jan 2017.
68. Barton FB, Rickels MR, Alejandro R, Hering BJ, Wease S, Naziruddin B, et al. Improvement in outcomes of clinical islet transplantation: 1999–2010. Diabetes Care. 2012;35(7):1436–45.
69. Senior PA, Kin T, Shapiro AMJ, Koh A. Islet transplantation at the University of Alberta: status update and review of progress over the last decade. Can J Diabetes. 2012;36:32–7.
70. Pepper AR, Gala-Lopez B, Ziff O, Shapiro AJ. Current status of clinical islet transplantation. World J Transplant. 2013;3(4):48–53.
71. Senior PAKT, Shapiro AMJ, Koh A. Islet transplantation at the University of Alberta: Status update and review of progress over the last decade. Can J Diabetes. 2012;36:32–7.
72. Ly TT, Nicholas JA, Retterath A, Lim EM, Davis EA, Jones TW. Effect of sensor-augmented insulin pump therapy and automated insulin suspension vs standard insulin pump therapy on hypoglycemia in patients with type 1 diabetes: a randomized clinical trial. JAMA. 2013;310(12):1240–7.
73. Shapiro AM. Strategies toward single-donor islets of Langerhans transplantation. Curr Opin Organ Transplant. 2011;16(6):627–31.
74. Thompson DM, Meloche M, Ao Z, Paty B, Keown P, Shapiro RJ, et al. Reduced progression of diabetic microvascular complications with islet cell transplantation compared with intensive medical therapy. Transplantation. 2011;91(3):373–8.

75. Ryan EA, Shandro T, Green K, Paty BW, Senior PA, Bigam D, et al. Assessment of the severity of hypoglycemia and glycemic lability in type 1 diabetic subjects undergoing islet transplantation. Diabetes. 2004;53(4):955–62.
76. Patrick AW, Campbell IW. Fatal hypoglycaemia in insulin-treated diabetes mellitus: clinical features and neuropathological changes. Diabet Med. 1990;7(4):349–54.
77. Gonder-Frederick LA, Clarke WL, Cox DJ. The Emotional, Social, and Behavioral Implications of Insulin-Induced Hypoglycemia. Semin Clin Neuropsychiatry. 1997;2(1):57–65.
78. Hathout E, Lakey J, Shapiro J. Islet transplant: an option for childhood diabetes? Arch Dis Child. 2003;88(7):591–4.

Diabetes in the Pediatric Surgical Patient

15

Ari J. Wassner and Michael S.D. Agus

Diabetes mellitus is a syndrome of persistent hyperglycemia due to impaired insulin production or action. Children with diabetes generally require the same types of surgical care as nondiabetic children, but the acute and chronic consequences of diabetes and its treatment require special considerations in their perioperative care. The annual incidence of diabetes in the United States is about 1/4000 children, but the worldwide incidence varies markedly by geographic location and ethnicity [1]. Compared to other comorbid conditions that pose particular surgical risks, diabetes is similar in incidence to cystic fibrosis (1/3500) and muscular dystrophy (1/3300), and much more common than acute leukemia (1/33,000). Moreover, the incidence of pediatric diabetes is rising. Thus, diabetes will be encountered frequently in pediatric surgical practice, and familiarity with the principles of its pathophysiology, treatment, and potential complications is critical for providing optimal surgical care to these patients.

A.J. Wassner · M.S.D. Agus (✉)
Department of Pediatrics, Harvard Medical School, Boston Children's Hospital, 300 Longwood Avenue, Boston, MA 02115, USA
e-mail: michael.agus@childrens.harvard.edu

A.J. Wassner
e-mail: ari.wassner@childrens.harvard.edu

Diagnosis

The normal range of random blood glucose values is approximately 60–140 mg/dL (4.0–7.8 mmol/L). Normal blood glucose is <100 mg/dL (5.6 mmol/L) in the fasting state, and <140 mg/dL (7.8 mmol/L) two hours after a glucose load. Persistent hyperglycemia above this range indicates abnormal glucose metabolism. The diagnosis of diabetes mellitus is defined by one or more of the following:

1. Classic symptoms of diabetes with blood glucose ≥ 200 mg/dL (11.1 mmol/L) (without respect to timing of last caloric intake);
2. Fasting blood glucose ≥ 126 mg/dL (7 mmol/L) (no caloric intake within 8 h);
3. Blood glucose ≥ 200 mg/dL (11.1 mmol/L) obtained 2 h after ingestion of a standard glucose load (1.75 g/kg, maximum 75 g);
4. Hemoglobin A1c (HbA1c) $\geq$ 6.5% (although this criterion may be less applicable in children than in adults).

All diagnostic criteria are based on plasma values performed in a laboratory; the diagnosis of diabetes cannot be made using "finger-prick" testing. Unless the diagnosis is clinically unequivocal (e.g., a patient presenting in diabetic ketoacidosis), abnormal values should be confirmed by repeat testing on a different day [2].

Typical symptoms of diabetes include polydipsia, polyuria, weight loss, fatigue, and malaise. Appetite may be increased due to the

D.J. Ledbetter and P.R.V. Johnson (eds.), *Endocrine Surgery in Children*,
DOI 10.1007/978-3-662-54256-9_15

insulin-deficient starvation state, but may also be decreased due to malaise and ketonemia. Hyperglycemia and glycosuria may lead to candidal infections of the genital area in toddlers and young children. A preceding viral illness is commonly reported prior to the onset of symptoms; such infections do not cause diabetes, but may trigger the appearance of symptoms due to increased hyperglycemia under the stress of illness or, in type 1 diabetes, increased immune-mediated beta cell destruction.

Pathophysiology and Classification

Normal Glucose Homeostasis

Glucose is the primary metabolic substrate used by most tissues to generate energy for cellular processes. Tissue uptake of glucose from the blood requires insulin, which is secreted from beta cells located within the pancreatic islets of Langerhans. Insulin secretion is regulated by blood glucose concentration, which is continuously sensed by beta cells. In response to a rise in blood glucose, beta cells release insulin to promote the uptake of circulating glucose into tissues.

Insulin is the primary hormone of the fed state, in which carbohydrate, protein, and fat that have just been consumed are available for disposition. The overall effect of insulin is to lower blood glucose. In the liver, insulin stimulates the conversion of glucose into glycogen, a storage form that serves as a short-term reserve of glucose. Insulin also decreases hepatic production of glucose by inhibiting both breakdown of glycogen (*glycogenolysis*) and synthesis of new glucose (*gluconeogenesis*). Finally, insulin promotes the storage of excess metabolic energy in the form of fat, and inhibits breakdown of triglycerides and release and oxidation of fatty acids.

In the normal fasting state, blood glucose is maintained by a number of mechanisms. Insulin secretion is suppressed when the blood glucose drops below about 70 mg/dL (3.9 mmol/L) [3]. At the same time, there is increased production of glucagon, epinephrine (adrenaline), growth hormone, and cortisol, which are often termed *counterregulatory hormones* because their effects on glucose metabolism oppose those of insulin. Under the influence of these hormones, hepatic glucose production and release are increased via gluconeogenesis; increased breakdown of glycogen occurs until stores are exhausted. Fat is broken down into free fatty acids, which are oxidized to provide energy for gluconeogenesis.

Ketones are small organic acids produced as a side product of fatty acid oxidation. Ketones serve an important role in normal fasting as an alternative metabolic substrate when glucose is scarce. Unlike many other tissues that can use other substrates as well (such as lactate or free fatty acids), the brain can effectively metabolize only glucose and ketones. Therefore, ketones are a critical alternative fuel for the brain during normal fasting or hypoglycemia. However, because ketones are acids, their accumulation can lead to metabolic acidosis. The most clinically important ketones are beta-hydroxybutyric acid and acetoacetic acid. Beta-hydroxybutyric acid can be measured in the serum, whereas acetoacetic acid is detected by the ketone assay on routine urinalysis.

Uncontrolled diabetes is, by definition, a state of inadequate insulin action. Although blood glucose is elevated, there is insufficient insulin action for glucose to be taken up by tissues, in effect mimicking a persistent state of starvation. Hyperglycemia above the threshold for renal glucose reabsorption causes glucosuria, osmotic diuresis, and polyuria. Urinary water loss leads to dehydration, which along with hyperosmolality due to hyperglycemia causes polydipsia. Weight loss occurs as ingested calories cannot be utilized and are excreted in the urine. At the same time, the metabolic consequences of starvation ensue. In the absence of insulin action, counterregulatory hormones increase, stimulating unregulated hepatic glucose production (which exacerbates hyperglycemia), fatty acid oxidation, and ketone production.

Type 1 Diabetes

Type 1 diabetes is the most common form of diabetes in children. It accounts for the vast majority (~90%) of pediatric diabetes overall, and almost all diabetes in children under 10 years of age, although type 2 diabetes has become increasingly common in older children and adolescents over recent years [1, 4]. Type 1 diabetes is characterized by profound insulin deficiency that, if untreated, inevitably results in severe hyperglycemia, ketoacidosis, and death. Although a number of alternative theories have been proposed, type 1 diabetes is widely believed to be caused by cell-mediated autoimmune destruction of pancreatic beta cells, leading to complete insulin deficiency. Autoantibodies to pancreatic antigens are markers of autoimmune beta cell damage and are present at diagnosis in nearly all patients with type 1 diabetes [5]. The pancreas has a large reserve of beta cells, and autoimmune beta cell destruction proceeds subclinically for months to years, becoming clinically evident only when residual beta cell function falls below the threshold needed to maintain euglycemia.

Type 2 Diabetes

Type 2 diabetes is caused by inadequate insulin action due to a combination of peripheral insulin resistance and decreased insulin secretion. Insulin resistance most often develops in the context of obesity and is a component of the metabolic syndrome. As insulin resistance emerges, insulin action becomes inadequate and intermittent hyperglycemia develops. Initially, beta cells compensate for peripheral insulin resistance by increasing insulin production. However, over time worsening insulin resistance and/or the strain of compensation causes beta cells function to decline. When insufficient insulin is produced to overcome insulin resistance, type 2 diabetes results. Thus, type 2 diabetes is caused by relative insulin deficiency, in contrast to the absolute deficiency that characterizes type 1 diabetes. For this reason, diabetic ketoacidosis is much less common in type 2 diabetes, although it can occur under physiologic stress such as surgery, injury, or infection.

Other Forms of Diabetes

Several other forms of diabetes fall outside the classification of type 1 and type 2 diabetes (Table 15.1). Although their pathogenesis is diverse, their common feature is inadequate insulin action, whether due to insufficient insulin production, insulin resistance, or a combination. The incidence of these conditions is rising in the pediatric population, and they are likely to be encountered increasingly in pediatric surgical practice. Indeed, diabetes may occur in any condition in which there is generalized loss of pancreatic function. Severe or recurrent pancreatitis may lead to loss of beta cell mass and diabetes. Similarly, patients may develop diabetes after complete or partial pancreatectomy,

Table 15.1 Common causes of diabetes mellitus in children

Type 1 (absolute insulin deficiency) A. Autoimmune B. Idiopathic
Type 2 (insulin resistance and relative insulin deficiency)
Genetic disorders of insulin secretion A. Monogenic diabetes B. Mitochondrial diabetes
Disorders of pancreatic function A. Cystic fibrosis B. Pancreatitis C. Trauma D. Post-pancreatectomy
Drug-induced diabetes A. Glucocorticoids B. Tacrolimus C. Cyclosporine D. Atypical antipsychotics
Endocrinopathies A. Cushing syndrome B. Pheochromocytoma C. Acromegaly D. Hyperthyroidism

Adapted from [2], with permission

depending on the amount of residual pancreatic function. Because of the redundancy of beta cell function, pancreatic damage or resection must be extensive to result in diabetes.

Cystic fibrosis-related diabetes (CFRD) is a common complication of cystic fibrosis, occurring in up to 50% of patients by age 30 [6]. Inspissation of pancreatic secretions causes progressive pancreatic injury that leads over time to beta cell loss and insulin deficiency. In addition, patients with cystic fibrosis may have frequent infections and may be treated with glucocorticoids, both of which contribute to insulin resistance. Since these patients generally maintain some insulin production, ketoacidosis is rare in CFRD. The presence of CFRD has been associated with decreased pulmonary function and increased mortality, risks that appear to improve with control of CFRD.

Numerous medications are associated with the development of diabetes. Glucocorticoids increase hepatic glucose production and insulin resistance, and chronic treatment (e.g., for severe asthma, inflammatory conditions, renal disease, or post-transplant immunosuppression) can result in diabetes. Tacrolimus and cyclosporine, frequently used in the post-transplant setting, can cause diabetes, possibly by causing direct injury to beta cells. Atypical antipsychotics such as olanzapine, quetiapine, and risperidone are associated with diabetes and are being prescribed to pediatric patients with increasing frequency.

Genetic forms of diabetes are increasingly being recognized. Monogenic diabetes (previously termed maturity onset diabetes of youth, or MODY) is a family of syndromes caused by single-gene defects in the molecular pathways of beta cell glucose sensing and insulin secretion. Mitochondrial diabetes is caused by mutations in mitochondrial proteins that are an integral part of these pathways. In general, all of these defects lead to inadequate insulin release in response to hyperglycemia. Monogenic and mitochondrial diabetes are generally less severe and slower in onset than type 1 diabetes. Some patients with monogenic or mitochondrial diabetes can be managed with oral hypoglycemic agents, but many require insulin therapy.

Treatment of Type 1 Diabetes

The overall goal of treatment in type 1 diabetes is to maintain a glycemic profile as close to normal as possible. Overall glycemic control is most often assessed by measuring the blood level of HbA1c, which has a direct relationship with average blood glucose over the preceding 4–12 weeks. HbA1c ranges from 4 to 5.6% in normal individuals, and a value $\geq$6.5% is consistent with diabetes. Improving glycemic control decreases the risk of long-term microvascular and macrovascular complications, but also increases the risk of hypoglycemia [7, 8]. Thus, ideal management of diabetes will achieve the tightest glycemic control possible while avoiding significant hypoglycemia. Consensus recommendations vary regarding optimal hemoglobin A1c at different ages [9, 10]. In general, a goal of HbA1c <7.5% is appropriate for children of all ages, but this goal may be adjusted upward in younger patients or in those with a history of significant hypoglycemia. The goal for older adolescents should approach the recommended target for adults (HbA1c <7%).

Patients with type 1 diabetes require continuous treatment with exogenous insulin because they have no endogenous insulin production. Complete omission of insulin can lead to diabetic ketoacidosis in a matter of hours. In the outpatient setting, insulin is administered subcutaneously according to a patient-specific regimen. Insulin regimens are variable, and for a given patient will depend on many characteristics including age, severity of disease, desired number of daily injections, daily schedule, predictability of eating, and the ability of the patient and/or caregivers to comply with the regimen. Therefore, only general principles and basic strategies of insulin management will be presented here.

Insulin Preparations and Regimens

Insulin is a 51-amino acid peptide hormone composed of an alpha- and a beta-chain linked by disulfide bonds. Insulin is synthesized in the pancreatic beta cell as a single polypeptide called pre-proinsulin, which contains both chains. As pre-proinsulin assumes its secondary and tertiary structures, the small peptide linking the alpha- and beta-chains (termed C-peptide) is cleaved. C-peptide is released from the beta cell along with insulin, and can be measured in the serum as a marker of endogenous insulin production.

In recent years, a number of new insulin preparations have significantly improved the flexibility of insulin regimens. Insulin preparations are generally classified according to their rapidity of onset and duration of action (Table 15.2). In general, the shorter acting an insulin preparation, the earlier its onset of action, the earlier and more pronounced its peak effect, and the shorter its duration of action [11–13]. *Rapid-acting insulin analogues* are convenient for meal coverage and correction of hyperglycemia and are increasingly used in this role in place of regular insulin, which has the same structure as the native insulin molecule and is considered *short-acting*. The sole *intermediate-acting insulin* is neutral protamine Hagedorn (NPH), which remains in wide use because its duration of action allows for convenient twice-daily dosing. *Long-acting insulin analogues* provide a nearly constant serum level of insulin; for this reason, they are a common choice to provide a basal level of insulin throughout the day, and have largely replaced older long-acting insulin preparations such as Lente and Ultralente.

If more than one insulin are given at the same time, they are often mixed and given as a single injection (with the exception of glargine and detemir, which cannot be mixed with other insulins). Premixed insulin preparations in fixed proportions are also available that may provide a simpler option for patients who have difficulty with several injections per day.

In a normal individual, the pancreas produces insulin at a low basal rate equivalent to about 0.01–0.02 units/kg/h [14]. Basal insulin is required even in the fasting state to supply the metabolic needs of tissues and to prevent unregulated hepatic production of glucose and ketones. When food is consumed, the ensuing rise in blood glucose triggers a sharp increase in

Table 15.2 Summary of insulin preparations

Insulin	Onset	Peak	Duration	Typical use
Rapid-acting				
Insulin aspart (Novolog®),	10–15 min	30–90 min	3–5 h	Prandial, correction
Insulin glulisine (Apidra®)	10–15 min	30–90 min	3–5 h	Prandial, correction
Insulin lispro (Humalog®)	10–15 min	30–90 min	3–5 h	Prandial, correction
Short-acting				
Regular insulin	30–60 min	2–4 h	5–8 h	Prandial, correction
Intermediate-acting				
NPH (isophane)	2–4 h	4–8 h	12–16 h	Basal, prandial
Long-acting				
Insulin detemir (Levemir®)	2–4 h	Peakless	16–20 h	Basal
Insulin glargine (Lantus®)	2–4 h	Peakless	20–24 h	Basal
Premixed preparations				
70% NPA/30% aspart	10–15 min	Biphasic	12–16 h	Basal/prandial
75% NPL/25% lispro	10–15 min	Biphasic	12–16 h	Basal/prandial
70% NPH/30% regular	30–60 min	Biphasic	12–16 h	Basal/prandial

NPA and NPL are intermediate-acting insulin analogues with similar profiles of action to NPH. *NPH* neutral protamine hagedorn; *NPA* neutral protamine aspart; *NPL* neutral protamine lispro insulin production that allows for disposition of ingested glucose. In type 1 diabetes, the goal of insulin therapy is to maintain the blood glucose as close to normal as possible by approximating the native pattern of basal and prandial insulin secretion. Thus, all insulin regimens consist of three components:

- *Basal insulin* regulates baseline hepatic glucose and ketone production;
- *Prandial insulin* is given at meals to dispose of ingested carbohydrate;
- *Correction doses* of insulin are given at predetermined intervals, if necessary, to correct hyperglycemia.

In the outpatient setting, insulin is administered subcutaneously, either as multiple daily injections, or by continuous infusion using an insulin pump.

A multiple daily injection regimen is one in which the patient administers a series of injections over the course of the day, using insulin syringes or an insulin pen. Such regimens follow two general patterns:

(i) *Split-Mixed Regimen*

This consists of fixed doses of insulin given at specified times of day. Basal insulin coverage is provided by NPH given twice daily (generally at breakfast and at dinner or bedtime). The morning dose of NPH also provides prandial coverage of lunch, since NPH has its peak effect 2–4 h after administration. Rapid- or short-acting insulin is given at breakfast and dinner for coverage of these meals. Correction doses for hyperglycemia are often incorporated by replacing fixed mealtime doses with a *sliding scale* of rapid-acting insulin, in which the insulin dose varies based on the blood glucose. A split-mixed regimen offers predictable dosage and timing of injections, fewer daily injections than other regimens, and usually does not require an injection at lunch, making it useful for young children with a consistent daily schedule or who would prefer not to receive an injection at school. Disadvantages include lack of flexibility; the fact that snacks are generally not covered with insulin; and that a peaking insulin (NPH) is given at bedtime, putting the patient at risk of nocturnal hypoglycemia. A simplification of this regimen uses a premixed insulin (which includes both NPH and a rapid- or short-acting insulin) given twice daily, at breakfast and dinner.

(ii) *Basal-Bolus Regimen*

This is more flexible and more closely mirrors physiologic insulin secretion. Basal insulin is provided by one or two daily doses of a long-acting insulin analogue, which provide a relatively constant insulin level. Prandial doses of a rapid-acting insulin analogue are given for any meal or snack based on its content: the patient determines the amount of carbohydrate to be consumed and calculates the appropriate dose of insulin using an *insulin:carbohydrate ratio* (e.g., 1 unit of insulin per 25 g of carbohydrate). To correct hyperglycemia, rapid-acting insulin analogue is given based on a *correction factor* (or *sensitivity factor*) and a target blood glucose. For example, a patient might receive a correction factor of 1 unit of insulin per 75 mg/dL that the blood glucose exceeds the target of 120 mg/dL. Since insulin sensitivity varies over the course of the day, a patient may have different insulin:carbohydrate ratios or correction factors at different times of day. Advantages of a basal-bolus regimen include closer approximation of physiologic insulin production and increased flexibility in meal timing and content, but at the expense of increased complexity and a greater number of injections per day.

Insulin Pumps

Continuous subcutaneous insulin infusion via an insulin pump is an increasingly common treatment modality for type 1 diabetes. An insulin pump is an automated infusion device that contains a reservoir of a rapid-acting insulin analogue. The device is connected directly or via flexible tubing to a small catheter inserted subcutaneously, and a computer program controls the administration of insulin. This setup allows continuous infusion of rapid-acting insulin analogue as well as bolus doses. The principles of insulin administration with a pump are identical to those of a basal-bolus regimen, but an insulin pump uses only rapid-acting insulin analogue rather than a combination of long- and rapid-acting preparations. Basal insulin is provided as a continuous infusion of rapid-acting insulin analogue, and this *basal rate* of infusion may vary over the course of the day. Prandial doses are given before meals and snacks using an insulin:carbohydrate ratio, and a correction factor is given for hyperglycemia.

Because of its precision and programmability, an insulin pump allows the most accurate approximation of physiologic insulin production of any currently available insulin regimen. It allows precise dosing and adjustment of the basal rate, insulin:carbohydrate ratio, and correction factor, all of which may vary by time of day, with exercise, or during illness. A pump provides great flexibility in meal and activity patterns, avoids the discomfort of multiple injections, and reduces the risk of hypoglycemia. In addition, "closed-loop" systems are being developed that will link an insulin pump to a continuous blood glucose monitor, with computer algorithms that mimic normal pancreatic function by adjusting insulin administration based on blood glucose. However, like any device, insulin pumps can experience mechanical, electrical, or software malfunctions that may cause failure of insulin delivery. Because rapid-acting insulin analogue has a short duration of action, interruption of insulin delivery by the pump can result in diabetic ketoacidosis within hours. Therefore, a patient on an insulin pump and her caregivers must check blood glucose frequently and remain constantly alert for the possibility of pump malfunction.

Blood Glucose Monitoring

Patients with type 1 diabetes must monitor their blood glucose frequently to achieve optimal diabetes control. At a minimum, blood glucose should be measured upon awakening in the morning, before each meal, and at bedtime. More frequent monitoring is necessary during periods of stress, illness, or under other circumstances that may precipitate either hyper- or hypoglycemia. Blood glucose monitoring is most commonly performed with a glucometer using capillary whole blood obtained by fingerstick. However, glucometers have limited precision, need frequent calibration to ensure accuracy, and depend on good user technique. Therefore, any blood glucose value measured by glucometer that is inconsistent with the clinical scenario should be repeated after addressing potential sources of error. In the inpatient setting, a laboratory measurement is useful if uncertainty remains.

Treatment of Type 2 Diabetes

Patients with type 2 diabetes differ from those with type 1 in that they continue to produce some endogenous insulin that is nevertheless insufficient to overcome their peripheral insulin resistance. Therefore, the primary treatment strategies for type 2 diabetes are directed at improving insulin sensitivity, with insulin therapy being reserved for patients who are unable to achieve adequate diabetes control with such measures. Improved control of type 2 diabetes decreases the risk of both microvascular and macrovascular complications, and treatment goals are equivalent to those for type 1 diabetes, including goals for HbA1c [15–17].

Lifestyle Modification

The first line of therapy in type 2 diabetes is lifestyle modification. Insulin resistance is closely related to obesity and can be markedly improved with sufficient weight loss. In addition to contributing to weight loss, increasing exercise has an independent effect on improving blood glucose and insulin sensitivity. Improving diet and exercise alone can be quite effective in improving HbA1c [18]. However, lifestyle modifications can be difficult to sustain and compliance is often poor, and many patients are unable to achieve adequate control of their diabetes by these means alone.

Metformin

In pediatric patients with type 2 diabetes who do not respond adequately to lifestyle modification, metformin is frequently the first medication that is initiated. Metformin's mechanism is action is not fully understood, but it appears to improve insulin sensitivity. It increases peripheral glucose uptake to some degree, but its effect is most pronounced in the liver, where increased insulin action leads to decreased gluconeogenesis. Metformin is given orally once or twice daily, and extended release formulations are available. The most common adverse effects of metformin are gastrointestinal symptoms, including nausea and diarrhea, which can often be avoiding by starting at a low dose and titrating up slowly.

The most worrisome potential adverse effect of metformin is lactic acidosis, which can be life-threatening. Because metformin is exclusively excreted by the kidney, the risk of lactic acidosis is increased in situations of reduced kidney function such as dehydration, shock, or renal insufficiency. Although lactic acidosis was described with an earlier related drug, phenformin, it is not clear whether metformin carries the same risk. A large meta-analysis failed to show any increased risk of lactic acidosis of metformin over other treatments for hyperglycemia in the ambulatory setting [19]. However, given the potential severity of this side effect, most experts continue to recommend caution around anesthesia and surgery, which may decrease renal perfusion and increase the risk of lactic acidosis. Therefore, metformin should be stopped 24 h prior to an elective procedure, and can be restarted postoperatively once adequate renal function has been ensured. Metformin should also be held prior to the administration of radiographic contrast that may impair kidney function.

Sulfonylureas and Meglitinides

These two classes of oral medications enhance endogenous insulin production by directly stimulating insulin release from the pancreatic beta cell. Meglitinides (rapeglinide, nateglinide) are short-acting and a given immediately before each meal. Sulfonylureas (glipizide, glyburide, gliclazide, glimepiride) have various durations of action, and may be taken one or more times daily. In part because of the adverse effect of hypoglycemia, sulfonylureas are used infrequently in children. Hypoglycemia is more common with longer acting formulations and in the setting of other risk factors such as decreased caloric intake, stress, or illness. Therefore, these medications should be stopped on the day of an elective surgical procedure.

Thiazolidinediones

Only two agents in this class, pioglitazone and rosiglitazone, are currently available routinely. Neither is approved for use in children, but they are used occasionally in older adolescents who do not tolerate metformin. Thiazolidinediones improve insulin sensitivity by interacting with peroxisome proliferator-activated receptor gamma (PPAR-γ) to increase glucose utilization and decrease glucose production. In adults, these agents are about as effective as metformin as monotherapy, but they are more expensive and have more associated adverse effects: in particular, rosiglitazone has been associated with an increased risk of cardiovascular events. Both agents rarely cause hepatitis, particularly in the setting of other risk factors. More commonly, thiazolidinediones cause weight gain, as well as fluid retention that can lead to peripheral edema and heart failure. These medications should be stopped on the day of an elective surgical procedure.

Insulin in Type 2 Diabetes

Patients with type 2 diabetes who are unable to achieve adequate control with lifestyle modifications and oral medication require insulin. However, practices vary as to the precise criteria for starting insulin therapy in pediatric patients with type 2 diabetes: persistent elevation of HbA1c, fasting or postprandial hyperglycemia, ketosis, or symptoms of diabetes despite oral therapy are all potential reasons to initiate insulin. The principles of insulin therapy are similar to those in type 1 diabetes, though there are important differences. First, due to their insulin resistance, individuals with type 2 diabetes generally require substantially higher doses of insulin than those with type 1 diabetes. Second, because patients with type 2 diabetes are not absolutely insulin deficient, they generally do not require continuous treatment with insulin to prevent ketoacidosis. The same types of insulin regimens are employed in type 2 diabetes as in type 1, with the exception that insulin pumps are infrequently used. Many patients achieve adequate control with only a basal dose of long-acting insulin analogue. Others use a correction factor (or sliding scale) of rapid-acting insulin analogue to correct hyperglycemia. Split-mixed insulin regimens for type 2 diabetes often consist of two daily injections of a premixed insulin preparation given before breakfast and dinner.

Complications of Diabetes

Diabetic Ketoacidosis (DKA)

DKA is a severe complication of diabetes that can be life-threatening if not detected and treated urgently. DKA is defined by the presence of the following:

1. Blood glucose ≥ 200 mg/dL
2. Ketones in the urine and serum
3. Metabolic acidosis, with arterial pH < 7.35, venous pH < 7.30, or bicarbonate <15 mg/dL.

Insulin suppresses glucose production by the liver (glycogenolysis and gluconeogenesis) and oxidation of fatty acids to ketones. When insulin action is insufficient in uncontrolled diabetes, these processes proceed unchecked. The liver produces excess glucose, and tissue uptake of glucose is reduced, leading to hyperglycemia. At the same time, the accumulation of ketones—which are organic acids—leads to metabolic acidosis. Dehydration is an invariable finding in DKA and an important factor in its pathogenesis. Factors contributing to dehydration include osmotic diuresis due to glycosuria, nausea and vomiting due to ketonemia, and respiratory losses due to compensation for metabolic acidosis. Dehydration decreases the glomerular filtration rate, which further worsens both hyperglycemia and ketonemia due to decreased excretion. As dehydration worsens, decreased tissue perfusion may lead to lactic acidosis that can further exacerbate metabolic acidosis.

The primary treatments for DKA are rehydration and insulin administration. During the therapeutic course these are titrated, along with appropriate electrolyte infusions, to steadily close the anion gap, resolve ketosis, and normalize blood glucose and electrolytes. Surgical intervention during DKA should be avoided if at all possible.

Hyperosmolar Hyperglycemic Syndrome (HHS)

It has long been recognized that patients with diabetes may develop a syndrome of severe hyperglycemia, hyperosmolality, and dehydration, but without the severe ketosis and metabolic acidosis that characterize diabetic ketoacidosis. This hyperosmolar hyperglycemia syndrome (HHS) is defined by:

1. Blood glucose >600 mg/dL
2. Serum osmolality >320 mOsm/kg
3. Absent or minimal ketones in urine or serum.

HHS is more common in obese patients, most of whom have type 2 diabetes, but it can occur in type 1 diabetes and has been reported in cystic fibrosis-related diabetes. HHS and DKA are thought to lie on a spectrum of deficient insulin action. While DKA occurs in the setting of severe insulin deficiency, HHS is thought to occur when insulin action is reduced to the point that it can suppress ketogenesis but not control hyperglycemia, which leads to osmotic diuresis and dehydration. As dehydration worsens, renal perfusion declines and less glucose is excreted, causing progressive hyperglycemia and hyperosmolality. Polydipsia may exacerbate hyperglycemia if the patient drinks glucose-containing beverages such as juice or soda.

Patients with HHS are profoundly dehydrated, but because hyperosmolality helps preserve intravascular volume, the true degree of dehydration may be difficult to assess clinically. Confusion, lethargy, and coma are frequent present when hyperosmolality is severe. Acidosis is uncommon (10–30%), and if present is due to lactic acidosis from decreased perfusion rather to ketoacidosis. Death occurs in up to 40% of cases and is usually caused by multiorgan failure due to hypovolemic shock, emphasizing the importance of early and aggressive volume resuscitation. Other complications include renal failure, rhabdomyolysis, hyperthermia, pancreatitis, hypokalemia, and hypophosphatemia. Treatment should take place in an intensive care setting and consists of fluid resuscitation with isotonic saline (at least 40 mL/kg initially), with administration of insulin only after the blood glucose has ceased to fall with further hydration [20].

Hypoglycemia

Hypoglycemia (blood glucose < 70 mg/dL or 3.9 mmol/L) is the most common acute complication of diabetes, and is generally caused by diabetes therapy rather than by the disease itself. Although hypoglycemia is occasionally caused by frank overdose of insulin or an oral insulin secretagogue, in the vast majority of cases hypoglycemia is due to a mismatch between insulin dose and carbohydrate intake. The most common precipitant is a decrease in carbohydrate intake without a corresponding adjustment of insulin doing, such as during a prolonged fast or a gastrointestinal illness. In the hospital setting, patients who are unable to eat in the perioperative period and do not receive sufficient carbohydrate by another route (e.g., intravenous dextrose) are at risk for hypoglycemia if their insulin dosing is not reduced accordingly.

Symptoms of hypoglycemia can be loosely classified as adrenergic or neuroglycopenic. Classic adrenergic symptoms of agitation, shakiness, weakness, pallor, diaphoresis, and nausea are caused by the release of epinephrine in response to hypoglycemia. Neuroglycopenic symptoms are due to the lack of sufficient glucose to sustain normal brain activity and include confusion, altered speech, lethargy, obtundation, or seizure. If hypoglycemia occurs repeatedly, habituation may occur with loss of the adrenergic response. *Hypoglycemia unawareness* due to lack of adrenergic symptoms puts patients at risk for severe life-threatening hypoglycemia, since they may not recognize hypoglycemia until the point of neuroglycopenia, at which point they may be unable to respond appropriately. Knowing that a patient has a history of hypoglycemia unawareness may influence monitoring for hypoglycemia in the inpatient setting.

Risk of Infection

Uncontrolled diabetes predisposes to infection in a number of ways. First, hyperglycemia impairs neutrophil chemotaxis and function. In patients with microvascular disease, decreased perfusion to injured areas may further impair the immune response as well as delay wound healing. With respect to surgical site infections, hyperglycemia may also interfere with collagen structure to impair wound healing and tensile strength. Historically, adults with diabetes have had a 10-fold higher rate of postoperative wound infections than those without diabetes [21]. Adults with a preoperative HbA1c above 7% have an overall twofold increased risk of postoperative infection, including wound infection, pneumonia, sepsis, and urinary tract infection [22]. Therefore, the degree of preexisting glycemic control has important implications for surgical planning in patients with diabetes. Postoperative glycemic control also affects the risk of infection (see Sect. 8).

Microvascular and Macrovascular Complications

Sustained hyperglycemia causes abnormal glycation of cellular proteins and metabolic alterations that damage endothelial cells. In patients with uncontrolled diabetes, progressive endothelial injury leads to a variety of vascular complications. Microvascular disease in the retina, glomerulus, and vasa nervorum manifests as diabetic retinopathy, nephropathy, and neuropathy, respectively. Changes in larger vessels lead to macrovascular complications such as atherosclerosis, myocardial ischemia, and stroke. These risks are further magnified by dyslipidemia and hypertension, which are more common in diabetic patients. Once established, the combination of peripheral neuropathy and vasculopathy increases the risk of lower extremity infections. Autonomic neuropathy can cause delayed gastic emptying and gastroparesis.

The risk of both microvascular and macrovascular complications depends on the magnitude and duration of hyperglycemia. These complications generally develop over the course of years, and are fortunately uncommon in children. Retinopathy, nephropathy, and mild neuropathy may be present if diabetes is severe and uncontrolled for a prolonged period. Dyslipidemia and hypertension are relatively common, but macrovascular complications and significant neuropathy (including gastroparesis) are very rare in children. Improved glycemic control (as assessed by lower HbA1c) has been demonstrated to decrease the risk of microvascular and macrovascular complications in both type 1 and type 2 diabetes [7, 8, 15–17].

Preoperative Evaluation

Planning for elective surgery in a patient with diabetes must take into account the type of diabetes, the degree of glycemic control, preexisting complications, and the complexity and duration of the surgical procedure. A patient with type 1 diabetes has absolute insulin deficiency and a higher risk of ketoacidosis than patients with other types of diabetes. Poor glycemic control increases the risk of postoperative infection, the likelihood of perioperative hyperglycemia (and accompanying risks of ketoacidosis or hyperosmolar hyperglycemia syndrome), and is associated with increased perioperative mortality [23]. Although there is no clear HbA1c threshold for these risks, it appears that risk of complications increases progressively with worsening diabetes control. Major surgery will affect glycemic control more than minor surgery, and requires a more intensive approach to perioperative glycemic management.

Elective surgery should occur when the patient's diabetes is under the best possible control, ideally with HbA1c in the goal range. However, many patients are not able to achieve such control, or to do so in a reasonable time frame, and a preoperative HbA1c near the goal range may be sufficient. Indeed, there is no clear consensus on acceptable ranges of preoperative HbA1c prior to elective surgery, but the following have been proposed: 7–9% for children under 5 years; 6–8.5% for those 5–13 years; and 6–8% for those over 13 years [24]. The more extensive the surgery, the more significant the perioperative risks and the need to ensure good glycemic control preoperatively. If control is not adequate, surgery should be deferred until the HbA1c has improved. When surgery must be performed as an emergency, glycemic control obviously cannot be assured, but a rapid preoperative evaluation can still assess perioperative needs and the risk of complications.

The preoperative history should include the patient's type of diabetes and its duration; treatment regimen, including insulin and/or oral medications; and last HbA1c measurement. A history of acute and chronic complications should be elicited, including ketoacidosis or hyperosmolar hyperglycemic syndrome, diabetes-related hospitalizations, nephropathy, neuropathy, and diabetes-related complications of any previous surgeries. A history of frequent hypoglycemia, as well as the patient's ability to recognize symptoms of hypoglycemia, should be elicited. The presence of associated conditions such as dyslipidemia, hypertension, and (in type

1 diabetes) hypothyroidism should also be assessed. The patient's primary diabetologist/endocrinologist should be identified, and communication between physicians regarding perioperative diabetes management is vital to ensure optimal perioperative diabetes care.

The physical examination should include routine vital signs, including blood pressure. Acanthosis nigricans indicates insulin resistance and may be present in overweight or obese individuals with any type of diabetes. In a patient with type 1 diabetes, an abnormal thyroid exam may indicate autoimmune thyroiditis. Areas of the skin where insulin is routinely injected should be examined for erythema that may suggest infection. Cutaneous lipohypertrophy or lipoatrophy due to repeated insulin administration may impair absorption of future insulin doses given at that site.

Preoperative laboratory studies specific to diabetes include HbA1c, blood glucose, and electrolytes. For patients taking metformin, renal function and liver transaminase should be measured. In patients in whom autoimmune thyroiditis is present or suspected, a thyroid stimulating hormone (TSH) may be measured; abnormal results should prompt consultation with the patient's diabetologist/endocrinologist prior to surgery.

General Principles of Perioperative Management

Diabetes Management in the Fasting Patient

Nearly all patients will be required to fast for some period prior to, during, and after surgery. Therefore, the principles of perioperative diabetes management are fundamentally those of managing diabetes in a fasting patient. These general principles can be applied to all phases of perioperative care, as well as to patients fasting for other reasons (e.g., illness, preparation for a diagnostic study, etc.). In this setting, a fasting patient is considered to be one who is not receiving enteral nutrition sufficient to meet minimum caloric and fluid needs. All patients treated with insulin are managed similarly while fasting regardless of their type of diabetes. Differences for diabetic patients who are not on insulin therapy are noted where appropriate.

Care of any fasting patient treated with insulin includes four basic elements:

1. Continuous infusion of intravenous glucose,
2. Frequent monitoring of blood glucose,
3. Continuous provision of basal insulin, and
4. Intermittent doses of rapid- or short-acting insulin to correct hyperglycemia.

Any patient who fasts for a prolonged period, whether or not he has diabetes, requires infusion of glucose to serve as metabolic substrate. Intravenous glucose should not be withheld simply due to the presence of diabetes, since this may lead to hypoglycemia. Infusion of fluid containing 5% dextrose (D5) at the standard maintenance rate for body mass is an appropriate starting point for most patients. The rate of infusion or concentration of dextrose may be increased if necessary to manage hypoglycemia. If hyperglycemia is present, in general it should be corrected with additional insulin rather than withholding glucose.

A fasting patient with diabetes should have his or her blood glucose monitored at minimum every 3–4 h. More frequent monitoring is necessary if significant hyper- or hypoglycemia is present. Monitoring every 30–60 min is appropriate if rapid fluctuations are possible, including intraoperatively or during an intravenous insulin infusion. Any patient with type 1 diabetes requires a continuous supply of basal insulin at all times, even while fasting, to avoid hyperglycemia, ketosis, and eventually ketoacidosis. Basal insulin is by definition that required for metabolic needs when the patient is not eating; therefore, if the patient's home dose of basal insulin has been properly determined, the same dose should be appropriate in the fasting state. Basal insulin preparations that provide continuous, peakless coverage (i.e., glargine, detemir, or insulin pump basal rates) generally require no dose adjustment for fasting. If the patient has persistent blood glucose values below 80 mg/dL (4.4 mmol/L) or above 250 mg/dL (13.9 mmol/L), the dose should be decreased or increased by 10–20%, respectively. Since NPH has a pronounced peak effect that may cause hypoglycemia if the patient does not eat, *NPH doses should be decreased by one third to one half during fasting*.

In addition to basal insulin, patients with diabetes require intermittent doses of rapid- or short-acting insulin to correct hyperglycemia. Rapid-acting insulin analogues are often preferred due to their fast onset and short duration of action. Rapid-acting insulin analogue should be given every 3–4 h as needed for hyperglycemia, using a correction factor based on the measured blood glucose at that time. The exact correction factor to be used is different for each patient and should be calculated and recommended by the treating endocrinologist. *Rapid-acting insulin analogue should not be given more frequently than every 3 h*, because hypoglycemia may result if a second dose is given while a prior dose is still acting (known as "dose stacking"). Occasionally, conventional basal insulin may be omitted and continuous insulin coverage provided using only frequent correction doses of a rapid-acting insulin analogue every 3–4 h. This approach is effective when greater dosing flexibility is desired, or when a long-acting preparation is not desirable (e.g., in an intensive care setting). However, this regimen requires close supervision, as a missed insulin dose will leave the patient without insulin coverage and vulnerable to rapid onset of ketoacidosis.

Using the above principles, the following general approach is a reasonable starting point in the majority of fasting patients with diabetes treated with subcutaneous insulin in any phase perioperative management:

- Infuse intravenous fluids containing 5% dextrose at the standard maintenance rate for body mass;
- Check blood glucose every 3 h (check hourly intraoperatively, or if using an insulin infusion);
- Ensure basal insulin coverage using a long-acting insulin analogue, NPH, or insulin pump basal rate (with any necessary dose adjustments);
- Correct hyperglycemia with rapid-acting insulin analogue every 3 h using a correction factor or sliding scale.

Patients with type 2 diabetes who are treated with insulin are managed similarly to those with type 1 diabetes. Intravenous dextrose and frequent blood glucose monitoring are required. Those on basal insulin should continue to receive it perioperatively, with dose adjustments if necessary as discussed above. Patients who receive only intermittent insulin at baseline can be managed effectively with repeated correction doses of rapid-acting insulin analogue every 3–4 h. Since hyperglycemia is exaggerated by the stress of surgery, patients who are controlled only on oral medication at baseline may require insulin perioperatively. For such patients, rapid-acting insulin analogue (0.1 unit/kg) may be used as an initial correction dose, with dose adjustments if needed based on the response.

Intravenous Insulin Infusions

Minor surgery often causes little disturbance in glycemic control, and most patients can be managed throughout their perioperative course with subcutaneous insulin. For major surgery, the metabolic changes are more significant and intravenous insulin infusion is preferred. Intravenous insulin should also be used whenever strict glycemic control is desired, or when poor perfusion may compromise absorption of insulin via the skin. Regular insulin is the recommended formulation for intravenous use; rapid-acting insulin analogues are equally effective, but are more expensive and have no advantage over regular insulin when given intravenously. Intravenous regular insulin has a short serum half-life (4–7 min) and therefore is best delivered as a continuous infusion, the rate of which can be finely titrated and rapidly adjusted with changes in the patient's condition. Drawbacks to an insulin infusion include the need for continuous intravenous access and very close monitoring of blood glucose to prevent hyper- or hypoglycemia. Because of the need for intensive monitoring, many institutions restrict the use of intravenous insulin infusions to operating rooms and critical care units.

An intravenous insulin infusion should be used intraoperatively for major surgery, including long (>2 h), complex, or extensive procedures that may cause rapid or significant fluctuations in blood glucose. The intravenous route should also be used if hemodynamic or temperature alterations are likely to compromise cutaneous perfusion. While on intravenous insulin, patients should receive an infusion of glucose-containing fluids (5–10% dextrose) to prevent hypoglycemia. When beginning an insulin infusion, regular insulin (1 unit/mL in normal saline) should be used at an initial rate of 1 unit per 5 g of dextrose in patients 12 years old or less, or 1 unit per 3 g of dextrose in patients older than 12 years [24]. It is important to take into account any prior subcutaneous insulin doses that may still be acting at the time the infusion is initiated. Blood glucose should be checked 30 min after initiation of the infusion or any adjustment in infusion rate, and then hourly. The rates of dextrose and insulin infusions should be adjusted to bring blood glucose into the target range (see below).

When transitioning a patient from intravenous to subcutaneous insulin, it is important to recall that the effect of intravenous insulin will dissipate rapidly, possibly before the onset of action of a subcutaneous preparation given at the time the infusion is stopped. Therefore, to ensure continuous insulin coverage, a subcutaneous dose of rapid- or short-acting insulin should be given 30 min prior to stopping the intravenous infusion.

Preparation for Surgery

In the case of elective surgery, preoperative management of diabetes is more dependent on the patient's degree of glycemic control than on whether the planned procedure is major or minor. Once a patient with diabetes has been deemed an appropriate candidate based on preoperative evaluation, preparation for the procedure does not vary significantly based on how extensive surgery will be. In all cases, however, coordination with the patient's diabetologist/endocrinologist is strongly encouraged to facilitate perioperative planning of diabetes care.

The majority of patients with diabetes can be admitted to the hospital on the day of their elective procedure. Preoperative overnight admission is necessary only in cases that require complex management of fluid and insulin, or if there is uncertainty about the degree of glycemic control or compliance with the diabetes regimen. However, since the risk of perioperative complications due to diabetes is related to long-term glycemic control and postoperative management, there is little rationale for admitting an otherwise stable patient for brief "optimization" of diabetes control prior to elective surgery. If glycemic control is poor, elective surgery should be delayed until adequate control is achieved. In the case of semi-elective surgery that cannot be delayed for the time required to improve glycemic control, it may be appropriate to proceed with surgery, with increased vigilance for possible complications.

An extended fast is generally required beginning the night before surgery. In patients treated with insulin, including all patients with type 1 diabetes, surgery should be scheduled as early in the day as possible—ideally as the first case—to avoid unnecessarily extending the fast and increasing the risk hypoglycemia. Since older children and adolescents customarily sleep through the night without eating or drinking, fasting overnight preoperatively does not generally require modification of overnight insulin coverage. The usual dose(s) of glargine, detemir, or NPH should be given the day prior to surgery, or the usual insulin pump basal rate(s) maintained. Preventing hypoglycemia on the morning of surgery is important because the patient will be "*nil per mouth*" (NPO) at that time. If the patient has a history of frequent morning blood glucose values below 100 mg/dL, the previous day's dose of basal insulin or the overnight insulin pump basal rate may be reduced by 20–30%. For infants who are still accustomed to feeding overnight, other adjustments to insulin may be required depending on the patient's age and the duration of fasting; the patient's endocrinologist should be consulted in such situations.

On the morning of surgery, the patient's blood glucose should be checked upon awakening. Hypoglycemia must be treated, preferably with glucose tablets or gel, or if necessary with a small amount of glucose-containing liquid, recognizing that this may interfere with the induction of anesthesia. The usual dose of basal insulin (glargine, detemir, or insulin pump basal rate) should be given. If NPH is used, the morning dose should be reduced by one third to one half on the morning of surgery. No rapid- or short-acting insulin should be given, unless needed to correct severe hyperglycemia ($\geq$400 mg/dL), which should be treated using the patient's rapid-acting correction factor. For patients treated with premixed insulin, the morning dose should be omitted; on admission, NPH alone should be given in the amount of 50% of the NPH component of the usual premixed dose.

On admission to the preoperative area, blood glucose and electrolytes should be measured and intravenous access established. The presence of ketones should be assessed either by urinalysis or by measuring serum beta-hydroxybutyric acid. An infusion of dextrose-containing fluids (normal saline, half-normal saline, or lactated Ringer's with 5% dextrose) should be started at the standard maintenance rate for body mass. If the blood glucose is greater than 250 mg/dL, a dose of rapid-acting insulin analogue may be given using the patient's correction factor (as long as no other rapid- or short-acting insulin has been given in the preceding 3 h).

Patients with type 2 diabetes treated with insulin should be managed equivalently to those with type 1 diabetes. Metformin should be stopped 24 h prior to elective surgery. Other oral diabetes medications should be stopped on the morning of the procedure.

When emergency surgery is required in a patient with diabetes, ensuring glycemic control is not possible in advance. Therefore, emergency surgery should proceed as clinically indicated, with additional attention to the risk of diabetes-related complications. Conditions that require urgent surgery often involve physiologic stress and/or systemic inflammation that may precipitate ketoacidosis or hypoglycemia. In the latter case, surgery may proceed as soon as hypoglycemia is corrected, generally with a bolus of intravenous dextrose followed by continuous infusion of dextrose-containing fluids. When a surgical emergency is complicated by diabetic ketoacidosis, the determination of how much to treat DKA before surgery can be difficult. Ideally, ketoacidosis should be completely resolved prior to surgery, including normalization of the anion gap, full rehydration, and correction of any electrolyte abnormalities (especially potassium). However, a balance must be struck between the severity of metabolic derangements and the urgency of operative intervention. It is important to remember that ketoacidosis itself increases insulin resistance, and patients in DKA or its aftermath often require more insulin than at baseline.

Perioperative Glycemic Control: Pathophysiology and Goals of Treatment

Stress and Glycemic Control

Even in patients without diabetes, hyperglycemia is a frequent complication of surgery. Any physiologic disturbance, even minor illness or psychosocial stress, can provoke the body's normal stress response, which includes the release of epinephrine, cortisol, glucagon, and growth hormone. These counterregulatory hormones raise blood glucose by increasing hepatic glucose production and as peripheral insulin resistance. Anesthesia and surgery also initiate a systemic inflammatory response with release of cytokines (e.g., tumor necrosis factor alpha, interleukin-6) that contribute to insulin resistance. These metabolic effects are sufficient to cause hyperglycemia even in normal individuals, of whom 25% will have hyperglycemia (>140 mg/dL or 7.8 mmol/L) intraoperatively [25]. Patients with diabetes cannot produce sufficient insulin even at baseline and are at even higher risk of perioperative hyperglycemia, which, if severe, can lead to diabetic ketoacidosis or hyperosmolar hyperglycemia syndrome. Therefore, all patients with diabetes require careful monitoring for hyperglycemia throughout the perioperative period. *Insulin doses often need to be increased perioperatively, sometimes substantially, to compensate for increases in glucose production and insulin resistance caused by the stress of surgery.* An initial dose increment of 5–10% is generally appropriate, with further increases as needed to achieve target glycemic control. Patients with type 2 diabetes may require insulin perioperatively even if they do not at baseline.

Adverse Effects of Perioperative Glucose Abnormalities

Although mild hyperglycemia is a normal physiologic response to significant illness, a great deal of evidence supports that uncontrolled hyperglycemia in the hospitalized patient—with or without a preexisting diagnosis of diabetes—is associated with a variety of adverse outcomes. In adults, hyperglycemia is associated with increased morbidity and mortality in critically ill patients with myocardial infarction, stroke, trauma, and sepsis, as well as in patients hospitalized with noncritical illness [26, 27]. In critically ill children, including those with trauma, burns, and septic shock, the magnitude and duration of hyperglycemia are similarly associated with increased morbidity, length of stay, and mortality [28–32]. In hospitalized children with noncritical illness, hyperglycemia has been associated with increased need for intensive care and longer length of stay, although not with increased mortality [33].

With specific reference to surgery, the majority of data linking perioperative hyperglycemia to adverse outcomes are derived from the cardiac surgical literature. In adult cardiac surgical patients, postoperative hyperglycemia is associated with increased risks of infection (including wound infections, pneumonia, and urinary tract infections), renal and hepatic dysfunction, and death [34, 35]. Studies of critically ill infants after repair of congenital heart disease show increased infection rates, length of stay, and mortality in those with postoperative hyperglycemia [36–40]. Little direct evidence exists about the effects of perioperative hyperglycemia in pediatric patients undergoing noncardiac surgery, or in pediatric surgical patients who are not critically ill. The precise level of glycemia at which perioperative risks begin to increase is not clear, but evidence supports a direct relationship, with more severe and prolonged hyperglycemia correlating with higher risk.

Since most studies of perioperative hyperglycemia have focused on the postoperative period, the role of intraoperative hyperglycemia is not as clearly understood. In adults there appears to be an association between intraoperative hyperglycemia and adverse outcomes including wound infection and mortality [41, 42]. An observational study of pediatric cardiac surgical patients found an increased risk of bacteremia in patients with intraoperative hyperglycemia, though mortality was not affected [43]. Thus, a relationship appears to exist between intraoperative hyperglycemia and morbidity, but causality has not been established and its importance is still unclear.

Goals for Perioperative Glycemic Control

Recognition of the risks of uncontrolled hyperglycemia has led to a great deal of investigation into whether glycemic control can reduce these risks, and if so, what is the ideal regimen to achieve this goal. In the last decade, a number of large studies and meta-analyses have evaluated varying regimens and target ranges of intensive glycemic control in critically ill adult populations. Most trials have compared an intervention group receiving an intravenous insulin infusion to maintain blood glucose in a near-normal target range with a control group received a conventional glycemic control regimen that varies among studies. Some studies have included surgical patients only, while others have included only medical patients or combinations of surgical and medical patients.

A promising early trial in surgical intensive care patients found a marked decrease in bacteremia, renal failure, and mortality in patients treated to near-normal blood glucose (80–110 mg/dL or 4.4–6.1 mmol/L) as compared to those with less strict control (180–200 mg/dL or 10–11.1 mmol/L) [44]. In contrast, a large randomized, controlled trial in a mixed medical/surgical cohort demonstrated increased mortality in patients treated to near-normoglycemia compared to those managed less aggressively [45]. Several other trials and meta-analyses of intensive glycemic control in surgical, medical, or mixed populations have produced inconsistent results regarding various morbidities and have not shown a convincing mortality benefit [46–53]. The first pediatric trial of intensive glycemic control evaluated a general pediatric intensive care population that included a majority (75%) of cardiac surgical patients. In this study, intensive glycemic control resulted in shorter length of stay, fewer infections, and fewer deaths [54]. Three subsequent large multicenter prospective randomized clinical trials, however, have since been completed which have uniformly shown no substantial benefit to glycemic control to similar targets of 80–100 mg/dL in critically ill children [55–57].

In contrast to any uncertainty regarding its possible benefits, evidence is unequivocal that intensive glycemic control carries an increased risk of hypoglycemia. In pediatric patients receiving such therapy, the incidence of severe hypoglycemia is as high as 25% [54], though much lower but nonzero in studies utilizing continuous glucose monitoring and a computer-driven algorithm [55, 57]. Since this hypoglycemia is iatrogenic due to insulin administration, it is more dangerous than physiologic fasting hypoglycemia because insulin suppresses ketogenesis and thus deprives the brain of its alternative metabolic substrate. Hypoglycemia in the intensive care setting is associated with complications of seizure, brain damage, and death in both adults and children [39, 58]. Moreover, compared to adults, children are at higher risk of hypoglycemia because of increased glucose utilization due to the large size of their brain relative to total body mass. Therefore, significant concern remains about the risk of hypoglycemia in children managed with intensive glycemic control with low blood glucose targets. Current best practice for critically ill children, therefore, is to manage glucose to a higher target of 150–180 mg/dL.

Though a great deal of data exists about glycemic control in critically ill adults, there are a number of limitations in applying this data to the routine perioperative care of children with diabetes. First, only a single trial of intensive glycemic control has been performed in children outside the neonatal period. Second, all trials have been conducted in critical care settings, and these results are difficult to generalize to the care of noncritically ill patients. Third, the majority of surgical patients studied (both adults and children) have undergone cardiac surgery, and potential differences between this population and patients undergoing other types of surgery have not been well characterized. Finally, studies of intensive glycemic control in surgical patients have focused on postoperative glycemic control, whereas data are more limited regarding the importance of intraoperative glycemic control. Observational studies have suggested a benefit of tight intraoperative glycemic control, but a randomized, controlled trial showed no benefit of maintaining near-normal intraoperative blood glucose over simply preventing severe hyperglycemia (>200 mg/dL or 11.1 mmol/L) [59].

In summary, uncontrolled postoperative hyperglycemia (>180 mg/dL) is clearly detrimental. Attempting to maintain normal blood glucose values may improve certain morbidities, but it does not clearly improve mortality and it markedly increases the risk of hypoglycemia. Therefore, based on the available data, consensus guidelines recommend a *postoperative blood glucose target range of 140–180 mg/dL (7.8–10 mmol/L)* [26]. It is possible that a lower, but still above-normal, target range (such as 126–140 mg/dL or 7–7.8 mmol/L) may confer more benefit while avoiding hypoglycemia, but this has not been prospectively evaluated [39]. Further studies are also necessary to assess the true benefits and risks of postoperative intensive glycemic control in the pediatric population. With regard to intraoperative management, although substantial observational evidence suggests that uncontrolled hyperglycemia is undesirable, the ideal blood glucose range is unknown. In the absence of clear data, current consensus guidelines for children with diabetes recommend maintaining *intraoperative blood glucose between 90 and 180 mg/dL (5–10 mmol/L)* [60].

Intraoperative Management

The stress of surgery can cause blood glucose to vary significantly, requiring close monitoring and frequent adjustments with insulin and infused dextrose. All patients should receive intravenous fluids with at least 5% dextrose. Monitoring of blood glucose should occur at least hourly during surgery. Any blood glucose value greater than 250 mg/dL (13.9 mmol/L) should prompt immediate measurement of ketones. Ketones greater than "trace" by urinalysis or serum beta-hydroxybutyrate greater than 0.6 mmol/L indicates evolving ketosis that requires administration of additional insulin to avoid the development of ketoacidosis. The optimal route of insulin administration depends on whether the surgery is major or minor, and should be discussed in advance with the anesthetist.

For major surgery, especially if expected to last over 2 h, an intravenous insulin infusion is recommended. The infusion should be started shortly before the procedure, along with a separate infusion containing 5–10% dextrose (see Sect. 6.2). Intraoperative blood glucose should be checked at least hourly, and the rates of infused dextrose and insulin adjusted to maintain blood glucose in the target range (90–180 mg/dL or 5–10 mmol/L).

For minor surgery, particularly that not requiring general anesthesia, patients can generally be managed intraoperatively with subcutaneous insulin. For patients on multiple daily injection regimens, basal insulin should be given prior to surgery, and a correction dose of rapid-acting insulin analogue given preoperatively if the blood glucose is elevated (section above). Intraoperative blood glucose should be checked at least hourly. If blood glucose is elevated above the target range, a subcutaneous injection of rapid-acting insulin analogue should be given based on the patient's correction factor, keeping in mind that *rapid-acting insulin analogue should be given no more frequently than every 3 h* due to its duration of action.

For patients using a subcutaneous insulin pump who are having minor surgery, the pump may be continued intraoperatively if several conditions are met. Subcutaneous (as opposed to intravenous) administration of insulin must be compatible with the specific patient and procedure. The planned surgery should be shorter than 2 h, to minimize the risk of malfunction of the pump or infusion set. A new pump infusion set must have been inserted within 24 h of the surgery. Both the pump and the infusion site must be placed in an area that is accessible to the anesthetist during the case, taking into account draping and any possible changes in patient positioning. Finally, the anesthetist must be comfortable with the technical aspects of administering insulin via the pump. If continued intraoperatively, the pump will provide basal insulin coverage. Correction doses for hyperglycemia may be given via the pump or as separate subcutaneous injections by syringe.

Postoperative Management

In the immediate postoperative period, patients may be unable to eat or drink for a variable amount of time depending on the nature and extent of their surgery. Until the patient has recovered from anesthesia, immediate postoperative care is identical to that provided intraoperatively, including infusion of fluids with dextrose, hourly blood glucose monitoring, and insulin management with either intravenous or subcutaneous insulin. Ketones should be measured in urine or serum in response to any glucose measurement greater than 250 mg/dL. The target range for blood glucose in the postoperative period is 140–180 mg/dL (7.8–10 mmol/L) (see above).

After minor surgery, most patients will resume oral intake shortly after recovering from anesthesia. For such patients, a prophylactic dose of a nonsteroid anti-emetic (such as ondansetron) should be considered during recovery: if the patient receives a dose of insulin in anticipation of eating and then cannot eat due to nausea, hypoglycemia may result. Steroid anti-emetics (such as dexamethasone) should be avoided if possible due to their side effect of hyperglycemia. Such patients should resume their home subcutaneous insulin regimen, including prandial and correction doses, as soon as they tolerate sufficient enteral intake to no longer require intravenous dextrose.

For a patient who has undergone major surgery, resumption of enteral nutrition may be delayed. Patients who are critically ill require an intravenous infusion for postoperative glycemic control. Otherwise, the patient may be able to transition to a subcutaneous regimen even if she remains fasting. In this case, she should continue to receive intravenous dextrose, blood glucose monitoring every 3–4 h, subcutaneous basal insulin, and subcutaneous correction doses every 3–4 h as needed for hyperglycemia above the target range. (Recall that doses of NPH should be reduced by one third to one half in a fasting patient.) Intravenous insulin should only be discontinued 30 min after a subcutaneous dose of rapid- or short-acting insulin has been given. Once the patient is able to tolerate oral intake, the usual home insulin regimen may be resumed, including prandial insulin doses. However, in a patient whose diet advances slowly, it may be necessary to reduce prandial doses proportionally to the amount of oral intake.

Patients who cannot tolerate enteral intake for an extended period may require total parenteral nutrition (TPN). Since in this situation dextrose is being infused continuously, ideal management would include a continuous infusion of insulin to match the infused glucose load. For the first 24 h after TPN is initiated, the usual basal insulin should be continued, and correction doses of rapid-acting insulin analogue should be administered every 3–4 h. The total daily amount of insulin needed for correction can then be added, as regular insulin, directly to the TPN mixture. The amount of insulin in the TPN can be adjusted daily based on blood glucose values. It is important to remember to review the amount of added insulin daily and adjust it in concert with any adjustment in dextrose concentration of the TPN.

Like any other postsurgical patient, discharge criteria for a patient with diabetes include the ability to tolerate sufficient enteral intake to maintain hydration and nutrition. In addition, the patient must have appropriate blood glucose levels on his or her home insulin regimen. In the case of minor surgery, these criteria are often met shortly after recovery from anesthesia, and the patient can be discharged from the postoperative care unit. For patients on oral diabetes medications, metformin may be restarted once adequate postoperative renal function is assured, and other medications may be restarted once the patient is tolerating adequate enteral intake.

References

1. Dabelea D, Bell RA, D'Agostino RB Jr, et al. Incidence of diabetes in youth in the United States. JAMA. 2007;297(24):2716–24.
2. Craig ME, Hattersley A, Donaghue KC. Definition, epidemiology and classification of diabetes in children and adolescents. Pediatr Diabetes. 2009;10 (Suppl 12):3–12.

3. Bolli GB, Fanelli CG. Physiology of glucose counterregulation to hypoglycemia. Endocrinol Metab Clin North Am. 1999;28(3):467–93.
4. Thunander M, Petersson C, Jonzon K, et al. Incidence of type 1 and type 2 diabetes in adults and children in Kronoberg, Sweden. Diabetes Res Clin Pract. 2008;82(2):247–55.
5. Bingley PJ. Clinical applications of diabetes antibody testing. J Clin Endocrinol Metab. 2010;95(1):25–33.
6. Betts P, Brink S, Silink M, et al. Management of children and adolescents with diabetes requiring surgery. Pediatr Diabetes. 2009;10(Suppl 12):169–74.
7. Diabetes Control and Complications Trial Research Group. The effect of intensive treatment of diabetes on the development and progression of long-term complications in insulin-dependent diabetes mellitus. N Engl J Med. 1993;329(14):977–86.
8. Nathan DM, Cleary PA, Backlund JY, et al. Intensive diabetes treatment and cardiovascular disease in patients with type 1 diabetes. N Engl J Med. 2005;353(25):2643–53.
9. American Diabetes Association. Diagnosis and classification of diabetes mellitus. Diabetes Care. 2010;33(Suppl 1):S62–9.
10. Rewers M, Pihoker C, Donaghue K, et al. Assessment and monitoring of glycemic control in children and adolescents with diabetes. Pediatr Diabetes. 2009;10(Suppl 12):71–81.
11. Bangstad HJ, Danne T, Deeb L, et al. Insulin treatment in children and adolescents with diabetes. Pediatr Diabetes. 2009;10(Suppl 12):82–99.
12. Mehta SN, Wolfsdorf JI. Contemporary management of patients with type 1 diabetes. Endocrinol Metab Clin North Am. 2010;39(3):573–93.
13. Miles HL, Acerini CL. Insulin analog preparations and their use in children and adolescents with type 1 diabetes mellitus. Paediatr Drugs. 2008;10(3):163–76.
14. Polonsky KS, Given BD, Hirsch L, et al. Quantitative study of insulin secretion and clearance in normal and obese subjects. J Clin Invest. 1988;81(2):435–41.
15. Holman RR, Paul SK, Bethel MA, et al. 10-year follow-up of intensive glucose control in type 2 diabetes. N Engl J Med. 2008;359(15):1577–89.
16. UK Prospective Diabetes Study (UKPDS) Group. Effect of intensive blood-glucose control with metformin on complications in overweight patients with type 2 diabetes (UKPDS 34). Lancet. 1998;352(9131):854–65.
17. UK Prospective Diabetes Study (UKPDS) Group. Intensive blood-glucose control with sulphonylureas or insulin compared with conventional treatment and risk of complications in patients with type 2 diabetes (UKPDS 33). Lancet. 1998;352 (9131):837–53.
18. Sigal RJ, Kenny GP, Wasserman DH, et al. Physical activity/exercise and type 2 diabetes. Diabetes Care. 2004;27(10):2518–39.
19. Salpeter SR, Greyber E, Pasternak GA, et al. Risk of fatal and nonfatal lactic acidosis with metformin use in type 2 diabetes mellitus. Cochrane Database Syst Rev 2010;4:CD002967.
20. Rosenbloom AL. Hyperglycemic hyperosmolar state: an emerging pediatric problem. J Pediatr. 2010;156 (2):180–4.
21. Cruse PJ, Foord R. A five-year prospective study of 23,649 surgical wounds. Arch Surg. 1973;107 (2):206–10.
22. Dronge AS, Perkal MF, Kancir S, et al. Long-term glycemic control and postoperative infectious complications. Arch Surg. 2006;141(4):375–80.
23. Noordzij PG, Boersma E, Schreiner F, et al. Increased preoperative glucose levels are associated with perioperative mortality in patients undergoing noncardiac, nonvascular surgery. Eur J Endocrinol. 2007;156(1):137–42.
24. Rhodes ET, Ferrari LR, Wolfsdorf JI. Perioperative management of pediatric surgical patients with diabetes mellitus. Anesth Analg. 2005;101(4):986–99.
25. Bower WF, Lee PY, Kong AP, et al. Peri-operative hyperglycemia: a consideration for general surgery? Am J Surg. 2010;199(2):240–8.
26. Moghissi ES, Korytkowski MT, DiNardo M, et al. American Association of Clinical Endocrinologists and American Diabetes Association consensus statement on inpatient glycemic control. Diabetes Care. 2009;32(6):1119–31.
27. Umpierrez GE, Isaacs SD, Bazargan N, et al. Hyperglycemia: an independent marker of in-hospital mortality in patients with undiagnosed diabetes. J Clin Endocrinol Metab. 2002;87(3):978–82.
28. Branco RG, Garcia PC, Piva JP, et al. Glucose level and risk of mortality in pediatric septic shock. Pediatr Crit Care Med. 2005;6(4):470–2.
29. Faustino EV, Apkon M. Persistent hyperglycemia in critically ill children. J Pediatr. 2005;146(1):30–4.
30. Srinivasan V, Spinella PC, Drott HR, et al. Association of timing, duration, and intensity of hyperglycemia with intensive care unit mortality in critically ill children. Pediatr Crit Care Med. 2004;5 (4):329–36.
31. Tuggle DW, Kuhn MA, Jones SK, et al. Hyperglycemia and infections in pediatric trauma patients. Am Surg. 2008;74(3):195–8.
32. Wintergerst KA, Buckingham B, Gandrud L, et al. Association of hypoglycemia, hyperglycemia, and glucose variability with morbidity and death in the pediatric intensive care unit. Pediatrics. 2006;118 (1):173–9.
33. Palacio A, Smiley D, Ceron M, et al. Prevalence and clinical outcome of inpatient hyperglycemia in a community pediatric hospital. J Hosp Med. 2008;3 (3):212–7.
34. Golden SH, Peart-Vigilance C, Kao WH, et al. Perioperative glycemic control and the risk of infectious complications in a cohort of adults with diabetes. Diabetes Care. 1999;22(9):1408–14.

35. Latham R, Lancaster AD, Covington JF, et al. The association of diabetes and glucose control with surgical-site infections among cardiothoracic surgery patients. Infect Control Hosp Epidemiol. 2001;22(10):607–12.
36. Falcao G, Ulate K, Kouzekanani K, et al. Impact of postoperative hyperglycemia following surgical repair of congenital cardiac defects. Pediatr Cardiol. 2008;29(3):628–36.
37. Polito A, Thiagarajan RR, Laussen PC, et al. Association between intraoperative and early postoperative glucose levels and adverse outcomes after complex congenital heart surgery. Circulation. 2008;118(22):2235–42.
38. Preissig CM, Rigby MR, Maher KO. Glycemic control for postoperative pediatric cardiac patients. Pediatr Cardiol. 2009;30(8):1098–104.
39. Ulate KP, Lima Falcao GC, Bielefeld MR, et al. Strict glycemic targets need not be so strict: a more permissive glycemic range for critically ill children. Pediatrics. 2008;122(4):e898–904.
40. Yates AR, Dyke PC 2nd, Taeed R, et al. Hyperglycemia is a marker for poor outcome in the postoperative pediatric cardiac patient. Pediatr Crit Care Med. 2006;7(4):351–5.
41. Duncan AE, Abd-Elsayed A, Maheshwari A, et al. Role of intraoperative and postoperative blood glucose concentrations in predicting outcomes after cardiac surgery. Anesthesiology. 2010;112(4):860–71.
42. Ouattara A, Lecomte P, Le Manach Y, et al. Poor intraoperative blood glucose control is associated with a worsened hospital outcome after cardiac surgery in diabetic patients. Anesthesiology. 2005;103(4):687–94.
43. O'Brien JE, Jr., Marshall JA, Tarrants ML, et al. Intraoperative hyperglycemia and postoperative bacteremia in the pediatric cardiac surgery patient. Ann Thorac Surg 2010;89(2):578–583; discussion 583–4.
44. Van den Berghe G, Wouters P, Weekers F, et al. Intensive insulin therapy in the critically ill patients. N Engl J Med. 2001;345(19):1359–67.
45. Finfer S, Chittock DR, Su SY, et al. Intensive versus conventional glucose control in critically ill patients. N Engl J Med. 2009;360(13):1283–97.
46. Annane D, Cariou A, Maxime V, et al. Corticosteroid treatment and intensive insulin therapy for septic shock in adults: a randomized controlled trial. JAMA. 2010;303(4):341–8.
47. Arabi YM, Dabbagh OC, Tamim HM, et al. Intensive versus conventional insulin therapy: a randomized controlled trial in medical and surgical critically ill patients. Crit Care Med. 2008;36(12):3190–7.
48. Brunkhorst FM, Engel C, Bloos F, et al. Intensive insulin therapy and pentastarch resuscitation in severe sepsis. N Engl J Med 2008;358(2):125–139.
49. Griesdale DE, de Souza RJ, van Dam RM, et al. Intensive insulin therapy and mortality among critically ill patients: a meta-analysis including NICE-SUGAR study data. CMAJ. 2009;180(8):821–7.
50. Marik PE, Preiser JC. Toward understanding tight glycemic control in the ICU: a systematic review and metaanalysis. Chest. 2010;137(3):544–51.
51. Preiser JC, Devos P, Ruiz-Santana S, et al. A prospective randomised multi-centre controlled trial on tight glucose control by intensive insulin therapy in adult intensive care units: the Glucontrol study. Intensive Care Med. 2009;35(10):1738–48.
52. Van den Berghe G, Wilmer A, Hermans G, et al. Intensive insulin therapy in the medical ICU. N Engl J Med. 2006;354(5):449–61.
53. Wiener RS, Wiener DC, Larson RJ. Benefits and risks of tight glucose control in critically ill adults: a meta-analysis. JAMA. 2008;300(8):933–44.
54. Vlasselaers D, Milants I, Desmet L, et al. Intensive insulin therapy for patients in paediatric intensive care: a prospective, randomised controlled study. Lancet. 2009;373(9663):547–56.
55. Agus MS, Steil GM, Wypij D, Costello JM, Laussen PC, Langer M, et al. SPECS study investigators. N Engl J Med 2012;367(13):1208–19. PMID:22957521.
56. Macrae D, Grieve R, Allen E, Sadique Z, Morris K, Pappachan J, Parslow R, et al. CHiP investigators. A randomized trial of hyperglycemic control in pediatric intensive care. N Engl J Med 2014;370(2):107–18. doi:10.1056/NEJMoa1302564. Erratum in: N Engl J Med 2014;370(15):1469. PMID:24401049.
57. Agus MS, Wypij D, Hirshberg EL, Srinivasan V, Faustino EV, Luckett PM, et al. HALF-PINT study investigators and the PALISI network. Tight glycemic control in critically Ill children. N Engl J Med 2017. doi:10.1056/NEJMoa1612348. [Epub ahead of print] PMID:28118549.
58. Krinsley JS, Grover A. Severe hypoglycemia in critically ill patients: risk factors and outcomes. Crit Care Med. 2007;35(10):2262–7.
59. Gandhi GY, Nuttall GA, Abel MD, et al. Intensive intraoperative insulin therapy versus conventional glucose management during cardiac surgery: a randomized trial. Ann Intern Med. 2007;146(4):233–43.
60. Betts P, Brink S, Silink M, et al. Management of children and adolescents with diabetes requiring surgery. Pediatr Diabetes. 2009;10(Suppl 12):169–74.

Part V
Bariatric Surgery

Assessing and Selecting Patients for Bariatric Surgery

16

Thomas H. Inge

The prevalence of obesity among children and adolescents is rapidly increasing and is associated with substantial medical and psychosocial morbidity [1, 2]. Current national estimates in the US, indicate that approximately one-third of adults are obese, while in the adolescent age group the prevalence of obesity is lower but has steadily risen over the decades from 4.6% in the late 1960s, to 14.8% in 2000, to 18.1% in 2008 [3]. Thus, it is critical that health professionals understand the risks of obesity and have the tools to initiate an action plan. Data indicate that essentially all children with a body mass index (BMI) above the 99th percentile become obese adults (BMI $\geq$ 30 kg/m^2) [1]. Since obese adults who were obese as children have more health complications and a higher mortality [4–7], it is reasonable to consider aggressive treatment options for mature adolescents to reduce the risk of morbidity and early mortality from obesity-associated disease [8–10].

Pediatric Obesity and Consequences

Of considerable concern is the problem of extreme obesity in youth, now estimated to affect 4% of children and adolescents [11]. Indeed, in the years 1999–2004, an estimated 4% of all pediatric age groups had a BMI $\geq$ 99th percentile. Minority groups demonstrated the greatest prevalence of extreme pediatric obesity (Blacks, 5.7% and Mexican Americans, 5.2%), while extreme obesity was found in 3.1% of Caucasians [11]. Longitudinally, nearly 90% of these extremely obese youth are expected to remain extremely obese, attaining an adult BMI of 35 kg/m^2 or greater [1].

Many studies in pediatric populations have demonstrated the health risks of obesity [12]. Youth with increased adiposity are at an increased risk of developing disturbances in glucose metabolism (including type 2 diabetes [13]), hypertension and dyslipidemia [14], obstructive sleep apnea [15], vascular dysfunction [16], gallbladder disease [17], menstrual irregularities and polycystic ovary syndrome [18], and later in life, a number of types of cancer [5].

Perhaps even more importantly, those youth with extreme obesity have accentuated odds for development of cardiovascular (CV) risk factors such as elevated blood pressure, dyslipidemia, and hyperinsulinemia [19]. The associations between elevated BMI and presence of CV risk factors appear markedly nonlinear, with impressive increases in the prevalence of multiple risk factors occurring only at very high BMI percentiles. For example, the prevalence of $\geq$3 risk factors climbs from 6%, to 7%, to 33% as BMI increases from the 90th, to the 95th, to the 99th percentile [1].

T.H. Inge (✉)
Akers Chair in Pediatric Surgery, Division of Pediatric Surgery, Adolescent Metabolic and Bariatric Surgery, Children's Hospital Colorado, 13123 East 16th Avenue, Box 323, Aurora, CO 80045-7106, USA
e-mail: thomas.inge@childrenscolorado.org

D.J. Ledbetter and P.R.V. Johnson (eds.), *Endocrine Surgery in Children*,
DOI 10.1007/978-3-662-54256-9_16

These health risks contribute to obesity-related increases in all-cause mortality. For extremely obese young adults (age 20–30), some estimates suggest that women may lose 5 and men 20 years of life due to carrying excess weight over a lifetime [20].

Treatment Approaches

Despite the fact that childhood obesity poses numerous immediate health risks and long-term consequences, there are few preventive and therapeutic strategies of proven effectiveness available. "Treatment" is intended to promote weight loss, reduce the risks of health problems, improve the quality of life, and, ultimately, extend survival. The categories of treatment include diet, exercise, behavioral modification, pharmacotherapy, and bariatric surgery. Behavioral weight management, which has been advocated for less extreme levels of obesity, results in poor rates of attendance and suboptimal weight reduction for youth with extreme obesity [21]. For adolescents with BMI values more than 40 kg/m^2, we found a 3% BMI reduction after one year of participation in a well-designed, multidisciplinary pediatric weight management program [22]. Indeed, based on the literature, poor weight loss results are expected for youth with extreme obesity [23, 24]. Beyond behavior-based treatment programs, there have been two drugs that achieved FDA approval for pediatric obesity treatment. Orlistat and sibutramine are agents which affect fat absorption and central serotonergic pathways, respectively. Pediatric studies have found that these drugs decrease BMI by 4 and 8% for orlistat and sibutrimine respectively in 12–24 months, but longer term data are not available [25, 26]. Moveover, the FDA has recently removed the most effective drug, sibutramine, from the US market due to adverse side effects. Therefore, noninvasive treatment options for obese youth, and particularly for morbidly obese youth, are quite limited, with generally poor treatment outcomes overall.

Bariatric Surgery

The immediate and future health and psychosocial effects of extreme obesity are concerning [27], and combined with lack of efficacy of most treatments, have prompted ever increasing consideration of bariatric surgery [28–30]. Indeed, the volume of pediatric (age ≤ 21) patients undergoing bariatric surgery tripled from the late 1990s to 2003, with an estimated 771 procedures per year in 2003 [31], rising to 2000 in 2004 [32, 33]. Statewide data from California indicates that rates of laparoscopic adjustable gastric banding increased 6.9-fold from 2005 to 2007 (1.5 per 100,000 population in 2007), while laparoscopic Roux-en-Y gastric bypass rates decreased slightly over the same time period [34]. Thus, the use of bariatric procedures in general appears to be steeply increasing in pediatric age groups over recent years, suggesting a need for appropriate assessment criteria prior to surgery and for prospectively and rigorously collected adolescent outcome data.

As of yet, the scientific evidence base is not sufficiently robust to allow a precise discrimination of which procedures are optimal for adolescents. Indeed, experts have broadly characterized the quality of evidence for effectiveness and safety of adolescent bariatric surgery as fair to poor for all procedures that have been reported [32]. Despite limitations in the evidence base, clinicians are faced with a need to manage myriad health problems in adolescents with extreme obesity and more recently, higher quality prospectively collected data have emerged documenting efficacy and safety of adolescent bariatric procedures [35–38]. Recommendations for assessment and selection of adolescent patients that are thoughtfully derived from our knowledge of obesity and bariatric surgery provide useful tools for those faced with sometimes difficult treatment decisions.

Preoperative Assessment

Screening of adolescents prior to bariatric procedures includes evaluation for the presence and severity of coexisting diseases, as well as assessment of the patient's and family's understanding and readiness for a major and life-changing procedure [39]. Recommended screening tests and evaluations that should be considered during the evaluation build on adult care paradigms [40] and are shown in Table 16.1. The preoperative assessment should include investigation into possible endogenous causes for obesity that may be amenable to treatment, as well as identification of any obesity-related health complications. Candidates for bariatric surgery should be evaluated by a multidisciplinary weight management team with adolescent experience, since this age group generally has medical and psychological needs that differ from morbidly obese adults. The rationale for the multidisciplinary assessment of potential bariatric candidates has been previously reviewed [41]. When applied to adolescent populations however, these teams should include a clinician with expertise in pediatric obesity, trained to detect obesity syndromes and obesity-related comorbid conditions that may require further evaluation and management. The team should also have expertise in pediatric psychology, nutrition, physical activity, nursing, and bariatric surgery [30, 39, 42–44]. One team member should have responsibility for coordinating each patient's care and ensuring follow-up and adherence to the prescribed preoperative medical and dietary regimen. Importantly, a social worker and medical subspecialists including endocrinology, pulmonary medicine, hepatology, cardiology, adolescent medicine, psychiatry, and gynecology should be readily available for consultation when questions arise. Surgeons participating in multidisciplinary adolescent bariatric teams should undergo subspecialty training in bariatric medical and surgical

Table 16.1 Recommended evaluation of an adolescent considering bariatric surgery

Clinical
• Comprehensive medial history and physical examination
• Anthropometrics: waist circumference, weight, height
• Systolic and diastolic blood pressure
• Tanner stage (≥ 4)
• Evaluation by pediatric psychologist or psychiatrist to screen for cognitive and psychiatric disorders, assess emotional maturity, decisional capacity and family support
Laboratory testing
• Fasting lipid profile
• Fasting insulin and glucose, hemoglobin A1C
• Oral glucose tolerance test (if elevated fasting glucose)
• Liver profile
• TSH
Other diagnostic evaluations
• Polysomnography (if symptoms of obstructive sleep apnea [snoring, daytime somnolence])
• Echocardiogram
• Electrocardiogram (and exercise stress test if prolonged QT interval)
• Urea breath test or endoscopy to exclude helicobacter pylori infection (if unexplained anemia or history of abdominal pain/ulcers)
• Abdominal US (if suspicion for gallstones or chronically elevated liver enzymes)
• Bone age (if needed to assess skeletal maturity)

care. The importance of proper training and experience in bariatric surgery for ensuring safe and effective bariatric care in the adolescent population cannot be understated.

Medical and psychiatric comorbidities, and family dysfunction identified during the preoperative screening assessment must be fully explored by appropriately trained specialists. It is not at all uncommon for this initial bariatric evaluation to discover numerous previously unidentified or poorly managed problems that require more indepth attention by specialists and thus close follow-up and coordination of care during the preoperative phase. The team must therefore have a plan for who on the team will be responsible for the active management or coordination of care for active health and psychosocial problems identified, since the adequacy of management of such problems may well bear on the ultimate success of the weight loss intervention. In the Surgical Weight Loss Program for Teens at Cincinnati Children's Hospital Medical Center, this time-intensive, but critical function is performed by an experienced nurse practitioner with expertise in adolescent medicine; a social worker (in conjunction with mental health workers as needed) then coordinates further assessment and management of psychosocial issues.

The final decision-making regarding whether to proceed with surgery must be made by the multidisciplinary team, taking into consideration both objective and subjective assessments of the severity of obesity and obesity-related comorbid conditions, risk of future health problems, failure to lose weight through more conventional means, psychosocial status and support, and patient and family readiness for surgery.

Patient Selection

Adults with a BMI ≥ 40 kg/m^2 or a 35 kg/m^2 with significant current comorbidities are considered candidates for weight loss surgery. In pediatrics, anthropometric features such as height, weight and BMI are usually described by percentile curves, based on a reference population. Thus in adolescents, BMI percentile curves will vary by age and gender. This creates some difficulty using an absolute BMI threshold during a period of continued linear growth. However, given that the reference data for extremely high BMI percentiles (e.g., >97th) are not reliable, using a percentile cutpoint for consideration of surgery may well overestimate the number of adolescents who need consideration of surgery [45]. Thus, it is prudent for the present time to use hard BMI values rather than percentiles for consideration of surgical intervention. As more information becomes available about the outcomes of weight loss surgery in adolescents, as well as the natural history and distribution of severe obesity in adolescents, it is possible that an age-specific threshold (percentile or z-score) will become more appropriate than a BMI threshold.

Table 16.2 Criteria for adolescent bariatric surgery

• BMI ≥ 35 kg/m^2 and a severe comorbidity that has significant short-term effects on health, such as severe obstructive sleep apnea, diabetes mellitus type 2, pseudotumor cerebri or severe and progressive steatohepatitis
• BMI ≥ 40 with other weight related medical and psychosocial comorbidities
• Physical maturity, defined as completing 95% of predicted adult stature based on bone age or reaching Tanner stage IV. This criterion is based on *theoretical* concerns that rapid weight loss after bariatric surgery might inhibit statural growth if an adolescent has not reached near adult height
• History of sustained efforts to lose weight through changes in diet and physical activity. There is no evidence that prolonged preoperative weight management programs enhance selection of patients for weight loss surgery. However, consistent attendance in such a treatment program may be a valuable indicator of the patient's ability to understand and adhere to medical and nutritional recommendations postoperatively, and provide information about the willingness of the family to support treatment efforts

Pratt et al. [44] (Table 16.2) have suggested that BMI criteria for weight loss surgery in adolescents include a BMI ≥ 35 kg/m^2 with one or more severe obesity-related disorders (e.g., type 2 diabetes mellitus, obstructive sleep apnea, pseudotumor cerebri, or severe steatohepatitis), or a BMI of ≥ 40 with more minor comorbidities (hypertension, dyslipidemia, mild steatohepatitis, significant impairment in quality of life, or arthropathy). These criteria build upon other work in the field [28, 43] and are reasonable, placing appropriate emphasis on the principle that surgery should only be considered when a strong medical or psychological rationale for the intervention can be documented.

It should be recognized that some findings during the initial evaluation may represent contraindications for surgery (Table 16.3), and that these criteria are only to be used as a starting point to select patients who are most likely to safely benefit from weight loss surgery. Crucial in the process is that the multidisciplinary team with pediatric expertise considers whether the patient and family have the ability and motivation to make lifestyle changes including consistent adherence to prescribed medical regimens (including preoperative use of micronutrient supplements). This process often takes months of regular visits to the clinic. The team should carefully consider during this evaluation phase whether the candidate demonstrates the ability to understand what dietary and physical activity changes will be required for optimal postoperative outcomes. Also, the team should consider whether there is evidence of mature decision-making, with appropriate understanding of potential risks and benefits of surgery, and whether the adolescent has support but not coercion from family members.

Reproductive Health Concerns

Since most (e.g., 75–80%) of the candidates presenting for bariatric surgery are female, gynecologic issues, fertility, and risk-taking behaviors are also important preoperative considerations. One-fourth of the adolescent girls seeking bariatric surgery are sexually active [46]. We have documented a 13% pregnancy rate among adolescents who underwent bariatric surgery, more than double the regional base rate [47]. Since most recommend avoidance of pregnancy for 12–18 months postoperatively [39], it is important that adolescent females undergoing bariatric surgery have comprehensive contraceptive counseling and be offered effective contraceptive options prior to surgery. In much the same way that contraception is strongly advised when prescribing potentially teratogenic medications such as isotretinoin (Accutane), we have found that with proper explanation and counseling, the majority (92%) of girls are willing to undergo intrauterine device placement at the time of bariatric surgery [46]. Additional benefit from the locally acting progestin within this device is the near cessation of menstrual blood loss in girl who may be at risk of iron deficiency after gastric restrictive surgery or bypass. Finally, the highly prevalent reproductive health concerns (including sexually transmitted disease prevention) among obese adolescent girls and boys should be addressed prior to surgery by a qualified healthcare provider.

Table 16.3 Contraindications for surgical weight loss procedures in adolescents include

• Medically correctable cause of obesity
• An ongoing substance abuse problem (within the preceding year)
• A medical, psychiatric, psychosocial, or cognitive condition that prevents adherence to postoperative dietary and medication regimens or impairs decisional capacity
• Current or planned pregnancy within 18 months of the procedure
• Inability on the part of the patient or parent to comprehend the risks and benefits of the surgical procedure

Conclusions

The recommendations contained herein regarding assessment and patient selection are intended to be a starting point based on the best judgement of medical and surgical specialists. Some studies that will validate these recommendations are underway, including the NIH funded, multicenter prospective Teen-LABS study (Teen-LABS.org) [48] and associated ancillary studies. As the evidence base related to adolescent bariatric surgery grows, so will the refinement in patient assessment guidelines.

References

1. Freedman DS, Mei Z, Srinivasan SR, Berenson GS, Dietz WH. Cardiovascular risk factors and excess adiposity among overweight children and adolescents: the Bogalusa Heart Study. J Pediatr. 2007;150 (1):12–7 e12.
2. Thompson DR, Obarzanek E, Franko DL, Barton BA, Morrison J, Biro FM, et al. Childhood overweight and cardiovascular disease risk factors: the National Heart, Lung, and Blood Institute Growth and Health Study. J Pediatr. 2007;150(1):18–25.
3. Ogden CL, Carroll MD, Curtin LR, Lamb MM, Flegal KM. Prevalence of high body mass index in US children and adolescents, 2007–2008. JAMA. 2010;303(3):242–9.
4. Whitaker RC, Wright JA, Pepe MS, Seidel KD, Dietz WH. Predicting obesity in young adulthood from childhood and parental obesity. N Engl J Med. 1997;337(13):869–73.
5. Must A, Jacques PF, Dallal GE, Bajema CJ, Dietz WH. Long-term morbidity and mortality of overweight adolescents. A follow-up of the Harvard Growth Study of 1922–1935. N Engl J Med. 1992;327(19):1350–5.
6. Sinaiko AR, Donahue RP, Jacobs DR Jr, Prineas RJ. Relation of weight and rate of increase in weight during childhood and adolescence to body size, blood pressure, fasting insulin, and lipids in young adults. The Minneapolis Children's Blood Pressure Study. Circulation. 1999;99(11):1471–6.
7. Vanhala M, Vanhala P, Kumpusalo E, Halonen P, Takala J. Relation between obesity from childhood to adulthood and the metabolic syndrome: population based study. BMJ. 1998;317(7154):319.
8. Inge TH. Bariatric surgery for morbidly obese adolescents: is there a rationale for early intervention? Growth Horm IGF Res. 2006;16 Suppl A:S15–9.
9. Daniels SR, Arnett DK, Eckel RH, Gidding SS, Hayman LL, Kumanyika S, et al. Overweight in children and adolescents: pathophysiology, consequences, prevention, and treatment. Circulation. 2005;111(15):1999–2012.
10. Garcia VF, DeMaria EJ. Adolescent bariatric surgery: treatment delayed, treatment denied, a crisis invited. Obes Surg. 2006;16(1):1–4.
11. Skelton JA, Cook SR, Auinger P, Klein JD, Barlow SE. Prevalence and trends of severe obesity among US children and adolescents. Acad Pediatr. 2009;9(5):322–9.
12. Must A, Strauss RS. Risks and consequences of childhood and adolescent obesity. Int J Obes Relat Metab Disord. 1999;23(Suppl 2):S2–11.
13. Pinhas-Hamiel O, Dolan LM, Daniels SR, Standiford D, Khoury PR, Zeitler P. Increased incidence of non-insulin-dependent diabetes mellitus among adolescents. J Pediatr. 1996;128(5 Pt 1):608–15.
14. Becque MD, Katch VL, Rocchini AP, Marks CR, Moorehead C. Coronary risk incidence of obese adolescents: reduction by exercise plus diet intervention. Pediatrics. 1988;81(5):605–12.
15. Kohler MJ, Thormaehlen S, Kennedy JD, Pamula Y, van den Heuvel CJ, Lushington K, et al. Differences in the association between obesity and obstructive sleep apnea among children and adolescents. J Clin Sleep Med. 2009;5(6):506–11.
16. Urbina EM, Kimball TR, McCoy CE, Khoury PR, Daniels SR, Dolan LM. Youth with obesity and obesity-related type 2 diabetes mellitus demonstrate abnormalities in carotid structure and function. Circulation. 2009;119(22):2913–9.
17. Barlow SE, Dietz WH. Obesity evaluation and treatment: expert committee recommendations. The Maternal and Child Health Bureau, Health Resources and Services Administration and the Department of Health and Human Services. Pediatrics. 1998;102(3): E29.
18. Pfeifer SM, Kives S. Polycystic ovary syndrome in the adolescent. Obstet Gynecol Clin North Am. 2009;36(1):129–52.
19. Berenson GS, Srnivasan SR. Cardiovascular risk factors in youth with implications for aging: the Bogalusa Heart Study. Neurobiol Aging. 2005;26 (3):303–7.
20. Fontaine KR, Redden DT, Wang C, Westfall AO, Allison DB. Years of life lost due to obesity. JAMA. 2003;289(2):187–93.
21. Zeller MH, Modi AC. Predictors of health-related quality of life in obese youth. Obesity (Silver Spring). 2006;14(1):122–30.
22. Lawson ML, Kirk S, Mitchell T, Chen MK, Loux TJ, Daniels SR, et al. One-year outcomes of Roux-en-Y gastric bypass for morbidly obese adolescents: a multicenter study from the Pediatric Bariatric Study Group. J Pediatr Surg. 2006;41(1):137–43; discussion 137–43.
23. Kalarchian MA, Levine MD, Arslanian SA, Ewing LJ, Houck PR, Cheng Y, et al. Family-based treatment of severe pediatric obesity:

randomized, controlled trial. Pediatrics. 2009;124 (4):1060–8.
24. Levine MD, Ringham RM, Kalarchian MA, Wisniewski L, Marcus MD. Is family-based behavioral weight control appropriate for severe pediatric obesity? Int J Eat Disord. 2001;30(3):318–28.
25. Gogakos A, Tzotzas TC, Krassas GE. Recent concepts of pharmacotherapy and bariatric surgery for childhood obesity: an overview. Pediatr Endocrinol Rev. 2009;7(2):83–94.
26. Wald AB, Uli NK. Pharmacotherapy in pediatric obesity: current agents and future directions. Rev Endocr Metab Disord. 2009;10(3):205–14.
27. Wake M, Canterford L, Patton GC, Hesketh K, Hardy P, Williams J, et al. Comorbidities of overweight/obesity experienced in adolescence: longitudinal study. Arch Dis Child. 2009;95(3):162–8.
28. Inge TH, Zeller MH, Lawson ML, Daniels SR. A critical appraisal of evidence supporting a bariatric surgical approach to weight management for adolescents. J Pediatr. 2005;147(1):10–9.
29. Ratcliff MB, Reiter-Purtill J, Inge TH, Zeller MH. Changes in depressive symptoms among adolescent bariatric candidates from preoperative psychological evaluation to immediately before surgery. Surg Obes Relat Dis. 2011;7(1):50–4.
30. Inge TH, Garcia V, Daniels S, Langford L, Kirk S, Roehrig H, et al. A multidisciplinary approach to the adolescent bariatric surgical patient. J Pediatr Surg. 2004;39(3):442–7; discussion 446–7.
31. Tsai WS, Inge TH, Burd RS. Bariatric surgery in adolescents: recent national trends in use and in-hospital outcome. Arch Pediatr Adolesc Med. 2007;161(3):217–21.
32. Treadwell JR, Sun F, Bruening W, Reston J, Noble M, Schoelles K, et al. Bariatric surgery in pediatric patients. In: 2007. http://www.hta.hca.wa.gov/documents/bariatric_pediatric.pdf. Accessed 21 Feb 2011.
33. Treadwell JR, Sun F, Schoelles K. Systematic review and meta-analysis of bariatric surgery for pediatric obesity. Ann Surg. 2008;248(5):763–76.
34. Jen HC, Rickard DG, Shew SB, Maggard MA, Slusser WM, Dutson EP, et al. Trends and outcomes of adolescent bariatric surgery in California, 2005–2007. Pediatrics. 2010;126(4):e746–53.
35. O'Brien PE, Sawyer SM, Laurie C, Brown WA, Skinner S, Veit F, et al. Laparoscopic adjustable gastric banding in severely obese adolescents: a randomized trial. JAMA. 2010;303(6):519–36.
36. Aikenhead A, Knai C, Lobstein T. Effectiveness and cost-effectiveness of paediatric bariatric surgery: a systematic review. Clinical Obesity. 2011:1–14.
37. Inge TH, Jenkins TM, Zeller M, Dolan L, Daniels SR, Garcia VF, et al. Baseline BMI is a strong predictor of nadir BMI after adolescent gastric bypass. J Pediatr. 2010;156(1):103–8 e101.
38. Varela JE, Hinojosa MW, Nguyen NT. Perioperative outcomes of bariatric surgery in adolescents compared with adults at academic medical centers. Surg Obes Relat Dis. 2007;3(5):537–40; discussion 541–32.
39. Inge TH, Krebs NF, Garcia VF, Skelton JA, Guice KS, Strauss RS, et al. Bariatric surgery for severely overweight adolescents: concerns and recommendations. Pediatrics. 2004;114(1):217–23.
40. Mechanick JI, Kushner RF, Sugerman HJ, Gonzalez-Campoy JM, Collazo-Clavell ML, Guven S, et al. American Association of Clinical Endocrinologists, The Obesity Society, and American Society for Metabolic & Bariatric Surgery Medical Guidelines for Clinical Practice for the perioperative nutritional, metabolic, and nonsurgical support of the bariatric surgery patient. Surg Obes Relat Dis. 2008;4(5 Suppl):S109–84.
41. Apovian CM, Cummings S, Anderson W, Borud L, Boyer K, Day K, et al. Best practice updates for multidisciplinary care in weight loss surgery. Obesity (Silver Spring). 2009;17(5):871–9.
42. Inge TH, Lawson L. Treatment considerations for severe adolescent obesity. Surg Obes Relat Dis. 2005;1(2):133–9.
43. Apovian CM, Baker C, Ludwig DS, Hoppin AG, Hsu G, Lenders C, et al. Best practice guidelines in pediatric/adolescent weight loss surgery. Obes Res. 2005;13(2):274–82.
44. Pratt JS, Lenders CM, Dionne EA, Hoppin AG, Hsu GL, Inge TH, et al. Best practice updates for pediatric/adolescent weight loss surgery. Obesity (Silver Spring). 2009;17(5):901–10.
45. Lenders CM, Wright JA, Apovian CM, Hess DT, Shukla RR, Adams WG, et al. Weight loss surgery eligibility according to various BMI criteria among adolescents. Obesity (Silver Spring). 2009;17 (1):150–5.
46. Hillman JB, Miller RJ, Inge TH. Menstrual concerns and intrauterine contraception among adolescent bariatric surgery patients. J Womens Health (Larchmt). 2011;20(4):533–8.
47. Roehrig HR, Xanthakos SA, Sweeney J, Zeller MH, Inge TH. Pregnancy after gastric bypass surgery in adolescents. Obes Surg. 2007;17(7):873–7.
48. Inge TH, Zeller M, Harmon C, Helmrath M, Bean J, Modi A, et al. Teen-longitudinal assessment of bariatric surgery: methodological features of the first prospective multicenter study of adolescent bariatric surgery. J Pediatr Surg. 2007;42(11):1969–71.

Bariatric Surgery in Children

17

Mansoor Ali Khan and Roger Ackroyd

Obesity refers to a condition of excess body fat. Over the last 30 years, there has been a dramatic increase in the incidence of obesity in children [1] and although an exact figure is difficult to quantify, largely due to difficulty in measuring total body fat in children, it is estimated that 18% of children in the USA [2] and about 1 million children in England are obese. Childhood obesity is also rising in other countries and it has been suggested that up to 22 million children under the age of five are overweight worldwide. As such, the rising prevalence of obesity is posing a serious short- and long-term public health crisis.

Etiology of Obesity

In order to determine the correct treatment, it is necessary to understand the etiological factors involved in childhood obesity. Although the fundamental basis for weight gain is an imbalance between caloric intake and output [2], it is unfortunately a more complex condition that is usually multi-factorial in origin (Table 17.1). In turn, it leads to wide-ranging comorbidities with clinical, psychosocial, and economic ramifications.

Genetic Predisposition

In some children, genetic factors in isolation may predispose to development of obesity; such conditions include genes that regulate appetite and metabolism, which even when exposed to normal calorific intake will predispose to obesity. Rare genetic conditions should be considered in children presenting at a very young age with obesity, e.g., Prader–Willi syndrome. Studies undertaken have demonstrated that children who are born to two obese parents are at higher risk of childhood obesity compared to children born to one obese parent [3]. Others have found that higher maternal weight entering pregnancy increases risk for obesity and its cardio-metabolic complications among offspring [4].

Recent studies have also demonstrated that when clinicians classify children by BMI categories and counsel about the risk for future obesity, they should recognize that greater height may be a marker for increased risk of adult overweight and obesity [5].

Endocrinopathies

The two main endocrine abnormalities implicated in the development of childhood obesity

M.A. Khan
Department of Surgery and Trauma, Imperial College London, London, UK
e-mail: manskhan@doctors.org.uk; Mansoor.Khan@imperial.nhs.uk; mkhan3@ic.ac.uk; mansoorkhan@nhs.net

R. Ackroyd (✉)
Department of General Surgery, Northern General Hospital, Herries Rd, Sheffield, South Yorkshire S5 7AU, UK
e-mail: roger.ackroyd@sth.nhs.uk; Roger.Ackroyd@sth.nhs.uk

D.J. Ledbetter and P.R.V. Johnson (eds.), *Endocrine Surgery in Children*,
DOI 10.1007/978-3-662-54256-9_17

Table 17.1 Obesity etiology

Congenital	Genetic predisposition
	Prader–Willi syndrome
Endocrine disorders	Cushing's disease/syndrome
	Hypothyroidism
Environmental	Hyperphagia
	Sedentary lifestyle

are Cushing's disease and hypothyroidism, although the link between obesity and the latter is weaker in children than adults.

Environmental Factors

Studies in the USA have reported an association between living in socially deprived areas and an increased incidence of childhood obesity. These results provide a new insight into the relationship between broader social and economic context and child obesity risk [6].

Previous studies suggested that breast-feeding may be protective against the development of childhood obesity. However, a recent randomized trial demonstrated that breast feeding does not reduce measures of adiposity at 6.5 years of age, and previous suggestions of protective effects against obesity may reflect confounding factors and selection bias [7]. Some studies have also demonstrated that early prenatal and postnatal growth patterns are important markers of risk of obesity later in life, with rapid neonatal weight gain a clear risk factor for obesity and metabolic syndrome in later childhood and adult life [8].

Lack of physical activity has also been implicated in causing obesity and cardio-metabolic risk in childhood. Studies undertaken have quantified these associations using objective physical activity measurements in children from different ethnic groups and demonstrated that efforts to increase activity levels in such groups would have equally beneficial effects [9]. Studies have also not surprisingly shown that limiting access to 'fast foods' could have beneficial effects on reducing childhood obesity [10].

Maternal depression and permissive parenting style are also potentially important risk factors in childhood obesity. It has been suggested that future research should clearly determine the correlation between these [11].

Psychological Factors

The impact of a child's temperament and the maternal perception of a child's BMI depend on the child's age. For example, children with a difficult temperament and insensitive mothers have a significantly higher risk for being overweight or obese during the school age phase, but not during early childhood. This may hold significant implications for childhood obesity prevention/intervention programs in which parents can be appropriately targeted [12]. Conduct problems in childhood are associated with being overweight and obese in young adulthood. Future studies should address the potential for interventions to reduce obesity risk in young adulthood for boys who manifest conduct problems early in life [13].

Management

The complex nature and multifactorial etiology of childhood obesity make it a difficult condition to manage. Management necessitates the use of a multidisciplinary team approach, reinforced by the limited systematic reviews of childhood obesity interventions that provide some practice-relevant information [14].

For young children who have no other health concerns, the goal of treatment may be weight maintenance rather than weight loss. For an obese child, maintaining weight whilst waiting to grow taller may be as difficult as losing weight is for older people. However, for older children or for younger children who have related health concerns, weight loss strategies are recommended.

Education

As overeating and a sedentary lifestyle are the two commonest factors directly attributable to the development of obesity, advice on diet and physical activity form the basis of any treatment offered to the patient. Physical activity not only burns calories, but also helps nutritional development of the child with resulting enhancement of both physical and mental health. Indeed, it has been shown that increased physical activity in childhood helps children maintain desirable weight during teenage years, regardless of the hormonal and emotional changes that occur during this period of life. Limiting time spent watching television and reducing recreational computer usage has both been deemed beneficial in increasing activity levels. Children should be encouraged to partake in any form of physical activity and this does not necessarily mean organized sporting activities. Children's activity levels often represent the activity levels of the parents, and as such, parents of obese children should also be encouraged to increase their activity levels.

Diet

Dietary factors play a significant role in contributing to obesity [10], with one of the largest drivers recognized as the increased consumption of sugar sweetened beverages over the past decade [15]. Parents have overall responsibility for the purchase, preparation, and location of consumption of food, and therefore play a major contributor role in prevention. Factors that may aid in weight reduction include:

- adequate fruit and vegetable intake
- limiting sweets and soft drinks
- limiting intake of 'fast food'

Delayed introduction of solids is associated with reduced odds of child overweight/obesity. Wider promotion of current infant feeding guidelines could have a significant impact on the rates of child overweight and obesity [16].

Psychological Input

Child and adolescent psychiatrists frequently encounter children who are obese and may be asked to work alongside primary care physicians and other specialists who treat youngsters with obesity. A multidisciplinary approach will allow optimal therapeutic recommendations for this population of patients and their families [17].

Medication

The two commonest prescriptions of weight loss drugs available for adolescents used to be sibutramine and orlistat. However, in January 2010, the Medicines and Healthcare products Regulatory Agency announced the suspension of the marketing authorisation for the obesity drug sibutramine (Reductil). This followed a review by the European Medicines Agency that concluded that the cardiovascular risks of sibutramine outweigh its benefits. Emerging evidence confirms an increased risk of nonfatal heart attacks and strokes with this medicine. Orlistat, which is approved for adolescents older than 12, prevents the absorption of fat in the intestines. Unfortunately, this can have the rather unpleasant side effect of problematic diarrhea and nutritional problems associated with fat malabsorption.

Surgery

Severe or morbid obesity, with a BMI exceeding 35–40, is often refractory to all therapies other than surgery. Bariatric or weight loss surgery is not generally recommended in childhood as it is fraught with ethical issues and the potential long-term benefits and complications of enteric diversion are not yet fully understood. On the other hand, it has been suggested that bariatric surgery in adolescents may have less complications and a shorter hospital stay than in adults [18]. The National Institute for Clinical Excellence (NICE) has outlined the exceptional circumstances that bariatric surgery is permitted in the UK:

1. The child/adolescent has achieved or nearly achieved physiological maturity
2. BMI ≥ 40 kg/m^2 or 35–40 kg/m^2 with other significant disease (e.g., type 2 diabetes, high blood pressure) that could be improved by weight loss
3. All appropriate nonsurgical measures have failed to achieve or maintain adequate clinically beneficial weight loss for at least 6 months
4. The child/adolescent is receiving or will receive intensive specialist management
5. The child/adolescent is fit for anesthesia and surgery
6. There is a commitment to the need for long-term follow-up.

Preoperative Assessment

The early manifestations of the comorbidities associated with obesity in adults are already present in severely obese children and should be addressed for their safe anesthetic management. Perioperative respiratory events are more frequent in overweight and obese patients [19] and therefore respiratory function should be optimized before surgery. Cardio-respiratory fitness should be optimized prior to bariatric surgery to potentially reduce postoperative complications [20]. Despite the excessive reserves of fat, obese patients are frequently nutritionally deficient related to poor dietary intake and this also poses major risks to postoperative recovery, especially in terms of wound healing.

Surgical Options

In broad terms, the options for operative management of obesity can be divided into restrictive procedures and malabsorptive procedures. These can be performed either as open or laparoscopic procedures [21], with the majority of weight loss procedures worldwide being conducted by latter approach.

The surgical intervention required depends on the eating habits of the patient. Patients who eat large volumes infrequently require restrictive procedures (gastric band/sleeve gastrectomy), whereas those who consume small amounts frequently require malabsorptive procedures (gastric bypass/duodenal switch).

Laparoscopic Gastric Band

A laparoscopic adjustable gastric band is an inflatable device that is placed around the proximal stomach to create a stoma which restricts the passage of food (Fig. 17.1). The proximal pouch rapidly fills creating a feeling of satiety and reducing the sensation of phagia.

Gastric bands are particularly useful for volume eaters, i.e., large meals or bulky foods. The restriction of the gastric band can be adjusted by a small access port placed under the skin. Saline is introduced or removed via this port to tighten or loosen the band and alter the volume of food allowed to pass. As the patient loses weight, there is a loss of perigastric fat, requiring adjustment of the band.

Unlike more open forms of weight loss surgery, gastric banding does not require cutting or removal of any part of the stomach and it is also reversible. Removal can be achieved as a laparoscopic procedure, after which the stomach usually returns to its normal pre-banded state. The postoperative stay for patients undergoing a laparoscopic band is usually 24 h, which is considerably less compared to other operative interventions.

The weight loss tends to be slower for patients who undergo a band insertion compared to malabsorptive procedures and once the band is removed, it is unfortunately not unusual for a person to gain weight again. On the other hand, unlike malabsorptive procedures, it is unusual for gastric band patients to experience any nutritional or micronutrient disturbances.

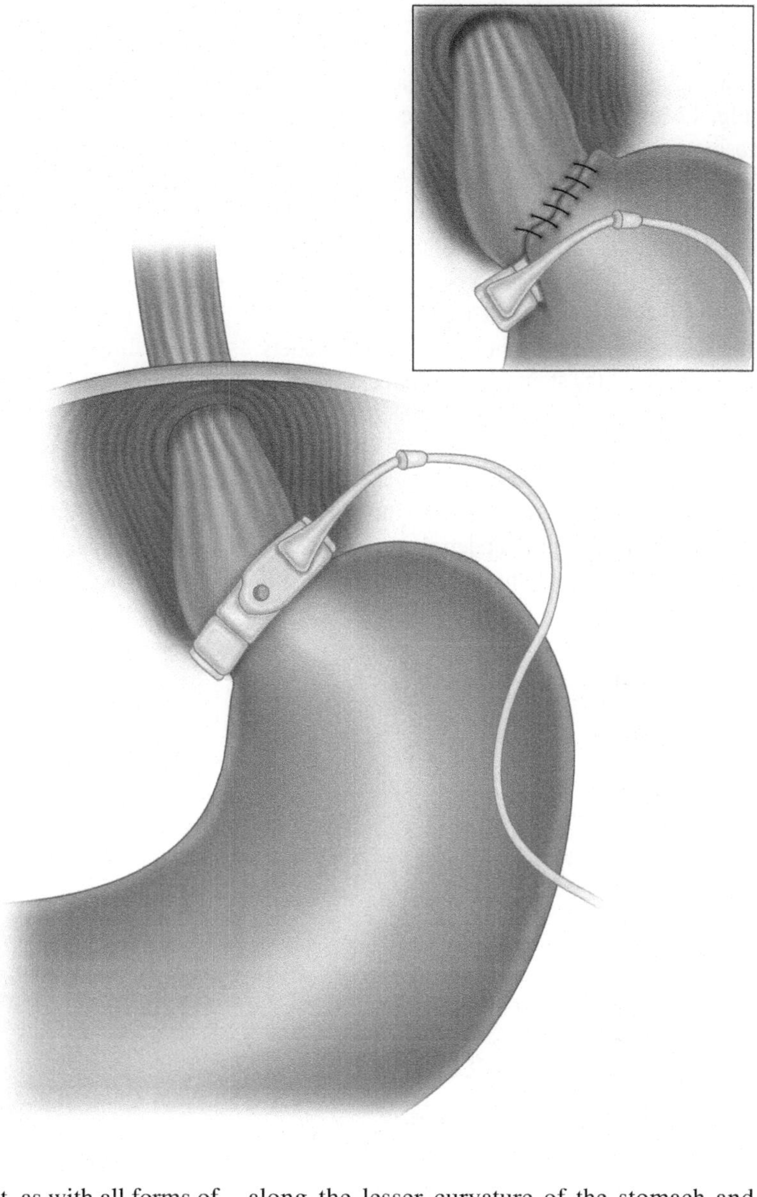

Fig. 17.1 Gastric band

It is important to note that, as with all forms of bariatric surgery, patients must carefully follow postoperative guidelines relating to diet, exercise, and band maintenance in order to maintain their weight reduction.

Laparoscopic Sleeve Gastrectomy

Sleeve gastrectomy is a procedure that involves reduction of the stomach capacity by over 80% (Fig. 17.2). A bougie is passed along the lesser curvature of the stomach and the stomach is then stapled along the line of the bougie to create a gastric conduit, with the remainder of the stomach being removed. Like gastric banding, this is a restrictive procedure, however, unlike a gastric banding it is not reversible. Studies have demonstrated that at 1-year follow-up, laparoscopic sleeve gastrectomy is a safe and effective option for bariatric surgery in children, achieving moderate weight loss and improvement of comorbidities [22, 23].

Laparoscopic Gastric Bypass

The laparoscopic roux-en-Y gastric bypass, (Fig. 17.3), is a combined restrictive and malabsorptive procedure. It was first performed in 1993 and is now the 'gold standard' operation. The procedure involves the creation of a proximal gastric pouch with a volume of approximately 30 ml. This creates a similar phenomenon to the previously mentioned gastric band pouch and sleeve gastrectomy in creating early satiety. The volume of the stomach remaining is less than in a sleeve gastrectomy with over 90% loss of volume. However, unlike the gastric band, where the pouch can be reversed, in gastric bypass surgery, the pouch is divided from the main body of the stomach. This is undertaken to prevent a fistula forming if the stomach was just 'partitioned'.

The small bowel is then divided approximately 0.5–1 m from the duodenal–jejunal flexure and a roux-en Y anastomosis is formed between 0.5 and 1 m further down the small bowel producing a degree of malabsorption.

The patient should have strict dietary guidelines, which include consumption of three small meals per day and avoidance of snacking, especially foods with high calorific content. Patients who undergo malabsorptive procedures require lifelong and extensive blood tests to check for deficiencies in life critical vitamins and minerals.

Gastric bypass is a safe and effective method of controlling body weight in morbidly obese children and adolescents [24]. A study of 25 patients undergoing childhood gastric bypass demonstrated that growth in height was not interrupted and no metabolic problems were encountered postoperatively.

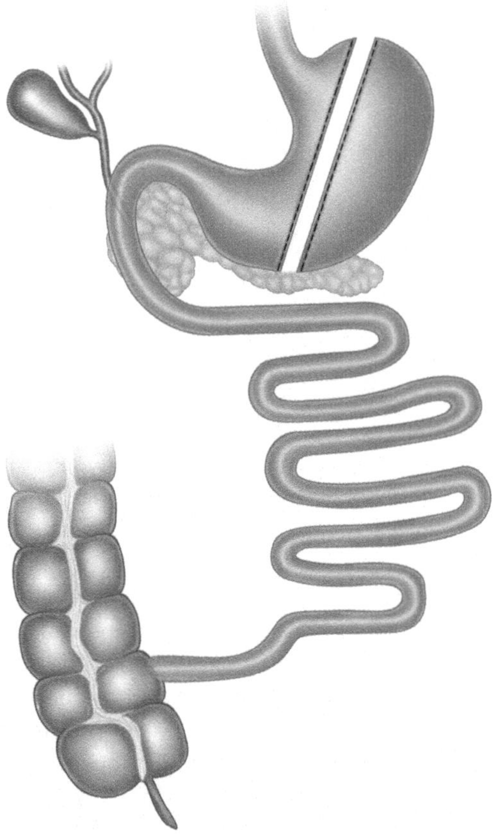

Fig. 17.2 Sleeve gastrectomy

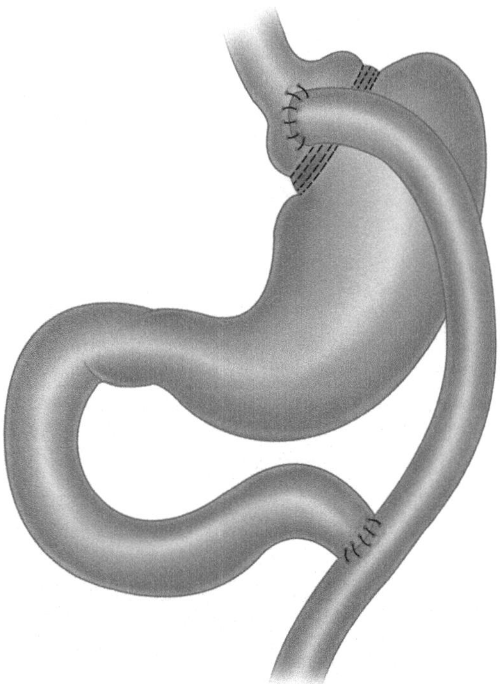

Fig. 17.3 Gastric bypass

Duodenal Switch

The duodenal switch procedure is also known as biliopancreatic diversion with duodenal switch. Like gastric bypass surgery it is a restrictive and malabsorptive procedure. Similar to the sleeve gastrectomy, a gastric conduit is fashioned along the lesser curve. The duodenum is then divided just beyond the pylorus. A roux-en-Y limb is then reconstituted to create common channel which is approximately 1 m from the ileocecal valve (Fig. 17.4).

The procedure is technically more demanding than a gastric bypass with associated higher complication rates. However, it has been shown to lead to superior weight loss in the super obese and it renders over 95% of patients with type II diabetes euglycemic.

Another advantage of the duodenal switch is that the pylorus between the stomach and small intestine is preserved, thereby preventing dumping syndrome, which is common after a gastric bypass.

Postoperative Complications

These can be divided into operative or nutritional complications (Table 17.2).

Operative Complications

The complications vary with the specific type of surgery, but include bleeding, infection, deep venous thromboembolism/pulmonary embolism, and gastrointestinal problems, such as dumping, vitamin/mineral deficiencies, vomiting (and nausea), staple line failure, stenosis (and bowel obstruction), ulceration, splenic injury, and

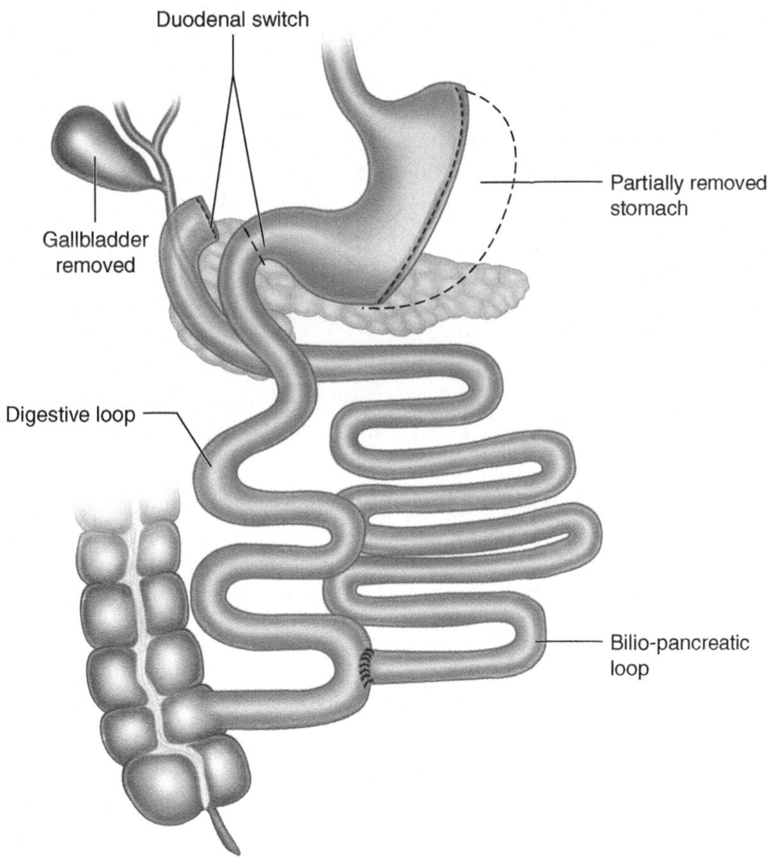

Fig. 17.4 Duodenal switch

Table 17.2 Complications of malabsorptive bariatric surgery

Complications of abdominal surgery	Complications of bypass procedure
Infection	Anastomotic leakage
Hemorrhage	Anastomotic stricture
Port site hernia	Anastomotic ulcer
Bowel obstruction	Dumping syndrome
Venous thromboembolism	Gallstones

perioperative death [25]. Specific complications of gastric banding include:

- Slipped band—manifesting with signs of obstruction or ischemia
- Band erosion into the gastric lumen—manifesting with pain or weight gain
- Port leakage—widening of the stoma and subsequent weight gain
- Port displacement
- Port site infection

Complications (and in turn mortality rates) are influenced by many factors, which can be either patient or surgeon related. Patient factors are largely dictated by preexisting risk factors such as heart disease, obstructive sleep apnea, diabetes mellitus, and other comorbidities. Surgeon-related complications are greater early in the surgeon's learning curve, and have been shown to be reduced in more experienced hands.

Nutritional Deficiencies

Calcium is normally absorbed in the duodenum. However, following bypass surgery the duodenum is out of continuity and routine supplementation with calcium citrate is therefore, recommended.

Similarly, the duodenum is the site for absorption of iron, however, unlike supplementation with calcium, ferrous supplementation has unpleasant side effects. It can cause considerable gastro-intestinal distress in normal doses, and some patients may not be able to tolerate this. In these cases where severe anemia may not be correctable, it may be necessary to administer parenteral iron.

Vitamin B_{12} requires intrinsic factor from the gastric mucosa to be absorbed. In patients with a small gastric pouch, there may be in sufficient amounts of intrinsic factor to permit absorption, even if oral supplementation is undertaken. In these patients vitamin B_{12} injections may be needed.

Protein malnutrition is a real risk with many patients requiring protein supplementation, especially during the early phases of rapid weight loss, to help prevent excessive loss of muscle mass.

Fat soluble vitamins (A, D, E, and K) deficiencies generally occur as a result of fat malabsorption and supplementation is often required.

Outcomes

The mortality rate among patients undergoing bariatric operations is generally quoted as between 0.05 and 2.0%. However, studies demonstrate that the mortality rate during hospitalization or within 30 days of surgery, underestimate the actual incidence. Bariatric surgery carries both short- and long-term risks [26].

Various publications have highlighted how mortality rates may be reduced. Surgeon-related factors have led to the establishment of standardized procedures. Full standardization of the gastric bypass procedure has demonstrated very low mortality and the low morbidity rates in certain institutions [27]. Long-term total mortality after gastric bypass surgery is significantly reduced, particularly deaths from diabetes, heart disease, and cancer [28].

Conclusions

Bariatric surgery has become an increasingly important method for managing medically complicated obesity. In patients who have undergone bariatric surgery, up to 87% of patients with type 2 diabetes mellitus develop improvement or resolution of their disease postoperatively. Patients who have undergone bariatric surgery require indefinite, regular follow-up care by physicians who need to follow laboratory parameters of macro and micronutrient malnutrition [29]. It has also demonstrated normalization of hyperlipidemia, hypertension, obstructive sleep apnea, and the risk of developing cancers is decreased [30].

As we now progress in the field of bariatric surgery, fewer complications, shorter hospital stays, and more evidence of successful weight loss consistently appears in the statistics that are published [31]. The long-term implications of bariatric surgery in children are not yet fully understood, and diligent long-term follow-up of all these patients is required to help determine this.

References

1. Joan CH, Debbie AL, Sue YSK. Childhood obesity. Lancet. 2010;375(9727):1737–48.
2. Browne AF, Inge T. How young for bariatric surgery in children? Semin Pediatr Surg. 2009;18(3):176–85.
3. Kopelman PG, Stock MJ. Clinical obesity in adults and children. 2nd ed. Malden: Blackwell Publication; 2005. p. 493.
4. Oken E. Maternal and child obesity: the causal link. Obstet Gynecol Clin North Am. 2009;36(2):361–77, ix–x.
5. Stovitz SD, et al. Child height and the risk of young-adult obesity. Am J Prev Med. 2010;38(1):74–7.
6. Greves Grow HM, et al. Child obesity associated with social disadvantage of children's neighborhoods. Soc Sci Med. 2010;71(3):584–91.
7. Kramer MS, et al. A randomized breast-feeding promotion intervention did not reduce child obesity in Belarus. J Nutr. 2009;139(2):417S–21S.
8. Cole TJ. Early causes of child obesity and implications for prevention. Acta Paediatr Suppl. 2007;96 (454):2–4.
9. Owen CG, et al. Physical activity, obesity and cardiometabolic risk factors in 9- to 10-year-old UK children of white European, South Asian and black African-Caribbean origin: the Child Heart and health Study in England (CHASE). Diabetologia. 2010;53(8):1620–30.
10. Mellor JM, Dolan CB, Rapoport RB. Child body mass index, obesity, and proximity to fast food restaurants. Int J Pediatr Obes. 2011;6(1):60–8.
11. Topham GL, et al. Maternal depression and socio-economic status moderate the parenting style/child obesity association. Public Health Nutr. 2010;13(8):1237–44.
12. Wu T, et al. Joint effects of child temperament and maternal sensitivity on the development of childhood obesity. Matern Child Health J. 2011;15 (4):469–77.
13. Duarte CS, et al. Child mental health problems and obesity in early adulthood. J Pediatr. 2010;156 (1):93–7.
14. Wolfenden L, et al. How useful are systematic reviews of child obesity interventions? Obes Rev. 2010;11(2):159–65.
15. Fletcher JM, Frisvold D, Tefft N. Taxing soft drinks and restricting access to vending machines to curb child obesity. Health Aff (Millwood). 2010;29 (5):1059–66.
16. Seach KA, et al. Delayed introduction of solid feeding reduces child overweight and obesity at 10 years. Int J Obes (Lond). 2010;32(10):1475–9.
17. Maloney AE. Pediatric obesity: a review for the child psychiatrist. Child Adolesc Psychiatr Clin N Am. 2010;19(2):353–70, x.18.
18. Boehm R, et al. Bariatric surgery in children and adolescents. Zentralbl Chir. 2009;134(6):532–6.
19. Veyckemans F. Child obesity and anaesthetic morbidity. Curr Opin Anaesthesiol. 2008;21(3):308–12.
20. McCullough PA, et al. Cardiorespiratory fitness and short-term complications after bariatric surgery. Chest. 2006;130(2):517–25.
21. Smith SC, et al. Open vs laparoscopic Roux-en-Y gastric bypass: comparison of operative morbidity and mortality. Obes Surg. 2004;14(1):73–6.
22. Till H, et al. Efficacy of laparoscopic sleeve gastrectomy (LSG) as a stand-alone technique for children with morbid obesity. Obes Surg. 2008;18(8):1047–9.
23. Scheimann A, et al. "Efficacy of laparoscopic sleeve gastrectomy as a stand-alone technique for children with morbid obesity" and "BioEnterics intragastric balloon for treatment of morbid obesity in Prader-Willi syndrome: specific risks and benefits". Obes Surg. 2009;19(5):671–2; author reply 673.
24. Soper RT, et al. Gastric bypass for morbid obesity in children and adolescents. J Pediatr Surg. 1975;10 (1):51–8.
25. Abell TL, Minocha A. Gastrointestinal complications of bariatric surgery: diagnosis and therapy. Am J Med Sci. 2006;331(4):214–8.

26. Goldfeder LB, Ren CJ, Gill JR. Fatal complications of bariatric surgery. Obes Surg. 2006;16(8):1050–6.
27. Dillemans B, et al. Standardization of the fully stapled laparoscopic Roux-en-Y gastric bypass for obesity reduces early immediate postoperative morbidity and mortality: a single center study on 2606 patients. Obes Surg. 2009;19(10):1355–64.
28. Adams TD, et al. Long-term mortality after gastric bypass surgery. N Engl J Med. 2007;357(8):753–61.
29. Koch TR, Finelli FC. Postoperative metabolic and nutritional complications of bariatric surgery. Gastroenterol Clin North Am. 2010;39(1):109–24.
30. Adams TD, et al. Cancer incidence and mortality after gastric bypass surgery. Obesity (Silver Spring). 2009;17(4):796–802.
31. Smiertka JK, Macpherson BH. Beyond bariatric surgery. Complications we fail to address. Obes Surg. 1996;6(4):377–81.

Further Reading

1. Agency for Healthcare Research and Quality and National Guideline Clearinghouse (NGC) Guideline Synthesis. Overweight and obesity in children and adolescents: assessment, prevention, and management, 2005, [online]. Available at: www.guidance.gov
2. National Health and Medical Research Council. Clinical practice guidelines for the management of overweight and obesity in children and adolescents, 2003, [online]. Available at: http://www.health.gov.au/internet/wcms/publishing.nsf/Content/obesityguidelines-guidelines-children.htm
3. National Institute for Clinical Excellence (NICE). CG43 Obesity: full guideline. 2006 [online] Available at: http://guidance.nice.org.uk/CG43

Part VI

Ovary, Testicles, and Fertility

18 Pathogenesis and Treatment of Disorders of Sexual Development

Rafael V. Pieretti and Patricia K. Donahoe

This chapter reviews the pathogenesis and treatment of Disorders of Sex Development (DSD). "Disorders of Sex Development" is a more comprehensive term than the older terms "Ambiguous Genitalia" or "Intersex" and covers a broad clinical spectrum of hormonal, metabolic, and chromosomal abnormalities resulting in abnormal genital development [1, 2]. Patients with DSD are best evaluated and treated by a multidisciplinary team of medical and surgical specialists. In this era of shared decision-making, the diagnosis and treatment plan must be thoroughly discussed with parents, with the goal of giving the child the most satisfactory quality of life possible. It is essential that surgeons taking care of these complex patients feel comfortable with all the available techniques, so they can achieve satisfactory anatomical and functional repairs that support either the male of female gender.

Developmental and Molecular Events Contributing to Normal Mammalian Sexual Differentiation

Normal sexual differentiation requires the appropriate chromosomal endowment (i.e., 46, XX for females and 46, XY for males) and a precise, sequential cascade of genetic, molecular, and morphologic events. Germ cells must accurately migrate to the hindgut and subsequently take up residence in the retroperitoneum, then condense in the urogenital ridge where they are required to induce the morphologic formation of either a testis or an ovary [3]. The gonad in turn produces steroid hormones and proteins. Receptors in local and more distant sites respond to the secreted hormones and proteins to activate signaling pathways and somatic gene responses, which lead to morphologic and biochemical changes resulting in the appropriate male or female phenotype [4].

A key site for early sexual development is the urogenital ridge, which is the origin of the undifferentiated gonad, the mesonephros, and the Wolffian and Müllerian ducts (Fig. 18.1) [1, 5]. The urogenital ridge arises from a thickening of the ventromedial aspect of the intermediate mesoderm between the early ectoderm and endoderm. A number of genes including the Wilms tumor (WT1) and steroidogenesis factor (SF-1) genes must be normally expressed in the urogenital ridge for the gonad and adjacent structures to form. For example, in mice, mutations in WT1 result in absence of the gonad and kidney [6] and in humans, mutations of WT1 are associated with

R.V. Pieretti (✉)
Department of Pediatric Surgery, MassGeneral Hospital for Children, 55 Fruit Street, Boston, MA 02114, USA
e-mail: rpieretti@gmail.com

P.K. Donahoe
Pediatric Surgical Research Laboratories, Massachusetts General Hospital, Boston, MA 02414, USA
e-mail: pkdonahoe@partners.org

D.J. Ledbetter and P.R.V. Johnson (eds.), *Endocrine Surgery in Children*,
DOI 10.1007/978-3-662-54256-9_18

abnormalities of the urogenital system seen in Denys–Drash syndrome, Frasier syndrome, and Wilms tumor associated with aniridia, GU malformations, and mental retardation (WAGR) syndrome [7]. Mutations in SF-1 in mice result in absence of gonads and adrenal glands [8] and produce similar phenotypes in humans [9].

Male and female primordial reproductive ducts coexist for a short period in all mammalian embryos. Müllerian ducts are the anlagen of the uterus, Fallopian tubes, and upper third of the vagina, and develop autonomously in the female in the absence of the testis. Wolffian ducts are the anlagen of the epididymis, vas deferens, and seminal vesicles, and require testosterone to develop. In the mouse, the Wolffian duct requires the action of PAX2 and PAX8, paired genes first discovered in *Drosophila.* Müllerian duct formation requires the activity of a series of secreted factors whose expression is directed by the WNT family of proteins [10, 11]. The Müllerian duct first forms by invagination of the coelomic epithelium which tubularizes under the influence of Wnt4, then elongates, as the epithelial cells migrate in close approximation to the Wolffian duct [12]. The Wolffian duct provides no cells, but its presence is essential for full elongation of the Müllerian duct to the distal urogenital sinus [13].

Primordial germ cells, the progenitors of the oocytes and spermatocytes, migrate to the urogenital ridge from outside the embryo [14]. They travel from the embryonic ectoderm, along the primitive streak, to the base of the allantois, the wall of the hindgut, and finally exit into the urogenital ridge, where they take up residence in the as yet undifferentiated gonad. Ectopic germ cells outside the urogenital ridge either fail to develop or form tumors [15, 16]. The migratory germ cell phenotype is controlled by integrins [17] and cKit signaling [18] and it is characterized by extensive mitosis [19]. The germ cells proliferate under the influence of Blimp-1 [20],

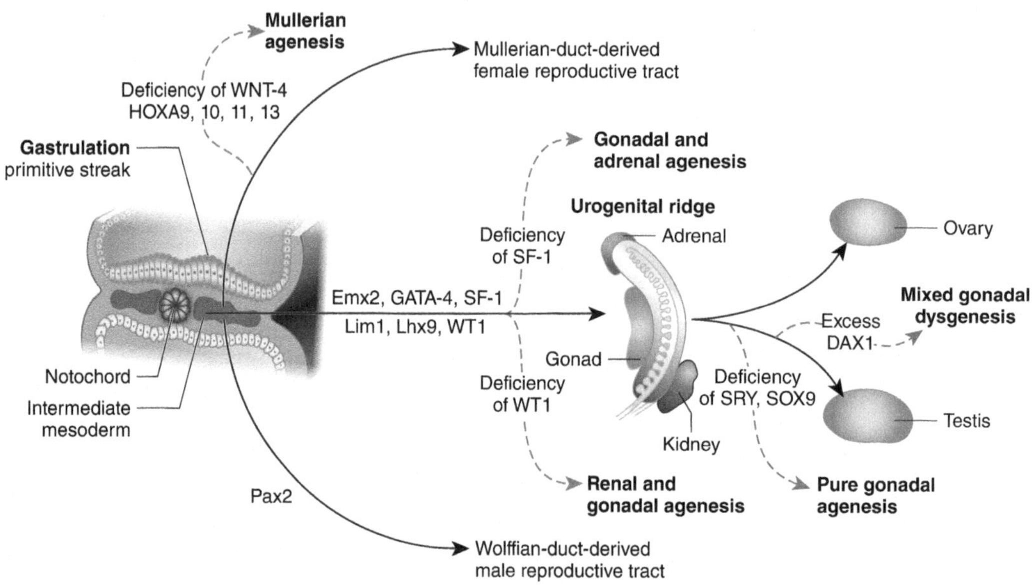

Fig. 18.1 Mutations in a number of genes can lead to a variety of syndromes of dysgenesis involving the Müllerian or Wolffian ducts, gonads, kidneys, and adrenal glands as a result of a deficiency or excess of the proteins shown. DAX1 denotes the gene duplicated in congenital adrenal hypoplasia on the X chromosome; Emx2, the empty spiracles homeobox gene; GATA-4, the gene encoding a protein that binds to a GATA DNA sequence; HOXA, homeobox protein; Liml, a homeobox gene important for limb development; Lhx9, a lim homeobox family member; Pax2, a paired box homeotic gene; SF-1, the gene for steroidogenic factor 1; SRY, the sex-determining region of the Y chromosome; SOX9, SRY homeobox 9; WNT-4, a protein that induces development of the Müllerian mesenchyma; and WT1, Wilms' tumor suppressor gene 1

BMP 2,4, and 8b, and Fragilis. Fragilis induces *Stella* that in turn induces the pluripotency genes *Oct/4*, *Sox2*, and *Nanog*. Germ cell expansion can be detected by expression of alkaline phosphatase and *Stella* [21, 22] as early as 3 weeks gestation in the human [23]. In addition to proliferation, the germ cells undergo imprint erasure imposed by DNA methylation and complex histone modification to reset epigenetic memory [24–26]. After entering the mesonephros, female germ cells enter meiosis in a characteristic anterior to posterior wave that is under the influence of retinoic acid mediated by the recently discovered gene, stimulated by Retinoic Acid 8 (*Stra8*). Since the testes degrade retinoic acid, *Stra8* is not expressed, meiosis is not initiated, and male germ cells remain arrested in the G0 phase of the cell cycle [27, 28].

The early, undifferentiated gonads exist as a primitive blastema of mesenchymal cells covered by coelomic epithelium. Testicular morphogenesis is initiated by a short burst of expression of the small transcription factors SRY, a master switch gene present on the short arm of the Y chromosome, and the SRY-related autosomal gene SOX 9 from chromosome 17q. The fact that full gonadal differentiation beyond the streak gonad stage requires the Y chromosome or the second X chromosome became evident in 1959 when the 45, X Turner phenotype was first recognized [29]. Subsequent cytogenetic studies localized the male differentiation region to the short arm of the Y chromosome [30, 31]. Later, a single-copy gene, the sex-determining region of the Y chromosome (SRY), was identified that encodes a DNA-binding protein, which is expressed in the gonadal ridge immediately before testis differentiation [32, 33]. When the SRY gene was transfected into XX female mouse embryos, a substantial proportion of these transgenic animals developed testes and assumed anatomic and functional male phenotypes [32, 34].

In addition to the Y chromosome, autosomal and X chromosome factors contribute to sex differentiation. For example, mutations on the long arm of chromosome 17q, found in cases of campomelic dysplasia associated with sex reversal [35–37], caused a defect in the SRY-related gene product, SOX 9, which contributes to sex differentiation. In addition, analysis of 46, XY sex-reversed females with intact SRY led to the discovery of the dosage-sensitive sex (DSS) reversal locus on the short arm of the X chromosome, duplication of which is required for female differentiation [38]. This region, which contains the gene *DAX1*, was then assumed to have a negative influence on testis differentiation because a double dose of the X chromosome is associated with dysgenesis of the testis. However, knockout of *DAX1* resulted in normal female gonadal development [39] which undermines the hypothesis that *DAX1* is responsible for ovarian differentiation. The only abnormality seen as a result of null mutation in *DAX1* occurs, counter intuitively, in the male, which displays abnormalities in spermatogenesis and spermatic cord formation [40]. Defects in the distal end of the short arm of chromosome 9p [41] and the distal end of the long arm of chromosome 10q [42] are also associated with sex reversal.

The genes responsible for ovarian development remain relatively obscure. Previously, the conventional wisdom was that the ovaries developed passively as a result of the absence of testicular determining genes. It is now clear that *Wnt-4* is associated with ovarian development, as homozygous inactivation of *Wnt-4* in females leads to masculinized gonads and an absence of the Müllerian ducts [11]. *Foxl2*, a forkhead transcription factor, is another gene that represses male development, allowing an XY gonad to develop as an ovary [43, 44]. Prenatal ovarian development also appears to be independent of steroid hormone action [45]. Taken together, it is now clear that ovarian differentiation is not simply a default pathway in the absence of testis differentiation [46].

The fetal testis develops seminiferous tubules with Sertoli cells surrounding germ cells and interstitial Leydig cells. The fetal testis produces two products required for further male differentiation, Müllerian Inhibiting Substance (MIS), which inhibits differentiation of the Müllerian duct [47], and testosterone, which stimulates Wolffian structures [47]. The external genital primordia develop autonomously into clitoris, labia minora, and labia majora. Complete differentiation of the external genitalia to phallus and scrotum requires reduction of testosterone to dihydrotestosterone by 5α-reductase [48]. The interaction of dyhydrotestoterone and androgen receptors causes lengthening of the phallus into a penis, fusing of the urogenital folds to form the penile urethra, and fusion of the labioscrotal swellings in the midline to form the scrotum. Autonomous female development can occur in the absence of ovaries.

The existence of a Müllerian inhibitor was proposed by Jost [47], who showed that testicular implants in female rabbit embryos stimulated the Wolffian duct but also caused regression of Müllerian ducts that could not be recapitulated by implants of testosterone alone. This regression is characterized morphologically by programmed cell death. Müllerian Inhibiting Substance (MIS) was purified [49, 50], and then used to clone the MIS gene [51, 52]. The bioactive C-terminal domain of MIS is homologous to a group of evolutionary conserved proteins, referred to as the transforming growth factor-ß (TGF-ß) family [52]. The MIS ligand binds to a heterologous receptor composed of at least two serine–threonine kinase transmembrane units, the type II receptor [53], which phosphorylates or activates the type I receptor [54], which in turn signals downstream via SMAD1/5/8 to initiate a series of molecular events that results in regression of the Müllerian ducts. MIS has been developed as an antiproliferative agent targeting tumors of Müllerian duct origin such as ovarian [23, 55], endometrial [56], cervical [57], cancers, as well as breast [58–60], and prostate [58] cancers. Abnormalities of the MIS gene itself or its receptors can result in the retained Müllerian duct syndrome, in which otherwise normal males, usually with undescended testes, have persistent Müllerian structures that have not undergone normal regression [61, 62].

Pathophysiology of Disorders of Sexual Differentiation (DSD)

There are three major categories of developmental aberrations that are responsible for the most common forms of Disorders of Sex Development (DSD) in newborns (Table 18.1). In the first category of DSD, the external genitalia of genetic females are masculinized by an excessive androgenic steroid production. In the second category of DSD, genetic males have deficient androgen production or action. The third category of DSD is notable for gonadal differentiation that is absent, incomplete, or asymmetrical [4]. It is important for physicians involved in the care of patients with DSD to understand the underlying pathophysiology so that they can make a timely and accurate diagnosis and be able to advise optimal treatment strategies.

46, XX DSD, Overandrogenization of the Genetic Female

In 46, XX DSD excessive androgens lead to virilization (or masculinization) of genetic females. Patients with 46, XX DSD were previously described as female pseudohermaphrodites or labeled with the diagnosis of congenital adrenal hyperplasia (CAH) or adrenogenital syndrome [63, 64]. The most common cause of excessive androgens is a defect in one of the P450 enzymes that in the adrenal gland convert progesterones to glucocorticoids and mineralocorticoids (Fig. 18.2). These enzyme abnormalities may occur in males and females but they cause ambiguous genitalia only in females.

In the human fetus adrenal differentiation occurs at 11 weeks gestation, after differentiation of the gonads and reproductive tract. Therefore, these enzyme defects lead to an excess androgen accumulation after 11 weeks gestation and affects the external genitalia that develop after that time —the genital tubercle and the urogenital folds. The genital tubercle normally forms the clitoris, but when exposed to excess androgens, develops as a penile structure. The urogenital folds, rather than developing as labia, acquire a bifid unfused or only partially fused scrotal appearance.

Mutations in the P450c21, or 21-hydroxylase gene, now known as CYP21 (Table 18.2), cause 90% of cases of CAH. The remainder of CAH cases are distributed among deficiencies of P450c11, 3ß-hydroxysteroid dehydrogenase,

Table 18.1 Disorders of sex development diagnosis and treatment

Disease	Diagnostic features	Physical examination phenotype	Gender assignment	Medical therapy	Surgical therapy
46, XX DSD (overandrogenized female) Congenital adrenal hyperplasia (adrenogenital syndrome)	Karyotype 46, XX electrolytes: K high, Na low Androgen high 17-hydroxyprogesterone high MIS 0 Sequence CYP21 Chromosomal FISH	Symmetrical gonads Clitoral hypertrophy Sinogram: UG sinus defect Enlarged labioscrotum	F	Hydrocortisone or cortisone acetate + Florinef Embryo selection from the blastocyst Steroid replacement in utero from 6 wk gestation	Perioperative stress steroids Clitoral reduction Vaginal exteriorization Labioscrotal reduction
46, XY DSD (Underandrogenized male) Testosterone deficiency	Karyotype 46, XY Testosterone low Sequence enzyme genes: 17-KS OH, P450scc, 3β-HSD, CYP17 FISH	Symmetrical, undescended, small testis Severe hypospadias No müllerian structures	If M	Presurgical testosterone stimulation Testosterone at adolescence	Hypospadias repair Prepenile scrotal repair Orchiopexy
		Predominant female phenotype if adolescence	If F	Estrogen/progesterone at	Gonadectomy
Androgen receptor deficiency Testicular feminization (complete androgen insensitivity)	Karyotype 46, XY Testosterone high MIS high Sequence androgen receptor gene FISH	Female phenotype No müllerian structures Normal testes Narrow male pelvic structures Sparce axillary and pubic hair	F	Estrogen/progesterone at adolescence	Infancy: gonadectomy, Adolescence: vaginal replacement
Reifenstein's syndrome (incomplete androgen insensitivity)	Karyotype 46, XY Testosterone normal MIS slightly elevated	As for testosterone if deficiency	If F	Estrogen/progesterone at adolescence	Infancy: gonadectomy, clitoral reduction, labioscrotal reduction Adolescence: vaginal replacement
	Sequence androgen receptor gene FISH CGH		If M	As for testosterone deficiency (above)	AS for testosterone deficiency (above)
5α-Reductase deficiency	Karyotype 46,XY Testosterone high DHT low MIS high	Severe hypospadias Symmetrical, undescended, normal testes Prepenile scrotum	M	Presurgical testosterone stimulation DHT replacement	Hypospadias repair Prepenile scrotal repair Prostatic and utricle opening

(continued)

Table 18.1 (continued)

Disease	Diagnostic features	Physical examination phenotype	Gender assignment	Medical therapy	Surgical therapy
	Sequence 5α-reductase type 2 gene FISH				
46, XY (complete gonadal dysgenesis)	Karyotype 46, XY Sequence candidate genes: SRY, SOX 9, DAX-1 Testosterone absent MIS absent FISH CGH	Phenotypic female Vagina present No gandas Symmetrical	F	Estrogen/progesterone at adolescence	Gonadectomy
45, X/46, XY (Ovotesticular DSD; MGD (mixed gonadial dysgenesis)	Karyotype 45, X/46, XY or 46, XY Testosterone low MIS low Sequence DAX-1 FISH CGH	Asymmetry of gonads: streak ovary and dysgenetc testis UG sinus Clitoral hypertrophy	If F	Estrogen/progesterone at adolescence	Clitoral recession Vaginal exteriorization Labioscrotal reduction Gonadectomy
			If M	Presurgical testosterone stimulation Testosterone at adolescence	
46 XY (90%) Ovotesticular DSD True hermaphrodite	Karyotype 46, XX Testosterone normal or low MIS normal or low CGH	Asymmetrical testis, ovary, or ovotestes UG sinus defect Clitoral hypertrophy	If F	Estrogen/progesterone at adolescence	Clitoral recession Vaginal exteriorization Labioscrotal reduction Preserve normal ovary or polar ovarian tissue
			If M	Presurgical testosterone stimulation Testosterone at adolescence	Staged hypospadias repair Prepenile scrotal repair Removal of müllerian structures Preserve vas and normal testis or central testicular tissue Orchiopexy? Prosthesis?

CGH comparative genomic hybridization; *DHT* dihydrotestosterone; *F* female; *FISH* fluorescent in situ hybridization; *M* male; *MIS* Müllerian inhibiting substance; *PCR* polymerase chain reaction; *UG* urogenital

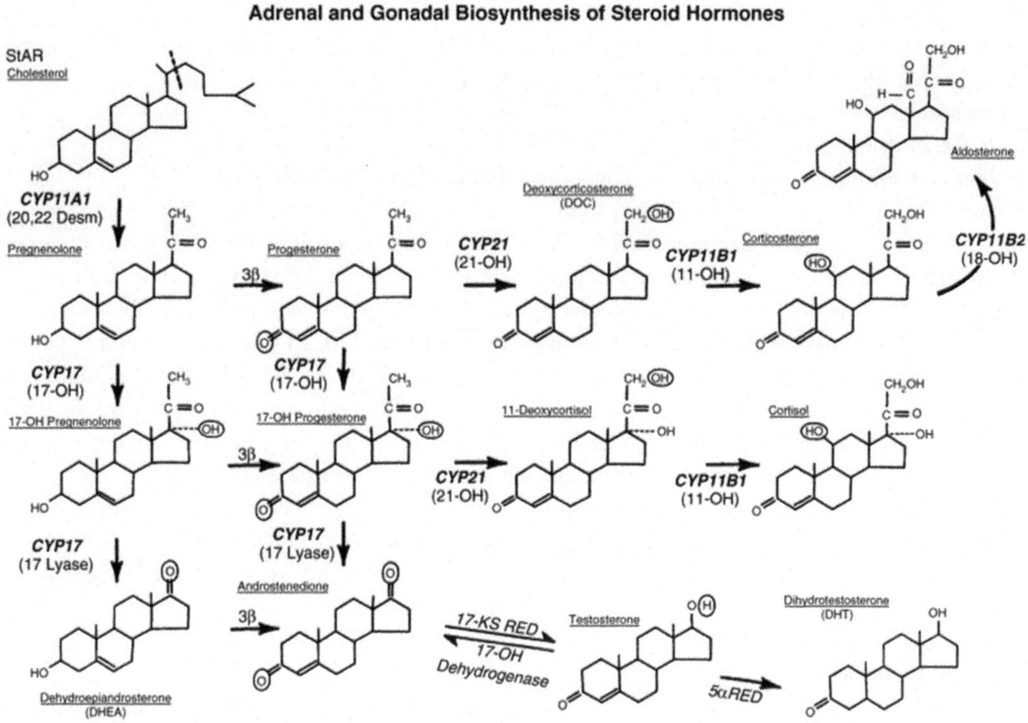

Fig. 18.2 Pathways of steroid hormone biosynthesis from cholesterol. New enzyme nomenclature is in *bold lettering*; old nomenclature is in *parentheses*. Enzymatic defects of CYP21, CYP11, or 3ß-hydroxysteroid dehydrogenase can lead to congenital adrenal hyperplasia. Deficiencies in testosterone production leading to a form of male pseudohermaphroditism can result from defects in CYP11A$_1$, CYP17, 3ß-hydroxysteroid dehydrogenase, and 17-ketosteroid reductase

Table 18.2 Steroid biosynthetic enzyme nomenclature

Old	New-protein	New-gene
Testis		
20,22-desmolase	P450scc (side chain cleavage)	CYP11A
17-hydroxylase	P450c17	CYP17
17-lyase	P450c17	CYP17
3β-hydroxysteroid	Same	Same
dehydrogenase (3ß-HSD)		
17-ketosteroid reductase	Same	Same
Adrenal		
21-hydroxylase	P450c21	CYP21
11-hydroxylase	P450c11	CYP11B1
18-hydroxylase	P450c11	CYP11B2

CYP17, or Steroid Acute Regulatory Protein (StAR), depending on the ethnic origin of the patient [4, 65, 66]. Rarely, 46, XX DSD results from exposure to exogenous androgens.

All the enzymatic defects of CAH result in deficient cortisol biosynthesis that stimulates the pituitary gland to increase corticotropin production. The increase in corticotropin stimulates the adrenal gland and leads to adrenal hyperplasia, elevated production of hormonal precursors proximal to the enzymatic defect, and preferential overproduction of androgenic steroids (Fig. 18.2). Elevations in 17-hydroxyprogesterone can be detected rapidly from a spot serum sample [67] which is mandatory in some states. Polymerase chain reaction (PCR), sequencing of known genes can be used to make this diagnosis in utero [4].

46, XY DSD, Undervirilization of the Genetic Male

Insufficient virilization (masculinization) of a 46, XY genetic male can occur because of insufficient androgen production, an androgen receptor deficiency, or an inability to convert testosterone to dihydrotestosterone. The three distinct subtypes of 46, XY DSD are reviewed below. 46, XY DSD was formerly known as male pseudohermaphroditism [68].

Testosterone Deficiency

Deficiency of androgen production can be caused by genetic defects of the enzymes [CYP11A1 (20,22 desmolase), CYP17 (17-hydroxylase or lyase), 3β-hydroxysteroid dehydrogenase (3ß-HSD), and 17β-hydroxysteroid dehydrogenase (17ß-HSD), or 17-ketosteroid reductase], which together and sequentially are responsible for the metabolism of cholesterol to testosterone (Fig. 18.2) [65]. When stimulated by chorionic gonadotropin patients with defects of these enzyme produce no (or only a minimal amount of) testosterone and because of testosterone deficiency, the penis may be small and hypospadiac [69]. In contrast, MIS levels are normal or high for their age and result in an absence of Müllerian structures. The testes may be undescended, small, or both.

Androgen Insensitivity

Androgen insensitivity is the most common cause of 46, XY DSD. Most abnormalities are caused by point mutations in the androgen receptor gene [70, 71]. However, not all patients with androgen insensitivity have a molecular defect in the androgen receptor gene. In these patients it is possible that the noncoding promoter, the 3′ untranslated region, or other transcription factors or their cofactors might be the cause of 46, XY DSD. There are two known isoforms of the androgen receptor. Type 2 is the predominant receptor in the external genitalia while the type 1 receptor is found in a multitude of other tissues [10].

The phenotype of androgen insensitivity can be mild or severe. The complete androgen insensitivity syndrome (CAIS), previously known as testicular feminization, results in a female phenotype even though the serum testosterone is high. MIS may be normal or, in some cases, considerably elevated, therefore Müllerian structures usually regress normally. The gonads are symmetrical and may be intra-abdominal or descended.

5α-Reductase Deficiency

Mutations of 5α-reductase type 2 genes lead to testosterone not being converted to the active hormone dihydrotestosterone in peripheral, particularly genital, target tissues [48, 72]. Normal dihydrotestosterone action in the genital area results in elongation and ventral closing of the penile raphe, which encloses the urethra and displaces the urethral orifice from the perineum to the tip of the penis [68] and in addition causes the labioscrotal folds to fuse to create scrotal sacs. The autosomal recessive 5α-reductase type 2 deficiency causes severe hypospadias associated with undescended testis, prepenile scrotum, and an enlarged prostatic utricle. The enzyme has binding sites for both testosterone and an NADPH cofactor. Point mutations in the NADPH cofactor have been associated with the defective phenotype of 46, XY DSD. The increase in activity of the 5α-reductase type 1 isoform at puberty produces a paradoxical virilization that may result in a change of sexual identity.

Abnormalities of Gonadal Development and Differentiation

Abnormalities of the sex chromosomes usually manifest as failed, incomplete, or asymmetrical gonadal differentiation. Patients with these disorders have either bilateral streak gonads, as in 46, XY pure gonadal dysgenesis DSD, or asymmetrical gonadal development, as in mixed gonadal dysgenesis (MGD) DSD or ovotesticular DSD (formerly termed true hermaphroditism).

46, XY Pure Gonadal Dysgenesis DSD

Patients with 46, XY pure gonadal dysgenesis DSD may have a defective Y chromosome [73]. Other causes of 46, XY pure gonadal dysgenesis DSD include mutations associated with camptomelic dysplasia, a severe disorder occurring in patients with a translocation in the distal arm of chromosome 9p near the SRY-related SOX 9 gene [35, 37], and mutations in WT1 associated with Frasier's syndrome [41]. The streak gonads in 46, XY pure gonadal dysgenesis DSD fail to develop bilaterally. They produce little or no testosterone so gonadotropin levels are compensatorily high. The streak gonads also produce no MIS so Müllerian duct structures are preserved resulting in a female phenotype.

Mixed Gonadal Dysgenesis (MGD) DSD

MGD DSD (also known as asymmetric gonadal dysgenesis) with a 45,X/46,XY karyotype is by far the most common of the chromosomal abnormalities causing DSD [4, 74]. The gonads are asymmetrical, most often with a small dysgenic testis on one side and a streak gonad on the other [75]. Most patients with this defect have retained Müllerian ducts. The small testis can produce enough testosterone to cause masculinization and hypertrophy of the clitoris. The vagina fails to migrate to the perineum and enters the urethra as a urogenital sinus (UGS) defect more distal to the bladder neck than seen in severe cases of CAH.

It is important to note that 40% of patients with MGD can have a 46, XY karyotype, and some have bilateral testes or streak ovaries. MGD is poorly understood at the molecular level [76]. The absence of the second X chromosome is in some way related to the early ovarian dysgenesis. The mosaicism of mixed gonadal dysgenesis results from the presence of at least two gonadal (chimeric) germ cell lines. The degree of testicular differentiation is determined by the percentage of cells expressing the XY genotype, which may also influence the degree of asymmetry. Loss of the Y chromosome can occur because of nondisjunction, the failure of paired chromosomes to migrate to opposite poles during cell division [1, 29, 77, 78].

Ovotesticular DSD

True ovotesticular DSD (previously known as true hermaphrodism) is rare, except among the Bantu in Southern Africa [79, 80]. More than 90% of these patients have a 46, XX karyotype. Asymmetry characterizes many of these patients, who have simultaneous ovarian and testicular differentiation without the dysgenesis characteristic of MGD. The etiology of ovotesticular DSD and the reason for the gonadal asymmetry remains an enigma. The testicular and ovarian tissue can be separated (i.e., an ovary on one side and a testis on the other), or can occur as ovotestis on both sides, or be combined only in one gonad as an ovotestis with a normal ovary or a testis on the other. When ovarian tissue and testicular tissue coexist in the same gonad, the testicular tissue is always central, and the ovarian

Table 18.3 Rapid diagnostic algorithm

Y Chromosome absent or abnormal		Y Chromosome present	
Gonadal symmetry	Gonadal asymmetry	Gonadal symmetry	Gonadal asymmetry
46, XX DSD[congenital adrenal hyperplasia]	Ovotesticular DSD	46, XY DSD	46, XX/46, XY MGD [Mixed gonadal dysgenesis]

These two diagnostic criteria—presence or absence of Y chromosome and gonadal symmetry or asymmetry—allow the rapid, accurate assignment of a patient into one of the four diagnostic categories with approximately 90% accuracy

tissue is polar [81]. Although early testicular differentiation occurs, spermatogenesis is not advanced [79], which may reflect the absence of other necessary Y-directed functions. The Müllerian structures are regressed on the side of the testicular tissue but retained on the side of the ovarian tissue and in the midline as well, with the vagina entering the distal urethra creating a UGS defect.

Diagnosis

A baby born with DSD must have a thoughtful yet expeditious evaluation to determine whether gender assignment can be made. An important goal is to minimize the immediate and long-term emotional trauma to the family and child and this is best accomplished by early referral to an experienced team of endocrinologists, geneticists, psychologists, and pediatric surgical specialists.

Although many syndromes can affect later sexual development, only four DSDs present at birth: (1) 46, XX DSD, formerly known as female pseudohermaphroditism, congenital adrenal hyperplasia (CAH) or adrenogenital syndrome [63, 64], which causes overandrogenization of a genetic female, (2) 46, XY DSD, previously termed male pseudohermaphroditism, which causes undervirilization of a genetic male, (3) MGD DSD mixed gonadal dysgenesis 45, X/46, XY, or (4) ovotesticular DSD, formerly known as true hermaphroditism. A child with pure gonadal dysgenesis, although having a 46, XY karyotype, is phenotypically female.

The diagnostic evaluation of patients with ambiguous genitalia is outlined in Table 18.1. Two screening criteria can be used to diagnose the infant as having one of the four disorders, symmetry and the presence of a Y chromosome (Table 18.3). The first diagnostic criterion is the physical finding of gonadal symmetry or asymmetry, and the second is sex chromosome determination. Gonadal symmetry is defined by the position each gonad relative to the external inguinal ring; i.e., gonads are symmetric when both are either above or below the external inguinal ring and gonads are asymmetric when one gonad is above the external ring and the other gonad is below the external inguinal ring. Gonads are symmetrical in 46, XX DSD and 46, XY DSD when a systemic biochemical defect influences both gonads equally. Gonadal asymmetry occurs in chromosomal abnormalities such as MGD (mixed gonadal dysgenesis) or ovotesticular DSD (true hermaphroditism), in which a predominant testis descends below the external ring and a predominant ovary remains above the external ring.

A detailed history and physical examination can be coupled and genetic testing to define the mutations or deletions known to cause defects in the four major categories and to define the DSD more fully. Subsequently, ultrasonography, magnetic resonance imaging, contrast radiography, and later panendoscopy, coupled with accurate laboratory analysis for disorders of enzymes affecting testosterone synthesis, should provide a definitive diagnosis and permit appropriate gender assignment with a high degree of accuracy.

The size of the penis and its location with respect to the scrotum should be carefully noted. Although the size of the phallus varies considerably, some guidelines are helpful [82, 69]. The average length of the penis is 3.5 ± 0.4 cm at term, 3.0 ± 0.4 cm at 35 weeks' gestation, and

2.5 ± 0.4 cm at 30 weeks' gestation. At term, a diameter of 1 cm is average. A penis smaller than 1.5 ± 0.7 cm in a full-term infants raises the possibility of female gender assignment, except in cases of 17-ketosteroid reductase or 5α-reductase deficiencies, when large body habitus or sex reversal at puberty, respectively, would favor male sex assignment. An early rectal examination permits detection of a uterus still enlarged under the influence of placental gonadotropin. The presence and severity of hypospadias should be noted. Palpation of the gonads can differentiate the firm testis from the softer ovotestis and differentiate a testis with an attached epididymis from an ovary in the inguinal position [4].

46, XX DSD Overandrogenization of the Genetic Female

If the patient is the proband for the family, the diagnosis of 46, XX DSD can be delayed but if a previous sibling has already manifested the disorder then genetic testing could permit prenatal diagnosis.

The condition presents in a wide clinical spectrum. The ovaries, uterus, and Fallopian tubes are normal. The vagina, however, is foreshortened because of failure to migrate to the perineum. Instead the vagina usually merges with the urethra to form a urogenital sinus (UGS) distal to the bladder neck. However, a rare but significant subset of patients may have a verumontanum, with the urethrovaginal confluence quite close to the bladder neck [83]. These severely masculinized patients can also have an enlarged, placentally stimulated prostate, palpable at the level of the verumontanum.

The external genitalia are characterized by variable clitoral enlargement, ranging from trivial to severe. In severe cases patients have an almost normal male phallus. The labia can be masculinized to form either enlarged labioscrotal folds or, in the most severe cases, complete scrotal fusion. The disorder is systemic so the gonads are symmetric and because the ovaries are normal, the gonads never descend into the labioscrotal folds or fused scrotum [4, 84]. The karyotype is always 46, XX in females. MIS is undetectable and serum 17-hydroxyprogesterone is elevated. Androgen levels are also elevated. Concomitant production of melanocyte-stimulating hormone can darken the genitalia and breast areolae.

An infant with bilateral nonpalpable testes should have a rapid analysis for 17 hydroxyprogesterone (a screening test done in some states on all newborns) and a karyotype determination to identify the presence or absence of the Y chromosome. These tests should identify patients with 46, XX DSD who has CYP21 disorders that cause potential life-threatening hormonal deficiencies.

PCR with appropriate probes demonstrates point mutations in the P450c21 gene [85]. Electrolytes are often normal at birth, but when maternal steroids wane after 5–7 days, serum sodium levels may fall and serum potassium levels may become markedly elevated which if unattended, can lead to cardiac arrest. Hence, this disorder must be considered a medical emergency until treatment is commenced.

46, XY DSD, Undervirilization of the Genetic Male

Testosterone Deficiency

By definition, 46, XY DSD patients have deficient androgenization of the external genitalia with a 46, XY karyotype. If the disorder is caused by an enzymatic defect in the production of testosterone, patients have low basal serum testosterone, and stimulation by chorionic gonadotropin produces little or no increase in testosterone. Because the genes coding for the enzymes in the pathway have been cloned, PCR or direct sequencing can be performed to detect specific deficiencies. The testes may be small and are often bilaterally and symmetrically undescended. The penis is small, and hypospadias is usually severe. Since MIS is normal there are no detectable Müllerian structures. In some cases, the phenotype is completely female [69, 86]. Gender assignment is controversial. The size of the phallus plays a role, as it may be better to raise infants with a small, nonreconstructable phallus as females, whereas it is invariably preferable to raise those with a reasonably sized phallus as males, particularly if they respond to exogenous testosterone. Special consideration should be given to those rare children with 17-ketosteroid reductase deficiency, which may be better raised as males because of later large body habitus.

Androgen Insensitivity

Patients with severely dysfunctional androgen receptors have Complete Androgen Insensitivity Syndrome (CAIS), previously known as testicular feminization [87]. The phenotype is female and these children have been raised as females. No Müllerian structures are present because the normal testes produce high levels of biologically active MIS that regress the Müllerian ducts. The testes are usually in the inguinal region, and their firmness and attached epididymis distinguish them from ovaries. The karyotype is 46, XY. The androgen receptor is deficient and the normal testes to produces high levels of testosterone and MIS. PCR or sequencing of the androgen receptor gene can often pinpoint the molecular defect and provide the definitive diagnosis.

Partial Androgen Insensitivity Syndrome (PAIS) results in only partially masculinized 46, XY patients, with a wide variation in phenotype. As with testosterone-deficiency syndrome, the penis is small and hypospadiac. The testes may be small and are often undescended but symmetrical, and Müllerian structures are not present. The testosterone levels are normal, and MIS levels are elevated. Most abnormalities are caused by point mutations in the androgen receptor gene [70, 71]. Again, the size of the phallus can influence gender assignment.

5α-Reductase Deficiency

46, XY DSD can also result from a deficiency of 5α-reductase, which is responsible for the conversion of testosterone to dihydrotestosterone which acts on the genital area resulting in elongation and ventral closing of the penile raphe, with normal displacement of the urethral orifice from the perineum to the tip of the glans penis [68]. This process is abnormal in these patients, resulting in severe penoscrotal hypospadias. Normal and symmetrical testes can be either undescended or fully descended. The labioscrotal folds are also closed posteriorly to create partial or bifid scrotal sacs. The prostatic utricle is often quite enlarged. Again, the karyotype is 46, XY. Serum levels of testosterone are high, but levels of dihydrotestosterone are low. The MIS levels are normal and Müllerian structures are not present. PCR and full DNA sequencing can be used to genotype and to detect mutations in the 5α-reductase type 2 gene.

At puberty 5-α-reductase type I present in skin and other organs markedly increase resulting in a dramatic phenotypic conversion and it is now considered more appropriate to raise these children as males. It should be noted, however, that in this group, gender assignment involves the greatest dilemma in societies committed to two sexes, but not in societies that more readily accept assignment to a third sex [48, 88, 89].

Abnormalities of Gonadal Development and Differentiation

46, XY Pure Gonadal Dysgenesis

Patients with pure gonadal dysgenesis are born as phenotypic females and there are no questions of ambiguity. Amniocentesis with a 46, XY karyotype that does not produce the expected phenotype on fetal ultrasonography allows earlier diagnosis than was previously possible. Dorsal pedal edema and some Turner characteristics may be the only obvious somatic manifestations of the defect in otherwise normal females. Müllerian structures are present, but gonads are not palpable due to failure of gonadal differentiation. Dysgenesis of the gonad results in an absence of testosterone and MIS.

Mixed Gonadal Dysgenesis (MGD)

Patients with mixed gonadal dysgenesis are characterized by asymmetry, with a streak gonad on one side and a dysgenetic testis on the other. Because the testes are dysgenetic, testosterone and MIS levels may be low. They have retained Müllerian structures because of lack of MIS [74, 75, 90]. The clitoris is usually hypertrophied. The most common karyotype is 45, XO/46, XY, but 40% of patients have the 46, XY karyotype. There is a propensity for neoplastic transformation of the abnormal gonads to gonadoblastoma or seminoma (or both) [78, 91, 92], that may occur even in newborns. These tumors can cause gonadal torsion and apparent loss of a gonad that, in rare cases, leads to a unilateral dysgenetic testis or streak ovary. Because gonadoblastomas may occur at any age, gonadectomy and female reconstruction and rearing are the options usually chosen. There is a subgroup of 45, XO/46, XY patients that are diagnosed prenatally with normal external genitalia and raised as males indicating a spectrum of the disorder.

Ovotesticular DSD (True Hermaphroditism)

The molecular cause of this disorder remains enigmatic [79, 80]. Patients with this disease also have asymmetry, with a testis on one side and an ovotestis on the other; however, various other gonadal combinations can occur. If an ovotestis is present, then testicular tissue is central, and the ovarian tissue is polar [81]. Neoplastic transformation is not observed in these unique gonads. The Müllerian structures are regressed on the side of the testicular tissue but retained on the side of the ovarian tissue, as is the midline uterus with the vagina entering the urethra as a urogenital sinus defect. The clitoris is hypertrophied. The karyotype is 46, XX in 90% of cases; the levels of testosterone and MIS are low but can sometimes be normal. Although early testicular differentiation occurs, spermatogenesis is not evident [79], which may reflect the absence of other necessary Y-directed functions. The sex of rearing is dictated by the phenotype, which is in turn directed by the predominant gonad.

Medical Management

46, XX DSD, Overandrogenization of the Genetic Female

Masculinized females with 46, XX DSD (CAH) can be at profound risk for life-threatening complications including cardiac arrest early in life. Because maternal cortisone crosses the placenta and is released slowly from fat stores, the abnormal hormone profile of the infant and the clinical manifestations of adrenogenital crisis may not become apparent until 5–7 days after birth. Heightened clinical awareness and prompt, appropriate treatment with glucocorticoid replacement can prevent serious complications of acute adrenal insufficiency.

Fludrocortisone (9α-fluorocortisol) 0.05–0.2 mg/day is started in severely virilized infants and in those less virilized with a family history of salt wasting as part of 46, XX DSD (CAH). Recent evidence that even patients with milder virilizing hermaphroditism have subclinical aldosterone deficiency has led to more liberal use of fluorocortisone, although some clinicians follow electrolyte levels and plasma renin activity before starting such treatment.

An infant in adrenal crisis should be rehydrated with isotonic saline. After the first hour, half-strength saline in 5–10% dextrose should be administered. This regimen corrects plasma sodium and chloride imbalances rapidly, but hyperkalemia and acidosis are corrected more slowly. Dramatic elevation of plasma 17-hydroxyprogesterone can be used to monitor the effectiveness of treatment. Infants in adrenal crisis are treated with 25 mg hydrocortisone sodium succinate, whereas older children receive 50–100 mg. This preparation has both glucocorticoid and mineralocorticoid activity with the mineralocorticoid activity equivalent to 0.1 mg of fludrocortisone. A similar regimen is used for infants exposed to the stress of surgery. Parents are taught to recognize situations that contribute to adrenal insufficiency, such as high fever, exposure to hot environments, or surgery. Breast milk and prepared formulas are low in sodium, so supplement salt is given. Growth must be monitored carefully to void inadequate treatment dosing or over suppression and chronic adrenal insufficiency.

Prenatal diagnosis and treatment are now available [93, 94]. Since dexamethasone crosses the placenta it may be given to suppress the fetal adrenal gland and decrease fetal androgen production, thereby minimizing in utero virilization. Dexamethasone is initiated by the fifth or sixth week of gestation before the start of sexual differentiation. Later the sex of the fetus is determined the CYP21 gene can be analyzed for mutations so that treatment can be discontinued in males and unaffected females. Affected females can be treated to term. Currently, embryo selection or genetic manipulation can be done at the early blastocyst stage. Blastocysts with a normal CYP21 gene can be preselected for subsequent implantation if a previous pregnancy produced a child with the CYP21 mutation.

46, XY DSD, Undervirilization of the Genetic Male

46, XY DSD patients with poor penile development who have testosterone biosynthetic defects or androgen resistance may be considered for female gender assignment. However, for those with 5α-reductase or 17β-hydroxysteroid reductase deficiencies, it may not be appropriate to assign a gender at birth. Patients assigned to the female gender should receive early surgical correction of the external genitalia and gonadectomy but do not receive hormone therapy until puberty, at which time they will require estrogen and progesterone treatment. Vaginal replacement should be planned for late puberty.

If it is elected to assign these infants to the male gender, testosterone is given to confirm that the penis responds to androgens and to improve the size of the penis before surgery. Repair should be done before 1 year of age if the size of the phallus permits. This approach takes advantage of an early period of presumed enhanced sensitivity to androgens. Testosterone is often withheld before hypospadias repair to reduce postoperative hyperactivity that can accompany testosterone therapy. If the child requires staged procedures, testosterone therapy, if needed, can precede the second stage. Testosterone replacement is resumed at adolescence. Patients with 5 alpha-reductase deficiencies should receive dihydrotestosterone replacement, if available. Otherwise, replacement can be achieved by giving higher doses of testosterone to overcome the enzyme block.

Abnormalities of Gonadal Development and Differentiation

In patients with mixed gonadal dysgenesis MGD or ovotesticular disease assigned to the female gender, no steroidal replacement is required in childhood. However, if the child has been assigned to the male gender, presurgical testosterone stimulation of the penis may be required before hypospadias repair. Treatment does not recommence until adolescence. If the patient is assigned to the female gender, estrogen and progesterone replacement are also started at adolescence. Patients with 46, XY pure gonadal dysgenesis require neither surgical nor medical therapy as newborns, and estrogen and progesterone replacement begins at adolescence. Renal function must be followed carefully in patients with the various WT1 isoform defects. Adrenal replacement therapy may be complex in patients with SF-1 mutations characteristic of the adrenal hypoplasia congenital syndrome. Vaginal replacement should be planned for late puberty.

Surgical Treatment of Urogenital Sinus Anomalies and Disorders of Sexual Differentiation

Patients with DSD and UGS abnormalities present many challenges for the medical team caring for them and for their parents who must make decisions. It is critical that the sex of rearing not be biased by the skills of the surgeon, who must

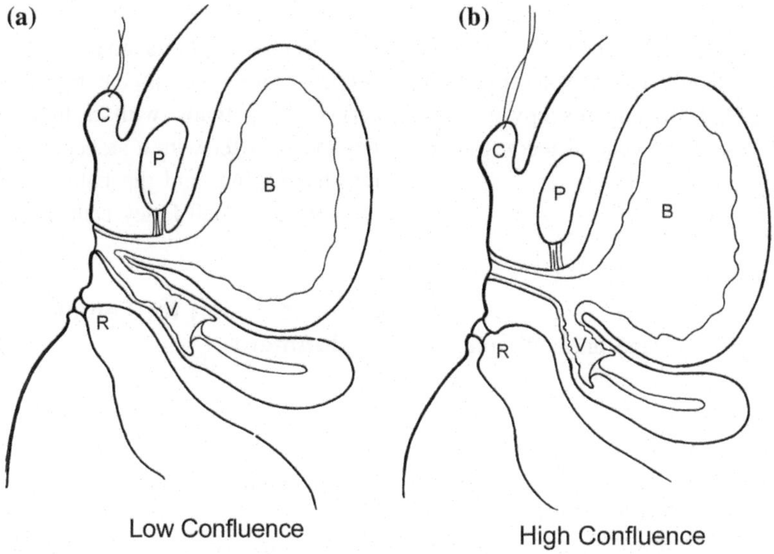

Fig. 18.3 **a** Low confluence urogenital sinus (*C* clitoris, *P* pubis, *B* bladder, *V* vagina, *R* rectum). **b** High confluence urogenital sinus (*C* clitoris, *P* pubis, *B* bladder, *V* vagina, *R* rectum). (From Pieretti RV, Donahoe PK. Disorders of sex development. In Coran AG, Adzick NS, Krummel TM, et al. (eds)., Pediatric Surgery, 7th ed. Philadelphia, PA: Elsevier, 2012, with permission.)

be equally capable at reconstructing the infant as male or female. There have been many significant advancements in the surgical options available to patients with DSD including those resulting from studies on clitoral innervation and new nerve-sparing clitoroplasty techniques [95–97]. Since these are relatively new techniques for treatment of females with CAH there is limited information on the long-term results of these operations on future sexual function and patient satisfaction [98].

Preoperative Evaluation of Anatomy

The preoperative evaluation of anatomy includes routine physical examination, a variety of imaging modalities, examination under anesthesia, and in some cases laparoscopy. Imaging studies that are particularly valuable include ultrasound, which is particularly good at visualizing the urinary tract and in most cases the uterus, vagina and gonads can be visualized, MRI of the pelvis. A specialized study specifically designed to evaluate children with DSD is a retrograde genitogram. When performed by an experienced radiologist and surgeon this study can identify the level of the junction of the urethra and vagina of a UGS and define its relation to the bladder neck and external sphincter in approximately 80% of the cases. This determination greatly facilitates the planning of the surgical procedure (Figs. 18.3a, b and 18.4).

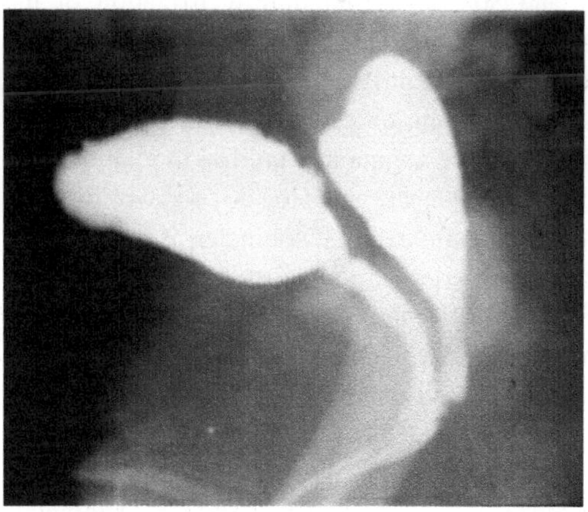

Fig. 18.4 Retrograde genitography showing a low confluence urogenital sinus in a patient with 46, XX DSD (CAH). (From Pieretti RV, Donahoe PK. Disorders of sex development. In Coran AG, Adzick NS, Krummel TM, et al. (eds)., Pediatric Surgery, 7th ed. Philadelphia, PA: Elsevier, 2012, with permission.)

Laparoscopy can be valuable for evaluation of pelvic organs and gonadal biopsy, as well as for therapeutic gonadectomy and resection of Müllerian structures [99, 100]. Laparoscopy is also a valuable tool to assist in eventual reconstruction procedures.

Preoperative Preparation

Preoperative mechanical and antibiotic preparation of the colon is important before pelvic reconstructive procedures. Patients with adrenal insufficiency taking steroids will need stress doses of steroids at anesthesia induction and during surgery, then for 2–3 days after surgery at double their usual oral dose, followed by a tapering back to baseline. Dosing after surgery often requires pediatric endocrinology consultation, as it is dependent on the patient's specific baseline requirements, the length and extent of surgery, and the expected length of hospitalization.

Surgical Reconstruction

Panendoscopy

Reconstructive procedures are preceded by a panendoscopy using a pediatric cystoscope with 0° and 30° optics. High flow irrigation of the urogenital sinus and probing with a 3 Fr. ureteral catheter can identify a very small vaginal orifice. It is important to precisely confirm the confluence of the vagina and urethra in relation with the bladder neck and to do so we use the verumontanum/external sphincter as a landmark. In our experience, the most accurate measurements are obtained by placing a 3 or 4 Fr. ureteral catheter with 1 cm markings alongside the cystoscope and under direct visualization put its tip at the bladder neck and then pull back and identify the junction of the UGS and measure the distance with the catheter markings. Anomalies with the junction at or above the verumontanum/external sphincter are considered high, and those below are considered low (Fig. 18.3a, b).

Patients with 46, XX DSD, MGD, and Ovotesticular DSD have a cervix at the most proximal part of the vagina. Patients with 46, XY DSD have either a small prostatic utricle or a deeper, more generous cavity with no proximal cervix. In patients with a high confluence a Fogarty catheter with a stopcock valve is passed into the vagina, and the balloon is inflated and secured to a small Foley catheter in the bladder.

Reconstruction for Female Gender Assignment

All 46, XX DSD newborns, should be assigned to the female gender, regardless of the extent of masculinization and have the appropriate reconstruction. Similar repairs can be used for selected patients who are not masculinized because of 46, XY DSD, MGD, or Ovotesticular DSD. The key components of a feminizing genitoplasty are clitoroplasty, labioplasty, and vaginoplasty. Surgical procedures should preserve clitoral sensation, and provide a female appearance and vagina that will allow painless sexual intercourse.

The timing of surgical reconstruction is controversial with some groups advocating delaying until the patient can make their own decisions [101]. As mentioned earlier most long-term outcome studies analyze the outcomes of older surgical procedures [102, 103] which may not be as relevant to newer techniques that are thought to result in an improved cosmetic appearance, have a lower complication rate, and are more likely to preserve sensation. Patients with a low confluence urogenital sinus can have reconstruction during infancy once they are metabolically stable and in most cases, we undertake an elective reconstruction at 3–6 months of age. We repair patients with higher confluences at 9–12 months of age.

Combined Clitoroplasty, Labioplasty, and Vaginoplasty

We recommend that the different components of surgical reconstruction should be incorporated into a single surgical procedure. The prepuce is used to create labia minora, the clitoris is reduced with preservation of sensation, and the labioscrotal swellings are used to fashion female appearing labia majora and to enhance the vaginoplasty. This approach is consistent with the recommendations from an international consensus statement on the management of children with DSD [64].

To optimize surgical exposure and elevate the perineum we place our patients in a hyperextended lithotomy position with the buttocks lying over and slightly beyond several folded towels. As previously described all procedures must begin with a panendoscopy.

Clitoroplasty

In cases with severe masculinization the clitoris is too large (sometimes resembling a penis) we recommend a clitoroplasty. Clitoroplasty techniques have evolved over time in an effort to preserve sensation for future orgasms, provide an acceptable appearance, and avoid painful erections. Clitoral resection and recession are no longer recommended. Kogan described a clitoroplasty with subtunical excision of the erectile tissue which has been used extensively and led to newer nerve-sparing techniques [104]. Baskin found that distribution of the sensory nerves of the clitoris is similar to the sensory nerves of the penis: they course under the pubic bone, come onto the top or dorsal aspect of the clitoris, and have circumferential branches from the dorsal neurovascular bundle. This makes a ventral approach to the corpora most likely to avoid nerve injury [105] (Fig. 18.5a). In Baskin's technique corporal tissue proximal to the bifurcation is left intact. This preserved erectile tissue may play an important role in sexual function.

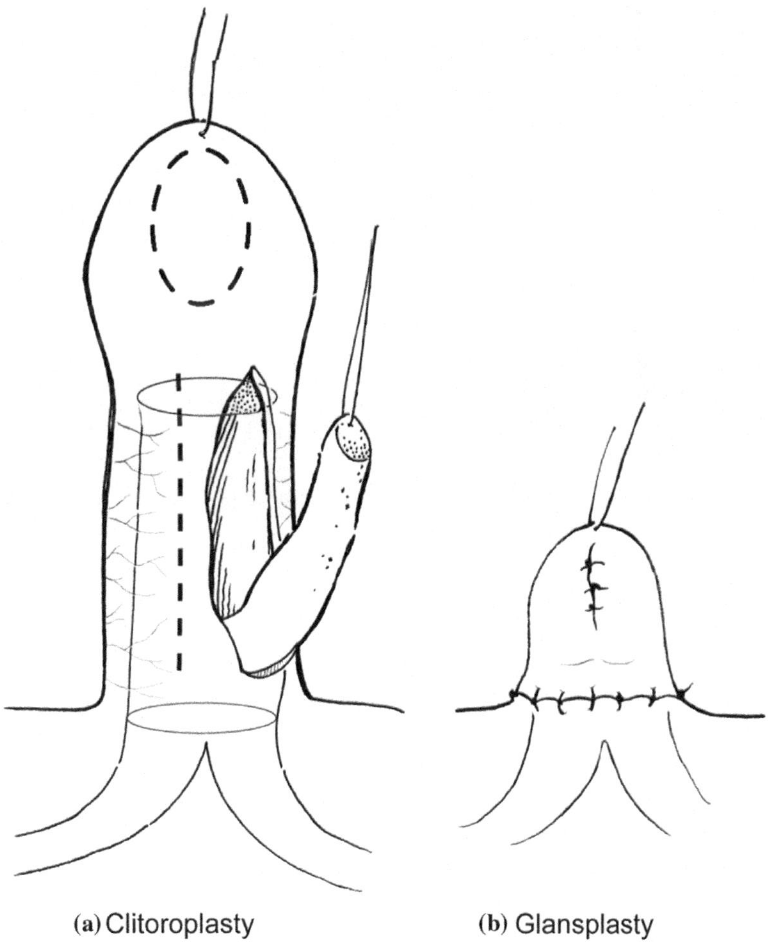

Fig. 18.5 **a** Excision of erectile tissue; also, an elliptical incision is outlined on the ventral aspect of the glans for glansplasty. **b** Completed clitoroplasty and glansplasty (body of the glans sutured to the corporal body stumps with absorbable sutures)

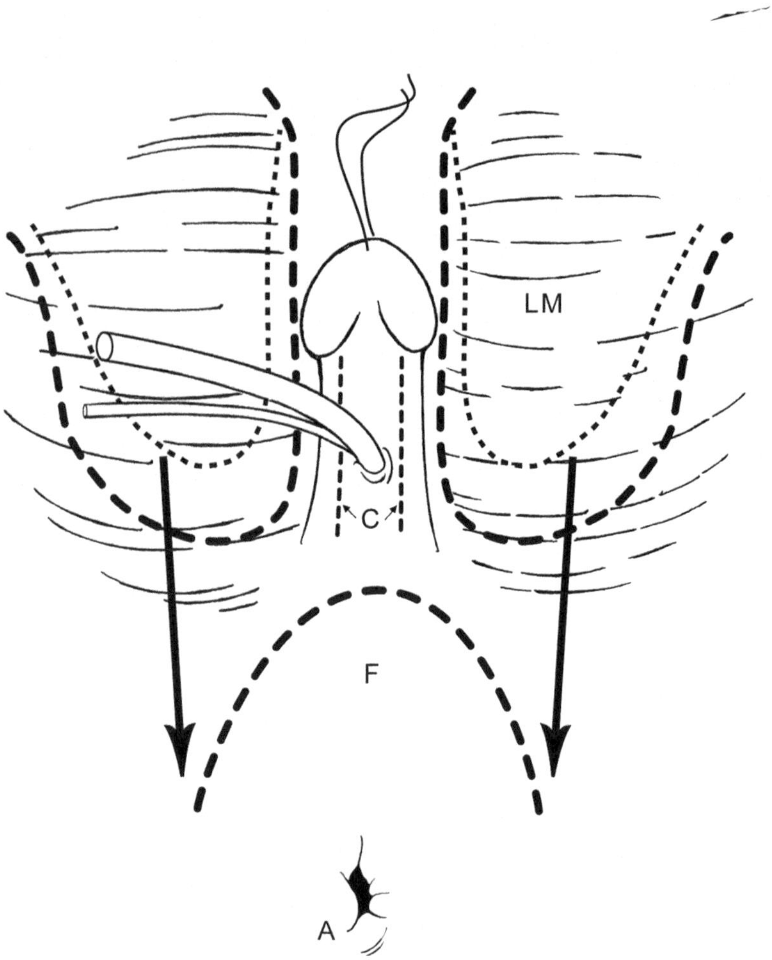

Fig. 18.6 Bilateral Y-V advancement of the labia majora. The flaps are cautiously defatted and moved posteriorly, besides the introitus to enhance the vaginoplasty. The medial aspects of the skin flaps are sutured to the lateral edges of the preputial skin mobilized during clitoroplasty, which became labia minora (*LM* labia majora, *C* clitoris, *F* flap). (From Pieretti RV, Donahoe PK. Disorders of sex development. In Coran AG, Adzick NS, Krummel TM, et al. (eds)., Pediatric Surgery, 7th ed. Philadelphia, PA: Elsevier, 2012, with permission.)

Our practice is to first perform panendoscopy as previously noted and place catheters into the bladder and vagina. Then a holding suture is placed in the glans, and two vertical incisions made, one on each side of the urethral plate (overlying the distal UGS), as one does for hypospadias surgery (Fig. 18.6). Prior injection of incisions with 1% lidocaine/1:200,000 epinephrine prevents excess bleeding.

The vaginoplasty is begun by outlining a wide-based inverted "U"-shaped perineal incision based on the anus with the apex of "U" at the level of the ischial tuberosities which will be the location of the vaginal opening (Fig. 18.6). The clitoris is degloved down to the peno-scrotal junction initially keeping the ventral strip of the urethral plate intact. Care is taken to leave a redundant segment of dorsal inner foreskin to allow the fashioning of a hooded prepuce for the clitoris and preserve an important source of sensation [105].

After degloving of the dorsal skin, the distal portion of the urethral plate/UGS is divided below the glans clitoris. The urethral plate/UGS is mobilized off the ventral aspect of the clitoral shaft downward to below the bifurcation of the corporal bodies. Next clitoral reduction is carried out. In most cases, a tourniquet is unnecessary although bleeding can be considerable in the older child. Longitudinal ventral incisions are made and the erectile tissue is dissected within the bodies (Fig. 18.5a). The body of the glans is sutured to the corporal body stumps with absorbable sutures (Fig. 18.5b). This step should, allow for painless engorgement of the proximally preserved corpora remnants with sexual activity.

In most cases we try to avoid reduction of the glans clitoris, aiming to preserve sensation, but, in patients with a large clitoris a wedge of glans tissue may be cautiously excised from its ventral aspect with careful re-approximation of the glans tissue (Fig. 18.5a, b).

The redundant dorsal tunica albuginea and neurovascular bundle are placed in a subcutaneous pocket above the pubic bone, folded and secured in place without impairing the neurovascular supply. The reduced clitoral shaft is covered with surrounding fatty tissue, fashioning a normal looking mons pubis. The preserved segment of dorsal foreskin should cover the glans partially, giving it a hooded appearance. The remainder of the dorsal prepuce is divided in the midline (Byars technique) and re-attached to the mucosal collar as with hypospadias repair. The preputial skin wings are rotated inferiorly and incorporated lateral to the urethral plate to create labia minora (Fig. 18.7).

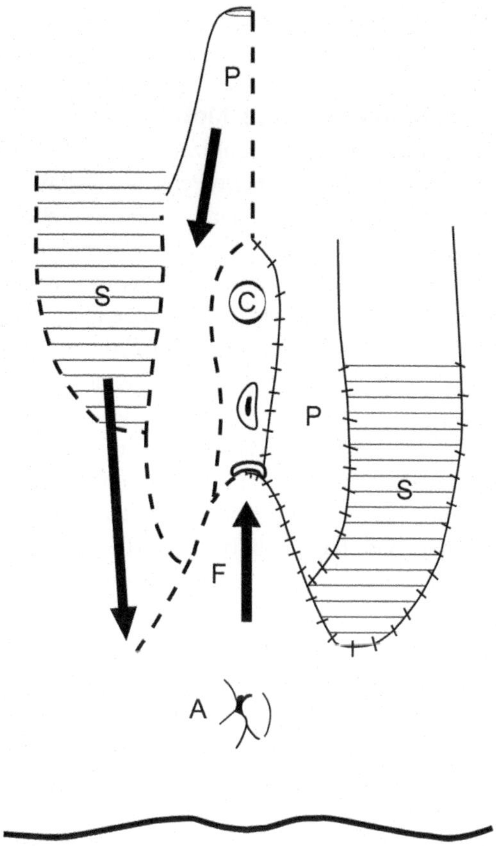

Fig. 18.7 Split prepuce used to create labia minora; labia majora Y-V plasty; flap vaginoplasty (*P* split prepuce, *S* labioscrotal fold, *C* clitoris, *F* flap). (From Pieretti RV, Donahoe PK. Disorders of sex development. In Coran AG, Adzick NS, Krummel TM, et al. (eds)., Pediatric Surgery, 7th ed. Philadelphia, PA: Elsevier, 2012, with permission.)

Labioplasty

Most girls with CAH have labioscrotal swellings that are more anterior than normal labia majora and significant skin rugation may also be present. The labioscrotal skin is moved posteriorly, adjacent to the vaginal introitus, by creating defatted and bilateral Y-V advancement flaps. The medial aspects of these flaps are sutured to the lateral edges of the prepucial skin flaps mobilized during clitoroplasty creating labia minora) (Fig. 18.7).

Vaginoplasty

The type of vaginoplasty is decided according with the anatomic location of the merging point of the vagina into the urethra. There are six types of vaginoplasty: cutback, flap, pull-through, total and partial urogenital sinus mobilization (TUM and PUM), and vaginal replacement.

Flap Vaginoplasty for Low Confluence UGS

Flap vaginoplasty is only indicated for cases with a low confluence UGS, because it does not bring the merging point of the vagina with the urethra any closer to the perineum. The technique is based on the description by Fortunoff and associates [106] and Hendren and Crawford [83] of a posterior inverted "U" flap of perineal skin based on the anus that is advanced to the posterior wall of normal caliber vagina. In flap vaginoplasty for low confluence UGS, there is no need to do a complete mobilization of the UGS. The UGS is dissected off the clitoral corpora and the dorsal wall is opened to create a more normal looking introitus. Later during labioplasty, the medial edge of the prepuce (labia minora) will be sutured to the outer edge of the opened, non-mobilized urethral plate/UGS (Fig. 18.7).

Vaginoplasty Using Urogenital Mobilization

Total Urogenital Sinus Mobilization

Total urogenital sinus mobilization (TUM) was described in 1997 by Alberto Peña as a technique to repair the UGS component of cloacal malformations [107]. Currently, total or partial urogenital sinus mobilization are used by most surgeons for UGS repair [108]. Urogenital sinus mobilization has the advantage of better visualization of the merging point of the urogenital sinus and it eliminates the need for vaginal separation, thus, markedly reducing the difficulty of the procedure. In this technique, the confluence is brought closer to the perineum and there is less need for skin flap mobilization. The posterior dissection is similar to that done for a pull-through or flap procedures, with, midline mobilization of the UGS off the rectum. The anterior dissection in cases requiring a total urogenital sinus mobilization is done past the pubourethral ligament, under the pubis, resulting in significant mobilization of the entire sinus, and in most cases the confluence can be brought more easily to the perineum (Fig. 18.3a, b).

Partial Urogenital Sinus Mobilization

Because of concerns of possible urinary incontinence and loss of clitoral sensation that might result from circumferential dissection of the UGS beyond the pubourethral ligament, Rink and colleagues proposed the use of a partial urogenital mobilization (PUM) where the anterior dissection stops at the pubourethral ligament aiming to avoid compromising the innervation to the bladder outlet and clitoris [109]. This procedure provides sufficient mobilization in all but cases of a very high confluence which require additional mobilization beyond the pubourethral ligament may be needed.

Alternatively, if the perineum cannot be reached without tension the vagina must be sharply dissected from the back wall of the bladder before the anastomosis to the inverted perineal "U" flap can be attempted. In these cases, the use of a prone position can facilitate the dissection of the vagina off the bladder. In cases requiring either total and partial urogenital sinus mobilization the distal segment of the vagina can be narrow and it is necessary to incise the posterior wall up to normal caliber vagina

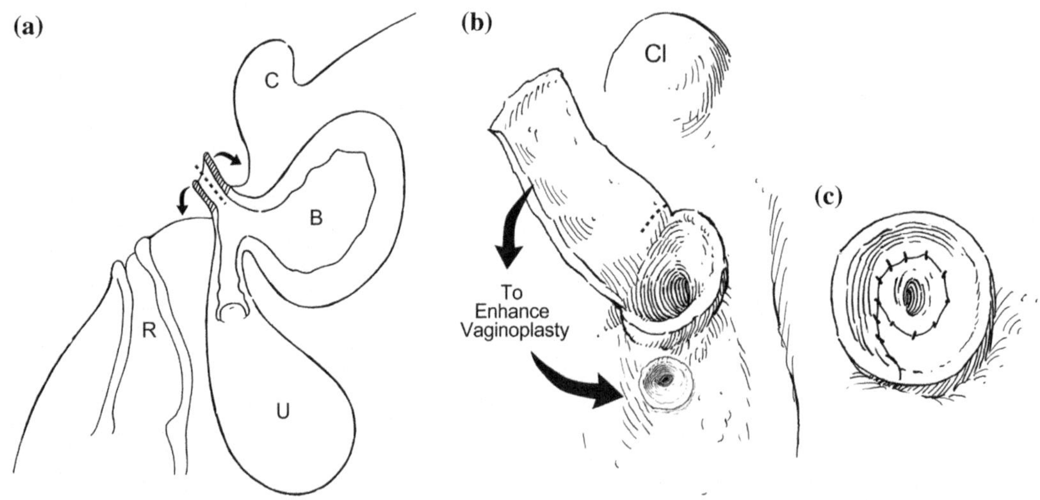

Fig. 18.8 **a** Use of the redundant sinus: split laterally to fashion a mucosa lined vestibule and/or to enhance the anterior vaginal wall. **b–c** Use of the redundant sinus: split laterally with spiral rotation of the flap to complete the vaginoplasty. (From Pieretti RV, Donahoe PK. Disorders of sex development. In Coran AG, Adzick NS, Krummel TM, et al. (eds)., Pediatric Surgery, 7th ed. Philadelphia, PA: Elsevier, 2012, with permission.)

and reconstruct the posterior vaginal wall with the inverted perineal "U" flap as previously described for a low vaginoplasty to avoid a vaginal stricture.

Splitting the Urogenital Sinus

As proposed by Rink, the urogenital sinus can be split to enhance the feminizing genitoplasty [109]. The common urogenital sinus can be split in the following manners: (1) In very low confluence cases, we do not mobilize the urogenital sinus but only incise it longitudinally on its ventral aspect up to confluence point; the lateral aspects of the opened sinus are sutured to medial aspects of the prepuce wings, thus, resulting in a more normal anatomical configuration, (2) The sinus can also be opened laterally to fashion a mucosa lined vestibule and to enhance the anterior wall (3) The sinus can be opened laterally, then, the incised sinus can be rotated to extend the vagina (Fig. 18.8a–c).

Pull-Through Vaginoplasty for Mid Level Vaginal Confluence

Before the advent of the urogenital sinus mobilization procedures, the majority of girls were reconstructed using a pull-through vaginoplasty as described by Hendren and Crawford [83]. Patients are prepped and draped to allow for rotation and supine or prone positioning. The operation begins with a panendoscopy and localization of the confluence and placement of catheters. An inverted perineal "U" flap is made, the urogenital sinus is exposed, and the vagina is mobilized circumferentially and meticulously separated off the bladder anteriorly [110]. The urethra is closed and a labial flap or an anterior island flap is connected to the anterior vagina (Fig. 18.9a–h).

In patients with a very high confluence we have found that having the patient in prone position improves visualization and exposure, allowing the vagina to be safely mobilized off the urogenital sinus and bladder [111]. The opening in the UGS can then be easily closed and the vagina is then mobilized circumferentially and brought to the perineum where it is sutured to the perineal skin flap as described for vaginoplasty (Fig. 18.10a–d).

Postoperative Care of the Female Patient

Postoperatively a small Foley bladder catheter is left indwelling for 3–4 days. The use of epidural anesthesia has improved pain management. Immobilization with a mermaid dressing in which the lower extremities are wrapped with stockinet prevents tension on the suture lines. A soft plastic foam or cotton is placed between the knees and ankles, and the anus is left exposed. The legs are loosely wrapped with an elastic bandage without covering the anus. The mermaid dressing is kept in place for 4–5 days to avoid thigh abduction, which puts tension on the suture line. A broad-spectrum antibiotic is used during the first 2 postoperative days and stress steroids given as needed.

Reconstruction for Male Gender Assignment

The treatment strategy for all patients assigned to the male gender is similar even though the underlying diagnoses may be different. Most of these patients have a (1) a small penis with penoscrotal, scrotal, or perineal hypospadias, (2) a severe ventral penile curvature, and (3) a partial or complete prepenile scrotum. Preoperative treatment with testosterone is often helpful in cases with a small penis.

Our preferred approach is to perform an one-stage hypospadias repair in patients with an adequate urethral plate, using the extended applications of the tubularized incised plate urethroplasty as described by Snodgrass [112]. In this technique the urethral plate is preserved. Degloving of the foreskin beyond the hypospadiac meatus into the scrotum is done which in many cases significantly corrects the ventral curvature. Additional ventral curvature correction is done as needed.

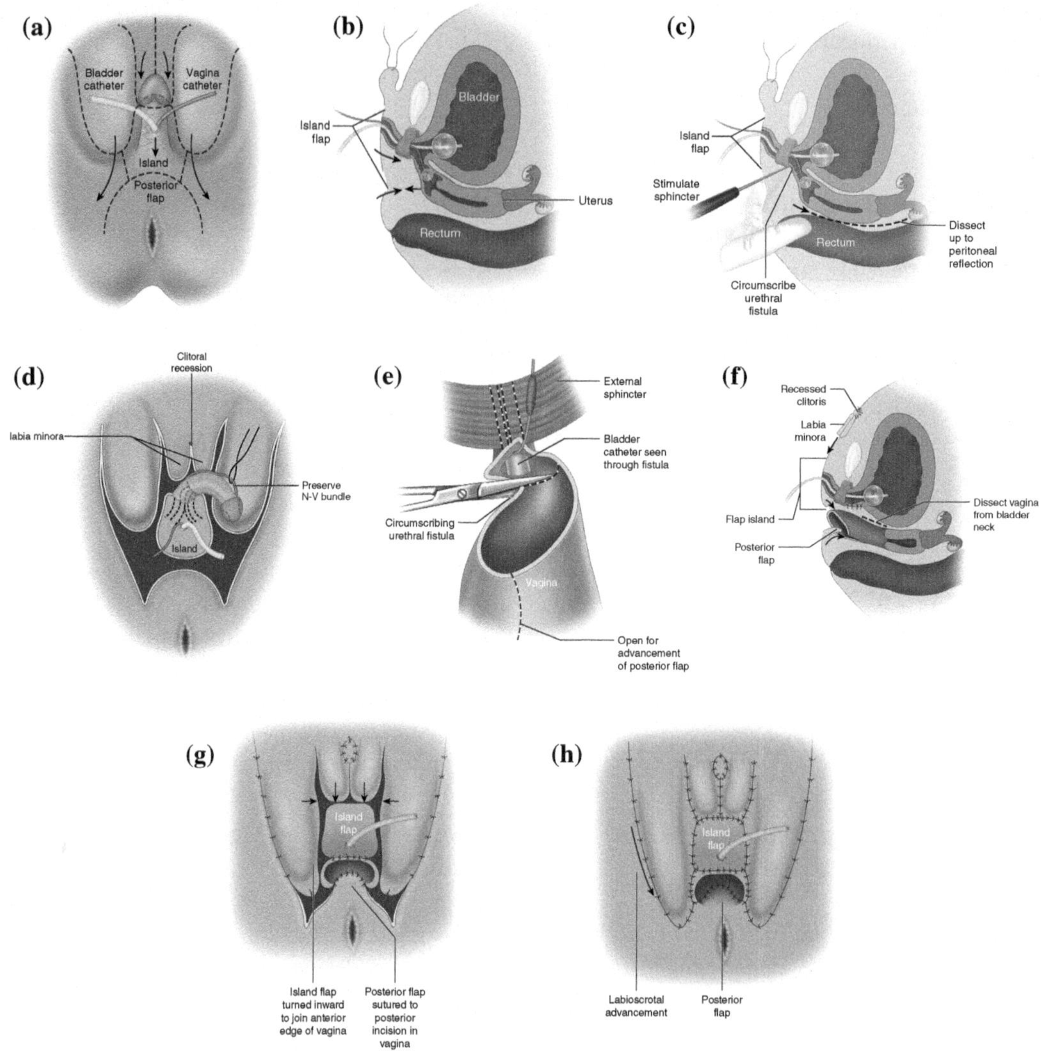

Fig. 18.9 a–h Pull-through vaginoplasty for mid-level vaginal confluence. **a** Locations of incisions viewed from the surgeon's perspective, from the perineum with the patient in the lithotomy position. **b** Sagittal view showing the *downward* and *inward* direction of movement of the anterior island flap (*right-pointing arrows*), and the *inward* position of the posterior flap. The *smaller arrow* shows the distance that must be traversed by the vagina, which has been separated from the urethra. **c** Dissection between the vagina and the rectum in a posterior direction and the beginning of the anterior separation of the vagina from the urethra. **d** Completely dissected flaps. **e** Separation of the vagina from the urethra. **f** Anterior plane of dissection behind the urethra and bladder. **g** Advancement of the labioscrotal flaps to cover defects, and *inward* rotation of the *anterior* island flap and the posterior U-flap to augment the introitus. **h** Completed reconstruction. (Adapted from Pieretti RV, Donahoe PK. Disorders of sex development. In: Coran AG, Adzick NS, Krummel TM, et al. (eds)., Pediatric Surgery, 7th ed. Philadelphia, PA: Elsevier, 2012, with permission.)

If the urethral plate cannot be preserved, a multistage repair is indicated. In some cases resection of the ventral tethering tissue and division of the urethral plate may not fully correct the ventral curvature and in these patients a dermal graft at the site of maximal concavity may be needed. The second stage, composite repair, is performed 6–9 months later; using an

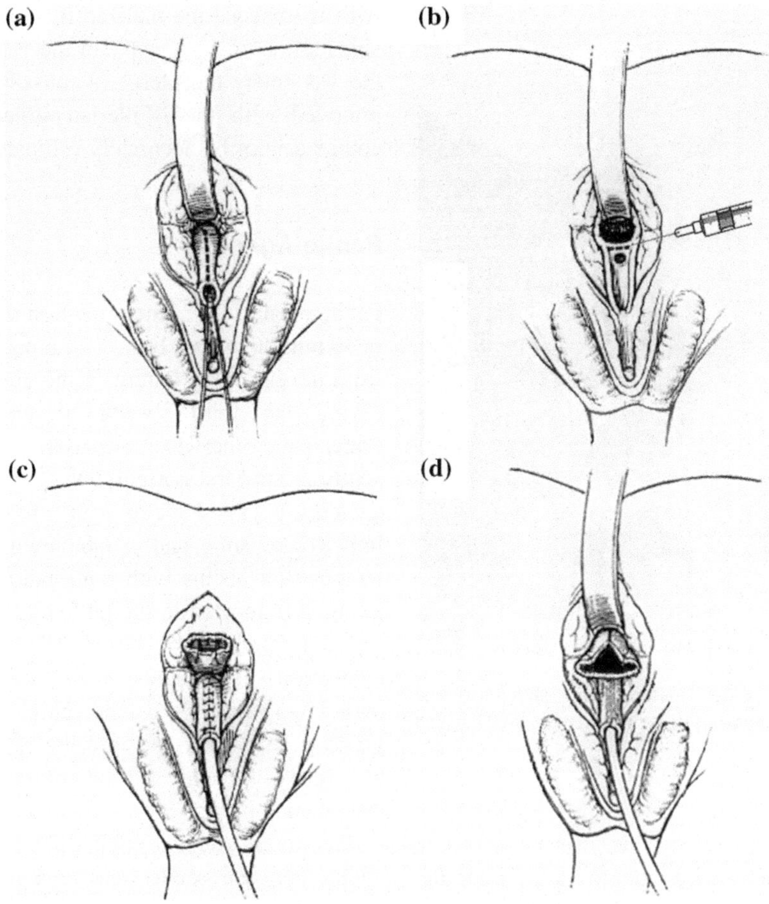

Fig. 18.10 a–d Posterior approach (use of the prone position to facilitate vaginal dissection). **a** The urogenital sinus is opened longitudinally on its posterior or dorsal surface up to the vaginal confluence. **b** A narrow malleable retractor is placed inside the vagina. The vagina is then lifted upward, which facilitates the separation of the vagina from the urethra and bladder neck. Injection of diluted epinephrine (1:200,000) helps the dissection of this fragile, *thin plane*. A small Beaver blade is useful for this difficult step. **c** The urethra is tubularized after the vagina has been separated. **d** The vagina is opened, and the U-flap is inserted to create an enlarged introitus

anterior tubularized incised plate urethroplasty combined with a posterior Thiersch-Duplay procedure (tubularization of local skin to fashion the new urethra). Also, the use of a buccal mucosa graft or an onlay island flap may be needed.

Penoscrotal Transposition

Partial or complete penoscrotal transposition is often found in cases with penoscrotal and perineal hypospadias. The least severe forms are known as bifid scrotum, prepenile scrotum, and shawl scrotum. The scrotoplasty should be delayed for six months or more after the hypospadias repair is completed, because the base of the flaps needed for the hypospadias repair must be divided and displaced during correction of the prepenile scrotum.

Removal of Müllerian Duct Remnants and Creation of a Neoseminal Vesicle

In patients with severe hypospadias, ovotesticular disease or mixed gonadal dysgenesis who have been assigned the male gender, retained Müllerian ducts can become quite enlarged (Fig. 18.11) leading to recurrent urinary tract

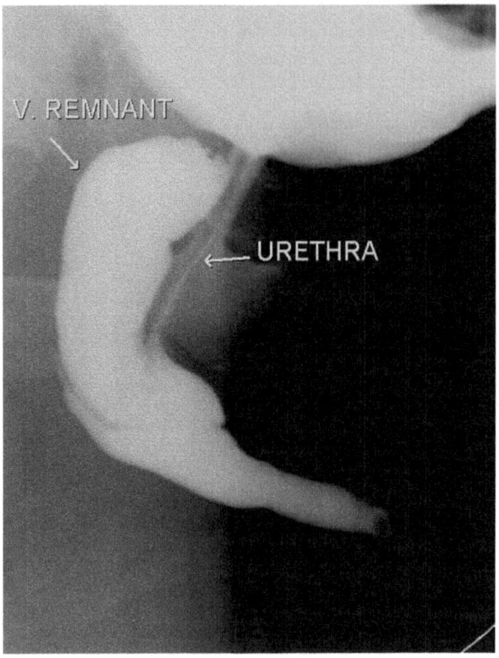

Fig. 18.11 Retrograde urethrogram showing and enlarged vaginal remnant in a patient with MGD reared as a male

infections, epididymo-orchitis, urinary retention, secondary incontinence due to urine trapping, and infertility. In such cases the Müllerian duct remnant should be removed.

Surgical treatment of Müllerian duct remnants is challenging, because of their close proximity to the ejaculatory ducts, pelvic nerves, rectum, vas deferens, and ureters. A number of surgical approaches have been described including transperitoneal, posterior with rectal retraction, anterior and posterior sagittal transrectal, transtrigonal, perineal, and transurethral fulguration, laparoscopic and robotic. We have successfully used the transtrigonal technique; however, the laparoscopic or robotic assisted procedures are less invasive and minimize possible damage to adjacent anatomical structures.

We have preserved the vas deferens if it courses within the outer wall of the dilated vagina [113]. The remainder of the Műllerian structures are removed, including the sometimes markedly dilated vagina. The strip of vaginal wall containing the vas deferens is tubularized with its mucosa internalized from the urogenital sinus to the point of entry of the vas deferens. If the vas enters the uterus, it must be divided or removed with the Müllerian structures, as its course cannot be accurately estimated.

Penile Agenesis

Penile agenesis is a rare condition occurring in 1 in 30 million births [114, 115]. It probably results from development failure of the genital tubercle during the fourth week of embryogenesis. Patients are otherwise normal 46 XY males. The scrotum appears normal and contains normal testicles [116]. Patients can present with an imperforate anus and a rectourethral fistula, a rectourethral fistula with a normal anus, or with the urethra located in the perineum inside a skin tag resembling a foreskin [114]. The diagnostic evaluation of patients with penile agenesis includes a renal ultrasound, pelvic MRI, retrograde urethrogram, and in cases associated with an imperforate anus, a distal colostogram trough the mucous fistula.

Parents of affected children face the difficult choice between gender reassignment and future reconstruction of penile agenesis. In the past gender reassignment was the most common choice, however, long-term follow-up of these patients has revealed that they are unhappy with the assigned female sex, and prefer to be males [117]. The alternative of penile reconstruction requires difficult and often multiple operations.

In adolescents and adults the most frequently used procedure for penile reconstruction is the microvascular transfer radial forearm flap, which is, a complex and rare operation performed only in highly specialized centers. The recent description by De Castro of a phalloplasty technique and complete urethroplasty using a quadrangle lower abdominal flap can bridge the interval between childhood and adolescence until a more definitive procedure can be undertaken [118].

We favor a staged surgical reconstruction. Cases with an associated imperforate anus and a rectourethral fistula require and urgent colostomy with a mucous fistula and a vesicostomy. Later a posterior sagittal rectourethral pull-through is performed and finally closure of the vesicostomy and colostomy. Patients born with a normal anus and a rectourethral fistula can be operated through a transperineal approach. We have used the quadrangle lower abdominal flap to fashion the neopenis in three patients, but we prefer a two-stage buccal mucosa urethroplasty to avoid or minimize complications.

Vaginal Agenesis

Vaginal agenesis is known as the Mayer-Rokitansky-Kuster-Hauser syndrome, it is a rare abnormality affecting approximately 1 in 5000–10,000 females. In this condition there is absence of the proximal portion of the vagina, resulting from failure of the sinovaginal bulbs to develop and form the vaginal plate.

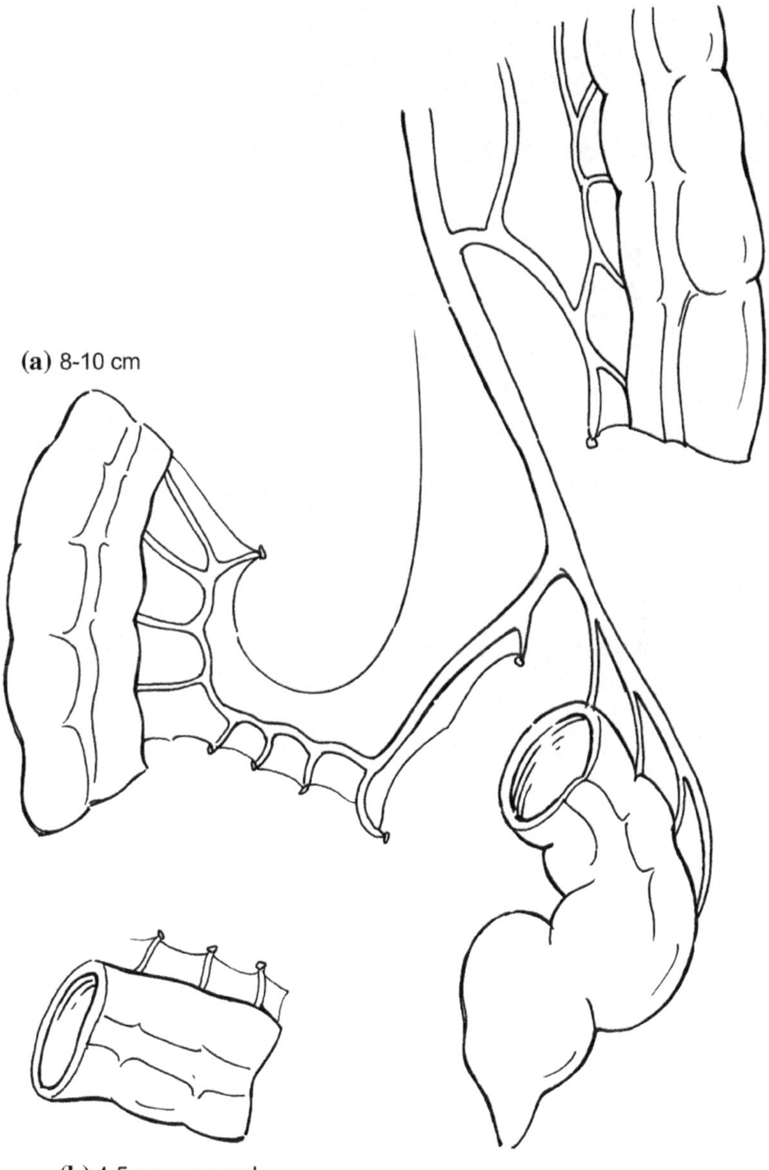

Fig. 18.12 **a** Fashioning of an 8-10 cm sigmoid sleeve. **b** A short distal sigmoid segment can be discarded to provide greater length on the mesenteric vascular pedicle so the neovagina can reach the perineum under no tension. (From Pieretti RV, Donahoe PK. Disorders of sex development. In: Coran AG, Adzick NS, Krummel TM, et al. (eds)., Pediatric Surgery, 7th ed. Philadelphia, PA: Elsevier, 2012, with permission.)

Two different types of Mayer-Rokitansky-Kuster-Hauser syndrome have been described; in the typical variety (type A) patients have symmetrical uterine remnants and normal Fallopian tubes. Cases with the atypical form (Type B) present with asymmetric uterine buds or abnormally developed fallopian tubes. The surgeon must be aware of the differences between the two types, because the majority of associated anomalies of other organs occur in type B patients [119, 120].

Skeletal anomalies are present in up to 12% of females affected with this condition, most commonly in type B cases, including patients with congenital fusion of the cervical vertebra known as the Klippel–Feil syndrome [121]. Duncan proposed the term MURCS association to describe the combination of Müllerian duct aplasia, renal aplasia, and cervicothoracic somite dysplasia [122].

Renal anomalies also present most frequently in patients with the type B variety [120]; these anomalies consist of either unilateral renal agenesis, horseshoe kidney, or ectopia of one or both kidneys which occurs in 74% of affected patients [123].

Vaginal atresia can be discovered at birth when the physical examination does not reveal a vaginal opening but most cases present later in life with primary amenorrhea. A few patients present with dyspareunia or failed intercourse. Physical examination reveals an absent vagina, but the hymen and a distal vaginal dimple or even an introitus are present since these structures are derived from the urogenital sinus. The diagnosis can be confirmed by pelvic ultrasound and magnetic resonance imaging.

Surgical Treatment of Vaginal Agenesis

Treatment of vaginal agenesis may be surgical or nonsurgical. Nonsurgical vaginal dilatation is possible in patients with a vaginal dimple or introitus. It consists of a program of daily, graduated, dilatations over several months and can result in a vagina that will permit intercourse. Once a satisfactory vaginal size is obtained, regular sexual intercourse can maintain an adequate vaginal cavity.

There have been many different techniques for vaginal construction that have been done for patients with vaginal agenesis including the fashioning of a skin neovagina, and the creation of an intestinal neovagina using sigmoid, cecum, or small intestine. Our preferred technique for vaginal replacement is to use a segment of distal sigmoid colon based on the left colic or superior hemorrhoidal vessels (Fig. 18.12a, b). A sigmoid neovagina has several advantages such as natural lubrication, less risk of excessive mucous production, less need for long-term dilations or stents, a lower risk of anastomotic stenosis. Most patients have normal sexual intercourse.

References

1. MacLaughlin DT, Donahoe PK. Sex determination and differentiation. N Engl J Med. 2004;350: 367–78.
2. Ahmed SF, Rodie M. Investigation and initial management of ambiguous genitalia. Best Pract Res Clin Endocrinol Metab. 2009;24:197–218.
3. Taketo T, Saeed J, Manganaro T, Takahashi M, Donahoe PK. Mullerian inhibiting substance production associated with loss of oocytes and testicular differentiation in the transplanted mouse XX gonadal primordium. Biol Reprod. 1993;49:13–23.
4. Federman DD, Donahoe PK. Ambiguous genitalia–etiology, diagnosis, and therapy. Adv Endocrinol Metab. 1995;6:91–116.
5. Arango NA, Donahoe PK. Sex differentiation in mouse and man and subsequent development of the female reproductive organs. Cambridge: Harvard Stem Cell Institute; 2010.
6. Hammes A, Guo JK, Lutsch G, Leheste JR, Landrock D, Ziegler U, Gubler MC, Schedl A. Two splice variants of the Wilms' tumor 1 gene have distinct functions during sex determination and nephron formation. Cell. 2001;106:319–29.
7. Reddy JC, Licht JD. The WT1 Wilms' tumor suppressor gene: how much do we really know? Biochim Biophys Acta. 1996;1287:1–28.
8. Lala DS, Rice DA, Parker KL. Steroidogenic factor I, a key regulator of steroidogenic enzyme expression, is the mouse homolog of fushi tarazu-factor I. Mol Endocrinol. 1992;6:1249–58.
9. Achermann JC, Ito M, Hindmarsh PC, Jameson JL. A mutation in the gene encoding steroidogenic factor-1 causes XY sex reversal and adrenal failure in humans. Nat Genet. 1999;22:125–6.

10. Parker KL, Schimmer BP, Schedl A. Genes essential for early events in gonadal development. Cell Mol Life Sci. 1999;55:831–8.
11. Vainio S, Heikkila M, Kispert A, Chin N, McMahon AP. Female development in mammals is regulated by Wnt-4 signalling. Nature. 1999;397:405–9.
12. Orvis GD, Behringer RR. Cellular mechanisms of Mullerian duct formation in the mouse. Dev Biol. 2007;306:493–504.
13. Carroll TJ, Park JS, Hayashi S, Majumdar A, McMahon AP. Wnt9b plays a central role in the regulation of mesenchymal to epithelial transitions underlying organogenesis of the mammalian urogenital system. Dev Cell. 2005;9:283–92.
14. Hacker N, Moore JG. Essentials of obstetrics and gynecology. Saunders; 1992.
15. Schneider DT, Schuster AE, Fritsch MK, Hu J, Olson T, Lauer S, Gobel U, Perlman EJ. Multipoint imprinting analysis indicates a common precursor cell for gonadal and nongonadal pediatric germ cell tumors. Cancer Res. 2001;61:7268–76.
16. Chang HL, Maclaughlin D, Donahoe PK. Somatic stem cells of the ovary and their relationship to human ovarian cancers. Harvard Stem Cell Institute; 2009.
17. Anderson R, Fassler R, Georges-Labouesse E, Hynes RO, Bader BL, Kreidberg JA, Schaible K, Heasman J, Wylie C. Mouse primordial germ cells lacking beta1 integrins enter the germline but fail to migrate normally to the gonads. Development. 1999;126:1655–64.
18. Buehr M, Gu S, McLaren A. Mesonephric contribution to testis differentiation in the fetal mouse. Development. 1993;117:273–81.
19. Tam PP, Snow MH. Proliferation and migration of primordial germ cells during compensatory growth in mouse embryos. J Embryol Exp Morphol. 1981;64:133–47.
20. Saitou M, Barton SC, Surani MA. A molecular programme for the specification of germ cell fate in mice. Nature. 2002;418:293–300.
21. McLaren A. Mammalian germ cells: birth, sex, and immortality. Cell Struct Funct. 2001;26:119–22.
22. Schnitzer JJ, Donahoe PK. Surgical treatment of congenital adrenal hyperplasia. Endocrinol Metab Clin North Am. 2001;30:137–54.
23. Ha TU, Segev DL, Barbie D, Masiakos PT, Tran TT, Dombkowski D, Glander M, Clarke TR, Lorenzo HK, Donahoe PK, Maheswaran S. Mullerian inhibiting substance inhibits ovarian cell growth through an Rb-independent mechanism. J Biol Chem. 2000;275:37101–9.
24. Hajkova P, Erhardt S, Lane N, Haaf T, El-Maarri O, Reik W, Walter J, Surani MA. Epigenetic reprogramming in mouse primordial germ cells. Mech Dev. 2002;117:15–23.
25. Seki Y, Yamaji M, Yabuta Y, Sano M, Shigeta M, Matsui Y, Saga Y, Tachibana M, Shinkai Y, Saitou M. Cellular dynamics associated with the genome-wide epigenetic reprogramming in migrating primordial germ cells in mice. Development. 2007;134:2627–38.
26. Kimmins S, Sassone-Corsi P. Chromatin remodelling and epigenetic features of germ cells. Nature. 2005;434:583–9.
27. Bowles J, Knight D, Smith C, Wilhelm D, Richman J, Mamiya S, Yashiro K, Chawengsaksophak K, Wilson MJ, Rossant J, Hamada H, Koopman P. Retinoid signaling determines germ cell fate in mice. Science. 2006;312:596–600.
28. Koubova J, Menke DB, Zhou Q, Capel B, Griswold MD, Page DC. Retinoic acid regulates sex-specific timing of meiotic initiation in mice. Proc Natl Acad Sci U S A. 2006;103:2474–9.
29. Ford CE, Jones KW, Polani PE, De Almeida JC, Briggs JH. A sex-chromosome anomaly in a case of gonadal dysgenesis (Turner's syndrome). Lancet. 1959;1:711–3.
30. Jacobs PA, Ross A. Structural abnormalities of the Y chromosome in man. Nature. 1966;210:352–4.
31. Page DC, Mosher R, Simpson EM, Fisher EM, Mardon G, Pollack J, McGillivray B, de la Chapelle A, Brown LG. The sex-determining region of the human Y chromosome encodes a finger protein. Cell. 1987;51:1091–104.
32. Koopman P, Munsterberg A, Capel B, Vivian N, Lovell-Badge R. Expression of a candidate sex-determining gene during mouse testis differentiation. Nature. 1990;348:450–2.
33. Sinclair AH, Berta P, Palmer MS, Hawkins JR, Griffiths BL, Smith MJ, Foster JW, Frischauf AM, Lovell-Badge R, Goodfellow PN. A gene from the human sex-determining region encodes a protein with homology to a conserved DNA-binding motif. Nature. 1990;346:240–4.
34. Koopman P, Gubbay J, Vivian N, Goodfellow P, Lovell-Badge R. Male development of chromosomally female mice transgenic for Sry. Nature. 1991;351:117–21.
35. Foster JW, Dominguez-Steglich MA, Guioli S, Kwok C, Weller PA, Stevanovic M, Weissenbach J, Mansour S, Young ID, Goodfellow PN, et al. Campomelic dysplasia and autosomal sex reversal caused by mutations in an SRY-related gene. Nature. 1994;372:525–30.
36. Tommerup N, Schempp W, Meinecke P, Pedersen S, Bolund L, Brandt C, Goodpasture C, Guldberg P, Held KR, Reinwein H, et al. Assignment of an autosomal sex reversal locus (SRA1) and campomelic dysplasia (CMPD1) to 17q24.3-q25.1. Nat Genet. 1993;4:170–4.
37. Wagner T, Wirth J, Meyer J, Zabel B, Held M, Zimmer J, Pasantes J, Bricarelli FD, Keutel J, Hustert E, et al. Autosomal sex reversal and campomelic dysplasia are caused by mutations in and around the SRY-related gene SOX9. Cell. 1994;79:1111–20.
38. Bardoni B, Zanaria E, Guioli S, Floridia G, Worley KC, Tonini G, Ferrante E, Chiumello G,

McCabe ER, Fraccaro M, et al. A dosage sensitive locus at chromosome Xp21 is involved in male to female sex reversal. Nat Genet. 1994;7:497–501.
39. Nef S, Parada LF. Cryptorchidism in mice mutant for Insl3. Nat Genet. 1999;22:295–9.
40. Hamza AF, Soliman HA, Abdel Hay SA, Kabesh AA, Elbehery MM. Total urogenital sinus mobilization in the repair of cloacal anomalies and congenital adrenal hyperplasia. J Pediatr Surg 2001;36:1656–8.
41. Barbaux S, Niaudet P, Gubler MC, Grunfeld JP, Jaubert F, Kuttenn F, Fekete CN, Souleyreau-Therville N, Thibaud E, Fellous M, McElreavey K. Donor splice-site mutations in WT1 are responsible for Frasier syndrome. Nat Genet. 1997;17:467–70.
42. Wilkie AO, Campbell FM, Daubeney P, Grant DB, Daniels RJ, Mullarkey M, Affara NA, Fitchett M, Huson SM. Complete and partial XY sex reversal associated with terminal deletion of 10q: report of 2 cases and literature review. Am J Med Genet. 1993;46:597–600.
43. Ottolenghi C, Omari S, Garcia-Ortiz JE, Uda M, Crisponi L, Forabosco A, Pilia G, Schlessinger D. Foxl2 is required for commitment to ovary differentiation. Hum Mol Genet. 2005;14:2053–62.
44. Schmidt D, Ovitt CE, Anlag K, Fehsenfeld S, Gredsted L, Treier AC, Treier M. The murine winged-helix transcription factor Foxl2 is required for granulosa cell differentiation and ovary maintenance. Development. 2004;131:933–42.
45. Couse JF, Hewitt SC, Bunch DO, Sar M, Walker VR, Davis BJ, Korach KS. Postnatal sex reversal of the ovaries in mice lacking estrogen receptors alpha and beta. Science. 1999;286:2328–31.
46. Uda M, Ottolenghi C, Crisponi L, Garcia JE, Deiana M, Kimber W, Forabosco A, Cao A, Schlessinger D, Pilia G. Foxl2 disruption causes mouse ovarian failure by pervasive blockage of follicle development. Hum Mol Genet. 2004;13:1171–81.
47. Jost A. Recherches sur la differenciation sexuelle de l'embryon du lapin. Arch Anat Microsc Morphol Exp. 1947;36:271–315.
48. Imperato-McGinley J, Guerrero L, Gautier T, Peterson RE. Steroid 5alpha-reductase deficiency in man: an inherited form of male pseudohermaphroditism. Science. 1974;186:1213–5.
49. Budzik GP, Powell SM, Kamagata S, Donahoe PK. Mullerian inhibiting substance fractionation by dye affinity chromatography. Cell. 1983;34:307–14.
50. Picard JY, Josso N. Purification of testicular anti-Mullerian hormone allowing direct visualization of the pure glycoprotein and determination of yield and purification factor. Mol Cell Endocrinol. 1984;34:23–9.
51. Cate RL, Mattaliano RJ, Hession C, Tizard R, Farber NM, Cheung A, Ninfa EG, Frey AZ, Gash DJ, Chow EP, et al. Isolation of the bovine and human genes for Mullerian inhibiting substance and expression of the human gene in animal cells. Cell. 1986;45:685–98.
52. Cate RL, Donahoe PK, MacLaughlin DT. Mullerian inhibittory substance fractionation by dye affinity chromatography. In: Sporn MB, Roberts AB, editors. Handbook of experimental pharmacology. Berlin: Springer; 1990.
53. Teixeira J, He WW, Shah PC, Morikawa N, Lee MM, Catlin EA, Hudson PL, Wing J, Maclaughlin DT, Donahoe PK. Developmental expression of a candidate mullerian inhibiting substance type II receptor. Endocrinology. 1996;137:160–5.
54. He WW, Gustafson ML, Hirobe S, Donahoe PK. Developmental expression of four novel serine/threonine kinase receptors homologous to the activin/transforming growth factor-beta type II receptor family. Dev Dyn. 1993;196:133–42.
55. Masiakos PT, MacLaughlin DT, Maheswaran S, Teixeira J, Fuller AF Jr, Shah PC, Kehas DJ, Kenneally MK, Dombkowski DM, Ha TU, Preffer FI, Donahoe PK. Human ovarian cancer, cell lines, and primary ascites cells express the human Mullerian inhibiting substance (MIS) type II receptor, bind, and are responsive to MIS. Clin Cancer Res. 1999;5:3488–99.
56. Renaud EJ, MacLaughlin DT, Oliva E, Rueda BR, Donahoe PK. Endometrial cancer is a receptor-mediated target for Mullerian inhibiting substance. Proc Natl Acad Sci U S A. 2005;102:111–6.
57. Barbie TU, Barbie DA, MacLaughlin DT, Maheswaran S, Donahoe PK. Mullerian inhibiting substance inhibits cervical cancer cell growth via a pathway involving p130 and p107. Proc Natl Acad Sci U S A. 2003;100:15601–6.
58. Hoshiya Y, Gupta V, Segev DL, Hoshiya M, Carey JL, Sasur LM, Tran TT, Ha TU, Maheswaran S. Mullerian inhibiting substance induces NFkB signaling in breast and prostate cancer cells. Mol Cell Endocrinol. 2003;211:43–9.
59. Segev DL, Ha TU, Tran TT, Kenneally M, Harkin P, Jung M, MacLaughlin DT, Donahoe PK, Maheswaran S. Mullerian inhibiting substance inhibits breast cancer cell growth through an NFkappa B-mediated pathway. J Biol Chem. 2000;275:28371–9.
60. Segev DL, Hoshiya Y, Stephen AE, Hoshiya M, Tran TT, MacLaughlin DT, Donahoe PK, Maheswaran S. Mullerian inhibiting substance regulates NFkappaB signaling and growth of mammary epithelial cells in vivo. J Biol Chem. 2001;276:26799–806.
61. Belville C, Josso N, Picard JY. Persistence of Mullerian derivatives in males. Am J Med Genet. 1999;89:218–23.
62. Hoshiya M, Christian BP, Cromie WJ, Kim H, Zhan Y, MacLaughlin DT, Donahoe PK. Persistent Mullerian duct syndrome caused by both a 27-bp deletion and a novel splice mutation in the MIS type

II receptor gene. Birth Defects Res A Clin Mol Teratol. 2003;67:868–74.
63. White PC, New MI. Molecular genetics of congenital adrenal hyperplasia. Baillieres Clin Endocrinol Metab. 1988;2:941–65.
64. Lee PA, Houk CP, Ahmed SF, Hughes IA. Consensus statement on management of intersex disorders. Int Consens Conf Intersex Pediatr. 2006;118: e488–500.
65. Miller WL. Steroid 17alpha-hydroxylase deficiency–not rare everywhere. J Clin Endocrinol Metab. 2004;89:40–2.
66. Pang S. Congenital adrenal hyperplasia. Endocrinol Metab Clin North Am. 1997;26:853–91.
67. Pang S, Pollack MS, Loo M, Green O, Nussbaum R, Clayton G, Dupont B, New MI. Pitfalls of prenatal diagnosis of 21-hydroxylase deficiency congenital adrenal hyperplasia. J Clin Endocrinol Metab. 1985;61:89–97.
68. Donahoe PK, Crawford JD, Hendren WH. Management of neonates and children with male pseudohermaphroditism. J Pediatr Surg. 1977;12: 1045–57.
69. Grumbach MM, Hughes IA, Conte FA. Disorders of sex differentiation. In: Larsen PR, Kronenberg HM, Melmed S, Polonsky KS, editors. Williams textbook of endocrinology. Philadelphia: WB Saunders; 2003. p. 842–1002.
70. Lubahn DB, Joseph DR, Sullivan PM, Willard HF, French FS, Wilson EM. Cloning of human androgen receptor complementary DNA and localization to the X chromosome. Science. 1988;240:327–30.
71. Tilley WD, Marcelli M, Wilson JD, McPhaul MJ. Characterization and expression of a cDNA encoding the human androgen receptor. Proc Natl Acad Sci U S A. 1989;86:327–31.
72. Walsh PC, Madden JD, Harrod MJ, Goldstein JL, MacDonald PC, Wilson JD. Familial incomplete male pseudohermaphroditism, type 2. Decreased dihydrotestosterone formation in pseudovaginal perineoscrotal hypospadias. N Engl J Med. 1974; 291:944–9.
73. Koopman P. Sry and Sox9: mammalian testis-determining genes. Cell Mol Life Sci. 1999;55: 839–56.
74. Robboy SJ, Miller T, Donahoe PK, Jahre C, Welch WR, Haseltine FP, Miller WA, Atkins L, Crawford JD. Dysgenesis of testicular and streak gonads in the syndrome of mixed gonadal dysgenesis: perspective derived from a clinicopathologic analysis of twenty-one cases. Hum Pathol. 1982;13: 700–16.
75. Donahoe PK, Crawford JD, Hendren WH. Mixed gonadal dysgenesis, pathogensis, and management. J Pediatr Surg. 1979;14:287–300.
76. Ito M, Yu R, Jameson JL. DAX-1 inhibits SF-1-mediated transactivation via a carboxy-terminal domain that is deleted in adrenal hypoplasia congenita. Mol Cell Biol. 1997;17:1476–83.
77. Engle E, Forbes A. Cytogenetic and clinical findings in 48 patients with congenitally defective or absent ovaries. Medicine 1965;44:135–164.
78. Manuel M, Katayama PK, Jones HW Jr. The age of occurrence of gonadal tumors in intersex patients with a Y chromosome. Am J Obstet Gynecol. 1976;124:293–300.
79. Donahoe PK, Crawford JD, Hendren WH. True hermaphroditism: a clinical description and a proposed function for the long arm of the Y chromosome. J Pediatr Surg. 1978;13:293–301.
80. van Niekerk WA. True hermaphroditism: an analytic review with a report of 3 new cases. Am J Obstet Gynecol. 1976;126:890–907.
81. Nihoul-Fekete C, Lortat-Jacob S, Cachin O, Josso N. Preservation of gonadal function in true hermaphroditism. J Pediatr Surg. 1984;19:50–5.
82. Flatau E, Josefsberg Z, Reisner SH, Bialik O, Iaron Z. Letter: penile size in the newborn infant. J Pediatr. 1975;87:663–4.
83. Hendren WH, Crawford JD. Adrenogenital syndrome: the anatomy of the anomaly and its repair. Some new concepts. J Pediatr Surg. 1969;4:49–58.
84. Donahoe PK, Schnitzer JJ. Evaluation of the infant who has ambiguous genitalia, and principles of operative management. Semin Pediatr Surg. 1996;5:30–40.
85. White PC, New MI. Genetic basis of endocrine disease 2: congenital adrenal hyperplasia due to 21-hydroxylase deficiency. J Clin Endocrinol Metab. 1992;74:6–11.
86. Grumbach MM, Conte FA. Disorders of sexual differentiation. In: Wilson JD, Foster DW, editors. Williams textbook of endocrinology. Philadelphia: WB Saunders; 1985. p. 312–401.
87. Wilson JD, Harrod MJ, Goldstein JL, Hemsell DL, MacDonald PC. Familial incomplete male pseudohermaphroditism, type 1. Evidence for androgen resistance and variable clinical manifestations in a family with the Reifenstein syndrome. N Engl J Med. 1974;290:1097–103.
88. Andersson S, Berman DM, Jenkins EP, Russell DW. Deletion of steroid 5 alpha-reductase 2 gene in male pseudohermaphroditism. Nature. 1991;354:159–61.
89. Imperato-McGinley J, Zhu YS. Androgens and male physiology the syndrome of 5alpha-reductase-2 deficiency. Mol Cell Endocrinol. 2002;198:51–9.
90. Federman DD. Abnormal sexual development: a genetic and endocrine approach to differential diagnosis. Philadelphia and London; 1967.
91. Scully RE. Gonadoblastoma. A review of 74 cases. Cancer. 1970;25:1340–56.
92. Muller J, Skakkebaek NE, Nielsen OH, Graem N. Cryptorchidism and testis cancer. Atypical infantile germ cells followed by carcinoma in situ and invasive carcinoma in adulthood. Cancer. 1984;54:629–34.
93. David M, Forest MG. Prenatal treatment of congenital adrenal hyperplasia resulting from

21-hydroxylase deficiency. J Pediatr. 1984;105: 799–803.
94. Pang SY, Pollack MS, Marshall RN, Immken L. Prenatal treatment of congenital adrenal hyperplasia due to 21-hydroxylase deficiency. N Engl J Med. 1990;322:111–5.
95. Baskin LS, Erol A, Li YW, Liu WH, Kurzrock E, Cunha GR. Anatomical studies of the human clitoris. J Urol. 1999;162:1015–20.
96. Baskin LS. Fetal genital anatomy reconstructive implications. J Urol. 1999;162:527–9.
97. Akman Y, Liu W, Li YW, Baskin LS. Penile anatomy under the pubic arch: reconstructive implications. J Urol. 2001;166:225–30.
98. Crouch NS, Liao LM, Woodhouse CR, Conway GS, Creighton SM. Sexual function and genital sensitivity following feminizing genitoplasty for congenital adrenal hyperplasia. J Urol. 2008;179: 634–8.
99. Yu TJ, Shu K, Kung FT, Eng HL, Chen HY. Use of laparoscopy in intersex patients. J Urol. 1995;154:1193–6.
100. Lima M, Aquino A, Domini M, Ruggeri G, Libri M, Cimador M, Pelusi G. Laparoscopic removal of mullerian duct remnants in boys. J Urol. 2004;171:364–8.
101. Diamond M. Pediatric management of ambiguous and traumatized genitalia. J Urol. 1999;162:1021–8.
102. Sotiropoulos A, Morishima A, Homsy Y, Lattimer JK. Long-term assessment of genital reconstruction in female pseudohermaphrodites. J Urol. 1976;115:599–601.
103. Creighton SM, Minto CL, Steele SJ. Objective cosmetic and anatomical outcomes at adolescence of feminising surgery for ambiguous genitalia done in childhood. Lancet. 2001;358:124–5.
104. Kogan SJ, Smey P, Levitt SB. Subtunical total reduction clitoroplasty: a safe modification of existing techniques. J Urol. 1983;130:746–8.
105. Schober JM, Meyer-Bahlburg HF, Ransley PG. Self-assessment of genital anatomy, sexual sensitivity and function in women: implications for genitoplasty. BJU Int. 2004;94:589–94.
106. Fortunoff S, Lattimer JK, Edson M. Vaginoplasty technique for female pseudohermaphrodites. Surg Gynecol Obstet. 1964;118:545–8.
107. Pena A. Total urogenital mobilization–an easier way to repair cloacas. J Pediatr Surg. 1997;32:263–7; discussion 267–8.
108. Ludwikowski B, Oesch Hayward I, Gonzalez R. Total urogenital sinus mobilization: expanded applications. BJU Int. 1999;83:820-2.
109. Rink RC, Metcalfe PD, Kaefer MA, Casale AJ, Meldrum KK, Cain MP. Partial urogenital mobilization: a limited proximal dissection. J Pediatr Urol. 2006;2:351–6.
110. Donahoe PK, Hendren WH 3rd. Perineal reconstruction in ambiguous genitalia infants raised as females. Ann Surg. 1984;200:363–71.
111. Leslie JA, Cain MP, Rink RC. Feminizing genital reconstruction in congenital adrenal hyperplasia Indian. J Urol. 2009;25:17–26.
112. Snodgrass W, Yucel S. Tubularized incised plate for mid shaft and proximal hypospadias repair. J Urol. 2007;177:698–702.
113. Donahoe PK. Neoseminal vesicle created from retained Mullerian duct to preserve vas as in male infants. J Pediatr Surg. 1988;23:272–4.
114. Skooj S, Belman A. Aphallia its classification and management. J Urol. 1989;141:589.
115. Evans JA, Erdile LB, Greenberg CR, Chudley AE. Agenesis of the penis: patterns of associated malformations. Am J Med Genet. 1999;84:47–55.
116. Skandalakis JE, Gray S, Broecker B. The embryonic basis for the treatment of congenital anomalies. In: Skandalakis JE, Gray S, editors. Embryology for surgeons. Baltimore, MD: Williams & Wilkins; 1994. p. 773–7.
117. Meyer-Bahlburg HF. Gender identity outcome in female-raised 46, XY persons with penile agenesis, cloacal exstrophy of the bladder, or penile ablation. Arch Sex Behav. 2005;34:423–38.
118. De Castro R, Merlini E, Rigamonti W, Macedo A, Jr. Phalloplasty and urethroplasty in children with penile agenesis: preliminary report. J Urol. 2007;177:1112–6; discussion 1117.
119. Strubbe EH, Lemmens JA, Thijn CJ, Willemsen WN, van Toor BS. Spinal abnormalities and the atypical form of the Mayer-Rokitansky-Kuster-Hauser syndrome. Skeletal Radiol. 1992;21:459–62.
120. Strubbe EH, Willemsen WN, Lemmens JA, Thijn CJ, Rolland R. Mayer-Rokitansky-Kuster-Hauser syndrome: distinction between two forms based on excretory urographic, sonographic, and laparoscopic findings. AJR Am J Roentgenol. 1993;160:331–4.
121. Duncan PA. Embryologic pathogenesis of renal agenesis associated with cervical vertebral anomalies (Klippel-Feil phenotype). Birth Defects Orig Artic Ser. 1977;13:91–101.
122. Duncan PA, Shapiro LR, Stangel JJ, Klein RM, Addonizio JC. The MURCS association: Mullerian duct aplasia, renal aplasia, and cervicothoracic somite dysplasia. J Pediatr. 1979;95:399–402.
123. Griffin JE, Edwards C, Madden JD, Harrod MJ, Wilson JD. Congenital absence of the vagina. The Mayer-Rokitansky-Kuster-Hauser syndrome. Ann Intern Med. 1976;85:224–36.

Testis Embryology, Anatomy and Physiology

19

John Hutson

Testicular descent to the scrotum is one of the main hallmarks of male sexual differentiation. It is a complex, multi-staged process with the different stages controlled by separate hormones [1–3]. The testis was not originally descended in vertebrates, but during the evolution of mammals the position of the male gonad has been relocated to the outside of the abdominal cavity. In most modern mammals the testis is now located in a perineal scrotum. By contrast, the scrotum in modern marsupials, such as the Kangaroo and Wallaby, is located in a pre-penile position directly over the external inguinal ring [4]. Scrotal location of the testis is required to provide a specialised, low-temperature environment for optimal physiological function [5].

Testicular Embryology

Early Sexual Development

Before 7–8 weeks of development, gonadal position in males and females is identical. At around this time, activation of the gene on the Y chromosome, known as SRY, triggers the development of the gonad leading to the testis [6, 7]. The genes controlling this process are still mostly unknown, but recent research has identified a number of these genes [6]. Early differentiation of the Sertoli Cells produces the glycoprotein hormone known as Müllerian inhibiting substance (MIS), also known as anti-Müllerian hormone (AMH). MIS/AMH causes regression of the Müllerian ducts that would otherwise form the fallopian tubes, uterus and upper vagina [8]. Testosterone produced by the Leydig cells not only enters the circulation, but also is secreted down the Wolffian duct to cause preservation of the duct itself so that it can continue to differentiate into the epididymis, vas deferens, and seminal vesicle.

The mesonephros regresses just before gonadal development so that the developing testis is left on a mesorchium, which is a peritoneal fold originally covering the urogenital ridge. Cranially, there is a thickening of the peritoneal fold that forms the cranial suspensory ligament. Caudally, the genito-inguinal ligament, also known as the gubernaculum, anchors the urogenital ridge to the inguinal abdominal wall.

J. Hutson (✉)
Department of Paediatrics, University of Melbourne, Melbourne, Australia
e-mail: john.hutson@rch.org.au

J. Hutson
Department of Urology, Royal Children's Hospital, Melbourne, Australia

J. Hutson
Douglas Stephens Surgical Research Laboratory, Melbourne Royal Children's Hospital, Murdoch Children's Research Institute, 50 Flemington Road, Parkville, VIC 3052, Australia

D.J. Ledbetter and P.R.V. Johnson (eds.), *Endocrine Surgery in Children*,
DOI 10.1007/978-3-662-54256-9_19

Transabdominal Testicular Migration

Between 8 and 15 weeks of development the Leydig cells also produce androgens and another hormone, known as insulin-like hormone 3 (INSL3), which causes the enlargement of the caudal end of the gubernaculum [9, 10]. This "swelling reaction" in the gubernaculum of the male holds the testis close to the future inguinal canal during enlargement of the abdominal cavity. By contrast, in the female, the ovary ascends relatively in the abdominal cavity because the female gubernaculum elongates in proportion to the body, as there is no swelling reaction. INSL3 is a newly described hormone, which is an analogue of insulin and relaxin, and is also known as relaxin-like factor [11]. INSL3 was discovered in 1999 when a transgenic mouse with a mutant INSL3 gene was found to have intrabdominal testes [9, 10]. Synthetic INSL3 stimulates the rodent gubernaculum in organ culture, and this is augmented by both testosterone and Müllerian inhibiting substance [12]. The receptor for INSL3 (LGR8 or RFX7) is localised to the gubernaculum during this critical time [13]. Although it is now accepted that INSL3 is the primary hormone controlling the transabdominal phase of testicular descent, it is a relatively uncommon cause of cryptorchidism, as only a small number of children have been identified with mutations of INSL3 or its receptor [14].

Inguinal-Scrotal Testicular Migration

During the second phase of testicular descent, also known as the inguinoscrotal stage, the gubernaculum must migrate from the inguinal region to the scrotum [15]. This occurs between about 25 and 35 weeks of gestation. As the testis is an intra-peritoneal organ on a mesentery, the mesorchium, it must reach the scrotum in a diverticulum of the peritoneum, known as the processus vaginalis. The latter develops inside the gubernaculum as it is elongating towards the scrotum, thus allowing the intrabdominal foetal testis to reach a subcutaneous position within the scrotum. The processus vaginalis divides the gubernaculum into three separate parts. There is an inner central column or cord which attaches to the epididymis and testis, an outer rim containing the developing cremaster muscle, and a distal solid tip, known as the bulb of the gubernaculum [16] (Fig. 19.1).

The inguinoscrotal phase of testicular descent is controlled by androgen [17, 18]. Intriguingly, there is a critical window for androgen effects on this phase, which in a rodent animal model is actually during the transabdominal phase of testicular descent. In foetal rats, the critical time for androgen effects on the second phase of descent is day 16–19 of development [19]. We have hypothesised that this is the time when the central nervous system is masculinised, so that the genitofemoral nerve can direct migration of the gubernaculum by release of calcitonin gene-related peptide (CGRP) [2] (Fig. 19.2). CGRP is known to have several effects on the gubernaculum in rodent models [20]. It was initially shown to cause rhythmic contractility of the cremaster muscle within the gubernaculum, which is suspected to be important for orientation of the direction of migration [21]. It also stimulates mitosis in the tip of the gubernaculum and inhibits apoptosis [22, 23]. However, it was unknown what caused the otherwise inert genito-inguinal ligament to undergo metamorphosis into an actively migrating structure.

We have shown recently that the gubernaculum acquires properties similar to an embryonic limb bud, with development of an active proliferating zone in its tip [24]. In an embryonic limb bud, the trigger for outgrowth comes from the overlying skin known as the apical epidermal ridge [25]. This specialised skin triggers the underlying mesenchyme to begin growing. We wondered, therefore, whether the inguinal skin provided similar signals to the gubernaculum [26]. With this in mind, it is interesting to note that the inguinal skin in marsupials has very special properties similar to a limb bud, as this is the site of the breast development in females and the scrotum in males [4, 27]. Importantly, the gubernaculum in marsupials is attached to the mammary gland in females and the scrotum in males [28]. The ilio-marsupialis muscle in

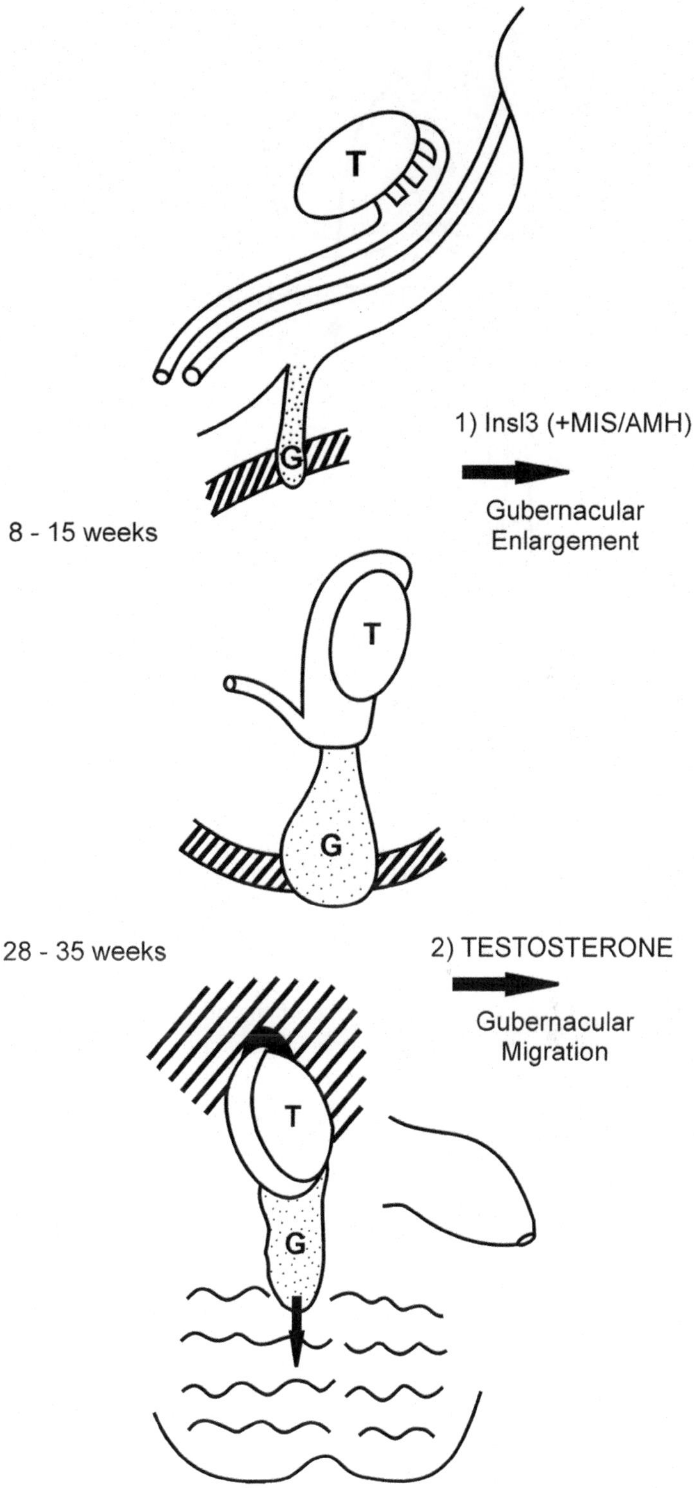

Fig. 19.1 The two stages of testicular descent. Between 8 and 15 weeks the gubernaculum or genito-inguinal ligament enlarges in male embryos under the action of Insl3 [augmented by MIS/AMH (?)]. This "swelling reaction" holds the testis near the groyne as the foetal abdomen enlarges, leading to transabdominal descent relative to the ovarian position. In the inguinoscrotal phase, the gubernaculum migrates out of the external inguinal ring, across the pubic bone and into the scrotum. The testis descends inside the processus vaginalis, which is a peritoneal diverticulum developing inside the gubernaculum. The inguinoscrotal phase is controlled by androgen

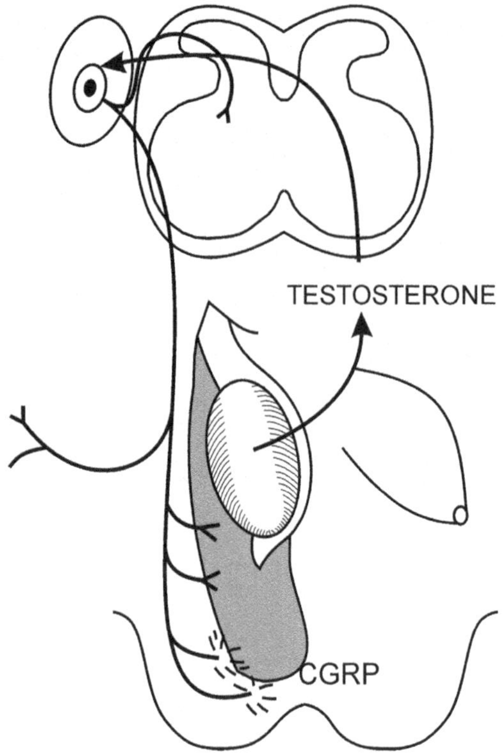

Fig. 19.2 The genitofemoral nerve hypothesis proposed that testosterone acted only indirectly on the gubernaculum by masculinising the genitofemoral nerve, which then produces a specific neurotransmitter (later identified as calcitonen gene-related peptide, CGRP) that is released from the nerve terminals to control gubernacular migration

marsupials is the female homologue of the cremaster muscle, and functions as a suspensory muscle of the nipples.

Relationship Between Gubernaculum and Mammary Bud

This intriguing relationship between the gubernaculum and the mammary gland in the marsupials stimulated us to look more closely at the embryonic rodent to see if there was a link between the gubernaculum and the mammary gland. When we examined the foetal rat and mouse, we found that there was an embryonic mammary bud immediately superficial to the gubernaculum in the inguinal region [29] (Fig. 19.3). In addition, the genitofemoral nerve supplied not only the gubernaculum but also mammary bud [30]. This raised the possibility that the mammary bud may supply signals to the underlying gubernaculum in a way similar to that seen in an embryonic limb bud. We have recently shown that there is expression of hoxa10 and fgf10 in the gubernaculum and the subcutaneous tissue forming the mammary fat pad [31].

At the time that we were investigating the role of the mammary gland and we were also trying to determine the site of androgen receptors that lead to masculinisation of the genitofemoral nerve. Initially, we had assumed that the receptors would be in the nerve itself [32]. As it is the sensory branches of the genitofemoral nerve that are most important for triggering gubernacular development, we looked for androgen receptors in the dorsal root ganglion. To our surprise, there are no androgen receptors in the dorsal root ganglion of the rat until after the critical window of androgen sensitivity on day 19 of foetal development [29]. In addition, there were no androgen receptors in the motor branches of the nerve at this time as well. When we looked at the gubernaculum, we were also surprised to find no androgen receptors until day 19 of development. However, the mammary buds and the adjacent mammary fat pad immediately outside the gubernaculum contained abundant androgen receptors during the critical window of androgen sensitivity [29]. Taking all these findings together, it is quite likely that androgens masculinise the genitofemoral nerve via the target organ, which in this case is the mammary fat pad. This would require the target organ to release a trophic factor that stimulates development of the nerves, which then produce calcitonin gene-related peptide, which is released from the sensory branches of the nerve to control migration of the gubernaculum (Fig. 19.4). There is some precedent for the possibility that target organs may stimulate androgen-sensitive development of the nerves, as the spinal nucleus of the bulbocavernosus is masculinised by a trophic effect from the muscle itself. In this case the trophic factor is brain-derived neurotrophic factor (BDNF) [33]. Whether a similar trophic factor is present in the mammary bud remains to be seen.

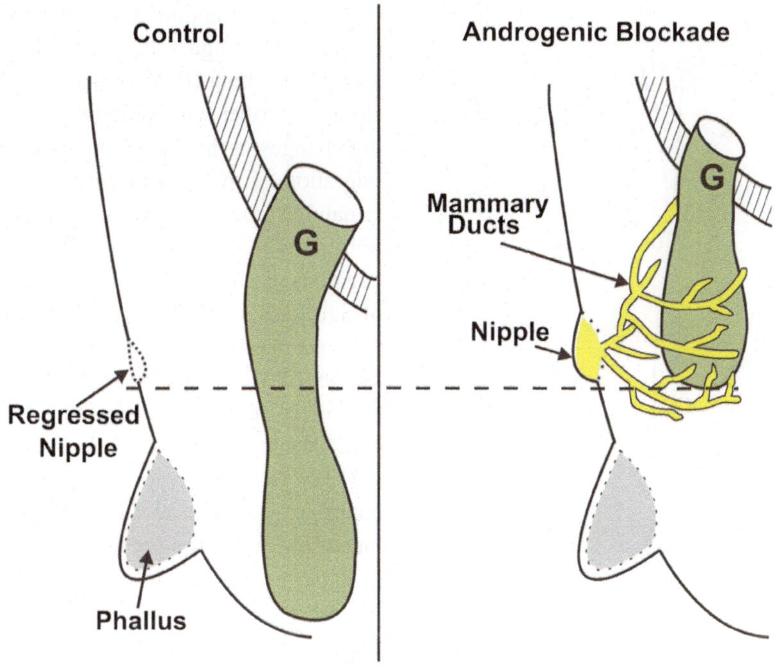

Fig. 19.3 Schema showing normal gubernacular migration from the external inguinal ring to the scrotum in rodents. Note the gubernaculum bypasses the regressing mammary bud and the phallus to reach the scrotum. After androgen blockade (with prenatal flutamide exposure), not only is gubernacular migration impaired, but also the mammary bud persists, and mammary ducts surround the gubernaculum [31]. (From Balic A, Nation T, Buraundi S, et al. Hidden in plain sight: the mammary line in males may be the missing link regulating inguinoscrotal testicular descent. J Pediatr Surg 45(2):414–8; discussion 418, with permission.)

Migration of the gubernaculum through the mammary fat pad requires remodelling of the tissues. We have recently identified that there are some matrix enzymes which are present in the mammary fat pad of the male that are likely to be involved in remodelling to allow gubernacular migration [Churchill et al. 2011]. Once the gubernaculum has reached the scrotum further remodelling is required so that the gubernaculum will become attached to the inside of it. In addition, the proximal processus vaginalis normally obliterates so that the testis can reside in a separate peritoneal cavity within the scrotum.

Patho-Embryology of Abnormal Testicular Descent

Failure of the swelling reaction during the first phase of testicular descent is a relatively rare cause of cryptorchidism. As mentioned previously, only a small number of children with cryptorchidism have been identified with mutations of the gene for INSL3 [14]. In addition, the mechanical process during the first phase of descent is relatively simple, merely requiring stimulation of the gubernaculum to enlarge, thereby anchoring the testis to the future inguinal canal. Given the relative simplicity of these mechanical events, it is not surprising that abnormalities of this process are a relatively rare cause of undescended testis.

By contrast, abnormalities of the inguinoscrotal phase of testicular descent would be expected to be common, given the complexity of the migration process and the large number of regulatory factors that must be involved. The precise location of the defects which lead to undescended testis in most children remain unknown, but we would anticipate that they will

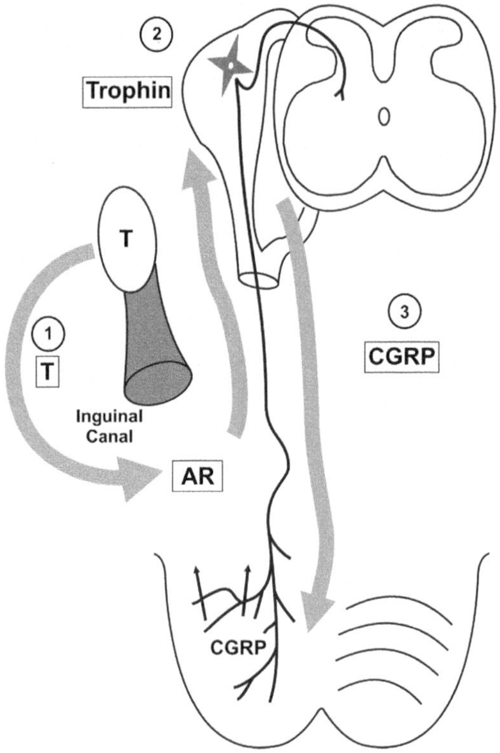

Fig. 19.4 Schema showing our current proposal for how androgens regulate inguinoscrotal descent. In the first step, testosterone (T) acts on androgen receptors (AR) in the inguinal region just outside the inguinal canal and along the mammary line. These androgen-sensitive cells of the mammary line produce a trophic factor that alters the genitofemoral nerve development to produce CGRP, which stimulates and regulates gubernacular migration

reside in the complex migratory process. Further research is required in this area to identify the abnormalities. Finally, failure of remodelling of the connective tissue after migration of the gubernaculum, to allow it to become attached to the inside of the scrotum, may predispose to perinatal torsion.

Anatomy of the Testis

The inguinal canal is formed by the abdominal muscles differentiating around the gubernaculum, which is embedded in the abdominal wall at the site of the future canal [34, 35]. Initially, the inguinal canal is straight, but becomes progressively oblique as the abdominal wall enlarges. During childhood, the inguinal canal remains only 1 cm in length until about 10 years of age, when it begins to elongate further with pubertal development causing changes in the shape of the pelvis [36]. After migration of the gubernaculum is complete, the remaining mesenchyme differentiates into the fibrous layers of the spermatic cord. The processus vaginalis should have obliterated fully by 6 months of age [37], which allows the spermatic cord to elongate in proportional to growth of the boy. The failure of the processus vaginalis to obliterate completely prevents elongation of the spermatic cord, leading to an acquired undescended testis [37, 38]. Acquired cryptorchidism has remained a controversial issue [39–42] (Fig. 19.5) but there is increasing general agreement that it is common [43].

The scrotal testis remains within its satellite peritoneal cavity, the tunica vaginalis, on a short mesentery, the mesorchium. This provides the testis with considerable mobility, but the mesentery is short enough to prevent testicular torsion. In boys where the mesentery of the testis is abnormally long there is a higher risk of torsion, which is most likely after the onset of puberty when the testis has enlarged.

When the testis fails to descend, it is important to remember that the primary abnormality is failure of gubernacular migration. This leaves the testis in the groin, but still within its tunica vaginalis, so that it is quite mobile within its peritoneal cavity. The external inguinal ring is usually quite a narrow opening after the testis has passed through it, however, when the testis is inside the inguinal canal the external ring is usually widely open. This can be determined on physical examination as a palpable triangular defect in the external oblique aponeurosis.

In most instances the cryptorchid testis is relatively normal, but becomes progressively dysplastic with the passage of time, secondary to the detrimental effects of the abnormal high temperature. In only a small percentage of cases is the testis itself abnormal, such as in children with disorders of sex development with primary testicular dysplasia.

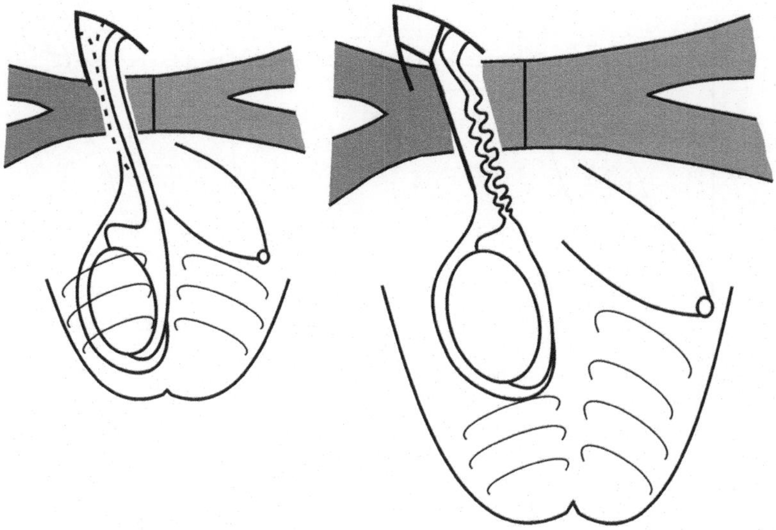

Fig. 19.5 In acquired cryptorchidism the persistence of the obliterated processus vaginalis (or an abnormal cremaster muscle in cerebral palsy) prevents normal elongation of the spermatic cord between birth and puberty. The net effect is the appearance of a descended testis gradually retracting out of the scrotum, when the testis is probably just stationary as the scrotum grows further away from the groin with age

Physiology of the Testis

During foetal development the testis produces several hormones to control its own development. These include MIS/AMH to trigger regression of the Müllerian ducts, INSL3 to stimulate the swelling reaction of the gubernaculum, and testosterone to stimulate regression of the cranial suspensory ligament and migration of the gubernaculum (see Fig. 19.1). Initially hormone production is independent of the hypothalamic-pituitary axis, and was thought to be autonomous. However, there is now evidence that the placenta may stimulate testicular hormones between 8 and 15 weeks of development [44].

After birth the testis is initially quiescent, but after about 2 months of age it begins responding to hypothalamic and pituitary hormones [45, 46]. This leads to postnatal surges in testosterone and MIS/AMH, and possibly other hormones, which collectively control postnatal germ cell development (Fig. 19.6). At birth the germ cell in the testis is a neonatal gonocyte, which resides in the centre of the tubule. Somewhere between 3 and 6 months of age, the gonocyte transforms into a type-A spermatogonium, which resides under the Sertoli cells on the basement membrane of the testicular tubule. Over the next 3 to 4 years, the spermatogonia mature further and eventually migrate back into the centre of the tubule where they become primary spermatocytes. The primary spermatocytes thereafter remain quiescent until puberty, when they mature further into spermatids with the onset of sexual maturation.

When the testis is cryptorchid, the gonocyte fails to transform into a spermatogonium, probably secondary to cellular dysfunction caused by the abnormal temperature [47–49]. Where there are insufficient spermatogonia, which are now thought to be the stem cells for subsequent spermatogenesis, there is a risk of subsequent infertility if there is no treatment [50]. The gonocytes which fail to transform would normally undergo apoptosis, which is probably a normal evolutionary process to eliminate abnormal gonocytes that contain some potential mutation [51]. In cryptorchidism the gonocytes did not undergo apoptosis in the normal manner, presumably also caused by abnormal temperature, and they are therefore left stranded in the postnatal testis. It is

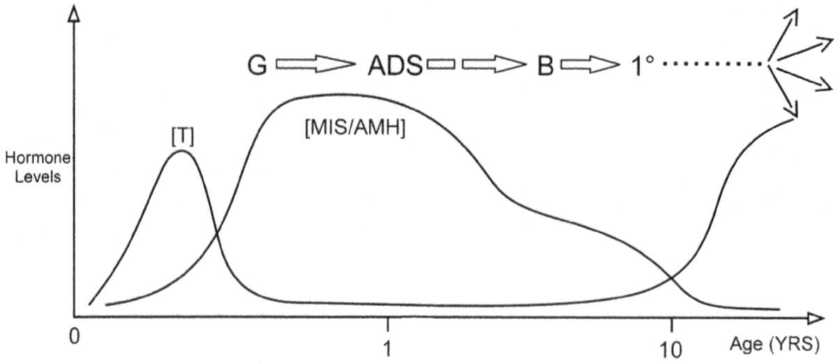

Fig. 19.6 Normal postnatal testicular hormone production relative to germ cell development. Schema showing "minipuberty" in 2–6-month-old boys with a transient peak in androgen production, followed by a sustained peak in MIS/AMH production till puberty. The postnatal gonocyte (G) transforms into a type-A dark spermatogonium (ADS) in the first year, possibly triggered by these hormonal changes. Later the germ cells mature into type B spermatogonia (B) and then into primary spermatocytes (1°), which is the resting germ cells until spermatogenesis is triggered at puberty

these persisting gonocytes which are thought to undergo progressive mutation which might eventually lead to carcinoma-in-situ and eventually malignant degeneration [52].

References

1. Barteczko KJ, Jacob MI. The testicular descent in human. Origin, development and fate of the gubernaculum Hunteri, processus vaginalis peritonei, and gonadal ligaments. Adv Anat Embryol Cell Biol. 2000;156:III–X, 1–98.
2. Hutson J, Hasthorpe S. Testicular descent and cryptorchidism: the state of the art in 2004. J Pediatr Surg. 2005;40:297–302.
3. Hutson JM, Hasthorpe S, Heyns CF. Anatomical and functional aspects of testicular descent and cryptorchidism. Endocr Rev. 1997;18(2):259–80.
4. Renfree MB, Harry JL, Shaw G. The marsupial male: a role model for sexual development. Philos Trans R Soc Lond B Biol Sci. 1995;350(1333):243–51.
5. Zorgniotti A. Temperature and environmental effects on the testis. New York: Plenum Press; 1991.
6. Bernard P, Harley VR. Wnt4 action in gonadal development and sex determination. Int J Biochem Cell Biol. 2007;39(1):31–43.
7. Sinclair AH, Berta P, Palmer MS, et al. A gene from the human sex-determining region encodes a protein with homology to a conserved DNA-binding motif. Nature. 1990;346(6281):240–4.
8. MacLaughlin DT, Donahoe PK. Sex determination and differentiation. N Engl J Med. 2004;350(4):367–78.
9. Nef S, Parada LF. Cryptorchidism in mice mutant for Insl3. Nat Genet. 1999;22(3):295–9.
10. Zimmermann S, Steding G, Emmen JM, et al. Targeted disruption of the Insl3 gene. Mol Endocrinol. 1999;13(5):681–91.
11. Ivell R, Einspanier A. Relaxin peptides are new global players. Trends Endocrinol Metab. 2002;13 (8):343–8.
12. Kubota Y, Temelcos C, Bathgate R, et al. The role of insulin 3, testosterone, Mullerian inhibiting substance and relaxin in rat gubernacular growth. Mol Hum Reprod. 2002;8:900–5.
13. Fu P, Layfield S, Ferraro T, et al. Synthesis, conformation, receptor binding and biological activities of monobiotinylated human insulin-like peptide 3. J Pept Res. 2004;63(2):91–8.
14. Ferlin A, Zuccarello D, Garolla A, et al. Hormonal and genetic control of testicular descent. Reprod Biomed Online. 2007;15(6):659–65.
15. Heyns C. The gubernaculum during testicular descent in the human fetus. J Anat. 1987;153:93–112.
16. Wensing C. Testicular descent in some domestic mammals. I. Anatomical aspect of testicular descent. Proc Kon Nederlande Akad Von Wetenschappen. 1968;71:423–34.
17. Hutson J. A biphasic model for the hormonal control of testicular descent. Lancet. 1985;2(8452):419–20.
18. Hutson J. Testicular feminisation—a model for testicular descent in mice and men. J Pediatric Surg. 1986;21:195–8.
19. Welsh M, Saunders PT, Fisken M, et al. Identification in rats of a programming window for reproductive tract masculinization, disruption of which leads to hypospadias and cryptorchidism. J Clin Invest. 2008;118(4):1479–90.
20. Hutson J. Pathophysiology of testicular descent: updates from experimental models. Asian J Surg. 1999;22(2):131–5.
21. Park W-H, Hutson J. A new inbred rat strain (TS) with suprainguinal ectopic testes: a model for

human cryptorchidism. Pediatr Surg Int. 1991;6:172–5.
22. Chan JJ, Farmer PJ, Southwell BR, et al. Calcitonin gene-related peptide is a survival factor, inhibiting apoptosis in neonatal rat gubernaculum in vitro. J Pediatr Surg. 2009;44(8):1497–501.
23. Yong EX, Huynh J, Farmer P, et al. Calcitonin gene-related peptide stimulates mitosis in the tip of the rat gubernaculum in vitro and provides the chemotactic signals to control gubernacular migration during testicular descent. J Pediatr Surg. 2008;43(8):1533–9.
24. Huynh J, Shenker NS, Nightingale S, et al. Signalling molecules: clues from development of the limb bud for cryptorchidism? Pediatr Surg Int. 2007;23(7):617–24.
25. Muneoka K, Han M, Gardiner DM. Regrowing human limbs. Sci Am. 2008;298(4):56–63.
26. Veltmaat JM, Mailleux AA, Thiery JP, et al. Mouse embryonic mammogenesis as a model for the molecular regulation of pattern formation. Differentiation. 2003;71(1):1–17.
27. Coveney D, Shaw G, Hutson JM, et al. The development of the gubernaculum and inguinal closure in the marsupial *Macropus eugenii*. J Anat. 2002;201(3):239–56.
28. Griffiths M, Slater E. The significance of striated muscle in the mammary glands of marsupials. J Anat. 1988;156:141–56.
29. Nation TR, Balic A, Southwell BR, et al. The hormonal control of testicular descent. Pediatr Endocrinol Rev. 2009;7(1):22–31.
30. Balic A, Nation T, Buraundi S, et al. Hidden in plain sight: the mammary line in males may be the missing link regulating inguinoscrotal testicular descent. J Pediatr Surg 2010;45(2):414–8; discussion 418.
31. Nightingale SS, Western P, Hutson JM. The migrating gubernaculum grows like a "limb bud". J Pediatr Surg. 2008;43(2):387–90.
32. Schwindt B, Farmer P, Watts L, et al. Localization of calcitonin gene-related peptide (CGRP) within the genitofemoral nerve (GFN) in immature rats. J Pediatr Surg. 1999;34:986–91.
33. Al-Shamma HA, Arnold AP. Brain-derived neurotrophic factor regulates expression of androgen receptors in perineal motoneurons. Proc Natl Acad Sci U S A. 1997;94(4):1521–6.
34. Biasutto SN, Repetto E, Aliendo MM, et al. Inguinal canal development: the muscular wall and the role of the gubernaculum. Clin Anat. 2009;22(5):614–8.
35. Niikura H, Okamoto S, Nagase S, et al. Early development of the human gubernaculum revisited. Clin Anat. 2008;21:547–57.
36. Parnis SJ, Roberts JP, Hutson JM. Anatomical landmarks of the inguinal canal in prepubescent children. Aust N Z J Surg. 1997;67(6):335–7.
37. Clarnette T, Hutson J. The genitofemoral nerve may link testicular inguinoscrotal descent with congenital inguinal hernia. Aust NZ J Surg. 1996;66(9):612–7.
38. Clarnette T, Lam S, Hutson J. Ventriculo-peritoneal shunts in children reveal the natural history of closure of the processus vaginalis. J Pediatr Surg. 1998;33:413–6.
39. Agarwal PK, Diaz M, Elder JS. Retractile testis–is it really a normal variant? J Urol. 2006;175(4):1496–9.
40. Donaldson K, Tong S, Washburn T, et al. Morphometric study of the gubernaculum in male estrogen receptor mutant mice. J Androl. 1996;17(2):91–5.
41. Guven A, Kogan BA. Undescended testis in older boys: further evidence that ascending testes are common. J Pediatr Surg. 2008;43(9):1700–4.
42. Redman JF. The ascending (acquired undescended) testis: a phenomenon? BJU Int. 2005;95(9):1165–7.
43. Wohlfahrt-Veje C, Boisen KA, Boas M, et al. Acquired cryptorchidism is frequent in infancy and childhood. Int J Androl. 2009;32(4):423–8.
44. Kaplan SL, Grumbach MM, Aubert ML. The ontogenesis of pituitary hormones and hypothalamic factors in the human fetus: maturation of central nervous system regulation of anterior pituitary function. Recent Prog Horm Res. 1976;32:161–243.
45. Baker SS, Liptak GS, Colletti RB, et al. Constipation in infants and children: evaluation and treatment. A medical position statement of the North American Society for Pediatric Gastroenterology and Nutrition. J Pediatr Gastroenterol Nutr. 1999;29(5):612–26.
46. Gendrel D, Roger M, Job J-C. Plasma gonadotropin and testosterone values in infants with cryptorchidism. J Pediatr. 1980;97:217–20.
47. Hadziselimovic F, Huff D. Gonadal differentiation–normal and abnormal testicular development. Adv Exp Med Biol 2002;511:15–21; discussion 21–3.
48. Huff D, Fenig D, Canning D, et al. Abnormal germ cell development in cryptorchidism. Karger. 2001;55:11–7.
49. Mieusset R, Fonda P, Vaysse P, et al. Increase in testicular temperature in case of cryptorchidism in boys. Fertil Steril. 1993;59:1319–21.
50. Ong C, Hasthorpe S, Hutson JM. Germ cell development in the descended and cryptorchid testis and the effects of hormonal manipulation. Pediatr Surg Int. 2005;21(4):240–54.
51. Giwercman A, Hansen L, Skakkebaek N. Initiation of sperm production after bilateral orchiopexy: clinical and biological implications. J Urol. 2000;163:1255–6.
52. Jorgensen N, Rajpert-De-Meyts E, Graem N, et al. Expression of immunohistochemical markers for testicular carcinoma in situ by normal human fetal germ cells. Lab Invest. 1995;72:223–31.

Surgical Considerations of Testicular Maldescent

20

John Hutson

Normal Postnatal Development of the Testis

Immediately after birth, the testis is physiologically quiescent, while the cells readjust to the sudden change in temperature from the 37 °C environment of the uterus to the 33 °C of the neonatal scrotum. The germ cells, known as neonatal gonocytes, are large cells occupying the centre of the seminiferous cords, and surrounded by Sertoli cells, which are aligned along the basement membrane. Outside the cords, the Leydig cells, which were actively producing testosterone prenatally, become inactive [1].

In the first few weeks postnatally, many testes not already in the scrotum will continue their descent to reach a scrotal position. In boys born prematurely before testicular descent is normally complete this process is common, but it also occurs frequently in term babies. This "delayed descent" postnatally accounts for the difference in incidence of undescended testes being reported as 4–5% at birth, but only 1–2% at 6–12 months [2, 3].

Testes that arrive late in the scrotum may not reach the most dependent part, and remain "high scrotal", which is thought to be a risk factor for later need for orchidopexy [2, 3]. In addition late-descending testes are known to carry a higher risk than fully descended testes at term of being undescended later in childhood, the so-called acquired undescended testis [3] (see below).

After the testis has descended, the proximal processus vaginalis is programmed to close, leaving the testis inside a small satellite peritoneal cavity within the hemiscrotum. By study of the frequency of hydrocele in babies with hydrocephalus and ventriculoperitoneal shunts, we were able to show a steep decline in frequency of hydrocele after 6 months of age, consistent with this being the upper limit of normal time of closure [4].

At 2–3 months of age the neonatal hypothalamus begins producing gonadotrophin-releasing hormone which triggers the pituitary gland to secrete luteinising hormone (LH) and follicle-stimulating hormone (FSH), which produces a sudden surge in the gonadotrophin blood levels between 3 and 6 months of age [5, 6]. The postnatal testis, which presumably has now adapted to its new low-temperature environment, secretes high levels of testosterone [7]. The serum androgen levels between 3 and 6 months of age are transiently similar to early puberty, and hence this brief postnatal hormone surge is

J. Hutson (✉)
Department of Paediatrics, University of Melbourne, Melbourne, Australia
e-mail: john.hutson@rch.org.au

J. Hutson
Department of Urology, Royal Children's Hospital, Melbourne, Australia

J. Hutson
Douglas Stephens Surgical Research Laboratory, Melbourne Royal Children's Hospital, Murdoch Childrens Research Institute, 50 Flemington Road, Parkville, VIC 3052, Australia

D.J. Ledbetter and P.R.V. Johnson (eds.), *Endocrine Surgery in Children*,
DOI 10.1007/978-3-662-54256-9_20

known as "mini-puberty" [7]. By 6 months the androgen levels are falling, and then remain extremely low throughout the rest of childhood until the onset of adolescent sexual maturation.

Another hormone that increases during "mini-puberty" is Müllerian inhibiting substance (MIS), or anti-Müllerian hormone (AMH). MIS/AMH levels increase in the blood at about 4 months of age, and remain high until about 1 year; they then decline gradually until 10–11 years of age when they fall suddenly to low levels at the onset of puberty [8, 9]. The function of MIS/AMH throughout childhood is unknown, but it is quite possible that it has a role in maintaining testicular physiology in its prepubertal state. Beyond puberty and with the onset of the blood–testis barrier, the Sertoli cells continue to secrete MIS/AMH, but most of it is now exocrine rather than endocrine, and is found in the seminal fluid. It is likely to have functions in maintaining the sperm, although this remains to be investigated.

It has been proposed that the primary function of "mini-puberty" is to initiate postnatal germ cell development, and it has been assumed that this is regulated by testosterone [10]. However, this is likely to be a more complex situation, as germ cell development is initially normal in neonatal TFM mice with complete androgen insensitivity and is responsive to AMH/MIS [11]. Which hormone (or hormones) controls postnatal germ cell development remains to be determined, and could have important therapeutic implications for improving fertility outcomes in cryptorchidism.

Germ cell development after birth is now recognised as a key event in both normal testicular maturation and in cryptorchidism. It was initially assumed that no germ cell development occurred until puberty, as the postnatal testis appeared completely inactive compared with postpubertal spermatogenesis. Certainly with regard to the speed of spermatogenesis in adolescence, the postnatal testis seemed completely inert, yet it has been gradually appreciated that key developmental changes were occurring, but at a much slower rate than after puberty. The neonatal gonocytes slowly migrate to the periphery of the spermatic cords at 3–6 months of age to make contact with the basement membrane. They then take on the morphology of type-A spermatogonia, which are now thought to be the so-called adult-dark spermatogonia (AD-S) of the postpubertal testis. These latter cells are considered to be the stem cells for spermatogenesis [12–14]. The AD-spermatogonia gradually develop into B-spermatogonia and then primary spermatocytes, which appear at 3–4 years of age and occupy the centre of the tubercle, as did the neonatal gonocyte just after birth.

Studies of the total germ cell numbers in the postnatal testis show that the lowest numbers are at 1–2 years of age, as it appears that not all postnatal gonocytes transform into AD-spermatogonia [6]. Given the importance of the stem cell population for subsequent fertility, it is quite likely that there is a screening process occurring, such that any germ cell that does not have optimal genetics or physiology is directed to undergo apoptosis rather than transformation. This could be the first step in "survival of the fittest", by only selecting the "best" gonocytes for reproduction (Fig. 20.1).

Postnatal Development in Cryptorchidism

In babies with cryptorchidism the postnatal hormone production by the testis is suppressed [15, 16], and the development of germ cells is interrupted at the first step postnatally, transformation of the gonocytes into AD-spermatogonia

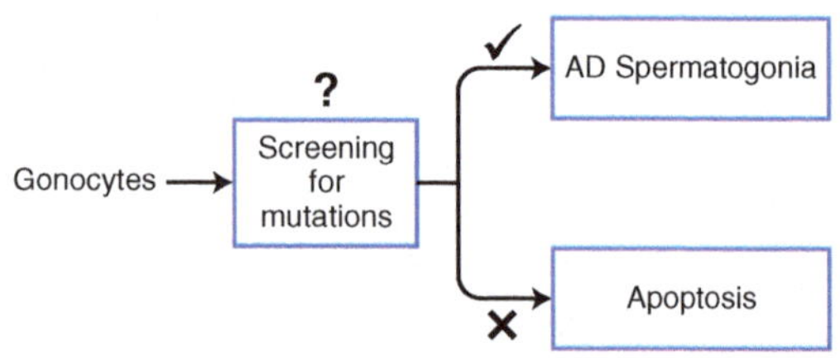

Fig. 20.1 Gonocyte transformation in the first year of life is an incomplete process, with many germ cells failing to transform and then undergoing apoptosis. It is quite possible that this is a sorting mechanism to select the "best" germ cells to become spermatogenic stem cells

[17, 18]. Whether this failure is related to innate genetic errors in the cryptorchid testis, or secondary to the abnormally high postnatal temperature of the misplaced organ, is unknown, but a secondary anomaly seems more likely [19]. Moreover, the entire management of undescended testes is based precisely on this premise, that the postnatal dysfunction is secondary to the position, and hence reversible with orchidopexy.

Many germ cells that fail to transform into AD-spermatogonia, probably secondary to the abnormal temperature interfering with cellular function, also fail to undergo apoptosis. This is likely to leave a cohort of gonocytes in the testicular tubules well beyond their normal time, and we suspect that they are the origin of the subsequent carcinoma-in-situ (CIS) cells after puberty, as they carry the same enzymatic markers [20]. The CIS cells are thought to be the origin of seminomas in previously cryptorchid men [21–23].

Timing of Orchidopexy

Surgical correction of testicular malposition is based on the assumption that postnatal dysfunction is secondary to abnormal temperature, and hence reversible with orchidopexy. Given that gonocyte transformation to AD-spermatogonia is deranged, orchidopexy should aim to correct this and hence should be performed within the first year of life. The exact optimal time remains unknown.

In the first 3 months after birth in term babies about half the testes not in the scrotum initially will descend. Beyond 12 weeks after term delayed descent becomes rare, therefore timing of orchidopexy should take this into account [24–26]. Also, there is widespread agreement amongst anaesthetists that elective surgery should be delayed until about 6 months, when day surgery is known to be safe, and it is well beyond the neonatal period where there remain some doubts about the long-term effects of general anaesthesia. Taken together, these factors lead to 6 months being our current recommended age for orchidopexy for congenital cryptorchidism, which allows for delayed testicular descent and hopefully is early enough to permit postnatal germ cell maturation before it is too late.

Unfortunately, there are no randomised, controlled trials showing the value of orchidopexy at 6 months of age, given the long lag-time before fertility can be measured. There are, however, promising recent studies using testicular growth (measured by ultrasonography) as a very early surrogate for later fertility. By measuring testicular volume, Kollin et al. [27] have shown that surgery at 9 months is significantly better than at 3 years of age.

The gradual reduction in recommended age for orchidopexy over the past few decades has revealed a second group of cryptorchid testes that present later in childhood. We now understand that these are probably acquired rather than congenital, and that they have some differences in aetiology and outcome.

Acquired Cryptorchidism

The first reports of possible acquired cryptorchidism appeared in the 1970s [28] but more widespread recognition of this phenomenon did not occur until the 1990s [29–32], when a group of children undergoing surgery at 5–10 years of age appeared despite an earlier recommended age for orchidopexy. Initially it was assumed that this was caused by delayed diagnosis of congenital cryptorchidism, however, it gradually became more obvious that in fact it was more likely the first presentation of acquired cryptorchidism.

There is now general acceptance that acquired cryptorchidism is not only a real entity, but also that it is quite common [33]. In some hospital audits, it makes up about half of all the orchidopexies being performed [34]. Prior to recognition of this variant, such children were probably diagnosed as having "retractile testes" [35–37]. The aetiology of acquired cryptorchidism remains uncertain, but may be related to minor androgen deficiency and failure of the processus vaginalis to obliterate completely after birth [30]. Persistence of a fibrous remnant of the processus vaginalis is likely to prevent elongation of the spermatic cord, so that as the boy grew and the scrotum become further away from the external inguinal ring, the testis would be left behind and appear to gradually ascend out of the scrotum [29] (see Fig. 19.5 in Chap. 19).

As the testis is intra-scrotal during the first year, we might anticipate that as a result of normal postnatal germ cell maturation, the gonocytes should have disappeared, and that the AD-spermatogonia should be present in adequate numbers. This would be predicted to lead to a low risk of malignancy, if abnormal gonocytes really are the origin of seminomas in previously cryptorchid testes.This is consistent with recent long-term follow-up of men with previous acquired cryptorchidism, showing no increased incidence of malignancy, but some suppression of fertility [38]. Given the potential prognosis of acquired cryptorchidism, many authors recommend orchidopexy once the testis no longer reaches the scrotum.

Indications for Treatment

The scrotum is a specialised, low-temperature environment which allows optimal postnatal development of the gonocytes and postpubertal spermatogenesis [39]. The temperature of the scrotum is 33 °C, which means that intraabdominal testes are 4 °C away from optimal physiology and intracellular functioning, which is the likely reason for secondary dysplasia. Temperature-dependent dysgenesis is proposed to cause progressive loss of the spermatogonia, leading to subsequent poor sperm counts, while any residual gonocytes might eventually mutate into a seminoma.

Successful surgical placement of the testis into the scrotum is dependent not only on the assumption that the damage is secondary rather than a primary disorder of the testis, but also that early intervention can prevent and/or reverse this. Additionally orchidopexy aims to overcome the cosmetic deformity.

Hormonal treatment has been controversial, since it was first introduced in the 1940s. In the 1970s and 1980s, gonadotrophins or analogues of gonadotrophin-releasing hormone were recommended for making the testis descend, but randomised, controlled trials have failed to substantiate the initial claims of success [40]. In recent years, hormone therapy has made a comeback as a way of improving germ cell development after orchidopexy [41].

However, this new use for hormones has been very controversial [42, 43], with non-randomised studies in support, but no randomised trial available [44] that really provides an evidence base. As a result, hormone therapy should be avoided until there is definitive evidence of its efficacy.

Surgical Management

The choice of surgical approach depends on the type or location of the cryptorchid testis. Congenital undescended testes can be categorised into palpable and impalpable, with standard inguinal orchidopexy for the former and laparoscopy for the latter. For acquired cryptorchidism the scrotal approach described by Bianchi is useful [45], and some surgeons would recommend this approach for many palpable congenital undescended testes.

Inguinal Orchidopexy

After an inguinal incision the testis within the tunica vaginalis is mobilised and the inguinal canal opened (Fig. 20.2). The distal attachment of the gubernaculum is divided and the cremaster muscle stripped off the spermatic cord (Fig. 20.3). The vas deferens and the testicular vessels are carefully separated from the processus vaginalis, (Fig. 20.4) which is transfixed and ligated at the internal inguinal ring (Fig. 20.5). The retroperitoneal space cranial to the internal ring is opened up so that the vas and particularly the vessels can be freed up from fibrous adhesions preventing stretching out their length. This is usually enough to achieve adequate length, but occasionally the cord structures need to be

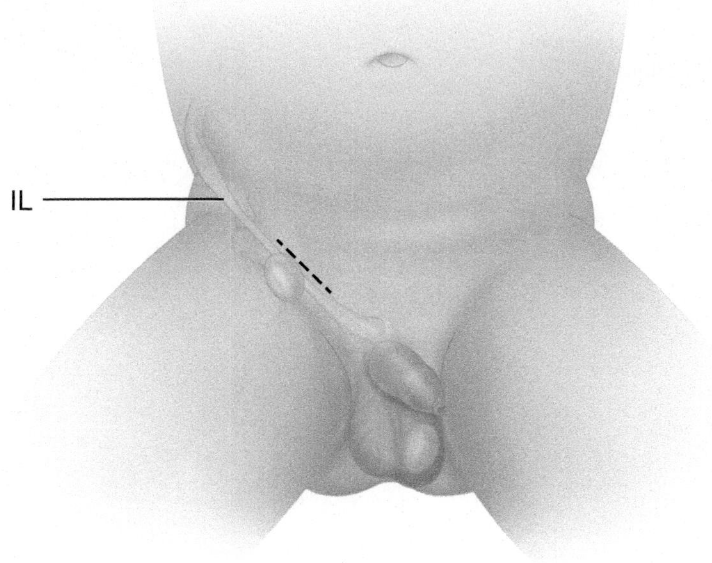

Fig. 20.2 Inguinal skin crease incision

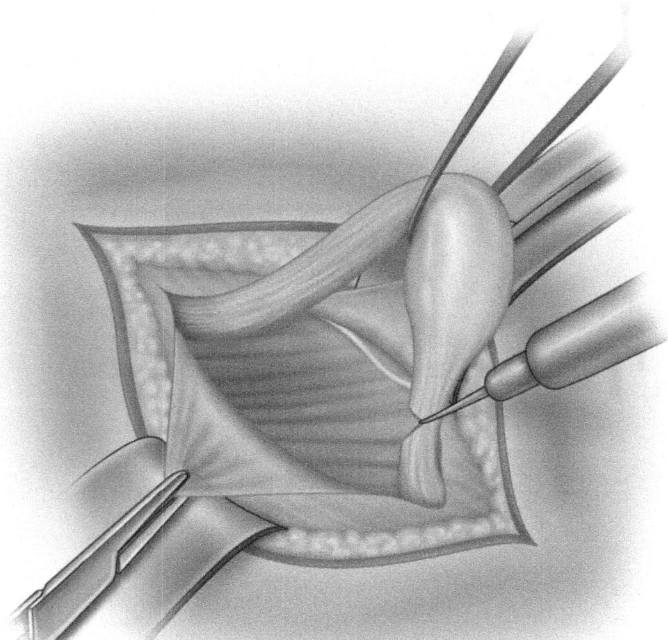

Fig. 20.3 The cremaster muscle fibres are stripped off the cord, allowing the gubernacular attachment to be divided

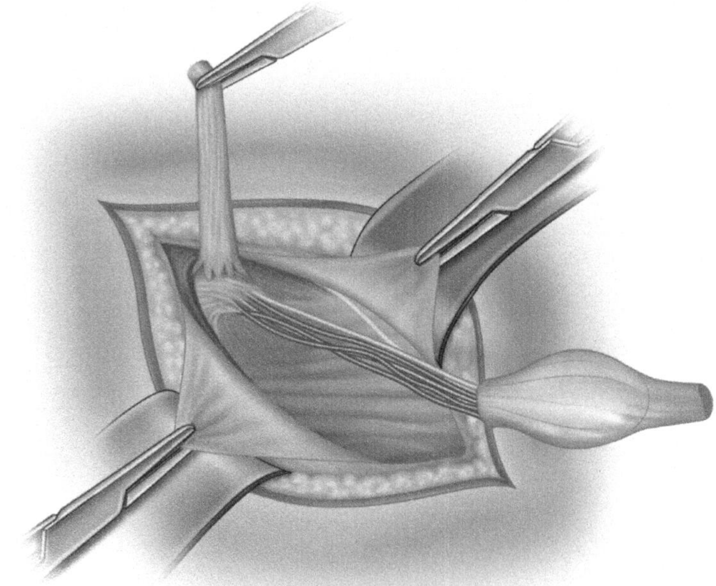

Fig. 20.4 The sac is stretched over the index finger while dissecting forceps gently brush off the other cord structures

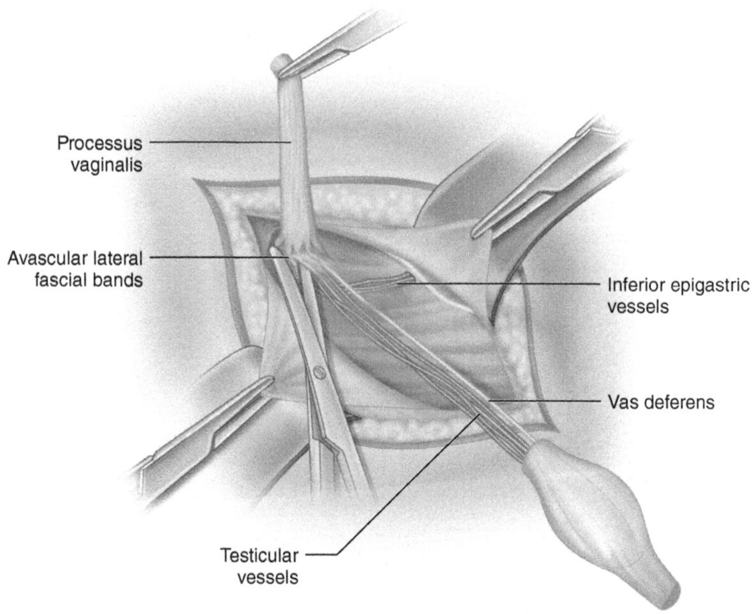

Fig. 20.5 Once separated from the vas deferens and vessels, the sac is transfixed and ligated at the internal inguinal ring

brought down medial to the inferior epigastric vessels, either by buttonholing the transversalis fascia or by ligating and dividing the vessels to pull the cord medially (Fig. 20.6).

The subcutaneous path to the scrotum is made by blunt dissection, usually with a finger (Fig. 20.7), and the scrotum is opened to develop a dartos pouch large enough for the testis. An

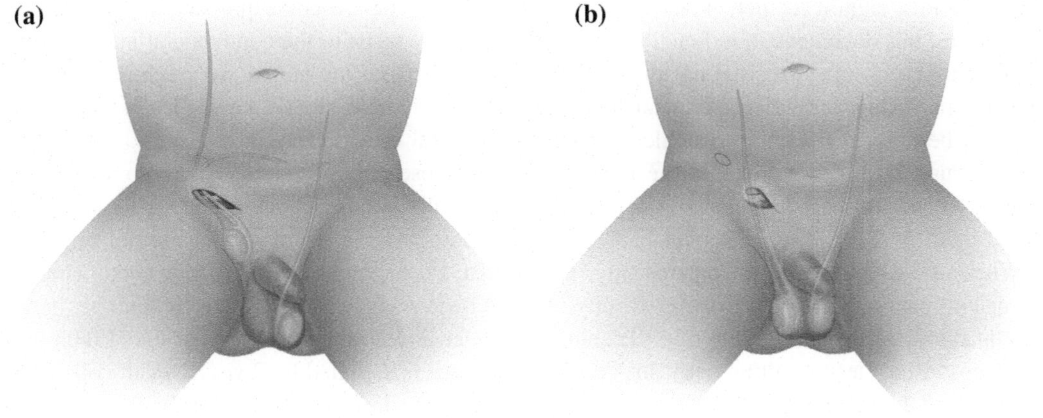

Fig. 20.6 **a** Transposition of the cord structures medial to the inferior epigastric vessels (known as the Prentiss manoeuvre) allows the spermatic cord to take a more direct path to the external ring. **b** The Prentiss manoeuvre increases the relative length of the spermatic cord by at least 1cm, even in infants.

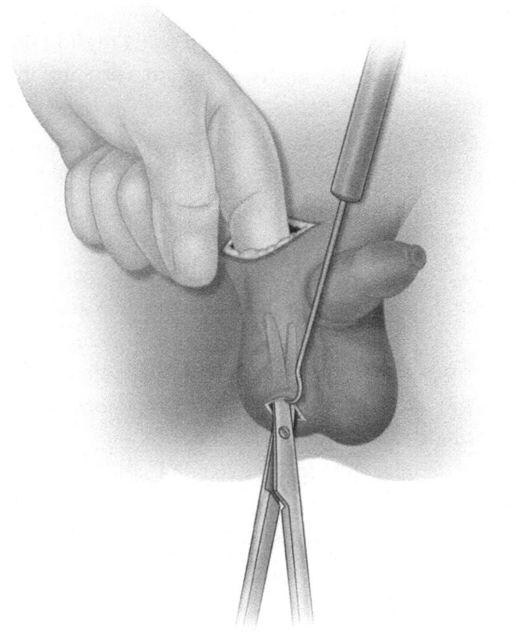

Fig. 20.7 A finger is used to create a passage to the scrotum by blunt dissection and the scrotum is opened

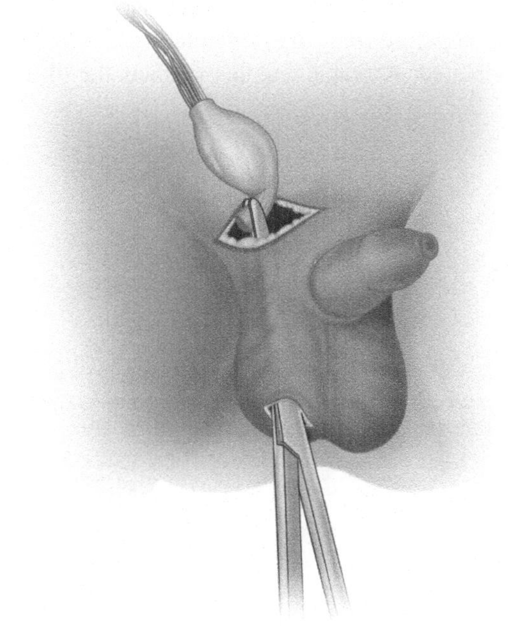

Fig. 20.8 After ensuring no twist in the spermatic vessels, the testis is pulled to the scrotum

artery forceps is passed through the scrotal incision and pushed up to the inguinal incision, guided by the finger. Taking care not to twist the spermatic cord, the testis is pulled down to the scrotal incision (Fig. 20.8). The tunica vaginalis is opened and any appendages removed (this prevents exploration for acute scrotum later in childhood) and the testis sutured to the scrotal septum. After closure of the inguinal canal and Scarpa's fascia, both skin incisions are closed.

Laparoscopic Orchidopexy

The laparoscope is inserted through an umbilical trocar and the presence and location of the testis identified. In a significant percentage of impalpable testes, this documents blind-ending vessels in the retroperitoneum, consistent with the vanishing testis, likely caused by perinatal torsion. This may be associated with an atrophic remnant, which is usually a tiny nodule in the scrotum. Whether or not this needs excision via a small scrotal incision remains controversial.

When the testis is found at laparoscopy, the key determinant for treatment is the proximity of the gonad to the internal inguinal ring. 'Peeping' or 'Peep-a-Boo' testes sitting just inside the internal ring are usually amenable to straightforward orchidopexy, with or without some laparoscopic mobilisation (Fig. 20.9).

Two extra small trocars are placed, one on each side, to allow working instruments. The peritoneum is divided with a wide margin around the testis, allowing the testicular vessels to be mobilised. A simple test that predicts the likely success of laparoscopic primary orchidopexy is to pull the testis to the contralateral inguinal ring (Fig. 20.10). If the gonad can reach the opposite side, then there should be sufficient length for successful orchidopexy in one stage.

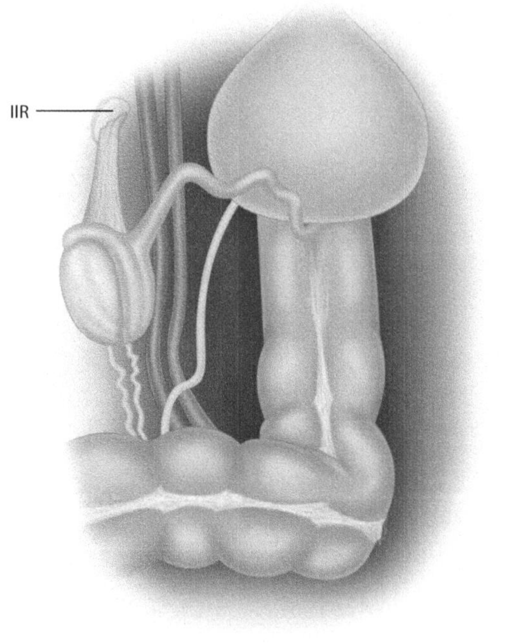

Fig. 20.9 The laparoscopic appearance of an intra-abdominal testis. The canal is often open and contains a gubernacular remnant. The testis is proximal to the ring on a short mesorchium with obvious vas and vessels

In those circumstances where the testis does not reach the other canal, usually when the testis is more remote from the ipsilateral inguinal canal, a decision needs to be made about whether a Fowler–Stephens operation should be done. Fowler and Stephens showed in the 1960s that the testis is supplied by 3 vessels with collaterals around the testis and epididymis: the testicular artery, the cremasteric artery, and the artery to the vas deferens [46]. This allows transection of the testicular vessels above the area of collaterals, thereby allowing the testis to be supplied by the other 2 vessels (Fig. 20.11). This procedure has become a useful way to bring a testis high in the abdominal cavity to the scrotum, despite the testicular artery being too short. The Fowler–Stephens manoeuvre can be done at the same time as orchidopexy, but many surgeons would do orchidopexy at a second stage, after allowing the collateral vessels to enlarge (Fig. 20.12). The 2-stage orchidopexy is usually done with an interval of about 6 months between the stages.

In a single-stage laparoscopic orchidopexy, the testicular vessels are mobilised with a wide margin of peritoneum. The scrotum is opened to make a dartos pouch, and then a long artery or laparoscopic forceps is passed through the inguinal incision and up to the external inguinal ring. Using blunt dissection, the instrument is passed through the back of the inguinal canal, taking care to avoid the inferior epigastric vessels laterally and the bladder medially. The testis is grasped and pulled to the scrotum, and fixed there as in the standard operation.

For the 2-stage procedure, the peritoneum is opened just below where the spermatic vessels appear below the colon and clipped or ligated. No mobilisation is carried out until the second stage, a few months later, when the testis is brought to the scrotum as described for the one-stage procedure.

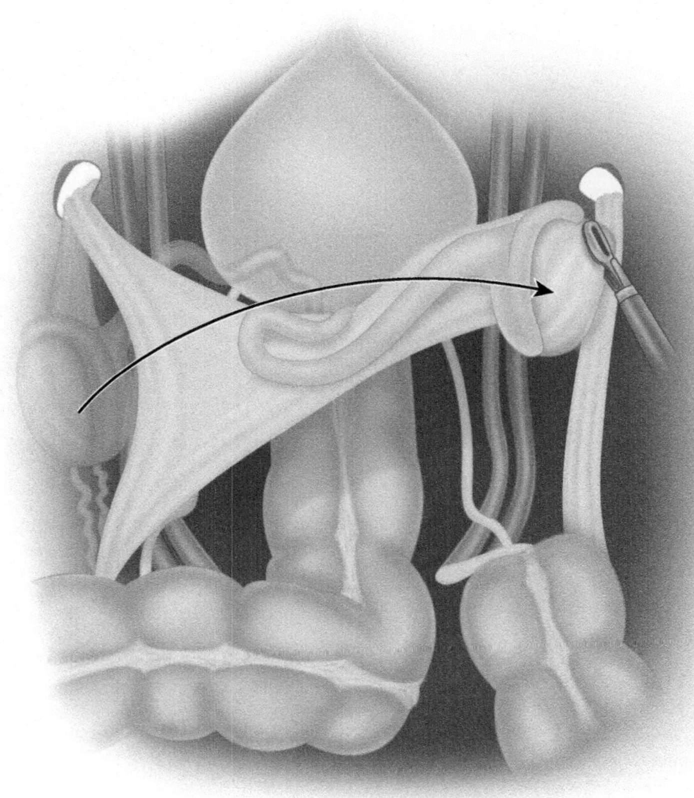

Fig. 20.10 A simple test for whether single-stage orchidopexy is feasible is to pull the testis to the contralateral side. If it reaches in to the opposite inguinal ring then orchidopexy should be straightforward

Scrotal Orchidopexy

A high scrotal incision is made, as originally described by Bianchi at the junction between the neck of the scrotum and pubic skin, or transversely in the upper scrotum. The testis is delivered through the wound and held under traction by an artery forceps. The scrotal connective tissue is stripped off and the cremasteric and external spermatic fascial layers are separated from the remaining cord structures, leaving the vessels, vas deferens and the processus vaginalis, which may be patent (more likely in congenital UDT). The processus is separated from the vas and vessels as for standard orchidopexy and herniotomy, and this is usually possible right up to and through the external inguinal ring by retraction of the upper wound margin. Retroperitoneal dissection, however, is not usually possible, so scrotal orchidopexy is best reserved for those testes that can be pulled to the upper scrotum under anaesthesia. Transfixation/ligation of the processus and anchoring the testis in a dartos pouch is similar to that in standard orchidopexy.

Outcomes of Orchidopexy

Short-Term Outcomes

The testis is located in the scrotum at 1-year follow-up in about 90% of patients, with a small risk of retraction or minor atrophy and occasional complete testicular atrophy. Intra-abdominal testes have a lower success, in the order of 80–85%, although most series do not include those atrophic testes that were excised [47]. The age at surgery does not appear to be a significant factor in the final scrotal location of a reasonable sized testis, as long as the operation is done by trained paediatric surgeons [27, 48].

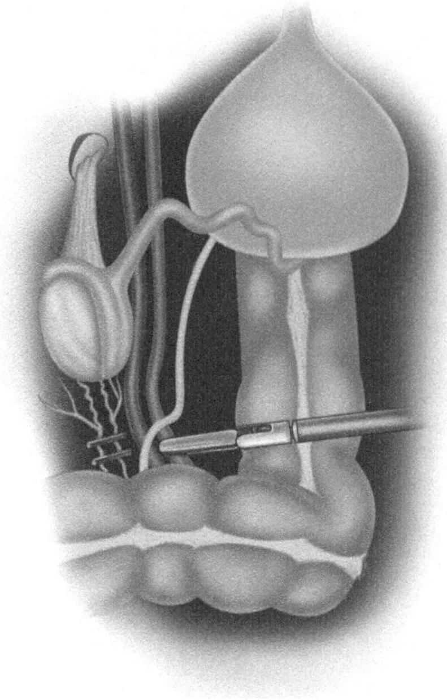

Fig. 20.11 For a first stage of the Fowler–Stephens procedure the colon is mobilised to expose the proximal gonadal vessels, remote from the testis. The vessels are then clipped or ligated

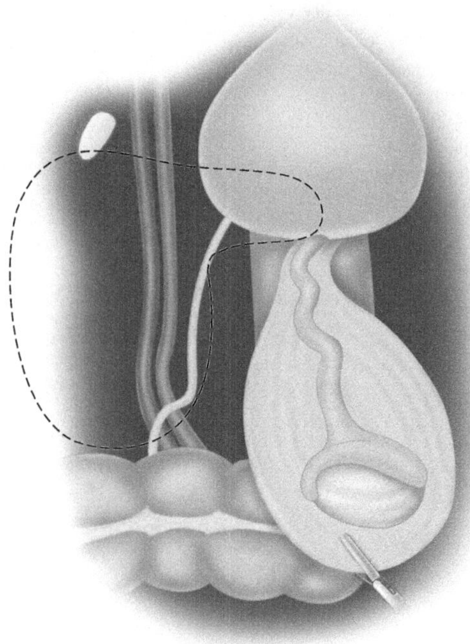

Fig. 20.12 In a single orchidopexy (or the second stage of a Fowler–Stephens operation) the peritoneum is divided widely around the testis to preserve collaterals between the gonadal vessels and the artery of the vas

Long-Term Outcomes

For both malignancy and possible infertility, most studies describing long-term results include patients operated on at a much older age than currently recommended. Moreover, because of the 30-year lag-time between surgery and follow-up, most studies arise from an era before acquired cryptorchidism was identified and characterised. This means that follow-up studies currently being published do not represent the optimal evidence about current practice, but merely record previous history.

If operation in the first year really does matter, by allowing normal germ cell development, then it will still be some time before we get long-term results. At present the prognosis for malignancy is a 5–10 fold increased risk (based on orchidopexies of both congenital and acquired undescended testes done at a median of 10 years of age). The prognosis for fertility from a similar cohort is about 60–70% fertile for men with previous unilateral cryptorchidism, but only about 30% fertile for men after bilateral orchidopexy.

It is not yet known whether these figures will be significantly improved or not by early surgery, although there is now some preliminary evidence that surgery at 9 months is significantly better than operation at 3 years of age [27]. The percentage of undescended testes with a primary disorder is unknown, but it is thought by most authors to be a small number. For the time being, we need to continue early intervention on the assumption that our increasing knowledge of postnatal germ cell maturation will lead to improved outcomes.

References

1. Ong C, Hasthorpe S, Hutson JM. Germ cell development in the descended and cryptorchid testis and the effects of hormonal manipulation. Pediatr Surg Int. 2005;21(4):240–54.

2. John Radcliffe Hospital Cryptorchidism Study Group. An apparent substantial increase since 1960. BMJ 293:1401.
3. John Radcliffe Hospital Cryptorchidism Study Group. Boys with late ascending testes: the source of patients with "retractile" testes undergoing orchidopexy. BMJ. 1986;293:789.
4. Clarnette TD, Lam SK, Hutson JM. Ventriculo-peritoneal shunts in children reveal the natural history of closure of the processus vaginalis. J Pediatr Surg. 1998;33(3):413–6.
5. Gendrel D, Roger M, Job JC. Plasma gonadotropin and testosterone values in infants with cryptorchidism. J Pediatr. 1980;97(2):217–20.
6. Hadziselimovic F. Cryptorchidism: management and implications. In: Hadziselimovic F, editor. Berlin: Springer; 1983.
7. Kaiserman KB, Nakamoto JM, Geffner ME, et al. Minipuberty of infancy and adolescent pubertal function in adrenal hypoplasia congenita. J Pediatr. 1998;133(2):300–2.
8. Baker M, Metcalfe S, Hutson J. Serum levels of Mullerian inhibiting substance in boys from birth to 18 years, as determined by enzyme immunoassay. J Clin Endocrinol Metab. 1990;70:11–5.
9. Baker ML, Hutson JM. Serum levels of Mullerian inhibiting substance in boys throughout puberty and in the first two years of life. J Clin Endocrinol Metab. 1993;76(1):245–7.
10. Hadziselimovic F, Hocht B, Herzog B. Infertility in cryptorchidism is linked to the stage of germ cell development at orchidopexy. Horm Res. 2007;68 (1):46–52.
11. Zhou B, Watts LM, Hutson JM. Germ cell development in neonatal mouse testes in vitro requires Mullerian inhibiting substance. J Urol. 1993;150(2 Pt 2):613–6.
12. Huff DS, Hadziselimovic F, Snyder HM 3rd, et al. Histologic maldevelopment of unilaterally cryptorchid testes and their descended partners. Eur J Pediatr. 1993;152(Suppl 2):S11–4.
13. Huff DS, Hadziselimovic F, Snyder HM 3rd, et al. Postnatal testicular maldevelopment in unilateral cryptorchidism. J Urol 1989;142(2 Pt 2):546–8; discussion 572.
14. Huff DS, Wu HY, Snyder HM 3rd, et al. Evidence in favor of the mechanical (intrauterine torsion) theory over the endocrinopathy (cryptorchidism) theory in the pathogenesis of testicular agenesis. J Urol 1991;146(2 Pt 2):630–1.
15. Farrer JH, Sikka SC, Xie HW, et al. Impaired testosterone biosynthesis in cryptorchidism. Fertil Steril. 1985;44(1):125–32.
16. Yamanaka J, Baker M, Metcalfe S, et al. Serum levels of Mullerian inhibiting substance in boys with cryptorchidism. J Pediatr Surg. 1991;26(5):621–3.
17. Hadziselimovic F, Huff D. Gonadal differentiation–normal and abnormal testicular development. Adv Exp Med Biol 2002;511:15–21; discussion 21–3.
18. Huff DS, Fenig DM, Canning DA, et al. Abnormal germ cell development in cryptorchidism. Horm Res. 2001;55(1):11–7.
19. Mieusset R, Fonda P, Vaysse P, et al. Increase in testicular temperature in case of cryptorchidism in boys. Fertil Steril. 1993;59:1319–21.
20. Jorgensen N, Rajpert-De Meyts E, Graem N, et al. Expression of immunohistochemical markers for testicular carcinoma in situ by normal human fetal germ cells. Lab Invest. 1995;72(2):223–31.
21. Giwercman A, Grindsted J, Hansen B, et al. Testicular cancer risk in boys with maldescended testis: a cohort study. J Urol. 1987;138(5):1214–6.
22. Giwercman A, Muller J, Skakkebaek NE. Carcinoma in situ of the testis: possible origin, clinical significance, and diagnostic methods. Recent Results Cancer Res. 1991;123:21–36.
23. Giwercman A, Muller J, Skakkeboek NE. Cryptorchidism and testicular neoplasia. Horm Res. 1988;30(4–5):157–63.
24. Pettersson A, Richiardi L, Nordenskjold A, et al. Age at surgery for undescended testis and risk of testicular cancer. N Engl J Med. 2007;356(18):1835–41.
25. Ritzen EM, Kollin C. Management of undescended testes: how and when? Pediatr Endocrinol Rev. 2009;7(1):32–7.
26. Thorup J, Cortes D. Surgical treatment and follow up on undescended testis. Pediatr Endocrinol Rev. 2009;7(1):38–43.
27. Kollin C, Karpe B, Hesser U, et al. Surgical treatment of unilaterally undescended testes: testicular growth after randomization to orchiopexy at age 9 months or 3 years. J Urol 2007;178(4 Pt 2):1589–93; discussion 1593.
28. Myers NA, Officer CB. Undescended testes: congenital or acquired? Aust Paediatr J 1975;11: 76–80.
29. Clarnette TD, Hutson JM. Is the ascending testis actually 'stationary'? Normal elongation of the spermatic cord is prevented by a fibrous remnant of the processus vaginalis. Pediatr Surg Int. 1997;12 (2/3):155–7.
30. Clarnette TD, Rowe D, Hasthorpe S, et al. Incomplete disappearance of the processus vaginalis as a cause of ascending testis. J Urol. 1997;157(5):1889–91.
31. Fenton E, Woodward A, Hutson J. The ascending testis. Pediatr Surg Int. 1990;5:6–9.
32. Smith A, Hutson JM, Beasley SW, Reddihough DS. The relationship between cerebral palsy and cryptorchidism. J Pediatr Surg. 1989;24(12)
33. Guven A, Kogan BA. Undescended testis in older boys: further evidence that ascending testes are common. J Pediatr Surg. 2008;43(9):1700–4.
34. Donaldson KM, Tong SY, Hutson JM. Prevalence of late orchidopexy is consistent with some undescended testes being acquired. Indian J Pediatr. 1996;63(6):725–9.
35. Agarwal PK, Diaz M, Elder JS. Retractile testis–is it really a normal variant? J Urol. 2006;175(4):1496–9.

36. Hack WW, Sijstermans K, van der Voort-Doedens LM, et al. The high scrotal ("gliding") testis revised. Eur J Pediatr. 2007;166(1):57–61.
37. Redman JF. The ascending (acquired undescended) testis: a phenomenon? BJU Int. 2005;95(9):1165–7.
38. Cortes D, Thorup JM, Visfeldt J. Cryptorchidism: aspects of fertility and neoplasms. A study including data of 1335 consecutive boys who underwent testicular biopsy simultaneously with surgery for cryptorchidism. Horm Res. 2001;55(1):21–7.
39. Zorgniotti A. Temperature and environmental effects on the testis. Adv Exp Med Biol. 1991;286:1–335.
40. deMuinck Keizer-Schrama SMPF, Hazebroek FW, Matroos AW, et al. Double-blind, placebo-controlled study of luteinising-hormone-releasing-hormone nasal spray in treatment of undescended testes. Lancet. 1986;1(8486):876–80.
41. Hadziselimovic F. Successful treatment of unilateral cryptorchid boys risking infertility with LH-RH analogue. Int Braz J Urol 2008;34(3):319–26; discussion 327–8.
42. Ritzen EM, Bergh A, Bjerknes R, et al. Nordic consensus on treatment of undescended testes. Acta Paediatr. 2007;96(5):638–43.
43. Thorsson AV, Christiansen P, Ritzen M. Efficacy and safety of hormonal treatment of cryptorchidism: current state of the art. Acta Paediatr. 2007;96(5):628–30.
44. Hutson JM, Balic A, Nation T, et al. Cryptorchidism. Semin Pediatr Surg. 2010;19(3):215–24.
45. Bianchi A, Squire B. Trans-scrotal orchidopexy: orchidopexy revisited. Pediatr Surg Int. 1989;4:189.
46. Fowler R, Stephens FD. The role of testicular vascular anatomy in the salvage of high undescended testes. Aust N Z J Surg. 1959;29:92–106.
47. Papparella A, Parmeggiani P, Cobellis G, et al. Laparoscopic management of nonpalpable testes: a multicenter study of the Italian Society of Video Surgery in Infancy. J Pediatr Surg. 2005;40(4):696–700.
48. Wilson-Storey D, McGenity K, Dickson JA. Orchidopexy: the younger the better? J R Coll Surg Edinb. 1990;35(6):362–4.

Testicular Torsion

21

Daniel W. Colliver and David F.M. Thomas

Testicular torsion (also termed torsion of the spermatic cord) occurs when the testis twists around the axis of the spermatic cord with consequent vascular occlusion and ischemia. If uncorrected, torsion progresses to infarction and testicular atrophy. Although the peak incidence is in adolescence, testicular torsion can occur at any age from intra-uterine life to late adulthood. This chapter will combine a summary of the pathophysiology and outcome of testicular torsion with an account of the clinical aspects of diagnosis and management.

Aetiology

Anatomy

Two patterns of testicular torsion are recognized, according to whether the testis twists within the confines of its coverings (intra-vaginal torsion—Fig. 21.1) or whether the testis and its coverings twist in their entirety—extra-vaginal torsion (Fig. 21.2). Extra-vaginal torsion is largely, if not wholly confined to intra-uterine or early postnatal life and although historically termed "neonatal" torsion it has become increasingly evident that with very rare exceptions this is an intra-uterine event.

The intra-vaginal pattern has been traditionally ascribed to a predisposing anatomical variant termed the "bellclapper" deformity, shown in Fig. 21.3a, b. However, whilst the concept of "horizontal lie" and the "bell clapper testis" are long established in conventional teaching, it is important to appreciate that the distinction between "horizontal" and "normal" orientation of the testis is inherently subjective. The reproducibility of this finding and the existence of "horizontal lie" as a distinctive anatomical variant have never been objectively validated in studies of patients and age-matched normal controls. The bell clapper deformity has, however, been the subject of a formal autopsy study reported by Caesar and Kaplan [1]. The relevant anatomical features of 101 testes were documented in series of 51 consecutive postmortem examinations in subjects ranging in age from 1 day to 75 years at the time of death. On the basis of the anatomical relationship between the testis and attachment of the tunica vaginalis these authors found that 12% of all testes demonstrated the "bell clapper" deformity. They concluded that whilst this subset of the population may be at risk for torsion "other factors in addition to anatomic predisposition must be involved". Similar findings were reported by Ishizuka et al. [2]. In males with normally descended testes the

D.W. Colliver
Department of Paediatric Surgery and Urology, Queens Medical Centre, Derby Road, Nottingham NG7 2UH, UK
e-mail: Daniel.colliver@nuh.nhs.uk; daniel.colliver@hotmail.com

D.F.M. Thomas (✉)
Department of Paediatric Urology, Leeds Teaching Hospitals, University of Leeds, Leeds General Infirmary, Great George Street, Leeds LS1 3EX, UK
e-mail: d.f.m.thomas@outlook.com

D.J. Ledbetter and P.R.V. Johnson (eds.), *Endocrine Surgery in Children*,
DOI 10.1007/978-3-662-54256-9_21

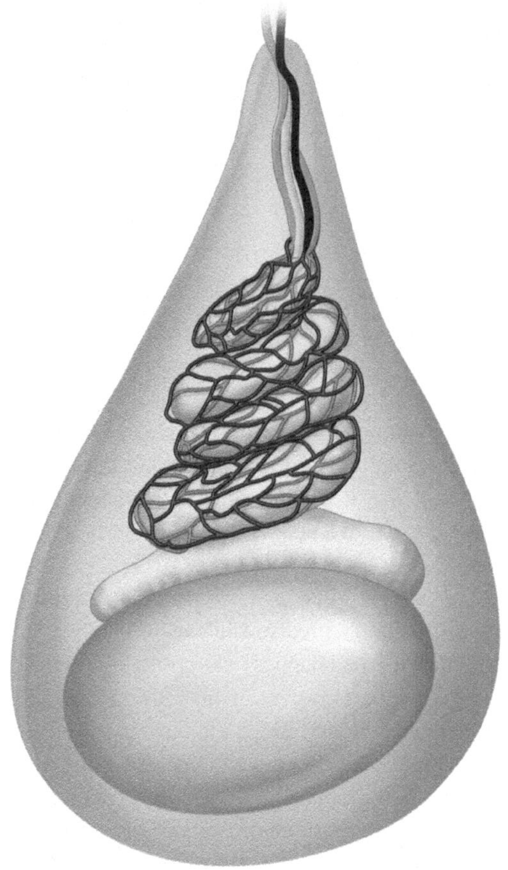

Fig. 21.1 Intra-vaginal torsion

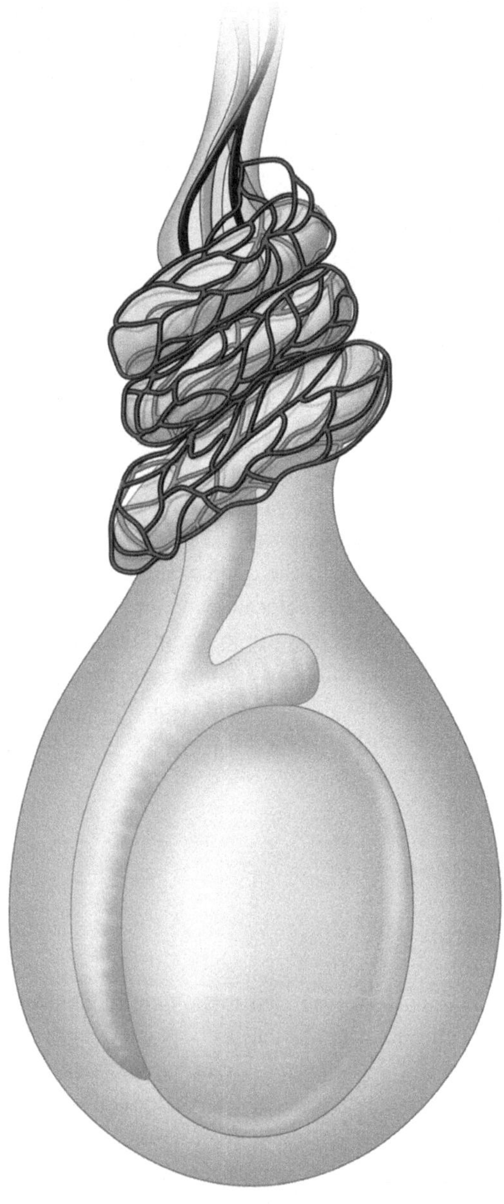

Fig. 21.2 Extra-vaginal torsion

"bell clapper" deformity almost certainly represents one end of the spectrum of normal anatomical development rather than a distinct pathological entity. It is unclear why a small percentage of such individuals experience torsion, whilst the majority of do not.

Genetic Factors

The familial occurrence of testicular torsion is well documented in the literature, with particular emphasis on siblings (notably identical twins) [3, 4]. It is seems likely that this does reflect agenuine genetic basis in affected families since the incidence is greater than might be expected by chance. The mechanism(s) whereby the expression of genetic factors lead to an increased predisposition to torsion is entirely unknown.

Precipitating Factors

A number of precipitating factors have been implicated, including trauma, recent exercise and

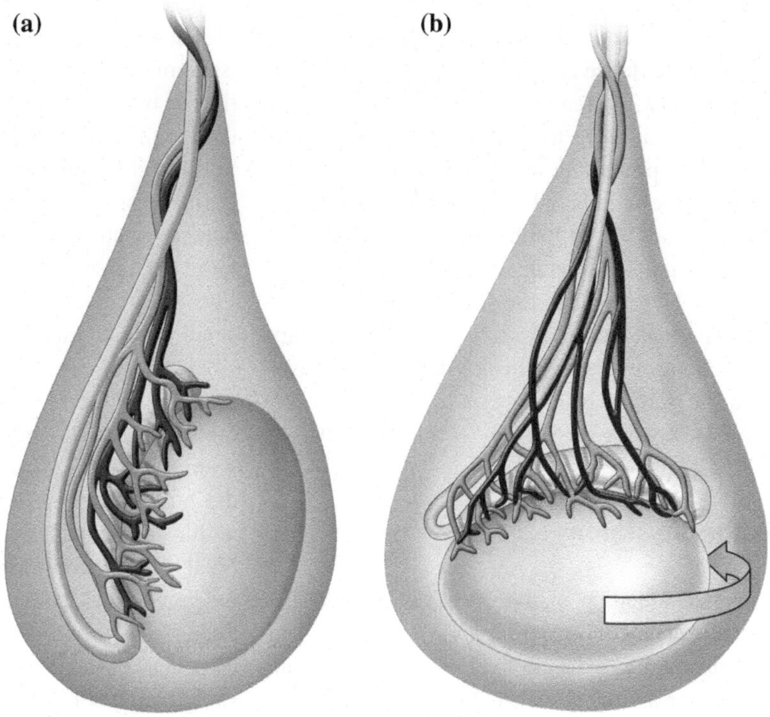

Fig. 21.3 a Normal lie. b The bellclapper deformity

cold weather. In the series reported by Williamson [5], a history of trauma (e.g. sporting injury) and recent exercise was noted in 8 and 11% of cases, respectively. However, it is difficult to assess their significance as precipitating factors since exercise and sporting injury are relatively common events in the lives of adolescents and young adults. In the majority of instances no obvious precipitating factor can be identified and Williamson observed that "sometimes, the onset of symptoms occurred during sleep."

Incidence

In the absence of reliable population-based data it is very difficult to derive an accurate figure for the true incidence of testicular torsion. From their analysis of 670 patients treated in Bristol, United Kingdom, between 1960 and 1984 Anderson and Williamson [6] calculated the annual incidence in their local population as 1 per 3942 males under the age of 25 years. The incidence figure of 1:4000 has been widely cited in subsequent publications.

Data collected prospectively by the Department of Health for England over an 11-year period from 1994 to 2005 indicated that the number of hospital admissions in England for "surgery for testicular torsion" in patients aged 0–17 years remained broadly constant over this period averaging 1010 hospital admissions per annum (range 884–1127) [7]. An approximation based on these Department of Health data and the annual birth rate in England yields an estimated incidence which is broadly consistent with Anderson and Williamson's figure, i.e. 1:3000 to 1:4000. With regard to neonatal torsion an incidence of 6:100,000 (1:17,000) was reported by John et al. [8] who analyzed data from the Mersey region of the United Kingdom collected over a 13-year period. The very limited published evidence does not identify any obvious geographical variation or difference between racial groups.

Testicular torsion is characterized by a bi-modal age distribution. A small peak is observed in the newborn period but the condition occurs most commonly during adolescence, with the peak incidence around 15 years of age. In the age range 13–21 years testicular torsion has been reported to account for at least 90% of all cases of acutely presenting scrotal pathology [9]. By contrast, the differential diagnosis in pre-pubertal boys is more varied, with torsion of the Hydatid of Morgagni accounting for approximately 50% of cases. Nevertheless, torsion of the testis is also an important cause of acute scrotal pathology throughout childhood constituting 34% of cases of acute scrotal pathology in a series of boys aged 0–12 years reported by Nour et al. [10].

Pathophysiology

Our understanding of the events occurring at a vascular and cellular level is largely derived from experimentally induced torsion in rat, porcine and canine animal models [11–15]. These studies have demonstrated that 720° torsion reliably produces complete cessation of perfusion, whereas the degree of ischemia produced by less severe degrees of experimentally induced torsion is more variable.

There appears to be some degree of inter-species variation in the timescale of ischemic tissue damage but whether this reflects differences in vascular anatomy or genuine differences in susceptibility of seminiferous tissue to ischemia is unclear. Nevertheless, it seems reasonable to assume that the consequences of 720° torsion observed in pigs and dogs can be reliably extrapolated to man.

Mechanisms of Tissue Damage

Ischemia

Spermatogenesis is an extremely active process capable of generating approximately 100–200 million sperm per day [16]. This high level of metabolic activity is mirrored in correspondingly high rates of oxygen consumption by the germinal epithelium and in its marked vulnerability to periods of ischemia. The tissues comprising the testis exhibit preferential sensitivity to ischemia with the germ cell population being the first to be lost, followed by the Sertoli cells and the Leydig cells [15]. Because the germ cells and Sertoli cells comprise most of the volume of the normal testis the extent of any reduction in testicular volume can be regarded as a sensitive indicator of severity of ischemic tissue damage. The testis receives its blood supply by long, small calibre artery with a relatively high vascular resistance. As a consequence, capillary pressure in the testis is only marginally higher than the venous pressure and oxygen tension within the testis is low, particularly in relation to the high metabolic demands of spermatogenesis within the adult testis. Whilst this may be beneficial in conferring protection against oxygen-radical mediated damage to sperm DNA under normal perfusion it may also explain why testicular tissue is so susceptible to relatively short periods of ischemia.

Bergh et al. [12] found that even a 30% reduction in perfusion was sufficient to induce cell death of spermatogonia and early primary spermatocytes in the adult rat testis. Heindel et al. [13] documented reductions in sperm production and testicular weight in rats following 720° torsion maintained for as little as one hour—despite subsequent restoration of perfusion to levels comparable to those prior to the induction of torsion. In addition to its duration, the severity of torsion appears to be an important determinant of outcome. Heindel et al. [13] found that experimentally induced unilateral torsion of 720° or more had a significant impact on subsequent fertility, whereas no effect was observed following torsion of 360°.

Reperfusion Injury

In addition to tissue damage mediated by ischemia, further damage occurs as a consequence of reperfusion injury following de-torsion and restoration of blood supply to the testis. Reactive oxygen species, such as H_2O_2, OH, and O_2, and reactive nitrogen species (RNS) such as NO and

ONOO have a well-recognized potential to cause cellular injury and one of the key enzymes involved in early reperfusion injury is thought to xanthine oxidase [17–19].

The administration of exogenous antioxidants, including selenium, l-carnitine and others has been shown to reduce the severity of testicular damage in experimentally induced torsion in animal models [20–25]. Inhibition of xanthine oxidase by allopurinol has also been shown to exert a protective effect [26, 27]. To date, the use of these and other agents to ameliorate testicular damage has been limited to experimental models but it is possible that anti oxidant therapy might find a role in clinical practice in the future—particularly when the testis is left in situ following de-torsion.

The Contralateral Testis

A history of unilateral torsion is associated with an increased probability of impaired spermatogenesis in the "healthy" contralateral testis.

Although this phenomenon has been studied both clinically and experimentally, the possible mechanisms remain unclear and published findings have sometimes been inconsistent or frankly contradictory. Nevertheless, there is a sufficient evidence to pose the theoretical question of whether it might be more beneficial for fertility to remove a potentially salvageable testis (to protect spermatogenic function in the contralateral testis) rather than leave it in situ?

A detailed analysis of evidence is beyond the scope of this chapter but the possible mechanisms of impaired spermatogenesis can be summarized as follows.

Reduced Perfusion

On the basis of a number of experimental studies [28–32], it has been postulated that changes in perfusion which have been observed in the contralateral testis occur in response to toxic vasoactive agents released into the circulation from the affected testis. This occurs particularly at the time of de-torsion when the arterial perfusion and venous drainage are restored to ischemic testicular tissue.

AutoImmune Damage

Seminiferous tissue is immunologically privileged and any breach of the blood-testis barrier incurs the risk of antigens being exposed to the immune system—thus invoking an autoimmune response. This phenomenon has been demonstrated following experimental torsion in rats [33] and, in addition it has been shown that immune mediated damage to the contralateral testis can be ameliorated by administration of immunosuppressive agents, including Dexamethasone and Cyclosporine [24, 25]. The clinical significance (if any) of auto-antibodies in man is unclear. Mastrogiacomo et al. [34] reported the presence of circulating agglutinating antibodies in 20% of 25 patients evaluated 6 months to 7 years after torsion but found no correlation between the presence of these antibodies and sterility. The reported incidence of detectable antisperm antibodies varies considerably in different series and some authors have been unable to identify auto-antibodies in any of their patients despite using standardized laboratory techniques [35]. In a study of the late outcome of pre-pubertal testicular torsion, Puri et al. reported that, of patients who were married, all had fathered one or more children. In unmarried patients, semen analysis was normal in 10 out of 13. Anti sperm antibodies were not found in any of their patients. These authors concluded that pre-pubertal torsion does not cause autosensitization or diminished fertility [36].

Congenital Dysplasia

Biopsy findings have suggested that the impairment in semen quality in men with a history of unilateral testicular torsion might be explained by pre-existing congenital dysplasia in the contralateral "healthy" testis. Hagen and associates reported abnormal histological appearances in 30 out of 34 biopsies of contralateral testes obtained at the time of surgery for torsion [37]. Likewise, Anderson and Williams [38] found pre-existing histological damage in 20 out of 35 patients, prompting them to conclude that "testes prone to torsion already show impaired spermatogenesis".

Reduced Germ Cell Mass

Can the reduction in semen quality observed in men who have undergone orchidectomy for torsion simply be explained by a quantitative reduction in seminiferous tissue? Ferreira and associates assessed the semen quality of 54 men aged between 19 and 42 years who had previously undergone unilateral orchidectomy for a variety of different indications including torsion. A significant and comparable reduction in sperm concentration was observed in all groups regardless of the indication for unilateral orchidectomy [39].

In summary, whilst follow-up studies in men with a history of torsion have consistently demonstrated evidence of impaired semen quality the causative mechanism(s) remain unclear.

Clinical Presentation

Torsion characteristically presents with severe pain of sudden onset accompanied by tenderness and swelling of the testis. The pain is often referred to the ipsilateral inguinal region and/or lower abdominal quadrant thus creating the potential for an erroneous diagnosis of appendicitis when right sided-or gastroenteritis in the case of left-sided torsion. This confusion may be compounded by a history of vomiting, which is feature of around 40% of cases of torsion. Examination of the testes should therefore be included as a mandatory part of the clinical examination of any child or adolescent presenting with sudden onset inguinal or lower abdominal pain.

It is important to note, however, that less than half of patients present with the classic "full house" of symptom and physical signs. Confusingly, pain may sometimes be minimal or absent in the early stages of torsion—particularly in younger children.

The key clinical findings consist of acute tenderness and swelling of the affected testis—which may be lying in an elevated position within the scrotum as a consequence of cremasteric contraction and physical shortening of the twisted cord. Inflammatory changes in the scrotal skin then ensue, in response to ischemia and the onset of necrosis within the underlying testis.

Differential Diagnosis

Testicular torsion accounts for around 90% of all cases of acute scrotal pathology in adolescents [9] and for this reason surgical exploration should be undertaken urgently unless there is convincing evidence of an alternative diagnosis. By contrast, the differential diagnosis is wide ranging in the pre-pubertal age group and encompasses the following;

Torsion of Hydatid of Morgagni (Torsion of a Testicular Appendage)

This typically presents with pain that is less severe, more localized and more insidious in onset than torsion of the testis. In a minority of cases, hemorrhagic infarction of the Hydatid of Morgagni is associated with visible discolouration—the so-called "blue dot" or "blue pea" sign. Although pathognomonic, this sign is more frequently absent or masked by edema and erythema of the overlying scrotal skin. An experienced clinician can often diagnose the condition on clinical grounds (with confirmation by ultrasonography if available). It is important to stress, however, that if the diagnosis cannot be established with certainty, urgent surgical exploration is indicated to exclude testicular torsion. Surgery may also be considered if the symptoms are slow to resolve on conservative management.

Epididymo-Orchitis

This diagnosis should be viewed with caution unless there is strong supportive evidence such as clear evidence of frank urinary infection and/or history of an underlying abnormality such as persistent Mullerian remnant or neuropathic bladder. Epididymo-orchitis is accompanied by marked tenderness, testicular tenderness and scrotal erythema. Other features may include fever, urinary symptoms and systemic ill health. Examination of the urine usually identifies evidence of infection. By contrast to testicular torsion the appearances on Doppler ultrasound are characterized by hyperemia rather than absent perfusion.

Idiopathic Scrotal Edema

This distinctive condition of unknown aetiology is virtually confined to young children. In contrast to the other causes of scrotal swelling and erythema in this age group, idiopathic scrotal edema typically gives rise to remarkably little pain or distress.

For the experienced clinician, the diagnosis rarely causes difficulty but where appropriate the use of scrotal ultrasonography will reliably distinguish idiopathic scrotal edema from other forms of acute scrotal pathology.

Other Causes

Other causes of acute scrotal pathology in the pre-pubertal age range include incarcerated hernia, acute hydrocele, Henoch–Schonlein vasculitis, and mumps orchitis. In adolescents the main differential diagnosis at the younger end of this age range is torsion of the hydatid of Morgagni, whereas epididymo-orchitis (possibly in conjunction with sexually transmitted disease) should be considered in the mid to later teenage years.

Investigation

The principle "investigation" is urgent surgical exploration—particularly in the post pubertal age group (in whom testicular torsion accounts for more than 90% of cases of acute scrotal pathology). Diagnostic imaging may, however, play a role in pre-pubertal boys if the clinical picture points strongly to an alternative diagnosis (e.g. torsion of the hydatid of Morgagni, epididymo-orchitis). However, if there is any suspicion of torsion, urgent exploration is still indicated in this age group.

Doppler ultrasonography is the modality of choice, but this investigation is operator-dependent and it may be difficult, if not impossible, to obtain urgently on an "out of hours basis". Surgical exploration should never be delayed to facilitate ultrasonography if the clinical evidence raises the possibility of testicular torsion. Isotope imaging using intravenous Pertechnetate, labelled with Technetium-99M is of historical interest only and plays no useful role in current practice.

Management

Attempted external manual de-torsion is neither desirable nor feasible in children or adolescents. Time is of the essence and appropriate anesthetic precautions should be taken rather than defer induction of anesthesia because of recent oral intake. Following delivery of the testis (via a midline or scrotal compartment incision) and de-torsion, a decision must be taken on whether to conserve or remove the testis. Relevant factors include; duration of the clinical history, appearance of the testis and presence or absence of arterial bleeding on incision of the tunica albuginea. Some authors have used intra-operative Doppler ultrasonography [40–42], but this does not appear to offer any significant advantage over clinical criteria in predicting potential viability. However, one study found a strong correlation between testicular parenchymal homogeneity or heterogeneity and viability or non-viability, respectively [42].

The available evidence suggests that where doubt exists it is preferable to err on the side of orchidectomy. If the decision is taken to conserve the testis, fixation of the testis to the scrotal wall and the septum is performed using non-absorbable sutures at three sites (three point fixation). A similar technique is employed for prophylactic fixation of the contralateral testis (to obviate the risk of asynchronous contralateral torsion).

Outcome

Viability and Testicular Atrophy

Unlike the experimental situation, it is often difficult, if not impossible, to accurately determine the severity of torsion in the clinical setting. Sessions et al. [43] reported a salvage rate of 62% for testes with a median degree of torsion of 360° compared with 38% when the median degree of torsion was 540°. However, these results were derived from retrospective chart review and experience suggests that, in practice, the degree of rotation is not usually documented with such precision—if at all. Moreover "salvage" rates cited in this study were largely based on the surgical assessment of potential viability at exploration, with only very limited outcome data. Nevertheless, these findings, coupled with extensive evidence derived from experimental studies indicate that the extent and timescale of ischemic injury in man is determined by the severity of torsion as well as its duration. Progression from ischemic necrosis to involution and atrophy extends over many months and published "salvage" rates based solely upon the assessment of potential viability by the operating surgeons (often relatively junior surgeons) may be highly misleading. For example, Krarup found that 68% of testes judged to be salvageable at the time of surgery were "more or less atrophied" when reassessed after a mean of 4.5 years [44]. In a follow-up study in boys aged 0–12 years (which excluded neonatal torsion), Macnicol found that virtually every testis which had been judged to be viable at exploration within 7–12 h of the onset of symptoms, subsequently underwent atrophy. Even when exploration was undertaken within 6 h, a third of "salvaged" testes had atrophied when assessed at two years [45]. Atrophy is not an "all or none" phenomenon and testes which retain some viability may nevertheless be significantly reduced in volume. Thomas et al. [46] assessed 67 patients at a median interval of 4 years after torsion and found that of those testes conserved at the time of exploration 85% subsequently demonstrated some degree of atrophy. Anderson and Williamson reported that 41% of salvaged testes demonstrated varying degrees of atrophy at 3–6 months [6].

Numerous studies have attempted to identify a critical "window" (duration of history) for the preservation of viability. Saxena et al. [47] reported that orchidectomy was performed in only 9% in boys presenting in less than 6 h compared with 56% in those with a history exceeding 6 h. As with most retrospective studies, however, the authors provided no follow-up data or information on the atrophy rate in the 44% of testes retained in boys whose history exceeded 6 h. The 6 h "window" identified by these authors must therefore be regarded as a measure of their decision-making at the time of exploration rather than a reliable predictor of viability. Bartsch et al. [48] cited an 8 h "cut off". Whilst their study did have the benefit of follow up, analysis of their data reveals that the 8 h figure cited by the authors is very misleading. All the normal-sized viable testes in their series had, in fact, been operated on within 4–6 h of the onset of symptoms. Only two testes had been operated upon in the period 6–8 h, both of which were abnormal (20 and 80% atrophy) on follow up.

Reviewing the published evidence, Drlik and Kocvara [49] concluded that it is "commonly accepted" that salvage declines sharply with symptom duration exceeding 6 h. Whilst this statement may apply to paediatric surgeons and urologists, it is clear that many clinicians have an inaccurate impression of the timescale of potential viability.

In summary, there has been uncritical acceptance of the flawed methodology and conclusions that characterize much of the clinical literature. A more critical appraisal of the evidence indicates that the best prospect of conserving a viable, normal-sized testis lies in restoring perfusion within 4–6 h of the onset of torsion. Varying degrees of complete or partial atrophy can be expected when surgical exploration is delayed until 6–8 h. Furthermore, after 6 h the outcome is probably determined to a large extent by the severity of torsion. In cases of 720° torsion there probably little realistic prospect of conserving any viable testicular tissue after 6–8 h. Preservation of a viable, normal-sized testis after 8–10 h (or longer) can occur occasionally but such cases almost certainly reflect incomplete or intermittent vascular occlusion or spontaneous resolution of the torsion.

It is not known whether the pre-pubertal human testis is more (or less) susceptible to ischemia than the adult testis. The very limited evidence coupled with anecdotal experience indicates that torsion is associated with a considerably higher rate of testicular loss in the pre-pubertal age group. However, it seems likely that the poorer outcomes are a consequence of greater diagnostic delay and a lack of awareness of torsion in young children amongst doctors—rather than any intrinsic difference in the sensitivity of the testis to ischemia.

Fertility and Semen Quality

The weight of published evidence consistently points to a significant reduction in semen quality in men with a history of testicular torsion. Krarup investigated the semen quality of 19 men of whom 11 had undergone orchidectomy, with conservation of the testis in eight. In this study only 1 patient (5%) had normal parameters of semen quality [44]. Bartsch et al. evaluated semen quality in two specimens obtained from 30 patients with a history of pre and post pubertal torsion. Semen quality was normal in 15 patients, doubtful in 3 and "pathological" in 12 patients [48]. Thomas et al. [46] assessed 67 patients at a median of 4 years after torsion and found abnormal semen in 86% of patients tested. Subsequent studies have yielded similar findings. Arap et al. evaluated the outcome of 24 patients of whom 15 had undergone orchidectomy whilst the testis had been conserved in nine. Sperm count and sperm morphology (assessed by WHO and the Kruger criteria) were impaired in both groups when compared with fertile controls, with the greatest impairment being observed in men whose testis had been conserved [35]. By contrast to the reasonably extensive literature on semen quality the impact of torsion on paternity (the actual ability to father children) does not appear to have been formally studied. When writing this chapter, searching the PubMed database with the keywords "testis", "torsion" and "paternity" failed to identify a single publication.

Endocrine Function

Experimental studies indicate that hormone-secreting Leydig cells are considerably more resistant to ischemia than germ cells and Sertoli cells [12, 15]. Thus, a testis that has undergone partial atrophy due to loss of germ cell volume may nevertheless be capable of contributing to endocrine function. However, this is difficult to quantify against a background of normal hormone production by the contralateral testis. A number of long-term studies have confirmed that levels of testosterone are consistently within the normal range—regardless of whether the affected testis was conserved or removed [35, 50, 51]. Likewise levels of gonadotrophic hormones FSH and LH within the normal reference range have also been reported in the majority of studies.

Romeo et al. investigated hormone function in a series of 20 pubertal patients with a previous history of torsion and found normal levels of testosterone, FSH and LH, when compared with healthy controls. Inhibin B levels were, however, significantly reduced compared with controls although there was no difference between orchidectomy and preservation of the testis [51]. Inhibin B is a marker of Sertoli cell function [52] and a reduced level is likely to be indicative of defective spermatogenesis or germ cell depletion in torsion patients.

Neonatal Torsion

This is a misnomer, since, with rare exceptions, torsion presenting in the first day or two of life is an intra-uterine event. Indeed, the antenatal diagnosis of testicular torsion by ultrasonography has been the subject of case reports [53].

Typically it presents as a firm, irregular swelling and overlying discoloration, which is evident at birth or the first 24–48 h of life. Ultrasound reveals enlargement of the testis and epididymis surrounded by hemorrhagic fluid and varying degrees of edema of the surrounding scrotal tissue. Absence of perfusion is confirmed on colour Doppler.

Previously, "neonatal" torsion was managed in a similar fashion to other age groups, namely by urgent surgical exploration and fixation of the contralateral testis. The 1990s saw a shift of approach prompted by a better appreciation of the natural history of neonatal torsion and recognition that exploration is invariably a futile exercise. Burge reported a series of 30 cases over a 20-year period, without encountering a single viable testis [54]. John et al. [8] reported a zero salvage rate in a series of 24 patients and other authors have reported a similar experience.

A more conservative approach has therefore evolved which uses ultrasonography to confirm the diagnosis and monitor the process of involution and atrophy. However, Baglaj and Carachi [55] reported three cases of bilateral torsion in their centre over a 20-year period and, in addition, identified a further 45 cases of bilateral neonatal torsion on a literature search. Kaye [56] and associates reported one case of bilateral torsion in a series of 16 neonates, whilst Djahangiriam et al. [57] reported a 5% incidence of bilaterality and Al-Salem [58] reported an incidence of 9%. Thus, the incidence of bilateral torsion appears to be considerably higher than would be expected simply by chance, suggesting that extra-vaginal torsion may be associated with an underlying anatomical abnormality which poses a risk to the contralateral testis.

It is also apparent that torsion can very rarely occur as a genuine neonatal event. Sorensen and associates published 10 cases occurring in infants under 30 days of age in whom the testis had previously seemed normal when examined during the course of routine neonatal examination. A 40% salvage rate was reported in this small series of patients [59].

On the basis of this published evidence a rethink of the current conservative approach to the management of neonatal torsion may now be justified—particularly with regard to prophylactic fixation of the contralateral testis. There do not appear to have been any long-term studies of exocrine and endocrine function following neonatal torsion as opposed to torsion occurring in later childhood or adolescence. In the absence of any evidence to the contrary, it seems reasonable to assume that endocrine function is normal in the longer term.

Parallels with long-term data for unilateral congenital cryptorchidism would suggest that, whilst sperm density (sperm count) might be decreased, the prospects for paternity are likely to be normal or only marginally reduced. Any decision regarding implantation of a testicular prosthesis is best deferred until adolescence.

References

1. Caesar RE, Kaplan GW. Incidence of the bell-clapper deformity in an autopsy series. Urology. 1994;44(1):114–6.
2. Ishizuka E, et al. A classification for intravaginal torsion of the testis. Eur Urol. 1988;15(1–2):108–12.
3. Lisk CH, Wilding RP. Torsion of the testicle in homozygous twins. Br J Urol. 1984;56(5):544–5.
4. Gorbonos A, Cheng EY. Perinatal testicular torsion in siblings. J Pediatr Urol. 2007;3(6):514–5.
5. Williamson RC. Torsion of the testis and allied conditions. Br J Surg. 1976;63(6):465–76.
6. Anderson JB, Williamson RC. Fertility after torsion of the spermatic cord. Br J Urol. 1990;65(3):225–30.
7. Tanner S. Trends in children's surgery in England. Arch Dis Child. 2007;92(8):664–7.

8. John CM, et al. Neonatal testicular torsion—a lost cause? Acta Paediatr. 2008;97(4):502–4.
9. Ben-Chaim J, et al. Etiology of acute scrotum at surgical exploration in children, adolescents and adults. Eur Urol. 1992;21(1):45–7.
10. Nour S, MacKinnon AE. Acute scrotal swelling in children. J R Coll Surg Edinb. 1991;36(6):392–4.
11. Lievano G, Nguyen L, Radhakrishnan J, Fornell L, John E. New animal model to evaluate testicular blood flow during testicular torsion. J Pediatr Surg. 1999;34(6):1004–6.
12. Bergh A, Collin O, Lissbrant E. Effects of acute graded reductions in testicular blood flow on testicular morphology in the adult rat. Biol Reprod. 2001;64(1):13–20.
13. Heindel RM, et al. The effect of various degrees of unilateral spermatic cord torsion on fertility in the rat. J Urol. 1990;144(2 Pt 1):366–9.
14. Becker EJ Jr, Turner TT. Endocrine and exocrine effects of testicular torsion in the prepubertal and adult rat. J Androl. 1995;16(4):342–51.
15. Smith GI. Cellular changes from graded testicular ischemia. J Urol. 1955;73(2):355–62.
16. Johnson L, Petty CS, Neaves WB. Further quantification of human spermatogenesis: germ cell loss during postprophase of meiosis and its relationship to daily sperm production. Biol Reprod. 1983;29(1):207–15.
17. Jezek P, Hlavata L. Mitochondria in homeostasis of reactive oxygen species in cell, tissues, and organism. Int J Biochem Cell Biol. 2005;37(12):2478–503.
18. Zangar RC, Davydov DR, Verma S. Mechanisms that regulate production of reactive oxygen species by cytochrome P450. Toxicol Appl Pharmacol. 2004;199(3):316–31.
19. Kumagai A, et al. Xanthine oxidase inhibitors suppress testicular germ cell apoptosis induced by experimental cryptorchidism. Mol Hum Reprod. 2002;8(2):118–23.
20. Avlan D, et al. The protective effect of selenium on ipsilateral and contralateral testes in testicular reperfusion injury. Pediatr Surg Int. 2005;21(4):274–8.
21. Ozkan KU, et al. The effect of zinc aspartate pretreatment on ischemia-reperfusion injury and early changes of blood and tissue antioxidant enzyme activities after unilateral testicular torsion-detorsion. J Pediatr Surg. 2004;39(1):91–5.
22. Abasiyanik A, Dagdonderen L. Beneficial effects of melatonin compared with allopurinol in experimental testicular torsion. J Pediatr Surg. 2004;39(8):1238–41.
23. Gulmez I, et al. Effect of testicular torsion on the contralateral testis and prevention of this effect by prednisolone. Eur Urol. 1987;13(5):340–3.
24. Jeong SJ, et al. Preventive effects of cyclosporine a combined with prednisolone and melatonin on contralateral testicular damage after ipsilateral torsion-detorsion in pubertal and adult rats. J Urol. 2010;184(2):790–6.
25. Mogilner JG, et al. Effect of dexamethasone on germ cell apoptosis in the contralateral testis after testicular ischemia-reperfusion injury in the rat. Fertil Steril. 2006;85(Suppl 1):1111–7.
26. Akgur FM, et al. The effect of allopurinol pretreatment before detorting testicular torsion. J Urol. 1994;151(6):1715–7.
27. Kehinde, E.O., et al., Allopurinol provides long-term protection for experimentally induced testicular torsion in a rabbit model. BJU Int. 2005;96(1):175–80.
28. Carden DL, Granger DN. Pathophysiology of ischaemia-reperfusion injury. J. Pathol. 2000;190(3):255–66.
29. Harrison RG, et al. Mechanism of damage to the contralateral testis in rats with an ischaemic testis. Lancet. 1981;2(8249):723–5.
30. Kizilcan F, et al. Ipsilateral and contralateral testicular blood flows during unilateral testicular torsion by 133Xe clearance technique. Int Urol Nephrol. 1992;24(5):515–20.
31. Kolettis PN, et al. Acute spermatic cord torsion alters the microcirculation of the contralateral testis. J Urol. 1996;155(1):350–4.
32. Nguyen L, et al. Effect of unilateral testicular torsion on blood flow and histology of contralateral testes. J Pediatr Surg. 1999;34(5):680–3.
33. Kosar A, et al. Immunologic aspect of testicular torsion: detection of antisperm antibodies in contralateral testicle. Eur Urol. 1999;36(6):640–4.
34. Mastrogiacomo I, et al. Immunological and clinical study of patients after spermatic cord torsion. Andrologia. 1982;14(1):25–30.
35. Arap MA, et al. Late hormonal levels, semen parameters, and presence of antisperm antibodies in patients treated for testicular torsion. J Androl. 2007;28(4):528–32.
36. Puri P, Barton D, O'Donnell B. Prepubertal testicular torsion: subsequent fertility. J Pediatr Surg. 1985;20(6):598–601.
37. Hagen P, et al. Testicular dysplasia causing disturbance of spermiogenesis in patients with unilateral torsion of the testis. Urol Int. 1992;49(3):154–7.
38. Anderson JB, Williamson RC. The fate of the human testes following unilateral torsion of the spermatic cord. Br J Urol. 1986;58(6):698–704.
39. Ferreira U, et al. Comparative study of the fertility potential of men with only one testis. Scand J Urol Nephrol. 1991;25(4):255–9.
40. Arda, I.S., Ozyaylali, I. Testicular tissue bleeding as an indicator of gonadal salvageability in testicular torsion surgery. BJU Int. 2001;87(1):89–92.
41. Cimador M, et al. Predictors of testicular viability in testicular torsion. J Pediatr Urol. 2007;3(5):387–90.
42. Kaye JD, et al. Parenchymal echo texture predicts testicular salvage after torsion: potential impact on the need for emergent exploration. J Urol. 2008;180(4 Suppl):1733–6.

43. Sessions AE, et al. Testicular torsion: direction, degree, duration and disinformation. J Urol. 2003;169(2):663–5.
44. Krarup T. The testes after torsion. Br J Urol. 1978;50 (1):43–6.
45. Macnicol MF. Torsion of the testis in childhood. Br J Surg. 1974;61(11):905–8.
46. Thomas WE, et al. Testicular exocrine malfunction after torsion. Lancet. 1984;2(8416):1357–60.
47. Saxena AK, Castellani C, Ruttenstock EM, Höllwarth ME. Testicular torsion: a 15-year single-centre clinical and histological analysis. Acta Paediatr. 2012;101(7):e282–6.
48. Bartsch G, et al. Testicular torsion: late results with special regard to fertility and endocrine function. J Urol. 1980;124(3):375–8.
49. Drlík M, Kočvara R. Torsion of spermatic cord in children: a review. J Pediatr Urol. 2013;9(3):259–66.
50. Anderson MJ, et al. Semen quality and endocrine parameters after acute testicular torsion. J Urol. 1992;147(6):1545–50.
51. Romeo C, et al. Late hormonal function after testicular torsion. J Pediatr Surg. 2010;45(2):411–3.
52. Stewart J, Turner KJ. Inhibin B as a potential biomarker of testicular toxicity. Cancer Biomark. 2005;1(1):75–91.
53. Herman A, et al. Antenatal sonographic diagnosis of testicular torsion. Ultrasound Obstet Gynecol. 2002;20(5):522–4.
54. Burge DM. Neonatal testicular torsion and infarction: aetiology and management. Br J Urol. 1987;59 (1):70–3.
55. Baglaj M, Carachi R. Neonatal bilateral testicular torsion: a plea for emergency exploration. J Urol. 2007;177(6):2296–9.
56. Kaye JD, et al. Neonatal torsion: a 14-year experience and proposed algorithm for management. J Urol. 2008;179(6):2377–83.
57. Djahangirian O, Ouimet A, Saint-Vil D. Timing and surgical management of neonatal testicular torsions. J Pediatr Surg. 2010;45(5):1012–5.
58. Al-Salem AH. Intrauterine testicular torsion: a surgical emergency. J Pediatr Surg. 2007;42(11):1887–91.
59. Sorensen MD, et al. Perinatal extravaginal torsion of the testis in the first month of life is a salvageable event. Urology. 2003;62(1):132–4.

Testicular Tumors in Children

22

Yaser El-Hout and Darius J. Bägli

There is a growing body of evidence that shows testicular tumors in prepubertal children and infants to be distinct clinically from testicular tumors in adults, or even adolescents, where more benign pathologies are being encountered in younger patients. With testicular tumors in children being relatively rare, this observation culminated with scattered small case series, in addition to centralized tumor registries, for example, the Prepubertal Testis Tumor Registry by the Section of Urology of the American Academy of Pediatrics (1980) and national oncology trials namely, the Children's Oncology Group in the USA, the German Society of Pediatric Oncology, and the Children's Cancer Study Group in the UK. This has led to fine-tuning in the management of prepubertal testicular tumor by showing radical surgery to be unnecessarily aggressive. This has led in a shift in the paradigm of management in pediatric testicular tumors, where more testis-sparing surgery is being performed without compromising safety and prognosis, hence reducing morbidity of adjuvant treatment that is skipped.

Epidemiology

Testicular tumor incidence follows a bimodal age distribution, peaking at around two years of life then during early adulthood [1]. Prepubertal testicular tumors account for 1–2% of pediatric solid tumors with an incidence of 0.5–2.0 per 100,000 children [2]. Mortality rates from pediatric testicular tumors are low, with one death per ten million per year. Prepubertal testicular cancer survival is about 99% at 5 years [3]. When looking into individual frequencies of pathologies, one has to be aware of inherent selection bias in underreporting benign cases to tumor registries leading to discordant reporting. Indeed, while earlier registry data showed more frequent malignant pathologies: 60% yolk sac tumors versus 40% benign and 25% teratoma [4], Pohl et al. surveyed four major pediatric centers in North America and found higher frequency of benign pathologies in unselected testicular lesions up to 75%, namely, 50% teratoma, 15% epidermoid cyst, 5% juvenile granulose cell tumors with less than 5% each of Leydig cell tumors, Sertoli cell tumors, and mixed gonadal stromal tumors. Malignant yolk sac tumors in this survey were only 15% [5].

Y. El-Hout
American University of Beirut Medical Center, PO Box: 11-0236, Riad El Solh, Beirut 1107 2020, Lebanon
e-mail: yelhout@aub.edu.lb

D.J. Bägli (✉)
Department of Surgery, Division of Urology, The Hospital for Sick Children, University of Toronto, 555 University Avenue, Toronto, ON M5G 1X8, Canada
e-mail: darius.bagli@sickkids.ca

D.J. Ledbetter and P.R.V. Johnson (eds.), *Endocrine Surgery in Children*,
DOI 10.1007/978-3-662-54256-9_22

Risk Factors and Associations

The exact causes for testicular cancers are not known. Few risk factors are identified that contribute to an increased incidence of testicular cancer while other associations are under study with no solid evidence in literature.

Cryptorchidism

The United States National Cancer Institute lists cryptorchidism, or undescended testicle, as a main risk factor for testicular cancer. Statistically, 5% of testicular cancers are associated with a history of cryptorchidism [6]. A cryptorchid testicle may be genetically and anatomically predisposed to abnormal structure and function, leading to testicular dysgenesis syndrome (TDS), which increases the risk for malignant degeneration, as well as poor semen quality and fertility implications [7]. In routine practice, most pediatric urologists would strive to perform orchidopexy prior to age 2, and would counsel families whose kids present with cryptorchidism about the risk of malignancy. Wood and Elder [8] found that the relative risk of testicular cancer in cryptorchidism is 2.75–8. Patients who undergo orchiopexy by ages 10–12 years have a relative risk for testicular cancer of 2–3, while patients who undergo orchiopexy after age 12 years or no orchiopexy are 2–6 times as likely to have testicular cancer as those who undergo prepubertal orchiopexy. A normally descended testis with contralateral cryptorchidism has no increased risk of testis cancer. Persistent inguinal or abdominal testes are at higher risk for seminoma (74%), while corrected cryptorchid or scrotal testicles that undergo malignant transformation are most likely to become nonseminomatous (63%).

Disorders of Sexual Differentiation

Patients with disorders of sex development (DSD), previously referred to as intersex disorders, are a unique subpopulation that is at an increased risk of gonadal tumors. DSD has been noted to be a main risk factor for type II germ cell tumors (GCT), namely, seminoma/dysgerminoma and non-seminoma (e.g., embryonal carcinoma, yolk sac tumor, choriocarcinoma and teratoma [9]. DSD male patients often have chromosomal abnormality that predisposes to genital ambiguity, hypovirilization, and a spectrum of gonadal dysgenesis. The prevalence of GCT is 15% in partial androgen insensitivity, but more than 30% in gonadal dysgenesis. Complete androgen insensitivity and ovotesticular DSD patients develop malignancies in 0.8 and 2.6%, respectively [10]. Recently, undifferentiated gonadal tissue has been implicated to be a precursor of gonadoblastoma. This transformation requires a defined region on the Y chromosome (the GBY region) which included the gene for testis-specific protein on the Y chromosome (TSPY) which is evolving as a marker for gonadoblastoma and GCT [11]. Aberrant TSPY expression increases protein synthesis, stimulates cell proliferation, and promotes tumorigenicity by binding to type B cyclins, enhancing an activated cyclin B-CDK1 kinase activity, resulting in a rapid G [2]/M transition in the cell cycle. Abnormal expression of TSPY gene in a DSD testis disrupts the normal cell cycle regulation leading to tumorigenesis [12].

Environmental Factors

Environmental factors are always connected to cancer formation, although in many cases the level of evidence is not compelling, with the data being largely mixed and inconclusive and the real accusable factors remaining elusive. Caucasians are more noted to develop testicular cancer than other ethnic groups. Additionally, there is a remarkable worldwide variation of testicular cancer incidence according to geographical region. For instance, while Denmark has among the highest incidence of testicular cancer in the world, the risk of testicular cancer was significantly lower among first generation immigrants to Denmark, versus men born in

Denmark to immigrant parents and Danish men with Danish parents [13]. The higher incidence of testicular cancer in the western world can be partly attributed to the rise in industrial chemicals over the last century. Prenatal exposure (or even during adolecense or adulthood) to such chemicals, namely, polychlorinated biphenyls, DDT, phthalates, hexachlorobenzene and other fat soluble organochlorines, may predispose to testicular cancer, as they were found in higher concentrations in mothers of males with testicular cancer [14]. A hypothesis, to explain why chemicals would influence testicular cancer development, is that they interfere with or mimic hormonal signaling pathways in utero or later, leading to aberrant development or differentiation, hence they are collectively termed, endocrine disrupting chemicals (EDC) [15]. Further studies have noted increased association with testicular cancer in obesity [16]. Maternal consumption of alcohol during pregnancy, but not smoking or coffee intake, was associated with higher risk of testicular cancer in their sons [17]. Recently, an association between marijuana use and GCT, particularly non-seminoma, was noted [18].

Microlithiasis

With the increased utility of ultrasonography in clinical medicine, the concern about testicular microlithiasis (TM) association with testicular cancer rose as microlithiasis is often an incidental finding affecting up to 14% of asymptomatic adult men and up to 2% of asymptomatic boys [19, 20]. Whenever this entity is diagnosed, it compels the clinician to provide follow-up, counseling and prognosis, namely because TM has been associated with certain genital pathologies: cryptorchidism in 10% [21], infertility in up to 23% [22], McCune–Albright syndrome in 60% [23], and testicular tumors in an alarming 45% [24]. TM is defined as foci of calcification within the seminiferous tubules that may represent tiny foci of dysgenetic tissue that could potentially progress into carcinoma in situ. Although the association of TM with tumor formation is mainly demonstrated in adults, only four scattered case reports were cited in children [25–28], making the association inconclusive. It is worth noting that testicular tumors have never been identified during prospective follow-up of a cohort followed up for TM, in either adults or children. Although some investigators found long-term follow-up of children with TM to be anxiety-provoking, not cost effective and with low yield [29], others still recommend ultrasound surveillance, physical examination and repeated patient education, with no well-defined protocols.

Clinical Presentation and Evaluation

History and Physical Examination

The most common presentation of testicular tumor is a painless testicular mass, noted in 88% in the Testis Tumor Registry. The parents maybe instrumental in detecting the mass, or it may be detected on a routine physical examination by the primary health care provider. Around 10–15% of patients would present with a coincidental or tumor-related hydrocele at presentation. A hydrocele may delay the diagnosis of a testis tumor. It is crucial, thus, to obtain an ultrasound in boys with a hydrocele precluding reliable palpation of the testicle. Pain is uncommon and may be due to acute bleed into the tumor or a rapid growth.

Physical examination is integral to the evaluation of a testicular mass and is performed with a broad differential diagnosis in mind to rule out a hernia, hydrocele, inflammatory/infectious orchitis (e.g., mumps), as well as the surgical emergency of acute testicular torsion. Physical examination reveals a hard mass in the testicular parenchyma. However, small masses deep in the parenchyma may be difficult to palpate, and would require sonographic assessment. Testicular masses must be differentiated from benign extratesticular lesions, whether benign (e.g., epididymal cyst) or malignant (e.g., rhabdomyosarcoma). The genitalia and other body parts should be carefully examined for signs of androgenization or feminization. Although metastatic disease at presentation is uncommon, examining groins, axillae and neck for lymphadenopathy, ausculting the lungs for abnormal sounds, eliciting bony pain and even a brief neurologic exam may yield positive findings in the rare occasion of metastasis and is considered good practice. Symptoms or signs of involvement at these anatomic locations guide subsequent radiographic evaluation.

Imaging and Other Diagnostics

An initial imaging with ultrasound remains the cornerstone evaluation of a testicular mass with a detection rate approaching 100%. High frequency window of 7.5–10 MHz can be beneficial in elucidating particular sonographic features of testicular versus paratesticular neoplasms [30] and while sonographic description of specific testicular tumors is available in radiologic literature, findings are too inconsistent to allow for a definitive diagnosis. Benign tumors are well demarcated with sharp borders and decreased Doppler signal. Epidermoid cysts have an echogenic rim with mixed echogenic or hypoechoic center [31]. Yolk sac tumors have homogeneous hypoechoic solid appearance, but may have other sonographic appearance. Ultrasound would also distinguish testicular tumors from extra-testicular lesions. The extent of testicular involvement can also be appreciated, a criteria that would be considered among others, if a testis-sparing surgery is contemplated.

Tumor markers are vital diagnostic clues in evaluating testicular tumors. Alpha feto-protein (AFP) is the most important marker in evaluating and following-up prepubertal testicular tumors. It is precursor protein of albumin, synthesized by the yolk sac and fetal liver and gut. AFP has a half- life of 5 days and is specific for yolk sac tumors, the main malignant tumor in this age group. Levels are elevated in 80–90% of children with a yolk sac tumor, and its preoperative elevation precludes testis-sparing surgery. The utility of AFP in infancy, however, can be confusing since an elevated level in a boy less than 1 year of age does not rule out the possibility of a benign tumor, like teratoma. AFP's known half-life of 5 days is attained around 4 months of life and is longer before that. Serum AFP would be normally as high as 50,000 ng/mL in neonates, 10,000 ng/mL by 2 weeks of age, and 300 ng/mL by age of 2 months [32]. While yolk sac tumor and teratoma elevate AFP, data from the Testis Tumor Registry did not show any teratoma diagnosed after 6 months of life to elevate AFP more than 100 ng/mL [4]. This observation highlights the decision-making to remove or spare the testis.

The other classical marker in testicular tumors is the beta subunit of the human chorionic gonadotropin (hCG) produced by the syncytiotrophoblast of the placenta. While this is useful in postpubertal and adult testicular tumors, it is not very useful in children, particularly because choriocarcinoma and embryonal carcinoma, both secreting hCG, are rare [33].

Because the majority of testicular tumors in prepubertal boys are, by and large, benign, the evolving strategy of evaluation is to defer metastatic workup until a tissue diagnosis is obtained at time of orchiectomy. This would spare the patient the unnecessary exposure to a CT scan if his pathology turns benign. Preoperative CT scan or MRI is warranted, however, if AFP is elevated, raising the suspicion of a yolk sac tumor. Because lung metastasis is present in 20% of yolk sac tumors, chest imaging is warranted.

Surgical Approach

Regardless of the eventual surgical management of testicular tumor by radical orchiectomy or testis-sparing surgery (partial orchiectomy or enucleation of tumor), the initial surgical approach and exposure is the same [34]. An ipsilateral inguinal incision is made along a Langer's line crease of minimal tension. The incisional length can be extended at surgeon's judgment to improve exposure, particularly to deliver large tumors. The incision is deepened using electrocautery through Scarpa's fascia to reach the external oblique aponeurosis. In younger patients, Scarpa's fascia is well developed and may be mistaken for the external oblique fasica. The external oblique fascia is sharply incised along its fibers to open the external inguinal ring, paying attention to preserve the underlying ilioinguinal nerve which provides cutaneous sensation to the inner aspect of the upper thigh. The spermatic cord is identified and bluntly dissected inferiorly to expose the pubic tubercle. Incising the cremasteric sheath longitudinally allows for easy isolation of the cord and precludes the need to repair the internal oblique which constitutes the canal floor and gives rise to the cremasteric fibers. The proximal spermatic cord is controlled with non-crushing clamp or a vessel loop/Penrose drain wrapped around it as a tourniquet. Theoretically, this prevents dissemination of potential malignant cells into bloodstream from testis manipulation, although little evidence supports this "ritual" practice. The scrotal neck is stretched and Scarpa's fascia incision may be extended while the testis is delivered out of the incision by gently pushing it out of the scrotum. This step may be challenging in large tumors. The gubernaculum is divided with electrocautry while carefully maintaining an intact tunica vaginalis covering the testis. At this point and according to the clinical scenario, the procedure can proceed as radical orchiectomy or a testis-sparing procedure.

Radical Orchiectomy

In the clinical scenario of a malignant tumor, almost invariably a yolk sac tumor evidenced by preoperative elevation of AFP, the above procedure is completed as a radical orchiectomy. The spermatic cord is doubly clamped, divided and the vas and vessels are doubly ligated above the internal inguinal ring level, using 2-0 or 3-0 nonabsorbable sutures cut sufficiently long. This allows identification and excision of the cord intraperitoneally, if later retroperitoneal lymph node dissection is undertaken. The testis and cord are sent in formalin for definitive pathological analysis. The abdominal defect is closed using absorbable sutures: the conjoined tendon may be reinforced by suturing it to the shelving edge of the inguinal ligament then the external oblique incision edges are closed together or imbricated. Scarpa's fascia is approximated and skin is closed in a running subcuticular fashion using absorbable sutures. No drain is necessary. Testicular prosthesis insertion in children is deferred until adolescence. Matching size prosthesis is offered in late adolescence for willing patients, old enough to consent and after near maximal compensatory growth of the contralateral testicle has occured.

Testis-Sparing Surgery

With one-third to up to 40% of prepubertal testicular tumors being benign, a growing trend is emphasizing testis-sparing surgery. Any prepubertal boy with age-adjusted normal AFP is a candidate of testis-sparing surgery. Other indications include small tumors less than 2.5 mm in diameter, a tumor in a solitary testis, bilateral malignant germ cell tumors or a non-germ cell tumor, regardless of size or laterality [35]. It has been observed that after partial orchiectomy for large benign tumors, a seemingly insignificant rim of normal tissue tends to get voluminous with follow-up, after the tumor is removed [36, 37].

For testis-sparing procedure, a cautious meticulous approach to potential malignancy is maintained. With the cord controlled, the testis is further draped to isolate it from the rest of the surgical field. The tunica vaginalis is opened and the testis is gently palpated for the tumor. Intraoperative ultrasound is useful to localize small tumors that are not convincingly palpable. A tunica albugenia incision is strategically done with knife in a way to allow access to the tumor with the least disruption of normal parenchyma. The tumor is enucleated or wedge-resected as feasible and sent for frozen section analysis. If the pathology is benign, the tourniquet is released and hemostasis of base of resection is ensured by suture ligatures and minimal bipolar cautery. The tunica albugenia is closed with fine running absorbable sutures. The testis is returned to scrotum in proper orientation and abdomen is closed. If frozen section analysis is suspicious for malignancy or is not conclusive, radical orchiectomy is completed as described above.

Staging

When pathology confirms a malignant tumor, further evaluation and adjuvant therapy may be needed. Therefore, staging of malignant tumors emerges as a method to categorize patients into treatment groups and to predict their prognosis. Although a classical TNM (tumor, nodes and metastasis) staging does exist for testicular cancer, it is infrequently used, owing to the declining utilization of radical retroperitoneal lymph node dissection (RRPLND) in pediatric patients because of evidence of limited added therapeutic benefit and significant potential long-term morbidity. However, other staging systems have been proposed, including a panel system of the Children's Oncology Group and Pediatric Cancer Group [38]. This staging system of testicular, as well as paratesticular tumors, employs pathology findings, imaging, and serial evaluation of tumor markers. Stage 1 includes local disease and normalization of markers after complete resection. Stage 2 is assigned for a trans-scrotal orchiectomy, microscopic disease in scrotum or cord less than 5 cm from proximal resection end, less than 2 cm retroperitoneal lymph node and/or persistent elevation of markers. Stage 3 includes retroperitoneal lymph node(s) larger than 2 cm in diameter and stage 4 represents distant metastasis. Of note, 80% of children with yolk sac tumor have stage 1 disease.

Types

Testicular tumors may be classified according to their histologic origin and their malignant potential.

Germ Cell Tumors

Teratoma

Teratoma is the most common benign prepubertal testicular tumor presenting at a median age of 1 year with a range of birth to 18 months. Teratomas consist of the combination of the three embryological germ-cell layers: ectoderm, mesoderm, and endoderm, giving rise to epithelium, cartilage, fat, bone, muscle, and neural elements, thus appearing heterogeneous sonographically. Cysts and calcifications on ultrasound are suggestive but are neither sensitive nor specific. Microscopically, prepubertal teratomas are predominantly mature, but immature teratomas (with embryonal or incompletely differentiated tissue, e.g., primitive neuroectoderm) have been reported [39].

Prepubertal teratoma is clinically and histologically distinct from its adult counterpart and is considered to have an almost universal benign behavior. While clinical metastasis is reported in 60% of adult teratoma [40, 41], only scattered case reports describe metastasis in prepubertal teratoma. Histologically, intra-tubular germ cell neoplasia (ITGCN) or carcinoma in situ is not found in seminiferous tubules of pediatric testes harboring teratoma, unlike the findings in adult testes with teratoma where 88% have ITGCN [42]. Even at a molecular level, adult teratoma shows complex cytogenetic aberrations that are not observed when prepubertal teratomas are subjected to conventional chromosomal or array-based hybridization studies [43], thus demonstrating the benign behavior of prepubertal teratoma. As such, testis-sparing surgery with excisional biopsy of teratoma is the only management required in prepubertal patients. However, in peripubertal boys with histologic evidence of pubertal changes, an orchiectomy should be performed because teratomas are potentially malignant in that age group, similar to adults. It is worth mentioning that malignant behavior of teratoma reported in literature, albeit rare, occurred with immature teratoma: one case of metastasis in a 3 month old boy with immature teratoma in a cryptorchid intra-abdominal testis [44], and 2 cases of somatic malignant neuroectodermal associated with testicular immature teratoma in a 20 month and 12 year boys [39].

Epidermoid Cysts

Epidermoid cysts may be related to well-differentiated teratomas and are benign regardless of age. They account for 3% of primary testicular tumors. They are of ectodermal origin, unlike teratomas that exhibit all three germ cell layers. On ultrasound, they appear as discrete intratesticular cystic masses with heterogeneous echogenic debris secondary to keratinized squamous epithelial deposits, Infrequently, they appear as homogeneous masses. Again, ultrasound findings are suggestive but never diagnostic. Testis-sparing surgery is sufficient, and epidermoid cysts are easily enucleated from surrounding testicular tissue [45], that never shows ITGCN [42]. Once pathology is confirmed, surveillance is not needed.

Yolk Sac Tumors

Yolk sac tumor is clinically important as it accounts for nearly all malignant prepubertal testicular tumors. The name yolk sac tumor has replaced numerous previous names that were confusing: clear-cell adenocarcinoma, extraembryonal mesoblastoma, mesoblastoma vitellinum, endodermal sinus tumor, juvenile embryonal carcinoma, orchioblastoma, and archenteronoma. Histologically, yolk sac tumors are yellow-gray, friable, predominantly solid tumors with a characteristic but highly variable range of histological patterns. Characteristic findings include focal areas of positive AFP immunostaining, prominent intracellular and extracellular hyaline globules, periodic acid-Schiff positive globules and Schiller–Duval bodies which are comprised of small central blood vessels surrounded by two layers of tumor cells [46].

Yolk sac tumors in prepubertal patients behave distinctly from their postpubertal counterparts. In children, they are predominantly pure in histology unlike in adults where they are mixed with other histological types. The majority of prepubertal tumors (85%) are stage 1 at presentation versus only 35% of postpubertal tumors [47]. Metastasis of yolk sac tumors follows a hematogenous spread, as 20% of prepubertal patients have lung metastases versus 4–6% of adults. While one-third of children with metastatic disease have it confined to the retroperitoneum, 50% have hematogenous spread without retroperitoneal involvement. As a result RRPLND, a critical adjuvant surgery in metastatic disease in adults, not as widely used in the management of metastatic disease in children [48]. Even at a molecular level, prepubertal yolk sac tumor behaves differently than its postpubertal counterpart. A chromosomal gain in the short arm of chromosome 12p has been noted in nearly all malignant adult germ cell tumors, a finding that is not demonstrated in prepubertal yolk sac tumor, yet it is characterized by other distinct changes on chromosomes 1, 6, and 20 [43].

Gonadal Stromal Tumors

Given the rarity of gonadal stromal tumors in children, as well as in adults, no rigorous guidelines are available to aid management, except for some case reports and small case series. The various types of stromal tumors are generally benign, though some tumors, particularly sertoli cell tumor, were shown to exhibit malignant behavior.

Sertoli Cell Tumor

Sertoli cell tumors account for 2% of primary prepubertal testicular tumors. Most available literature is dominated by data on adult patients. In a review of 60 cases of Sertoli cell tumors, only four patients were younger than 20 years, all being over 15 years old. In adult Sertoli cell tumors, 10% malignancy is cited [49]. However, the Prepubertal Testis Tumor Registry cites the median age of diagnosis of Sertoli cell tumor at 6 months, ranging from 4 months to 10 years, with no reported malignant behavior. Bilateral involvement is observed in 25% [50]. Around 10% of Sertoli cell tumors are hormonally active with precocious puberty and/or gynecomastia as presenting symptoms [51, 52]. Around 33% of Sertoli cell tumors (specifically, large-cell calcifying subtype) have associated endocrine abnormalities or genetic syndromes, namely, Peutz–Jeghers and Carney syndromes. Familial Peutz–Jeghers syndrome is autosomal dominant with mutations in STK11/LKB1 on chromosome 19p [53] and includes, in addition to Sertoli cell tumors, hamartomatous polyposis of gastrointestinal tract and mucocutaneous pigmentation. Carney syndrome is associated with myxoid lesions of skin, soft tissue and heart, cutaneous blue nevi, lentigines of the face and lips, Cushing's disease, pituitary adenoma, and schwannoma [54]. Awareness of familial disease inheritance is crucial in counseling patients and first degree relatives of potential significant morbidities.

Histologically, Sertoli cell tumors are yellow to gray, firm and well circumscribed with areas of hemorrhage and minor cysts in one-third of pathologies. Microscopically, a relatively acellular, vascular, fibrous to hyalinized stroma is common, with cells having a variable eosinophillic cytoplasm. Large-cell calcifying variant of Sertoli cell tumor is clinically and histologically distinct, being more multifocal, hormonally active and seen in pediatrics, yet invariably benign in patients less than 5 years old. Nonetheless, metastatic assessment is considered for large tumors, 5 cm in diameter or larger, with cellular atypia, increased mitotic activity, necrosis, vascular invasion or for Sertoli cell tumors in older children [55].

Leydig Cell Tumor

Leydig cell tumors are universally benign, presenting between 5 and 10 years of age with variable picture of precocious puberty. In fact, 10% of precocious puberty is attributed to Leydig cell tumor. Findings include an early growth spurt, frequent erections, external genitalia larger than the patient's peers, pubic, axillary and facial hair, acne, and deepening of the voice. Although common in adults with virilization, signs of feminization and gynecomastia are uncommon in children, presenting in up to 15% [2]. Differential diagnosis includes central nervous system lesions, adrenocortical carcinoma, and congenital adrenal hyperplasia (CAH). In the presence of a testicular mass, a Leydig cell tumor is the most likely diagnosis. Because virilization may manifest before a tumor is palpable, all boys with precocious puberty should undergo an ultrasound of the testicles to rule out a small tumor. Blood work shows an elevated testosterone level with low or normal FSH and LH levels. Normal levels of 17-hydroxyprogesterone exclude the diagnosis of CAH.

Leydig cell tumors are ideally managed by testis-sparing excision. Leydig cell tumors are well-circumscribed tan nodules, and exhibit diffuse sheets of large eosinophilic polygonal cells with Reinke crystals in around 40% [56]. Immunostaining is positive for vimentin and inhibin. Persistence of androgenic effects may be due to a contralateral tumor, but this is rare in children, yet difficult to detect on physical examination and better assessed by sonographic evaluation. With complete excision and absence of contralateral tumors, many children may proceed through premature puberty secondary to a "activated" hypothalamic–pituitary–gonadal axis. A pediatric endocrinology follow-up is prudent.

Juvenile Granulosa Cell Tumor

Juvenile granulosa cell tumors are the most common testicular tumors in neonates, presenting before the first 6 months of life. Of 22 newborns in the Prepubertal Testis Tumor Registry, 6 had juvenile granulosa cell tumors, 6 had yolk sac tumors, and 6 had undifferentiated stromal tumors [50]. Tumor architecture in juvenile granulosa cell tumor is distinct from yolk sac tumor, and is composed of sheets of granulosa-like cells in a nodular inter-mixed with cystic pattern. Unlike in yolk sac tumor, immunostaining is AFP negative and inhibin-alpha positive [57]. Chromosome analysis is recommended, as juvenile granulosa cell tumors are associated with mosaicism, genetic changes in Y chromosome and ambiguous genitalia [58, 59]. However, the tumor is benign and testis-sparing excision is curative. No cases of recurrent or metastatic disease have been reported to date.

Gonadoblastoma

Gonadoblastomas contain both germ cells and stromal cells including large germ cells resembling seminoma, sex cord non-germinal elements such as Sertoli or granulosa cells, and stromal elements such as Leydig cells [60]. Usually presenting in postpubertal patients, gonadoblastoma occurs almost exclusively in dysgenetic gonads of intersex disorders (streak gonads). Gonadoblastoma is more likely to occur in dysgenetic gonads or dysgenetic testes in patients with a Y chromosome or evidence of some Y chromatin. Gonadoblastomas occur in 3% of patients with true hermaphroditism, and 10–30% of patients with mixed gonadal dysgenesis or pure gonadal dysgenesis and an XY karyotype. Gonadoblastomas are bilateral in 40% of cases. Gonadoblastomas are often asymptomatic and detected incidentally when dysgenetic gonads are removed or present with virilization. Although gonadoblastomas are benign, overgrowth of the germinal components leading to a dysgerminoma (seminoma) occurs in 50% of cases, with 10% developing overt malignant tumors [61].

Gonadoblastomas are treated by radical orchiectomy. Any dysgenetic gonad in a child with a Y chromosome should be removed prophylactically in infancy or early childhood. Tumors are much less likely in patients who lack a Y chromosome, such as patients with Turner syndrome or XX patients with pure gonadal dysgenesis [62]. When malignant degeneration is present, a metastatic evaluation and appropriate follow-up are indicated. These tumors are radiosensitive and have a favorable prognosis. Choriocarcinoma or embryonal carcinoma are unfavorable elements, and impart a poor prognosis.

Others

Leukemia

Secondary malignancies of the testicle are rare, with acute lymphoblastic leukemia (ALL) being the most clinically relevant secondary malignancy. While only 2% of boys have overt clinical involvement of testicles at diagnosis, 20% would have microscopic testicular involvement with complete remission in a majority of them [38]. Patients with T-cell leukemia or with higher leukemia cell burdens are more susceptible to testicular involvement [63]. Pretreatment testicular biopsy is unnecessary because it does not predict patients who are prone to have persistent or relapsing disease, although with modern chemotherapy protocols, remission is more likely.

With classical protocols, approximately 10% of patients had relapse in testicles, presumably because testes represented privileged testicular-blood barrier sites from chemotherapy [64]. With modern ALL chemotherapy, testicular relapse now occurs in less than 1% of patients [65]. Post-chemotherapy biopsy in the absence of physical findings is no longer routine. In limited clinical scenarios, testicular enlargement persisting or occurring after chemotherapy should undergo biopsy to confirm testicular ALL. Positive testicular biopsies are invariably associated with relapse elsewhere and additional intensive systemic chemotherapy and radiation are initiated. In the rare scenario of unilateral testicular relapse, orchiectomy is considered, in an attempt to limit radiation dose to the contralateral testicle and attempt to preserve its endocrine function [66].

Hyperplastic Adrenal Rests

Adrenal rests are located along the spermatic cord and in the testicular hilum of newborns [67–69]. Although they regress in infancy, boys with congenital adrenal hyperplasia (CAH) may have prominent hyperpastic rests secondary to stimulation by high levels of adrenocorticotropic hormone (ACTH). Bilateral, nodular growths in the testes are noted, often mistaken for bilateral Leydig cell tumors, particularly with boys with mild unrecognized CAH and precocious puberty. The nodules of CAH are similar histologically to Leydig cell tumors, potentially complicating a definitive diagnosis. Any child presenting with precocious puberty and a testicular mass should undergo measurement of serum 17-hydroxyprogesterone, to distinguish these two entities. Testicular nodules associated with CAH are typically multifocal, including extratesticular involvement and have architecture similar to the adrenal cortex. Reinke crystals, pathognomonic of Leydig cell tumors, should be absent. Many, but not all, of these nodules resolve or significantly reduce in size in response to steroid replacement or an increase in steroid therapy. Orchiectomy should be avoided, unless the biopsy is suspicious or the adrenal rests are large.

Post-surgical Management and Prognosis

Post-surgical management is required for patients with malignant testicular tumors, i.e., yolk sac tumors. Stage 1 disease will be confirmed in 80% of those patients that undergo radical orchiectomy with complete resection of tumor, have normal imaging, and have normalization of AFP level. The overall recurrence risk is 20% with no therapy other than orchiectomy; therefore, patients with stage 1 disease are candidates for active surveillance with AFP every 2–3 months, plain chest radiographs every 2–3 months, and CT scans or MRI every 3–4 months for the first 2 years, although CT scans could be done every 6 months in the second year. After 2 years, if there is no evidence of recurrence, surveillance using all of these methods can be less frequent, since the risk is greatest in the first 2 years [70].

Historically, RRPLND was the most common form of adjuvant therapy for the treatment of yolk sac tumors; however, with the prevalent and reliable use of AFP to detect occult metastases and refinement of multiagent chemotherapy, the role of RRPLND to diagnose and treat metastatic disease in prepubertal patients has diminished. This is made further less attractive given the increased risk of bowel obstruction after laparotomy in children, the questionable feasibility of nerve sparing in prepubertal RRPLND and the lack of long-term functional data available regarding children undergoing RRPLND for testicular cancer. Given these factors, retroperitoneal surgery in children has been reserved for biopsy of radiographically equivocal nodes or for resection of a persistent retroperitoneal mass after chemotherapy, notwithstanding potential postoperative complications including bowel obstruction, wound infection, chylous ascites, and subsequent ejaculatory dysfunction.

Since their introduction in the 1970s, platinum-based chemotherapeutic agents have revolutionized adjuvant treatment of metastatic testicular cancers that show remarkable susceptibility across affected age groups. With modern protocols, overall survival of prepubertal testicular cancers approaches 100%. This has been demonstrated by multicenter-data reported from several collaborative groups from Europe and USA.

The German Society of Pediatric Oncology [71] showed that only 14 of 91 patients (15%) with stage 1 yolk sac tumors recurred after radical inguinal orchiectomy with observation alone. Recurrences were cured by chemotherapy alone. At time of orchiectomy, 5 patients presented with metastasis, 4 of whom were cured by chemotherapy. Chemotherapy included four courses of vinblastine, bleomycin, and cisplatin. A delayed RRPLND was done if viable tumor was seen after two courses. Additional three courses of etoposide, ifosfamide and cisplatin were also given.

The Italian Cooperative Study [72] included 36 patients with testicular tumors but a total of 95 pediatric patients with germ-cell tumors that were gonadal and extragonadal. Primary surgery followed by multiagent chemotherapy conferred a 100% survival for patients with testicular germ-cell tumors. The chemotherapeutic regimen was highly toxic with 3 therapy-specific mortalities.

The UK Children's Cancer Study Group [73] enrolled 63 patients with yolk sac tumors after orchiectomy. Stage 1 patients underwent surveillance, while stage 2 or higher patients received a multiagent chemotherapy including etoposide, carboplatin, and bleomycin. Eleven of 51(22%) patients in the surveillance group had recurrence, but all were cured by chemotherapy. All 22 patients with residual or metastatic disease were cured by chemotherapy.

Studies from the US Children's Oncology Group [74, 75] showed a recurrence rate of 18%

(11 of 63 patients) for stage 1 yolk sac tumors, with all recurrences and a stage 2 disease (14 patients) cured by chemotherapy. The group also showed that combination chemotherapy (etoposide and bleomycin) with high-dose cisplatin was more successful in lowering event-free survival (absence of relapse, progression, second malignancy, or death) than standard cisplatin doses, but overall survival was similar. Indeed, a higher number of deaths (6:1) for the high-dose cisplatin regimen warrants reserving it to higher risk disease [76].

Conclusion

This chapter shows that prepubertal testicular tumors behave differently from their adult counterparts in clinical behavior, histologic characteristics, and molecular biology. In the absence of an age-adjusted elevation in alpha feto-protein, the recommended initial surgical management is an inguinal exploration with excisional biopsy and frozen section analysis. The majority of patients will have a benign tumor and thus require no additional evaluation or adjuvant treatment. Patients with the most common malignancy, i.e., yolk sac tumor, will usually have stage 1 disease, reasonably managed with post-resection observation. The minority of patients with metastasis, or a stage 1 disease that progresses, will virtually all be cured with a multiagent platinum-based chemotherapeutic protocol with a refined safety profile. The overall outlook for pediatric patients with testicular tumors is optimistic in regards to survival, quality of life, and fertility preservation. This is brought forth by the evolving trend on reducing the morbidity of the surgery and the adjuvant therapies for these children.

References

1. Schneider DT, Calaminus G, Koch S, Teske C, Schmidt P, Haas RJ, Harms D, Göbel U. Epidemiologic analysis of 1442 children and adolescents registered in the German germ cell tumor protocols. Pediatr Blood Cancer. 2004;42:169–75.
2. Coppes MJ, Rackley R, Kay R. Primary testicular and paratesticular tumors of childhood. Med Pediatr Oncol. 1994;22:329–40.
3. Alanee S, Shukla A. Paediatric testicular cancer: an updated review of incidence and conditional survival from the surveillance, epidemiology and end results database. BJU Int. 2009;104:1280–3.
4. Ross JH, Rybicki L, Kay R. Clinical behavior and a contemporary management algorithm for prepubertal testis tumors: a summary of the prepubertal testis tumor registry. J Urol. 2002;168:1675–9.
5. Pohl HG, Shukla AR, Metcalfe PD, Cilento BG, Retik AB, Bagli DJ, Huff DS, Rushton HG. Prepubertal testis tumors: actual prevalence rate of histological types. J Urol. 2004;172(6 Pt 1):2370–2.
6. Thorup J, McLachlan R, Cortes D, Nation TR, Balic A, Southwell BR, Hutson JM. What is new in cryptorchidism and hypospadias—a critical review on the testicular dysgenesis hypothesis. J Pediatr Surg. 2010;45(10):2074–86.
7. Toppari J, Virtanen HE, Main KM, Skakkebaek NE. Cryptorchidism and hypospadias as a sign of testicular dysgenesis syndrome (TDS): environmental connection. Birth Defects Res A Clin Mol Teratol. 2010;88(10):910–9.
8. Wood HM, Elder JS. Cryptorchidism and testicular cancer: separating fact from fiction. J Urol. 2009;181 (2):452–61.
9. Looijenga LH, Hersmus R, de Leeuw BH, Stoop H, Cools M, Oosterhuis JW, Drop SL, Wolffenbuttel KP. Gonadal tumours and DSD. Best Pract Res Clin Endocrinol Metab. 2010;24(2):291–310.
10. Pleskacova J, Hersmus R, Oosterhuis JW, Setyawati BA, Faradz SM, Cools M, Wolffenbuttel KP, Lebl J, Drop SL, Looijenga LH. Tumor risk in disorders of sex development. Sex Dev. 2010;4(4–5):259–69.
11. Li Y, Tabatabai ZL, Lee TL, Hatakeyama S, Ohyama C, Chan WY, Looijenga LH, Lau YF. The Y-encoded TSPY protein: a significant marker potentially plays a role in the pathogenesis of testicular germ cell tumors. Hum Pathol. 2007;38 (10):1470–81.
12. Lau YF, Li Y, Kido T. Gonadoblastoma locus and the TSPY gene on the human Y chromosome. Birth Defects Res C Embryo Today. 2009;87(1):114–22.
13. Myrup C, Westergaard T, Schnack T, Oudin A, Ritz C, Wohlfahrt J, Melbye M. Testicular cancer risk in first- and second-generation immigrants to Denmark. J Natl Cancer Inst. 2008;100(1):41–7.
14. Hardell L., van Bavel B., Lindström G., Carlberg M., Charlotte Dreifaldt A., Wijkström H., Starkhammar H., Eriksson M., Hallquist A., Kolmert T. Increased concentrations of polychlorinated biphenyls, hexachlorobenzene, and chlordanes in mothers of men with testicular cancer. Environ Health Perspect. 2003;111(7):930–4.
15. Nori F, Carbone P, Giordano F, Osborn J, Figà-Talamanca I. Endocrine-disrupting chemicals and

testicular cancer: a case-control study. Arch Environ Occup Health. 2006;61(2):87–95.
16. Dieckmann KP, Hartmann JT, Classen J, Diederichs M, Pichlmeier U. Is increased body mass index associated with the incidence of testicular germ cell cancer? J Cancer Res Clin Oncol. 2009;135 (5):731–8.
17. Mongraw-Chaffin ML, Cohn BA, Anglemyer AT, Cohen RD, Christianson RE. Maternal smoking, alcohol, and coffee use during pregnancy and son's risk of testicular cancer. Alcohol. 2009;43(3):241–5.
18. Daling JR, Doody DR, Sun X, Trabert BL, Weiss NS, Chen C, Biggs ML, Starr JR, Dey SK, Schwartz SM. Association of marijuana use and the incidence of testicular germ cell tumors. Cancer. 2009;115(6):1215–23.
19. Serter S, Gumus B, Unlu M, Tunçyürek O, Tarhan S, Ayyildiz V, Pabuscu Y. Prevalence of testicular microlithiasis in an asymptomatic population. Scand J Urol Nephrol. 2006;40:212–4.
20. Peterson AC, Bauman JM, Light DE, McMann LP, Costabile RA. The prevalence of testicular microlithiasis in an asymptomatic population of men 18-35 years old. J Urol. 2001;166:2061–4.
21. Husmann DA. Cryptorchidism and its relationship to testicular neoplasia and microlithiasis. Urology. 2005;66:424–6.
22. Sakamoto H, Shichizyou T, Saito K, Okumura T, Ogawa Y, Yoshida H, Kushima M. Testicular microlithiasis identified ultrasonographically in Japanese adult patients: prevalence and associated conditions. Urology. 2006;68:636–41.
23. Wasniewska M, De Luca F, Bertillonnai S, Matarazzo P, Weber G, Crisafulli G, Valenzise M, Lala R. Testicular microlithiasis: an unreported feature of McCune-Albright syndrome in males. J Pediatr. 2004;145:670–2.
24. Furness PD III, Husmann DA, Brock JW III, Steinhardt GF, Bukowski TP, Freedman AL, Silver RI, Cheng EY. Multi-institutional study of testicular microlithiasis in childhood: a benign or premalignant condition? J Urol. 1998;160:1151–4.
25. McEniff N, Doherty F, Katz J, Schrager CA, Klauber G. Yolk sac tumor of the testis discovered on a routine annual sonogram in a boy with testicular microlithiasis. AJR Am J Roentgenol. 1995;164:971–2.
26. Arrigo T, Messina MF, Valenzise M, Rosano M, Alaggio R, Cecchetto G, Zirilli G, De Luca F. Testicular microlithiasis heralding mixed germ cell tumor of the testis in a boy. J Endocrinol Invest. 2006;29:82–5.
27. Drut R. Yolk sac tumor and testicular microlithiasis. Pediatr Pathol Mol Med. 2003;22:343–7.
28. Slaughenhoupt B, Kadlec A, Schrepferman C. Testicular microlithiasis preceding metastatic mixed germ cell tumor-first pediatric report and recommended management of testicular microlithiasis in the pediatric population. Urology. 2009;73(5):1029–31.
29. Dagash H, Mackinnon EA. Testicular microlithiasis: what does it mean clinically? BJU Int. 2007;99:157–60.
30. Benson CB, Doubilet PM, Richie JP. Sonography of the male genital tract. AJR Am J Roentgenol. 1989;153:705–13.
31. Shapeero LG, Vordermark JS. Epidermoid cysts of testes and role of sonography. Urology. 1993;41:75–9.
32. Wu JT, Book L, Sudar K. Serum alpha fetoprotein (AFP) levels in normal infants. Pediatr Res. 1981;15 (1):50–2.
33. Palmer JS, Morris K, Steinberg GD, Kaplan WE. Testicular, sacrococcygeal, and other tumors. In: Vogelzang NJ, Scardino PS, Shipley WU, Coffey DS, editors. Comprehensive textbook of genitourinary oncology. 2nd ed. Philadelphia: Lippincott Williams & Wilkins; 2000.
34. Hinman F Jr, Baskin LS. Radical orchiectomy. In: Hinman F Jr, Baskin LS, editors. Hinman's atlas of pediatric urologic surgery. 2nd ed. Philadelphia: Saunders Elsevier; 2009. p. 612–8.
35. Steiner H, Höltl L, Maneschg C, Berger AP, Rogatsch H, Bartsch G, Hobisch A. Frozen section analysis-guided organ-sparing approach in testicular tumors: technique, feasibility, and long-term results. Urology. 2003;62(3):508–13.
36. Shukla AR, Woodard C, Carr MC, Huff DS, Canning DA, Zderic SA, Kolon TF, Snyder HM 3rd. Experience with testis sparing surgery for testicular teratoma. J Urol. 2004;171(1):161–3.
37. Metcalfe PD, Farivar-Mohseni H, Farhat W, McLorie G, Khoury A, Bägli DJ. Pediatric testicular tumors: contemporary incidence and efficacy of testicular preserving surgery. J Urol. 2003;170(6 Pt 1):2412–5; discussion 2415–6.
38. Wu H, Snyder HM 3rd. Pediatric urologic oncology: bladder, prostate, testis. Urol Clin North Am. 2004;31:619–27.
39. Kato K, Ijiri R, Tanaka Y, Toyoda Y, Chiba K, Kitami K. Testicular immature teratoma with primitive neuroectodermal tumor in early childhood. J Urol. 2000;164:2068–9.
40. Carver B, Al-Ahmadie H, Sheinfeld J. Adult and pediatric testicular teratoma. Urol Clin North Am. 2007;34:245–51.
41. Bahrami A, Ro J, Ayala A. An overview of testicular germ cell tumors. Arch Pathol Lab Med. 2007;131:1267–80.
42. Manivel J, Reinberg Y, Nehans G, et al. Intratubular germ cell neoplasia in testicular teratomas and epidermoid cysts—correlation with prognosis and possible biologic significance. Cancer. 1989;64:715–20.
43. Harms D, Zahn S, Gobel U, et al. Pathology and molecular biology of teratomas in childhood and adolescence. Klin Padiatr. 2006;218:296–302.
44. Hasegawa T, Maeda K, Kamata N, et al. A case of immature teratoma originating in intra-abdominal

undescended testis in a 3-month-old infant. Pediatr Surg Int. 2006;22:570–2.
45. Walsh C, Rushton HG. Diagnosis and management of teratomas and epidermoid cysts. Urol Clin North Am. 2000;27(3):509–18.
46. Ulbright TM, Roth LM. Recent developments in the pathology of germ cell tumors. Semin Diagn Pathol. 1987;4:304–19.
47. Grady RW. Current management of prepubertal yolk sac tumors of the testis. Urol Clin North Am. 2000;27(3):503–9.
48. Grady RW, Ross JH, Kay R. Patterns of metastatic spread in prepubertal yolk sac tumor of the testis. J Urol. 1995;153(4):1259–61.
49. Gómez García I, Romero Molina M, López-García Moreno A, et al. Sertoli cell tumor, a rare testicular tumor, our experience and review of the literature. Arch Esp Urol. 2010;63(5):392–5.
50. Thomas JC, Ross JH, Kay R. Stromal testis tumors in children: a report from the prepubertal testis tumor registry. J Urol. 2001;166(6):2338–40.
51. Diamond FB Jr, Root AW, Hoover DL, Monteforte H. Hetero- and isosexual pseudoprecocity associated with testicular sex-cord tumors in an 8 year-old male. J Pediatr Endocrinol Metab. 1996;9(3):407–14.
52. Gabrilove JL, Freiberg EK, Leiter E, Nicolis GL. Feminizing and non-feminizing Sertoli cell tumors. J Urol. 1980;124(6):757–67.
53. McGarrity TJ, Amos C. Peutz-Jeghers syndrome: clinicopathology and molecular alterations. Cell Mol Life Sci. 2006;63(18):2135–44.
54. Washecka R, Dresner MI, Honda SA. Testicular tumors in Carney's complex. J Urol. 2002;167(3):1299–302.
55. Young R, Koelliker D, Scully R. Sertoli cell tumors of the testis, not otherwise specified: a clinicopathologic analysis of 60 cases. Am J Surg Pathol. 1998;22:709–21.
56. Al-Agha OM, Axiotis CA. An in-depth look at Leydig cell tumor of the testis. Arch Pathol Lab Med. 2007;131(2):311–7.
57. Shukla AR, Huff DS, Canning DA, et al. Juvenile granulose cell tumor of the testis: contemporary clinical management and pathological diagnosis. J Urol. 2004;171(5):1900–2.
58. Cortez J, Kaplan G. Gonadal stromal tumors, gonadoblastomas, epidermoid cysts, and secondary tumors of the testis in children. Urol Clin North Am. 1993;20:15–26.
59. Young R, Lawrence W, Scully R. Juvenile granulosa cell tumor—another neoplasm associated with abnormal chromosomes and ambiguous genitalia, a report of 3 cases. Am J Surg Pathol. 1985;9:737–43.
60. Cools M, Stoop H, Kersemaekers AM, et al. Gonadoblastoma arising in undifferentiated gonadal tissue within dysgenetic gonads. J Clin Endocrinol Metab. 2006;91(6):2404–13.
61. Cooper C, Cooper M, Carter J, Russell P. Gonadoblastoma progressing to dysgerminoma in a 55-year-old woman with normal karyotype. Pathology. 2007;39(2):284–5.
62. Bianco B, Lipay MV, Melaragno MI, Guedes AD, Verreschi IT. Detection of hidden Y mosaicism in Turner's syndrome: importance in the prevention of gonadoblastoma. J Pediatr Endocrinol Metab. 2006;19(9):1113–7.
63. Gajjar A, Ribeiro RC, Mahmoud HH, Sandlund JT, Liu Q, Furman WL, Santana VM, Crist WM, Rivera GK, Pui CH. Overt testicular disease at diagnosis is associated with high risk features and a poor prognosis in patients with childhood acute lymphoblastic leukemia. Cancer. 1996;78(11):2437–42.
64. Finklestein JZ, Miller DR, Feusner J, Stram DO, Baum E, Shina DC, Johnson DG, Gyepes MT, Hammond GD. Treatment of overt isolated testicular relapse in children on therapy for acute lymphoblastic leukemia. A report from the Children's Cancer Group. Cancer. 1994;73(1):219–23.
65. Jacobs JE, Hastings C. Isolated extramedullary relapse in childhood acute lymphocytic leukemia. Curr Hematol Malig Rep. 2010;5(4):185–91.
66. Arima K, Hasegawa D, Ogawa C, Kato I, Imamura T, Takusagawa A, Takahashi H, Kitagawa Y, Hori T, Tsurusawa M, Manabe A, Hosoya R. Detection of submicroscopic disease in the bone marrow and unaffected testis of a child with T-cell acute lymphoblastic leukemia who experienced "isolated" testicular relapse. Int J Hematol. 2009;90(3):370–3.
67. Srikanth MS, West BR, Ishitani M, Isaacs H Jr, Applebaum H, Costin G. Benign testicular tumors in children with congenital adrenal hyperplasia. J Pediatr Surg. 1992;27(5):639–41.
68. Ghazi AA, Hadayegh F, Khakpour G, Azizi F, Melby JC. Bilateral testicular enlargement due to adrenal remnant in a patient with C11 hydroxylase deficiency congenital adrenal hyperplasia. J Endocrinol Invest. 2003;26(1):84–7.
69. Erdogan S, Ergin M, Cevlik F, Yuksel B, Tuncer R, Tunali N, Polat S. Testicular adrenal rest hyperplasia due to 21-hydroxylase deficiency: a case report. Endocr Pathol. 2006;17(1):83–7.
70. Connolly JA, Gearhart JP. Management of yolk sac tumors in children. Urol Clin North Am. 1993;20:7.
71. Haas RJ, Schmidt P, Göbel U, Harms D. Testicular germ cell tumors an update—results of the German Cooperative Studies 1982–1997. Klin Paediatr. 1999;211:300–4.
72. Lo Curto M, Lumia F, Alaggio R, et al. Malignant germ cell tumors in childhood: results of the first Italian cooperative study "TCG 91". Med Pediatr Oncol. 2003;41:417–25.
73. Mann JR, Raafat F, Robinson K, et al. The United Kingdom Children's Cancer Study Group's second germ cell tumor study: carboplatin, etoposide, and bleomycin are effective treatment for children with malignant extracranial germ cell tumors, with acceptable toxicity. J Clin Oncol. 2000;18:3809–18.

74. Rogers PC, Olson TA, Cullen JW, et al. Treatment of children and adolescents with stage II testicular and stages I and II ovarian malignant germ cell tumors: a Pediatric Inter Group study—Pediatric Oncology Group 9048 and Children's Cancer Group 8891. J Clin Oncol. 2004;22:3563–9.
75. Schlatter M, Rescorla F, Giller R, et al. Excellent outcome in patients with stage I germ cell tumors of the testes: a study of the Children's Cancer Group/Pediatric Oncology Group. J Pediatr Surg. 2003;38:319–24.
76. Cushing B, Giller R, Cullen JW, et al. Randomized comparison of combination chemotherapy with etoposide, bleomycin, and either high-dose or standard-dose cisplatin in children and adolescents with high-risk malignant germ cell tumors: a Pediatric Inter group study—Pediatric Oncology Group 9049 and Children's Cancer Group 8882. J Clin Oncol. 2004;22:2691–700.

23 Ovarian Embryology, Anatomy, and Physiology Including Normal Menstrual Physiology

Nancy Sokkary and Jennifer E. Dietrich

This chapter reviews the embryology and anatomy of the ovary and adjacent structures and also reviews the physiology of ovarian function and menstruation. Familiarity with the anatomy and development of the ovary is essential to appreciate many of the pathological findings and malformations of the ovary discussed in other chapters. Familiarity with the anatomy and development of the ovary is also critical to understand the conduct of operations involving the ovary. Knowledge of ovarian and menstrual physiology is the necessary foundation to understand the normal gynecological health and the gynecological disorders of adolescent girls.

Embryology of the Ovary and Ovum

The development of the ovary and the ovum are intimately linked but can be considered as separate processes. Both the development of ovary and ovum begins early in embryogenesis and continues through birth, puberty, child-bearing years, and menopause.

N. Sokkary
Department of Pediatrics, UNM Children's Hospital, The University of New Mexico, 306 A San Pablo St SE, Albuquerque, NM 87108, USA

J.E. Dietrich (✉)
Department of Pediatric and Adolescent Gynecology, Texas Children's Hospital, 6620 Main St., Suite 1450, Houston, TX 77030, USA
e-mail: jedietri@bcm.tmc.edu

Embryology of the Ovary

By 4–5 weeks gestational age, the developing fetus begins the process of sexual differentiation. In fetuses with no testicular-determining-factor gene, the totipotent gonad becomes the female ovary [1, 2]. Specific genes such as WT-1, LIM-1, SF-1, and possibly DAX-1 also play role in ovarian development [3]. In fetuses predetermined for female development, the gonadal ridges ultimately become ovarian tissue [1, 2]. The gonadal ridges are located on the posterior wall of the peritoneal cavity next to the primitive mesonephros (Fig. 23.1). The primitive ovaries then migrate from what will be the upper abdomen to the pelvis through processes of chemotaxis and ligament attachment [1, 2].

The ligament that helps to guide each ovary into position is known as the gubernaculum, which in its primitive form is a cord of mesenchyme connected to the lower medial pole of the gonad. The gubernaculum then attaches to the uterus and ultimately becomes the fibrous bands of the utero-ovarian (or meso-ovarian or ovarian) ligament, which attaches the ovary to the lateral surface of the uterus, and the round ligament, which extends from the uterine horn (the junction of the uterus and the fallopian tube) through the internal inguinal ring to the mons pubis (Fig. 23.2) [4]. Another primitive ligament at the lateral-superior aspect of the gonad becomes the infundibulopelvic ligament or suspensory ligament of the ovary (Fig. 23.2). Ultimately, a normally positioned ovary lies below the pelvic brim within the "true" pelvis,

D.J. Ledbetter and P.R.V. Johnson (eds.), *Endocrine Surgery in Children*,
DOI 10.1007/978-3-662-54256-9_23

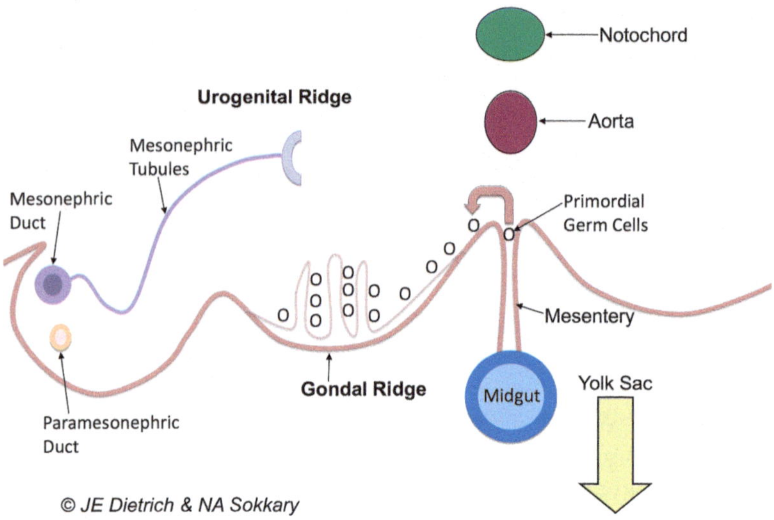

Fig. 23.1 Development of the ovary. Copyright JE Dietrich and NA Sokkary

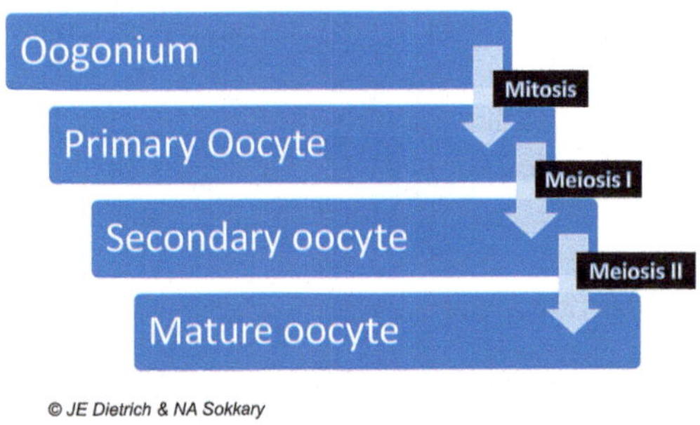

Fig. 23.2 Stages of oogonial development. Copyright JE Dietrich and NA Sokkary

suspended between the utero-ovarian and infundibulopelvic ligaments [4]. It is important to note that the process of ovarian development is completely independent of the Müllerian development of uterus, fallopian tubes, and vagina [1, 2].

Embryology of the Ovum

The development of a human egg, or ovum, capable of being fertilized is the result of a complex process that begins early in embryogenesis and proceeds through a series of orderly stages through sexual maturity. Primitive germ cells originate from the yolk sac endoderm and migrate to the gonadal ridges (Fig. 23.1). The gonadal ridges form primitive sex cords made of up of both ectoderm and mesenchyme [1]. Primitive germ cells in the sex cords give rise to oogonia (plural of oogonium) by 6–7 weeks gestational age [1]. With repeated divisions the number of oogonia peaks around 16–20 weeks gestational age when 6–7 million may be present. After this peak, a slow process of apoptosis of the oogonia ensues. Oogonia that do not undergo apoptosis are transformed to the 1–2 million oocytes (immature ova) that are present at birth. Through the specialized process of cell division called meiosis the diploid oogonium is transformed to a haploid mature oocyte (Fig. 23.3). The development of an oocyte occurs within a capsule of somatic cells in the cortex of the ovary known as a follicle. Each follicle typically contains only one oocyte [2]. Through a process of slow apoptosis, the number of oocytes decreases throughout life. By the reproductive years only 300,000–500,000 oocytes remain and of these, only 400–500 will become mature ovulatory follicles [1, 3].

The process of oocyte development begins prenatally with duplication of genetic material and formation of the primary oocyte that then undergoes begins meiosis I. The process of meiosis I is halted in prophase and primary oocytes remain in this state until menarche. During meiosis I there is recombination of

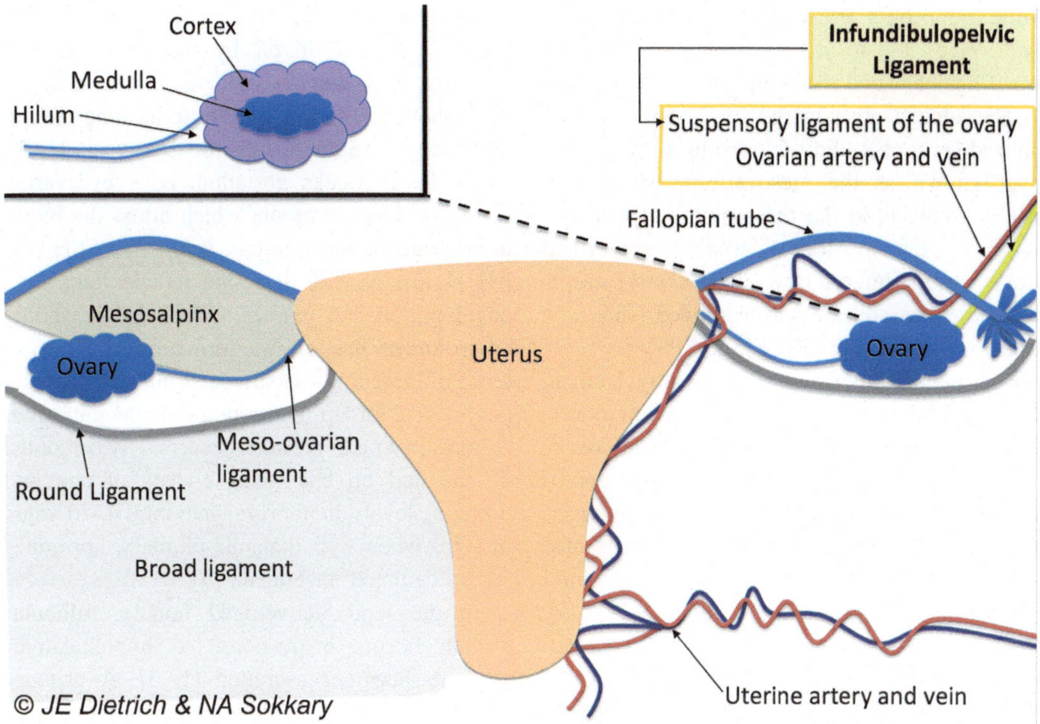

Fig. 23.3 Anatomy of the ovary. Copyright JE Dietrich and NA Sokkary

genetic material maternal between homologous chromosomes which increases genetic diversity. With menstruation meiosis I is completed and the genetic material of the primary oocyte is divided resulting in a secondary oocyte, and a polar body (a nonfunctional primordial entity) and meiosis II begins [1, 3]. The secondary oocyte remains frozen in meiosis II until fertilization when a mature ovum and another polar body is produced.

A primary oocyte is a complex structure made up of yolk, the germinal vesicle (the large nucleus of the primary oocyte before meiosis completed) and the germinal spot (the nucleolysis of the oocyte) [2]. Although made up of many complex parts, human oocytes are relatively fragile, measuring only 0.2 mm in diameter. Each has protective layers including a thick, transparent envelope known as the zona pellucida and an outer layer called the corona radiata [1, 2].

Anatomy of the Ovary and Adnexa

The ovaries, fallopian tubes, and broad ligament complexes make up the adnexa of the uterus. The ovary is normally located just posterior to the fallopian tube on the pelvic sidewall. The ovary is in close proximity to the fallopian tube, and is, in fact, connects the tube by a small muscular complex, known as the fimbria ovarica [5]. The position of the tube near the ovary allows "sweeping" motions of the fimbria of the fallopian tube to collect mature ova from the ovarian surfaces.

The blood supply to the ovary on each side is redundant with a continuous arcade of vessels to supply and support the adnexal structures [5]. Specifically, the ovarian arteries (originating from the renal artery on the left and the aorta on the right) located within the infundibulopelvic ligaments, supply the lateral aspect of the ovary, while Sampson's artery, within the round ligament, gives rise to arterial branches within the broad ligament and mesosalpinx.

The adnexa are covered by a series of specialized peritoneal folds. Closest to the ovary is a layer known as the mesovarium, which ultimately connects to the mesosalpinx. The continuity of the peritoneal folding (described previously in Embryology of the Ovary) means that the entire adnexa can be moved when one aspect is moved (Fig. 23.2) [5].

In a neonate, the ovary is typically 1 cm in diameter and weighs 250–350 mg. Commonly, the right ovary is slightly larger than the left ovary [1, 5]. From the neonatal period to the reproductive years, the ovary will ultimately increase its weight by 10 times. The ovary consists of 3 major portions—the outer cortex, the central medulla, and the ovarian hilum (Fig. 23.2) [1, 5]. The hilum is the point of attachment of the ovary to the mesovarium, the folds of peritoneum that tether the ovary to the body wall [1, 5]. The hilum contains blood vessels, nerves, and hilus cells. The hilar cells are the origin of certain types of ovarian tumors, such as Sertoli or Leydig cell tumors [5]. The outer cortex consists of the tunica albuginea, made up of cuboidal and germinal epithelium. The cortex of the ovary is responsible for follicle formation and is responsive to follicle stimulating hormone (FSH). The supporting network or stromal support tissues within the cortex have the ability to respond to luteinizing hormone (LH) or human chorionic gonadotropin (hCG). The central medulla is largely comprised of mesonephric cells without hormonally sensitive components [1, 5].

Physiology of the Ovary

The ovary has two main physiologic responsibilities: (1) the release of oocytes and (2) the production of steroid hormones [1]. Although Hippocrates, Soranus, and Galen all provided early descriptions of the ovary, it was not until the 1500s when Andreas Vesalius, a Professor of Surgery at the University of Padua, described ovarian follicles that we began to understand ovarian function [1, 3]. Ovarian function is a cyclical process driven by the hypothalamic-pituitary axis and is not static, but changes throughout a female's life, from the time of fetal development to the postmenopausal years [1, 3].

At 18–20 weeks gestation, cells in ovarian cortex develop receptors which allow the ovary to respond to the pituitary hormones FSH and LH [1, 3]. At this time, the female fetus may develop transient ovarian cysts. The hormonal environment that allows formation and persistence of these cysts usually lasts into the neonatal period and for up to 6 months of neonatal life. A hormonal nadir is usually reached by 6 months of age and no later than 2 years of age and hormone levels do not rise again until 4–10 years of age, when hypothalamic-pituitary hormones are upregulated once again [3].

In the reproductive-aged female, follicular growth occurs in response to hypothalamic-pituitary hormone secretion [1, 3]. A primary follicle is recruited, developing progressively into a preantral follicle, antral follicle, and subsequently, a preovulatory follicle (Fig. 23.4). At the time of full follicular maturation, when the follicular cyst may be 2 cm in diameter, and in response to peak LH and prostaglandin presence, ovulation occurs. It is during this time, that the first meiotic division is completed. The second meiotic division takes place only if a mature oocyte is fertilized. Increasing concentrations of FSH cause the granulosa cells of the follicle to increase production of estradiol [3]. Following ovulation the cells of the ruptured follicle reorganize and form a fluid-filled corpus luteum cyst with hypertrophied granulosa cells in the walls of the cyst. In the presence of low LH concentrations, the corpus luteum produces progesterone for a short time (approximately 14 days), but the corpus luteum rapidly ages and then regresses (Fig. 23.4). With corpus luteal regression, menses ensue [3].

Menarche

Menarche is the first menstrual cycle. The median age of menarche for girls in the United States

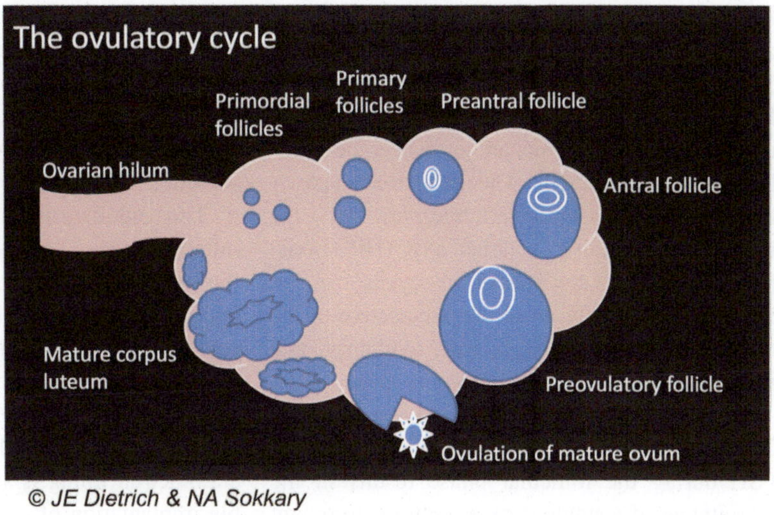

Fig. 23.4 The ovulatory cycle. Copyright JE Dietrich and NA Sokkary

is 12.43 years, with 10% starting by age 11.11 years and 98% starting by 13.75 years of age [6]. The age of menarche has steadily decreased from the 1800s to the mid-twentieth century, but has remained relatively stable over the last 40 years [6, 7]. The age at which an adolescent begins her menstrual cycle is dependent upon several factors including race, geographic location, and nutritional status. The American Academy of Pediatrics reviewed US statistics and found that there is some variation in the age of menarche based on ethnic background. For instance, black females begin menstruating at a median age of 12.02 years, Hispanic females at 12.25 years, and Caucasian females at 12.55 years [8]. It is also known that women in less developed countries tend to be older at menarche. For example, the mean age of menarche in Algeria is 14.3 years, and in Bangladesh, it is even higher at 15.8 years [7, 9]. Increased vegetable intake, decreased calorie consumption, and increased energy expenditure, at least in part, contribute to the older age of menarche in developing countries. These findings are probably related to observations that a body weight of 46 kilograms and a BMI of 17 seem to be a necessary prerequisite for menarche [6, 10].

The age of menarche can also be described in its relation to other elements of pubertal development. Most girls will have their first menstrual cycle 2–3 years after the onset of breast development (thelarche) and rarely before Tanner stage III breast development [6]. Menarche, along with the other parts of puberty, is dependent upon on a complex interplay of various hormones. Gonadotropin releasing hormone (GnRH) is a decapeptide that is released from the hypothalamus. Before the onset of puberty GnRH release is inhibited by other areas of the brain by incompletely defined mechanisms. During normal development, this inhibition is cyclicly interrupted and leads to the pulsatile secretion of GnRH which In turn leads to the pulsatile release of both follicle stimulating hormone (FSH) and Luteinizing hormone (LH) from the anterior pituitary [10, 11]. The amplitude and frequency LH and FSH release slowly increase as puberty approaches [11]. The resultant fluctuations eventually lead to the first menses [10]. Even before menarche, FSH begins to stimulate the conversion of androgens to estrogen.

The Menstrual Cycle

The first menses is usually 2–7 days in length but as one progresses in gynecologic years, cycle regulation increases, and the menses becomes shorter [6]. It takes approximately 14 months from the first menses to have a regular cycle. The average length between menstrual cycles is 34 days but may range from 21 to 45 days [12]. It may take 24 months for ovulation to occur and up to 12 years from menarche to become regularly ovulatory [6, 10]. The menstrual cycle is based on the intricate interplay of the hypothalamic-pituitary-ovarian axis (HPO axis) [10]. However, the menstrual cycle can be viewed more simply, from the perspective of the ovary, as divided into follicular, ovulatory, and luteal phases (Fig. 23.5) [10].

At the time of puberty, there may be as few as 250,000 surviving oocytes. A slow steady rise in FSH during the follicular phase results in the recruitment of a single oocyte within a dominant follicle. FSH also signals the granulosa, or follicular, cells to increase conversion of testosterone to estradiol [13]. During the follicular phase, granulosa cells continue to increase estrogen secretion, followed by a slow rise in progesterone toward the end of the follicular phase. When estrogen increases above a certain threshold, it has positive feedback on the hypothalamus to signal the pituitary to increase both LH and FSH [13]. Around day 14 of the menstrual cycle, approximately 24 h after peak LH secretion, ovulation, the release of the egg from the dominant ovarian follicle, occurs. If an oocyte is fertilized, then the syncytiotrophoblast component of the developing embryo secrets human chorionic gonadotropin (hCG) that signals the corpus luteum, the remnant of the dominant follicle, to continue progesterone production until the placenta takes over this essential support of the pregnancy [13, 14]. The increase in progesterone has a negative feedback on LH and FSH, thereby preventing selection of another dominant follicle during the luteal phase. If an oocyte is not fertilized, the corpus luteum will degenerate and estrogen and progesterone secretion will decrease [14].

The endometrium is also responsive to hormone changes. The increase in estrogen during the proliferative phase leads to increased endometrial thickness [14]. The glands and vessels of the endometrium during this phase proliferate and the endometrial lining increases from 3.5 to 5 mm in thickness [14]. During this time, when progesterone is the dominant hormone, the endometrial lining is stable and ready for possible implantation of a fertilized ovum. If implantation does not occur within 2 weeks of ovulation then the corpus luteum degenerates and progesterone levels fall. Falling progesterone levels result in shedding of the endometrial lining and menstrual bleeding. In addition, the loss of progesterone's inhibitory feedback signals to the HPO axis allows FSH and LH secretion from the anterior pituitary gland to resume and the cycle to repeat [12].

Abnormal Menses

Abnormal menstruation is a common finding in adolescent girls as it may take 2 years or more for menstrual cycles to become regular. Adolescents often experience oligomenorrhea (infrequent menses), metrorrhagia (bleeding between menses), and menorrhagia (heavy bleeding), all of which may be associated with an underlying

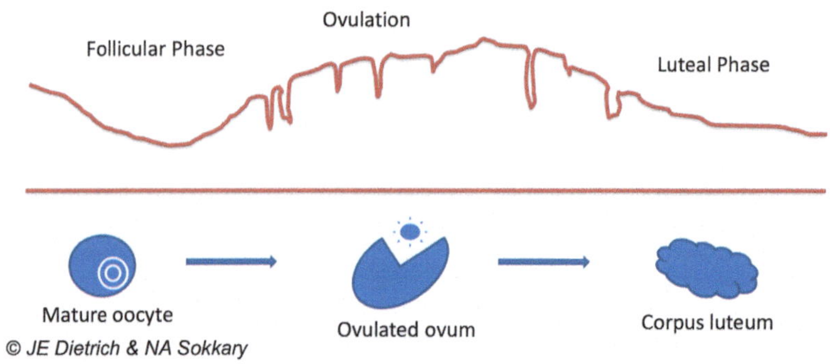

Fig. 23.5 Menstual cycle. Copyright JE Dietrich and NA Sokkary

gynecologic disorder or systemic disease [10]. For this reason, it is important to assess the timing, frequency, and flow of menses to determine if menses are normal [10, 15].

Amenorrhea and Oligomenorrhea

Amenorrhea is the absence of menstruation. Primary amenorrhea is delayed menarche and can be associated with normal or abnormal pubertal development. Secondary amenorrhea is the absence of menstruation after menarche has occurred. Oligomenorrhea is defined as greater than 35 days per cycle. Secondary amenorrhea in adolescents is usually defined as no menses for 6 months; however, most reports recommend beginning an evaluation after 3 months without menses, as more than 95% of adolescents will have a menses more frequently than every 3 months by their second gynecologic year [11, 15, 16]. The incidence of secondary amenorrhea among adolescents is 4% but oligomenorrhea is more common [14]. The etiologies of secondary amenorrhea and oligomenorrhea overlap with the most common causes being pregnancy and anovulation. Other etiologies include polycystic ovarian syndrome (PCOS), premature ovarian failure, eating disorders, congenital adrenal hyperplasia, ovarian and adrenal tumors, and prolactinomas [12, 16]. Furthermore, oligomenorrhea and secondary amenorrhea may also be the presenting symptom of a systemic conditions such as diabetes, Cushing's disease, hyper or hypothyroidism, and Turner's syndrome [12, 15].

Menorrhagia and Metrorrhagia

The amount of blood loss during menses can be difficult to assess, especially in adolescents. The normal blood loss during with each cycle is 30 ml but because most people cannot accurately estimate blood loss in milliliters it is usual to quantify menstrual blood loss using pad/tampon counts [6]. A pad count of greater than 6 per day is considered abnormal [6, 10]. Menorrhagia is usually defined as greater than 80 ml of blood loss per cycle or bleeding more than 7 days continuously. Metrorrhagia is bleeding with irregular intervals [9]. The combination of heavy menses with irregular bleeding is known as menometrorrhagia. The etiology of heavy menses in adolescents is often secondary to anovulatory cycles and less frequently related the presence of polyps or fibroids [10]. It is also important to consider bleeding disorders during the evaluation of irregular menses. For example, von Willebrand disease, which is by far the most common bleeding disorder encountered in menorrhagia, occurs in 1% of the general population, but is found in up to 16% of girls presenting to the emergency department with menorrhagia [6]. Finally, platelet dysfunction and hypothyroidism may present with menometrorrhagia, so investigation of these causes is warranted [15].

References

1. Speroff G, Kase NG. Clinical Endocrinology and Infertility. In: Speroff G, Kase NG, editors. The ovary, embryology and development. 6th ed. Philadelphia: Lippincott, Williams and Wilkins; 1999. p. 107–22.
2. Gray H. Anatomy of the human body. In: The ovum; 1918. p. 1–4. (epub, accessed 9 Jan 2010).
3. Sperling MA. Pediatric endocrinology. In: Sperling MA, editors. Puberty and its disorders in the female. 3rd ed. Philadelphia: Saunders Publishing; 2008. p. 530–43.
4. Dietrich JE, Hertweck SP, Bond S. Undescended ovaries: a clinical review. J Pediatr Adolesc Gynecol. 2007;20(2):57–60.
5. Rock JA, Thompson JD. Te Linde's operative gynecology. In: Rock JA, Thompson JD, editors. Principles of anatomy and perioperative considerations. 8th ed. Philadelphia: Lippincott Williams and Wilkins; 1997. p. 72–4.
6. American Academy of Pediatrics Committee on Adolescence and American College of Obstetricians and Gynecologists Committee on Adolescent Health Care. Menstruation in girls and adolescents: using the menstrual cycle as a vital sign. Pediatrics. 2006;118:2245–50.
7. Hermanson AD. Update on female pubertal development. Curr Opin Obstet Gynecol. 2002;14:475–81.
8. Sun S, Schubert C, Chumlea W, et al. National estimates of the timing of sexual maturation and racial differences among US children. Pediatrics. 2002;110:911–9.

9. Thomas F, Renaud F, Benefice E, de Meeus T, Guegan J. International variability of ages at menarche and menopause: patterns and main determinants. Hum Biol. 1997;73:271–90.
10. Emans S, Laufer M, Goldstein D, Gordon K. The physiology of puberty. In: Pediatric and adolescent gynecology. 5th ed. Philadelphia: Lippincott Williams and Wilkins; 2005. p. 120.
11. Popata V, Prodanova T, Calisb K, Nelsona L. The menstrual cycle a biological marker of general health in adolescents. Ann NY Acad Sci. 2008;1135:43–51.
12. Adams P. Menstruation in young girls: a clinical perspective. Obstet Gynecol. 2002;99:655–62.
13. Losos B, Raven H, Johnson G, Singer S. Biology. New York: McGraw-Hill; 2002. p. 1207.
14. Rosenthal M. Gynecology sourcebook. 3rd ed. Los Angeles: Lowell House; 1999. p. 21.
15. World Health Organization Task Force on Adolescent Reproductive. Health. World Health Organization multicenter study on menstrual and ovulatory patterns in adolescent girls. II. Longitudinal study of menstrual patterns in the early postmenarchal period, duration of bleeding episodes and menstrual cycles. J Adolesc Health Care. 1986;7:236–44.
16. Oriel K, Schrager S. Abnormal uterine bleeding: Am Family Phys. 1999;60(5):1371–80; discussion 1381–2.

Ovarian Tumours in Children

24

David F.M. Thomas

This chapter reviews ovarian tumours in foetuses, newborns, infants, children, and adolescents. Since the histologic diagnosis is usually uncertain before surgical biopsy or resection the clinical presentation, differential diagnosis, and evaluation of ovarian masses at different ages and the natural history of physiologic ovarian cysts is examined. Finally, specific ovarian neoplasms and their treatment is considered.

Fetal and Infant Ovarian Cysts

Aetiology and Incidence

The increasing use of prenatal ultrasound has led to the detection of fetal ovarian cysts in many pregnancies. These are functional cysts [1] arising in follicles stimulated by maternal oestrogen, placental human chorionic gonadotrophin (HCG), and fetal gonadotrophins [2]. They are more common in pregnancies complicated by maternal diabetes, toxaemia, or rhesus isoimmunisation [3]. Clinically, significant cysts with a diameter greater than two centimetres occur in 1 in 2500 pregnancies [4] and over 90% of newborn girls will have smaller ovarian cysts visible by ultrasound [5].

D.F.M. Thomas (✉)
Department of Paediatric Urology, Leeds Teaching Hospitals and University of Leeds, Leeds General Infirmary, Great George Street, Leeds LS1 3EX UK
e-mail: d.f.m.thomas@leeds.ac.uk

Pathology

Most neonatal follicular cysts resolve during the first year of life [6–8]. Ovarian torsion is more common with cysts larger than 4 cm in diameter and is usually a prenatal event. However, torsion has been associated with smaller cysts with a diameter down to 2.2 cm [9]. Torsion can lead to autoamputation of the ovary and fallopian tube [10]. Most of these free-floating abdominal masses slowly atrophy postnatally but a minority persist. Massive fetal ovarian cysts can be associated with polyhydramnios and pulmonary hypoplasia and can cause dystocia [11]. Neoplastic ovarian cysts in the foetus and newborn are extremely rare with only a single case report from 1945 [12].

Presentation and Differential Diagnosis

Most fetal and neonatal ovarian cysts are asymptomatic and detected on routine ultrasound exams. Simple follicular cysts appear as thin walled hypoechogenic cysts in the abdomen. Debris in the cyst suggests haemorrhage into the cyst or torsion (Fig. 24.1). Symptoms of pain and vomiting in a neonate or infant may be related to acute torsion, haemorrhage, or adhesions to adjacent small or large bowel [7]. Mortality related to haemorrhage or torsion has been reported in 3 infants [8, 13, 14].

The differential diagnosis of an intraabdominal cyst in a foetus or newborn includes renal and

D.J. Ledbetter and P.R.V. Johnson (eds.), *Endocrine Surgery in Children*,
DOI 10.1007/978-3-662-54256-9_24

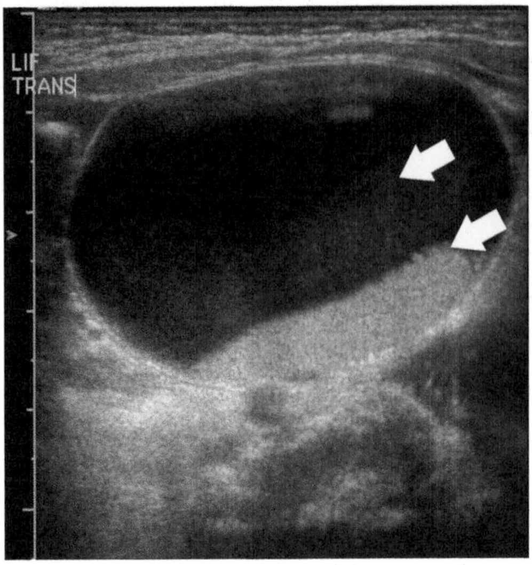

Fig. 24.1 Ultrasound of a one-month-old with antenatally diagnosed ovarian cyst, demonstrating layering of debris within a large thin walled cyst suggesting previous ovarian torsion. (Courtesy of Dr. Alistair Calder, Great Ormond Street Children's Hospital, London, UK.)

enteric duplication cysts and lymphatic malformations [15]. An absent ovary or a contralateral multicystic ovary increases the chances of the cyst being ovarian in origin. Enteric cysts have a thicker, two-layered wall on ultrasound examination.

Management

The criteria for intrauterine intervention are not well defined. Simple aspiration of larger cysts with a diameter of 5 cm or more [16, 17] may be followed by re-accumulation of fluid [9]. Massive cysts, which might obstruct labour, can be aspirated [11] before delivery. Bilateral ovarian cysts might be an indication for preterm delivery or intervention to prevent torsion [9].

Conservative management with serial ultrasound scans for asymptomatic unilateral neonatal cysts is recommended as most simple cysts will resolve spontaneously [18] and even some complex cysts containing debris will resolve leaving a follicular ovary with presumed function [5, 16]. Indications for intervention include a complex cyst with solid elements suggesting a neoplasm. In addition, cysts that do not resolve, and those with a diameter greater than 4 cm are at increased risk of torsion and intervention should be considered. Simple percutaneous aspiration is not recommended as a fatal outcome has been reported when a cyst of enteric origin was aspirated [19]. Reaccumulation of cyst fluid may occur because of stimulation by neonatal gonadotrophins, which peaks at 3–4 months post-natal age.

Surgical treatment is by laparoscopy which confirms the ovarian origin of the cyst and allows fenestration or excision by an intra- or extracorporeal technique [20–22]. Alternatively, an umbilical incision can be used for open surgery, as the neonatal ovary is very mobile [23, 24].

Post-operative Complications and Outcomes

Following surgery under a general anaesthetic, most newborns and infants make an uneventful recovery, establishing full feeds within 24–48 h. Reported wound complications include infection, mostly with staphylococcal organisms, port site hernias, and dehiscence with omental protrusion.

The ultimate functional outcome of a fetal ovarian cyst depends on its characterisation [8]. Simple cysts, which continue as simple cysts, have a good prognosis with 85% resolving spontaneously and leaving a functioning follicular ovary. However, complex cysts containing debris (see Fig. 24.1) have frequently undergone torsion and many will disappear on subsequent scans, with only 16% surviving as follicular ovaries. Approximately half of simple fetal ovarian cysts will become complex before birth [9], so that in neonates complex cysts outnumber simple cysts. Therefore, the prognosis for a fetal ovary containing a cyst of 2 cm or more in diameter is guarded, as the majority will become complex and either atrophy or be resected. For the rare case of bilateral ovarian cysts, preterm delivery or fetal intervention can be considered, although data from prospective trials is not available and the balance of the risks of intervention versus the risks of ovarian loss must be carefully considered.

Ovarian Cysts in Children

Aetiology and Incidence

The ovary in prepubertal girls is active with a low rate of maturation and involution of follicles [25] driven by intermittent release of pituitary gonadotrophins [26]. By ultrasound approximately 2% of girls under the age of 8 years will have small cysts, which may be bilateral. True precocious puberty with elevated levels of gonadotrophins may be the cause of multiple small cysts. However, cysts with a diameter over 1 cm may be hormonally active and associated with pseudoprecocious puberty [15]. In girls aged 2–5 years old, precocious puberty may be the presentation of the McCune–Albright Syndrome, with café-au-lait spots and polyostotic fibrous dysplasia occurring at a later age [25, 27].

With puberty the ovaries increase in size and multiple small cysts are common. The ultrasound appearance is often described as multicystic if the ovaries contain more than six follicles of greater than 4 mm diameter. These cysts result from the ovarian response to pulsatile gonadotrophin secretion [28]. A multicystic ovary should not be confused with a polycystic ovary, which is defined by the ultrasound appearance of 12 or more follicles measuring 2–9 mm in diameter. This can occur in 20% of healthy women but is also associated with the polycystic ovary syndrome [29]. This syndrome of ovarian dysfunction is managed medically by gynaecologists and endocrinologists without the need for surgical intervention.

The risk of malignancy in a prepubertal ovarian cyst is very low but cysts which persist and those with solid elements on imaging should be investigated and surgical excision considered (see the discussion of ovarian neoplasms later in the chapter).

Presentation and Management

Although most ovarian cysts are asymptomatic, pain can be triggered by torsion [30] or haemorrhage. Girls with signs of precocious puberty or uterine bleeding should undergo endocrine investigations and ovarian scanning. Tumour markers, serum α-fetoprotein (α-FP) and β-human chorionic gonadotrophin (β-HCG) should be measured and the ultrasound scan repeated after an interval of a few weeks. Most ovarian cysts in this age group will resolve spontaneously [31] but persistent, hormonally active, or symptomatic cysts should be excised by an ovarian sparing cystectomy preferably performed laparoscopically.

Outcome and Follow-Up

Histological examination of the excised tissue will confirm the diagnosis. Children with signs of precocious puberty or abnormal hormone production should be followed by a paediatric endocrinologist.

Ovarian Cysts in Adolescents

Aetiology and Incidence

Follicular cysts are common in adolescents. They are fluid-filled simple cysts, usually 2–3 cm in diameter that arise in the first half of the menstrual cycle. They and resolve in the second half of the cycle. However, if ovulation does not occur, they can grow to a very large volume. Corpus luteal cysts develop in the second half of the menstrual cycle and secrete progesterone. They can grow up to 6 cm in diameter before rupturing.

In addition to physiologic follicular and corpus luteum cysts the differential diagnosis of an ovarian cyst in an adolescent includes neoplasms, ectopic pregnancy, endometriosis, tubal anomalies, and the sequelae of sexually transmitted infections [25].

Presentation and Management

Irregular menses and pain secondary to rupture and haemorrhage are the common presentations. A palpable mass was reported in 14% of girls with ovarian cysts in one series [32]. Most follicular and corpus luteal cysts will resolve over 4–5 weeks, although larger cysts with diameters up to 8 cm may take 3 months to resolve.

The indications for surgical intervention include persistence of the cyst beyond 3 months, the risk of ovarian torsion (Fig. 24.2), symptoms that do not resolve, and solid elements on imaging suggestive of a neoplasm. Preservation of viable ovarian tissue is of paramount importance and consultation with an experienced adolescent gynaecologist may reduce the number of unnecessary oophorectomies [33]. Laparoscopy confirms the ovarian origin of the lesion. Since simple aspiration of the cyst leads to a high incidence of recurrence [34], cysts are best managed with fenestration of the cyst or cystectomy.

Torsion of the ovary is managed initially by derotation to assess tissue viability. Ischaemic and damaged ovarian tissue has remarkable potential for recovery, which can be assessed at a second laparoscopy delayed 2–3 weeks after derotation [35]. Definitive surgery for the ovarian cyst can be safely performed at the second laparoscopy. Fixation of the contralateral normal ovary is controversial, as the prevention of possible but rare future torsion must be balanced against adhesion formation impairing fertility [36, 37].

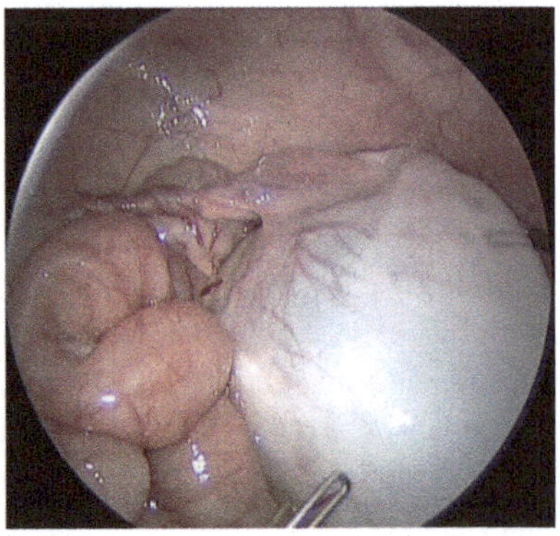

Fig. 24.2 Laparoscopic view of a neonatal ovarian cyst with torsion of the long ovarian pedicle

Endometriosis can occur in adolescents as well as in adults [38]. Endometriomas are blood-filled cysts arising in functioning endometrium within the ovary. The presence of altered blood gives a typical "chocolate cyst" appearance on ultrasound scanning and at surgery. The clinical presentation may be with acute pain secondary to ovarian torsion or haemorrhage but a more frequent presentation is with increasingly painful menstrual periods in an adolescent girl. The diagnosis is suggested by the appearances on ultrasound and confirmed at laparoscopy. The treatment is laparoscopic cystectomy and clearance of other pelvic endometrial deposits. If the endometriosis is extensive, a second laparoscopic procedure may be required after a 3 month course of hormonal suppression with gonadotrophin releasing hormone. Surgical intervention has been shown to relieve symptoms in the short term but there is little data on long-term outcomes and future fertility [39, 40].

Outcome

Histology of excised tissue will confirm the diagnosis. For functional cysts, fenestration has a low recurrence rate with the best chance of preserving ovarian tissue [3]. Cystectomy is required if a neoplastic cyst is suspected. Very large cysts and those with elevated tumour markers can be managed with open surgery through a Pfannenstiel incision. Ovarian preserving resections are the initial procedure of choice because malignant tumours are rare in cystic disease of the ovaries.

Ovarian Tumours

Incidence and Classification

The interest in ovarian tumours is related to their great variety rather than their incidence, which is only approximately 2–3 girls per 100,000 population annually [18, 41]. A tertiary paediatric surgical centre may only see a few patients a year with ovarian tumours, three-quarters of which are benign. Malignant ovarian tumours represent only 1% of childhood cancer [42]. However, there is a larger variety of tumours arising from the ovary than from any other organ (Table 24.1). Tumours arise from the three embryological cell lines found in the ovary, with germ cell tumours being the most common, accounting for 75% of ovarian neoplasms, followed by sex cord–stromal tumours, 15%, and finally, epithelial tumours, which usually present in adolescents, making up around 10% [43–45]. The very rare variants of germ cell tumours and metastatic tumours occurring in the ovary will not be discussed. The aetiology of these tumours is largely unknown, although gonadoblastomas, are associated with chromosome anomalies and the WT1 mutation of Frasier syndrome [46, 47].

Table 24.1 Classification of ovarian tumours in children

Germ cell tumours (75%)
• Dysgerminomas • Yolk sac tumours (endodermal sinus tumour) • Teratomas – Mature (Dermoids) – Immature – Embryonic • Choriocarcinoma • Gonadoblastoma • Embryonal carcinoma • Mixed germ cell tumours
Sex cord–stromal tumours (15%)
• Thecomas • Fibromas • Juvenile granulosa cell tumours • Sertoli–Leydig cell tumours (Arrhenoblastomas)
Epithelial tumours (10%)
• Serous – Benign – Borderline – Malignant • Mucinous – Benign – Borderline – Malignant • Endometrioid
Miscellaneous
• Lymphoma • Leukaemia • Metastatic tumours – Neuroblastoma – Rhabdomyosarcoma – Nephroblastoma

Pathology of Benign Ovarian Tumours

Thecomas occur rarely in the second decade, with some producing oestrogens and presenting with precocious puberty [48] and others containing androgen-producing lutein cells leading to virilisation [49]. These tumours may be calcified.

Fibromas are rare in childhood and can grow to a large size and be associated with ascites and pleural effusions (Meigs Syndrome). Fibromas have also been described in children with the basal cell nevus syndrome [50].

Gonadoblastomas contain mixed germ cell and sex cord–stromal cell elements and are frequently bilateral. They most often occur in phenotypically female patients with 46 XY or an XY mosaic karyotype [50]. Although benign, they arise in dysgenetic gonads and are associated with malignant ovarian germ cell tumours. Frasier syndrome is the association of nephropathy and gonadoblastoma in a phenotypic female with XY chromosomes and is associated with the WT1 gene [46].

Mature cystic teratomas (MCTs), also known as ovarian dermoid cysts, are the most frequently occurring ovarian tumours accounting for approximately 40% of all ovarian neoplasms in children. The cells are mostly diploid and arise in primordial germ cells which have entered meiosis [42]. All three germ layers may be present, with ectodermal elements predominating including teeth and hair (Fig. 24.3a and b). In children, these are benign tumours containing both solid tissue and cystic areas, with 10% occurring bilaterally. Late recurrent malignant germ cell tumours have been described in young adult women with a previously excised mature cystic teratoma [51].

Immature teratomas are less common than MCTs and contain immature neuroectodermal elements. A careful histological search has to be

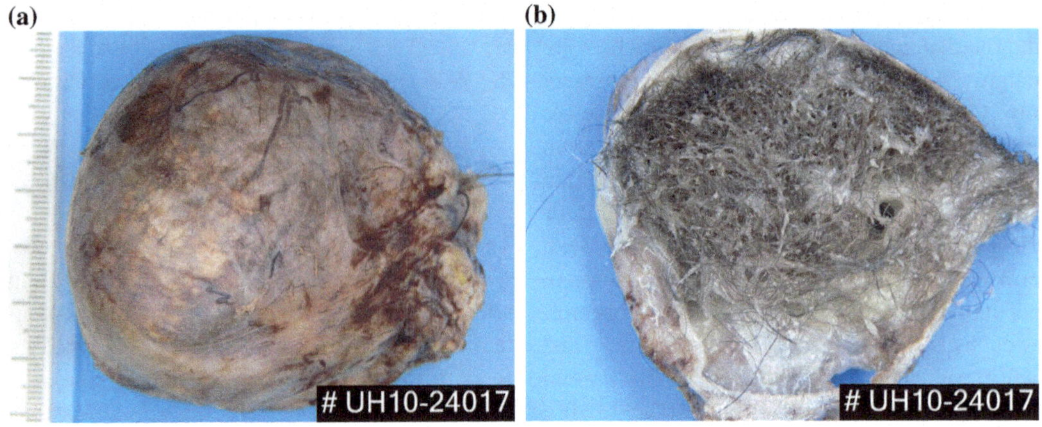

Fig. 24.3 An excised ovarian dermoid cyst (mature teratoma) **a** external surface **b** transected to demonstrate hair in the cyst. (Courtesy of Dr. Elizabeth Benjamin, University College London Hospital, London, UK.)

made within these tumours for yolk sac elements, which are potentially malignant.

Gliomatosis peritonei are nodules of glial tissue sited on the peritoneum or omentum and have been described in patients with immature ovarian teratomas. Studies suggest that these are metaplastic cells arising from peritoneal stem cells and not seeded from the ovarian tumour [52].

Pathology of Malignant Ovarian Tumours

Dysgerminomas represent 11% of paediatric ovarian tumours, making them the most common malignant ovarian tumour in children. They are analogous to testicular seminomas. They are solid tumours and are bilateral in up to 15% of patients [53]. Microscopically they consist of epithelioid cells and mature lymphocytes. In addition, multinucleated cells and syncytiotrophoblastic giant cells may be present and produce β-HCG [54]. Dysgerminomas are found in mixed germ cell tumours and can arise with gonadoblastomas in dysgenetic gonads. Dysgerminomas usually present as localised stage 1 disease [55] but metastases can be found in pelvic and retroperitoneal lymph nodes, with rare haematogenous spread to the liver, lungs and bone. Serum lactic dehydrogenase is a useful tumour marker for many of these tumours [56].

Yolk sac tumours or endodermal sinus tumours are the second most common malignant ovarian tumour in children, most often arising in post-menarchal teenage girls but also rarely occurring in younger girls [57]. These solid tumours contain undifferentiated embryonic cells which produce α-fetoprotein [58]. These are aggressive tumours which spread locally in the peritoneal cavity, via the lymphatics to retroperitoneal and pelvic lymph nodes, and via the bloodstream to the liver, lungs and brain [59].

Mixed germ cell tumours make up one-third of malignant germ cell tumours and contain more than one neoplastic germ cell element, mostly dysgerminomas, yolk sac tumours, immature teratomas, and the rarer germ cell malignancies. Malignant germ cell tumours may be aneuploid and may exhibit the isochromosome 12p [60, 61]. They can produce α-fetoprotein or β-HCG [57].

Juvenile granulosa cell tumours are the most common of the stromal sex cord tumours and account for up to 10% of ovarian malignant tumours in children and adolescents [62]. They have cystic and solid elements and secrete oestrogens [63]. Mixed granulosa and thecal cell tumours also occur [64]. They are hormonally active and usually present at an early stage before spread has occurred outside the ovary. Adults with the Peutz–Jeghers Syndrome have an increased risk of developing sex cord–stromal tumours [65].

Sertoli–Leydig tumours or arrhenoblastomas are rare malignant tumours of the ovary with the majority presenting before the age of 20 years [66] and most will produce androgens [49]. Production of α-fetoprotein has also been reported [67]. They have cystic and solid elements and are usually localised to the ovary at presentation.

Epithelial cell tumours are much less common in children and adolescents compared to adults and are classified into serous and mucinous subtypes. The majority are benign or borderline with low malignant potential [68]. Borderline epithelial tumours have varying nuclear atypia but lack stromal invasion and are more common in adolescents [45, 69]. Malignant adenocarcinomas are very rare in adolescents and children [57, 70, 71]. Borderline tumours spread locally in the pelvis and have a high incidence of bilaterality. Malignant epithelial tumours spread in the peritoneal cavity to retroperitoneal and pelvic lymph nodes and via the bloodstream to liver and lungs.

Lymphomas are rare ovarian tumours in Europe and America but are the most commonly described ovarian tumour in West African children [72].

Presentation of Ovarian Tumours

The majority of ovarian tumours will present with symptoms or clinical signs while a minority will be found incidentally on imaging at laparotomy or at laparoscopy [18]. Pain, usually described by children in the lower abdomen, is the most common symptom. Acute severe pain suggests ovarian torsion, while recurrent or chronic pain of less severity may be the result of haemorrhage into or rupture of the tumour [73]. Lower abdominal distension may be the only complaint at presentation. A palpable mass may be detected arising from the pelvis or in the lower abdomen, indicating a larger tumour with a diameter greater than 7 cm and a higher risk of malignancy [74]. Hormonally active ovarian tumours are rare and present with signs of precocious puberty, vaginal bleeding, or virilisation.

Investigations of Ovarian Tumours

Imaging starts with ultrasound scanning (Fig. 24.4) and colour flow Doppler to assess blood flow to the lesion and ovary but ultrasound

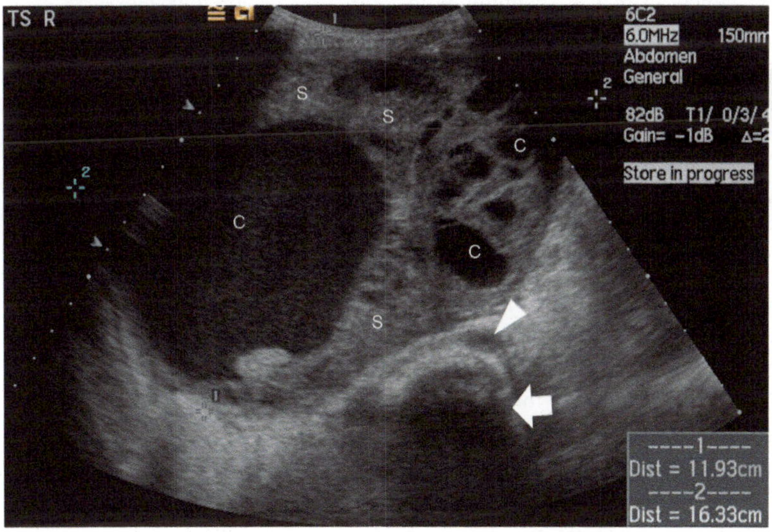

Fig. 24.4 Transverse abdominal ultrasound scan in a six year old girl presenting with an abdominopelvic mass and premature thelarche. The large mass contains cystic (c) and solid (s) elements. The *arrow points* to the spine and the *arrowhead* to the abdominal aorta. (Courtesy of Dr. Alistair Calder, Consultant Radiologist at Great Ormond Street Children's Hospital, London, UK.)

Table 24.2 Tumour markers

Tumour	Markers
Teratoma	α-FP
Yolk sac tumour	α-FP
Dysgerminoma	β-HCG and LDH-1
Choriocarcinoma	β-HCG
Embryonal carcinoma	α-FP and β-HCG
Sertoli–Leydig tumour	α-FP
Epithelial tumours	CA-125

α-FP α-fetoprotein, *β-HCG* β-human chorionic gonadotrophin, *LDH-1* lactic dehydrogenase, *CA-125* Cancer antigen 125

scanning does not always distinguish between benign and malignant lesions. However, lesions with an irregular outline, significant solid elements and a diameter greater than 7.5 cm have a higher risk of malignancy [74]. A smooth capsule and predominantly cystic structure increases the chances that the lesion is localised and benign [75].

MRI scanning provides better anatomical detail with differentiation between uterine and ovarian lesions [76–78]. Pathologically enlarged lymph nodes, ascites, and liver metastases may also be identified on magnetic resonance imaging. If vascular detail is required, more information will be gained from CT scanning with vascular contrast but at the biological cost of additional irradiation. CT scans of the chest will identify lung metastases and would be performed when staging the rare malignant ovarian tumours.

Tumour markers are useful but cannot distinguish between malignant and benign tumours [79]. Tumour markers may be elevated in benign and immature germ cell tumours but raised levels should always increase the suspicion of a malignant neoplasm. Table 24.2 indicates the tumour markers seen in ovarian tumours.

Girls with precocious puberty or signs of virilisation should have endocrine investigations, including pituitary gonadotrophins, oestradiol, progesterone, and testosterone levels. Ovarian cysts and tumours are uncommon causes of precocious puberty.

Surgery for Ovarian Tumours

Most ovarian tumours are managed by surgical excision with preservation of ovarian tissue whenever possible [80]. A staging procedure is appropriate when malignancy is suspected. Staging for germ cell tumours (Table 24.3) is

Table 24.3 Children's Oncology Group (COG) staging for ovarian germ cell tumours

Stage	Description
Ia	Limited to one ovary
Ib	Limited to both ovaries
II	Microscopic residual or positive lymph nodes <2 cm diam.
	Peritoneal evaluation and washings negative
	± Tumour markers
III	Lymph node involvement ≥2 cm diam.
	Gross residual tumour or biopsy of tumour only
	Visceral involvement (bladder, bowel, omentum)
	Peritoneal washings positive
	±Tumour markers
IV	Distant metastases, (usually liver or lungs)
Gliomatosis peritonei does not raise stage I or II disease to a higher stage	

From von Allmen D (2005) Malignant lesions of the ovary in childhood. Semin Pediatr Surg 14:100–5, with permission less invasive as no additional information is gained from sampling peritoneal tissue and lymph nodes which are palpably and macroscopically normal [81]. However, when malignant epithelial or sex cord–stromal tumours are suspected, sampling should include peritoneal, omental, and lymph node biopsies since metastatic spread tissue may be macroscopically and palpably normal (Table 24.4) [82, 83].

The characteristics of the tumour and the surgeon's experience will determine whether the surgical procedure is laparoscopic or open via a Pfannenstiel or lower midline incision. For tumours above 7.5 cm diameter and when imaging and tumour markers suggest a malignant tumour, an open operation is recommended. The incision has to be adequate to deliver malignant tumours intact, as aspiration of malignant cysts will increase by one the stage of the tumour. Laparoscopy with an ovarian preserving dissection is appropriate for smaller benign tumours [35, 74, 84].

Ascitic fluid or peritoneal washings should be collected for cytology before starting any dissection. Both ovaries should be inspected. Frozen section histology of biopsies is helpful in diagnosing borderline epithelial tumours without stromal invasion but is not recommended for germ cell tumours, where it can be misleading [83].

Torsed ovaries should be untwisted and inspected for viability and any underlying pathology. Malignant tumours account for less than 5% and benign tumours approximately 30% of torsed ovaries [85]. For ovaries of doubtful viability, detorsion alone and subsequent imaging is recommended. A second surgical procedure undertaken for ovaries suspected of harbouring neoplasms [35]. Even ovaries, which initially appear infarcted, have a remarkable ability to recover after the blood supply is restored.

For many tumours, it is possible to find a plane of dissection between the lesion and ovarian tissue adjacent to the hilum and an ovarian sparing operation can be safely performed for germ cell tumours [18, 43, 84]. A higher rupture rate is reported for germ cell tumours undergoing a laparoscopic cystectomy but, with copious washings of the pelvic cavity, chemical peritonitis and adhesions can be minimised [48]. For larger tumours and where no plane of dissection can be identified, a salpingo-oophorectomy is appropriate or an oophorectomy alone for germ cell tumours not involving the fallopian tube.

Careful inspection and excisional biopsy of lesions of the contralateral ovary are important as there is a significant risk of bilaterally in germ cell and epithelial tumours [53]. Staging for malignant germ cell tumours includes excisional biopsies of suspicious peritoneal and omental lesions and pathological lymph nodes (Table 24.3). Staging for malignant epithelial and sex cord–stromal tumours requires lymph node and peritoneal biopsies of pathological and macroscopically normal tissue (Table 24.4) [83].

In a small minority of patients, germ cell tumours will have spread and be fixed to adjacent organs. If complete tumour resection would result in extensive damage to surrounding normal

Table 24.4 Staging for malignant ovarian epithelial and sex cord–stromal tumours[a]

Stage	Description
Ia	Limited to one ovary, without lc features or malignant cells in washings
Ib	Limited to both ovaries, without lc features or malignant cells in washings
Ic	As above and with tumour on the surface or tumour ruptured, or malignant cells in washings
II	Spread to pelvic tissues
III	Peritoneal implants or involvement of omentum or small bowel outside the pelvis or positive inguinal or retroperitoneal lymph nodes
IV	Distant metastases to liver parenchyma, lungs or cytologically positive pleural effusion

[a]Based on recommendations of the International Federation of Gynecology and Obstetrics (FIGO) [100]

tissues then a biopsy should be taken and a tissue diagnosis established. Malignant germ cell tumours should then be treated with four courses of chemotherapy and imaging repeated to assess shrinkage. In many cases, excision of the tumour will be possible at a second laparotomy after chemotherapy.

Rare disorders of sex development (DSD) may result in a female child with an XY karyotype having intra-abdominal testes. The risk of malignancy in these gonads is increased, although the magnitude of that risk varies according to the diagnosis. In Swyer syndrome the lifetime malignancy risk is in the order of 30% and bilateral gonadectomy is recommended at the time of diagnosis [86]. Although these girls usually present with failure to enter puberty due to gonadal dysfunction, a small number will present with advanced germ cell tumours. However, girls with the Complete Androgen Insensitivity syndrome have a much lower risk of malignancy of between 2 and 5%, so removal of the gonads can be delayed until after the completion of puberty [87]. Long-term oestrogen replacement is required after gonadectomy, firstly to induce puberty and secondly to maintain normal female development.

Epithelial tumours are uncommon in children. Good outcomes depend on tumour clearance at the time of surgery. Borderline and benign tumours can be excised with ovarian sparing procedures [88, 89], but the very rare bilateral malignant cystadenocarcinoma may require a radical bilateral oophorectomy with an abdominal hysterectomy.

Careful haemostasis is essential before closing the abdomen or removing ports. Fixation of a single remaining ovary following oophorectomy is controversial, as the benefits of preventing future torsion must be balanced against the formation of adhesions reducing fertility [36].

Post-operative Course and Outcomes

Following major pelvic and abdominal surgery, patients must be observed carefully for signs of blood loss or sepsis. Inadvertent bowel damage during laparoscopic surgery can lead to delayed intestinal leakage and peritonitis. Surgical incisions and port sites should be inspected for signs of sepsis and incisional hernia. Teenage patients should be assessed pre-operatively for the need for deep vein thrombosis prophylaxis both during the procedure and post-operatively.

The majority of patients will have benign or stage 1 disease and will make a rapid and uneventful recovery. Laparoscopic surgery should lead to return to a full diet and full mobilisation within 36 h and the need for less post-operative analgesia compared with open surgery.

Patients are usually followed for a minimum of 2 years with ultrasound scans every six months to monitor the contralateral and any remaining ipsilateral ovary. The contralateral ovary is at risk of a metachronous tumour, particularly following excision of a germ cell or epithelial tumour. Patients who have a single remaining ovary should be counselled about their reduced fertility [90], although many successful pregnancies are reported following tumour excision, even with tumour spillage or following unilateral salpingo-oophorectomy and chemotherapy for malignant germ cell tumours [91].

Immature teratomas should be followed with regular imaging and measurements of serum α-fetoprotein. The finding of small foci of yolk sac tumour within the teratoma is not an indication for immediate chemotherapy. In one reported study of 44 immature teratomas in 1999, thirteen contained foci of yolk sac tumour but only one patient had a recurrent tumour after surgical excision alone [92]. This patient's recurrence was a yolk sac tumour and responded well to chemotherapy.

All malignant tumours must be accurately staged to plan appropriate chemotherapy regimens. As most cancers are stage l, it is important to avoid over treating these patients as surgery alone and careful follow-up with imaging and measurement of tumour markers is the recommended management.

Germ cell tumours are highly sensitive to cisplatin-based chemotherapy and stage II to IV disease is treated with four courses of bleomycin, etoposide and carboplatin [93] under the supervision of a paediatric oncologist [94]. Overall 4-year survival rates of 90% can be achieved with minimal drug toxicity, with good responses reported even in advanced stage disease [95].

Stage I stromal cell tumours are similarly managed with surgery alone, with the more advanced stages treated with a cisplatin-based chemotherapy regimen [75]. Lower grade tumours with fewer than 20 mitoses per high powered field respond well, with comparable outcomes to germ cell tumours. However the higher grade stromal tumours with spread beyond the ovary are less responsive and additional and more toxic agents may be required [96].

Patients with epithelial tumours should be managed similarly to adults with the same condition. For benign and borderline tumours, preserving fertility is the priority [69, 97]. This increases the incidence of recurrent borderline tumours but the patient may have completed one or two successful pregnancies before a second and more aggressive surgical excision is required [98]. The very rare malignant epithelial tumours in children may receive a cisplatin-based chemotherapy regimen but the long-term prognosis is poor with less than a 15% survival at 10 years [99].

The best outcomes are achieved when patients are managed by a multidisciplinary team including radiology, oncology, gynaecology [33], paediatric surgery, and endocrinology. All these patients should be treated in centres experienced in the management of tumours in children and adolescents. The aims are to successfully treat the tumour, while preserving future fertility and minimising drug toxicity.

Acknowledgements The authors wish to thank Dr. Alistair Calder, Consultant Radiologist at Great Ormond Street Children's Hospital for the images in Figs. 24.1 and 24.4 and Dr. Elizabeth Benjamin, Consultant Histopathologist, of University College London Hospital for the photographs reproduced in Fig. 24.3a and b.

References

1. Ben-Ami I, Kogan A, Fuchs N, et al. Long term follow up of children with ovarian cysts diagnosed prenatally. Prenat Diag. 2010;30:342–7.
2. Vogtlander MF, Rijntjes-Jacobs EG, van den Hoonaard TL, et al. Neonatal ovarian cysts. Acta Paediatr. 2003;92:498–501.
3. de Wilde RL. Recurrence of functional cysts after laparoscopic fenestration. Am J Obstet Gynecol. 1989;161:839.
4. Bryant AE, Laufer MR. Fetal ovarian cysts: incidence, diagnosis and management. J Reprod Med. 2004;49:329–37.
5. Luzzatto C, Midrio P, Toffalutti T, et al. Neonatal ovarian cysts: management and follow up. Pediatr Surg Int. 2000;16:56–9.
6. Brandt ML, Luks FI, Filiatrault D, et al. Surgical indications in antenatally diagnosed ovarian cysts. J Pediatr Surg. 1991;26:276–81.
7. Dolgin SE. Ovarian masses in the newborn. Semin Pediatr Surg. 2000;9:121–7.
8. Foley PT, Ford WD, McEwin R, et al. Is conservative management of prenatal and neonatal ovarian cysts justified? Fetal Diag Ther. 2005;20:454–8.
9. Galinier P, Carfagna L, Juricic M, et al. Fetal ovarian cysts, management and ovarian prognosis: a report of 82 cases. J Pediatr Surg. 2008;43:2004–9.
10. Houben C, Chu W, Cheung G, et al. Antenatal ovarian torsion; a "free floating" cyst. Ultraschall Med. 2008;29:311–3.
11. Heling KS, Chaoui R, Kirchmair F, et al. Fetal ovarian cyst; prenatal diagnosis, management and post-natal outcome. Ultrasound Obstet Gynecol. 2002;20:47–50.
12. Zeigler EE. Bilateral ovarian carcinoma in a thirty week fetus. Arch Pathol. 1945;40:279–82.
13. Havlik DM, Nolte KB. Sudden death in an infant resulting from torsion of the uterine adnexa. Am J Forensic Med Pathol. 2002;23:289–91.
14. Kasian GF, Taylor BW, Sugarman RG, et al. Ovarian torsion related to sudden infant death. CMAJ. 1986;135:1373.
15. Helmrath MA, Shin CE, Warner BW. Ovarian cysts in the pediatric population. Semin Pediatr Surg. 1998;7:19–28.
16. Bagalon P, Giorlandino C, Nahom A, et al. The management of fetal ovarian cysts. J Pediatr Surg. 2002;37:25–30.
17. Perrotin F, Potin J, Haddad G, et al. Fetal ovarian cysts: a report of 3 cases managed by aspiration. Ultrasound Obstet Gynec. 2000;16:655–9.
18. Cass DL, Hawkins E, Brandt ML, et al. Surgery for ovarian masses in infants, children and adolescents. J Pediatr Surg. 2001;36:693–9.

19. Puligandla PS, Laberge JM. Lethal outcome after percutaneous aspiration of a presumed ovarian cyst in a neonate. Semin Pediatr Surg. 2009;18:119–21.
20. Pantelli C, Minocha A, Kulkarni MS, et al. The role of laparoscopy in the management of adnexal lesions. Surg Laparosc Endosc Percut Tech. 2009;19:514–7.
21. Schenkman L, Weiner TM, Phillips JD. Evolution of the surgical management of neonatal ovarian cysts: laparoscopically assisted transumbilical extracorporeal ovarian cystectomy. J Laparoendo Adv Surg Tech. 2008;18:635–40.
22. van der Zee DC, van Sleumeren JC, Bax KM, et al. Laparoscopic approach to surgical management of ovarian cysts in the newborn. J Pediatr Surg. 1995;30:40–3.
23. Colby C, Brindle M, Moss RL. Minimally invasive laparotomy for treatment of neonatal ovarian cysts. J Pediatr Surg. 2001;36:868–9.
24. Lin J-Y, Lee Z-F, Chang Y-T. Transumbilical management of neonatal ovarian cysts. J Pediatr Surg. 2007;42:2136–9.
25. Strickland JL. Ovarian cysts in neonates, children and adolescents. Curr Opin Obstet Gynecol. 2002;14:459–65.
26. Miller D, Blake JM, Stringer DA, et al. Prepubertal ovarian cysts: 5 year experience. Obstet Gynecol. 1993;81:434–8.
27. Mauras N, Blizzard RM. The McCune–Albright syndrome. Acta Endocrinol Scand. 1986;279:207–17.
28. Stanhope R, Adams J, Jacobs HS, et al. Ovarian ultrasound assessment in normal children, idiopathic precocious puberty and during low dose pulsatile gonadotrophin releasing hormone treatment of hypogonadotrophic hypogonadism. Arch Dis Child. 1985;60:116–9.
29. Rotterdam ESHRE/ASRM sponsored PCOS consensus workshop group. Revised 2003 consensus on diagnostic criteria and long-term health risks related to polycystic ovary syndrome (PCOS) (2004) Human Reproduction 19:41–7.
30. Cass DL. Ovarian torsion. Semin Pediatr Surg. 2005;14:86–92.
31. Qublan HS, Abdel-hadi J. Simple ovarian cysts: frequency and outcome in girls aged 2–9 years. Clin Exp Obstet Gynecol. 2000;27:51–3.
32. Kanizsai B, Orley J, Szigetvari I, et al. Ovarian cysts in children and adolescents: their occurrence, behaviour and management. J Pediatr Adolesc Gynecol. 1998;11:85–8.
33. Hernon M, McKenna J, Busby G, et al. The histology and management of ovarian cysts found in children and adolescents presenting to a children's hospital 1991–2007: a call for more paediatric gynaecologists. BJOG. 2010;117:181–4.
34. Brandt ML, Helmrath MA. Ovarian cysts in infants and children. Semin Peditr Surg. 2005;14:78–85.
35. Karpelowsky JS, La Hei ER, Matthews K. Laparoscopic resection of benign ovarian tumors in children with gonadal preservation. Pediatr Surg Int. 2009;25:251–4.
36. Ns Crouch, Gyampoh B, Cutner AJ, et al. Ovarian torsion, to pex or not to pex? Case report and review of the literature. J Pediatr Adolesc Gynecol. 2003;16:381–4.
37. Nagel TC, Sebastian J, Malo JW. Oophoropexy to prevent sequential or recurrent torsion. J Am Assoc Gynecol Laparosc. 1997;4:495–8.
38. Stavroulis AI, Saridogan E, Creighton SM, et al. Laparoscopic treatment of endometriosis in teenagers. Eur J Obstet Gynecol Reprod Biol. 2006;125:248–50.
39. Adamson GD, Pasta DJ. Surgical treatment of endometriosis—associated infertility: meta-analysis compared with survival analysis. Am J Obstet Gynecol. 1994;171:1488–504.
40. Unger CA, Laufer MR. Progression of endometriosis in non-medically managed adolescents: a case series. J Pediatr Adolesc Gynecol. 2011;24:e21–3.
41. Lindfors O. Primary ovarian neoplasms in infants and children: a study of 81 cases diagnosed in Finland and Sweden. Ann Chir Gynaecol Suppl. 1971;177:1–6.
42. Castleberry RP, Cushing B, Perlman E, et al. Germ cell tumors. In: Pizzo PA, Poplack DG, editors. Principles and practice of pediatric oncology. 3rd ed. Philadelphia, PA: Lippincott-Raven; 1997. p. 921–45.
43. Brookfield KF, Cheung MC, Koniaris LG, et al. A population based analysis of 1037 malignant ovarian tumors in the pediatric population. J Surg Res. 2009;156:45–9.
44. Brown MF, Hebra A, McGeehin K, et al. Ovarian masses in children: a review of 91 cases of benign and malignant masses. J Pediatr Surg. 1993;28:930–2.
45. You W, Dainty LA, Rose GS, et al. Gynecologic malignancies in women aged less than 25 years. Obstet Gynecol. 2005;105:1405–9.
46. Gwin K, Cajaiba MM, Caminoa-Lizarralde A, et al. Expanding the spectrum of Frasier's syndrome. Pediatr Dev Pathol. 2008;11:122–7.
47. Shinoyama H, Nakajima M, Naka H, et al. A girl with bilateral ovarian tumours; Frasier syndrome. Eur J Pediatr. 2002;161:81–3.
48. Templeman C, Blenshevsky A, Fallat ME, et al. Non-inflammatory ovarian masses in girls and young women. Obstet Gynecol. 2000;96:229–33.
49. Young YH, Scully RE. Ovarian Sertoli-Leydig cell tumors: a clinic-pathologic analysis of 207 cases. Am J Surg Path. 1985;9:543–69.
50. Lack EE, Young RH, Scully RE. Pathology of ovarian neoplasms in childhood and adolescents. Pathol Ann. 1992;27:281–356.
51. Anteby EY, Ron M, Revel A, et al. Germ cell tumours of the ovary arising after dermoid cyst resection: a long term follow up study. Obstet Gynecol. 1994;83:605–8.
52. Ferguson AW, Katabuchi H, Ronnett BM, et al. Glial implants in gliomatosis peritonei arise from

normal tissue, not the associated teratoma. Am J Pathol. 2001;159:51–5.
53. von Allmen D. Malignant lesions of the ovary in childhood. Semin Pediatr Surg. 2005;14:100–5.
54. Song ES, Lee JP, Han JH, et al. Dysgerminoma of the ovary with precocious puberty: a case report. Gynecol Endocrin. 2007;23:34–7.
55. Ayhan A, Celik H, Taskiran C, et al. Oncologic and reproductive outcome after fertility-saving surgery in ovarian cancer. Eur J Gynecol Oncol. 2003;24:223–32.
56. Sheiko MC, Hart WR. Ovarian germinoma (dysgerminoma) with elevated serum lactic dehydrogenase: case report and review of the literature. Cancer. 1982;49:994–8.
57. Gribbon M, Ein SH, Mancer K. Pediatric malignant ovarian tumors: a 43 year review. J Pediatr Surg. 1992;27:480–4.
58. Kawai M, Furuhashi Y, Kano T, et al. Alpha-fetoprotein in malignant germ cell tumors of the ovary. Gynecol Oncol. 1990;39:160–6.
59. Cicin I, Saip P, Guney N, et al. Yolk sac tumours of the ovary: evaluation of clinicopathological features and prognostic factors. Eur J Gynecol Reprod Biol. 2009;146:210–4.
60. Cossu-Rocca P, Zhang S, Roth LM, et al. Chromosome 12p abnormalities in dysgerminoma of the ovary: a FISH analysis. Modern Pathology. 2006;19:611–5.
61. Ulbright TM. Gonadal teratomas: a review and speculation. Adv Anat Pathol. 2004;11:10–23.
62. Calaminus G, Wassalowski R, Harms D, et al. Juvenile granulosa cell tumors of the ovary in children and adolescents: results from 33 patients. Gynecol Oncol. 1997;65:447–52.
63. Chan LF, Storr HL, Scheimberg I, et al. Pseudo-precocious puberty caused by a juvenile granulosa cell tumour secreting androstenedione, inhibin and insulin-like growth factor-I. J Pediatr Endocronol Metab. 2004;17:679–84.
64. Fleming NA, de Nanassy J, Lawrence S, et al. Juvenile granulosa and theca cell tumor of the ovary as a rare cause of precocious puberty: case report and review of the literature. J Pediatr Adolesc Gynecol. 2010;23:2127–30.
65. Scully RE. Sex cord tumor with annular tubules. A distinctive ovarian tumor of the Peutz-Jeghers syndrome. Cancer. 1970;25:1107–21.
66. Schneider DT, Calaminus G, Wessalowski R, et al. Therapy of advanced ovarian juvenile granulosa cell tumor. Klin Pediatr. 2002;214:173–8.
67. Tetu B, Ordonez NG, Silva EG. Sertoli-Leydig cell tumor of the ovary with alpha-fetoprotein production. Arch Pathol Lab Med. 1986;110:65–8.
68. Tsai JY, Saigo PE, Brown C, et al. Diagnosis, pathology, staging, treatment and outcome of epithelial ovarian neoplasia in patients aged under 21 years. Cancer. 2001;91:2065–70.
69. Aggarwal A, Lucco KL, Lacy J, et al. Ovarian epithelial tumors of low malignant potential: a case series of 5 adolescent patients. J Pediatr Surg. 2009;44:2023–7.
70. Njim L, Moussa A, Saidani Z, et al. Bilateral ovarian borderline tumor in a four year old girl. J Pediatr Adolesc Gynecol. 2010;23:e1–4.
71. Shankar KR, Wakhlu A, Kokai GK, et al. Ovarian adenocarcinoma in premenarchal girls. J Pediatr Surg. 2001;36:511–5.
72. Mohammed A, Malami SA, Calvin B, et al. A histopathological study of ovarian neoplasms in children in Northern Nigeria. Afr J Paediatr Surg. 2010;7:75–7.
73. Iwata A, Matsubara K, Umemoto Y, et al. Spontaneous rupture of a benign ovarian cystic teratoma in a premenarchal girl. J Pediatr Adolesc Gynecol. 2009;22:e121–3.
74. Vaysse C, Delsol M, Carfagna L, et al. Ovarian germ cell tumors in children. Management, survival and ovarian prognosis. A report of 75 cases. J Pediatr Surg. 2010;45:1484–90.
75. Choudhary S, Fasih N, McInnes M, et al. Imaging of ovarian teratomas: appearances and complications. J Med Imaging Radiat Oncol. 2009;53:480–3.
76. Fedele L, Dorta M, Brioschi D, et al. Magnetic resonance evaluation of gynaecological masses in adolescents. Adolesc Pediatr Gynecol. 1990;3:83–8.
77. Iyer VR, Lee SI. MRI, CT and PET/CT for ovarian cancer detection and adnexal characterisation. Am J Roentgenol. 2010;194:311–21.
78. Stevens SK, Hricak H, Stern JL. Ovarian lesions: detection and characterisation with Gadolinium-enhanced imaging at 1.5 T1. Radiology. 1991;181:481–8.
79. Ruttenstock EM, Saxena AK, Schwinger W, et al. Pediatric ovarian tumors—dilemmas in diagnosis and management. Eur J Pediatr Surg. 2010;20:116–20.
80. Kennedy AW. Ovarian neoplasms in childhood and adolescents. Semin Reprod Endocrinol. 1988;6:79–90.
81. Billmire D, Vinocur C, Rescorla F, et al. Outcome and staging evaluation in germ cell tumors of the ovary in children and adolescents: an intergroup study. J Pediatr Surg. 2004;39:424–9.
82. Morice P, Joulie F, Camatte S, et al. Lymph node involvement in epithelial ovarian cancer: analysis of 276 pelvic and paraaortic lymphadenectomies. J Am Coll Surg. 2003;197:198–205.
83. Oltmann SC, Garcia NM, Barber R. Pediatric ovarian malignancies: how efficacious are current staging procedures? J Pediatr Surg. 2010;45:1096–102.
84. Savasi I, Lacy JA, Gerstle JT, et al. Management of ovarian dermoid cysts in the pediatric and adolescent population. J Pediatr Adolesc Gynecol. 2009;22:360–4.
85. Oltmann SC, Fischer A, Barber R, et al. Pediatric ovarian malignancy presenting as ovarian torsion: incidence and relevance. J Pediatr Surg. 2010;45:135–9.

86. Michala L, Goswami D, Creighton SM, et al. Swyer syndrome: presentation and outcomes. BJOG. 2008;115:737–41.
87. Cools M, Drop SLS, Wolffenbuttel K, et al. Germ cell tumors in the intersex gonad: old paths, new directions, moving frontiers. Endocr Rev. 2006;27:468–84.
88. Palomba S, Zupi E, Rosso T, et al. Comparison of two fertility sparing approaches for bilateral borderline ovarian tumours—a randomised controlled study. Hum Reprod. 2007;22:578–85.
89. Song T, Choi CH, Lee YY, et al. Pediatric borderline ovarian tumors: a retrospective analysis. J Pediatr Surg. 2010;45:1955–60.
90. Zanetta G, Bonazzi C, Grazia M, et al. Survival and reproductive function after treatment of malignant germ cell ovarian tumors. A review of 74 cases. Cancer. 2001;89:361–8.
91. Yoo SC, Kim WY, Yoon JH, et al. Young girls with malignant ovarian germ cell tumors can undergo normal menarche and menstruation after fertility sparing surgery and chemotherapy. Acta Obstet Gynecol Scand. 2010;89:126–30.
92. Cushing B, Giller R, Ablin A, et al. Surgical resection alone is effective treatment for ovarian immature teratoma in children and adolescents: a report of the pediatric oncology group and the children's cancer group. Am J Obstet Gynecol. 1999;181:353–8.
93. Stern JW, Bunin N. Prospective study of carboplatin-based chemotherapy for pediatric germ cell tumors. Med Pediatr Oncol. 2002;39:163–7.
94. Pantelli C, Curry J, Kiely E, et al. Ovarian germ cell tumours: a 17 year study in a single unit. Eur J Pediatr Surg. 2009;19:96–100.
95. Biswajit D, Patil CN, Sagar TG. Clinical presentation and outcome of pediatric ovarian germ cell tumors: a study of 40 patients. J Pediatr Hematol Oncol. 2010;32:e54–6.
96. Brown J, Shvartsman HS, Deavers MT, et al. The activity of taxanes in the treatment of sex cord-stromal ovarian tumors. J Clin Oncol. 2004;22:3517–23.
97. Kanut-Pektas M, Ozat M, Gungor T, et al. Fertility outcome after conservative surgery for borderline ovarian tumors: single center experience. Arch Gynecol Obstet. 2011;284:1253–8.
98. Morowitz M, Huff D, von Allmen D. Epithelial ovarian tumors in children: a retrospective analysis. J Pediatr Surg. 2003;38:331–5.
99. Lambert HE, Gregory WM, Nelstrop AE, et al. Longterm survival in 463 women treated for advanced epithelial carcinoma of the ovary. Int J Gynecol Cancer. 2004;14:772–8.
100. F.I.G.O. Committee on Gynecologic Oncology. Current FIGO staging for cancer of the vagina, fallopian tube, ovary and gestational trophoblastic neoplasia. Int J Gynecol Obstet. 2009;105:3–5.

Ovarian Torsion

25

Anne C. Fischer

Ovarian torsion is the twisting of the ovary on its vascular pedicle. Torsion first obstructs the lymphatic and venous drainage and as the twist tightens it may interrupt arterial inflow. Torsion leads to a distorted, swollen, and often hemorrhagic ovary that can become ischemic, eventually necrosis, and cause peritonitis.

Ovarian torsion can occur at any age. It is an uncommon problem in children and adolescents and is even less frequent in adult women. Ovarian torsion typically presents with acute lower abdominal pain, and the diagnosis is difficult because of the nonspecific symptoms and physical findings. In addition, imaging has only a limited ability to unequivocally confirm the diagnosis [1–3]. A high index of suspicion for ovarian torsion is necessary to make a timely diagnosis and institute early surgery that may save the ovary.

Historically, surgical treatment was thought to usually require an oophorectomy due both to the ischemia, which was thought to cause irreversible damage to the ovary, and to the distortion of the ovary, which was assumed to be secondary to an underlying pathologic process requiring resection. Newer data from larger studies has challenges those assumptions. First, follicular function has been shown to recover after detorsion of blue and even black ovaries that were clearly ischemic. Second, most ovarian torsions have been shown to occur in either normal ovaries or are associated with benign conditions that do not require oophorectomy [4–6]. These findings have led to a slow evolution of pediatric surgical practice away from routine oophorectomy toward a consensus of attempting ovarian salvage by simple detorsion [7–10].

Pathophysiology

Despite being attached to the pelvic sidewall by ligaments, the ovary has a fair amount of mobility that allows it to twist on its pedicle. Torsion of the ovary usually occurs with the torsion of the adjacent fallopian tube around the broad ligament and is known as adnexal torsion. Less commonly, there may be an isolated torsion of the ovary around its mesovarium attachment or isolated torsion of the fallopian tube around its mesosalpinx attachment. If ovarian torsion is not corrected in a timely fashion, then the lymphatics and veins and finally the arteries in the vascular pedicle are occluded with subsequent ischemia. Necrosis of the affected adnexa and peritonitis follow.

The ovary is classically thought to have a dual blood supply via the ovarian artery and the uterine artery. A dual blood supply might protect the ovary from ischemia during torsion. However, only 56% of ovaries have a dual blood supply while the ovarian artery alone supplies 40% of ovaries and the uterine artery alone supplies 4% of ovaries. In addition, adnexal

A.C. Fischer (✉)
Pediatric Surgery, 927 45th St Ste 301, West Palm Beach, FL 33407, USA
e-mail: annefischermdphd@gmail.com

D.J. Ledbetter and P.R.V. Johnson (eds.), *Endocrine Surgery in Children*,
DOI 10.1007/978-3-662-54256-9_25

torsion typically involves both vascular pedicles —the ovarian artery in the suspensory ligament and branches from the uterine artery contained in the ovarian ligament, so even ovaries with a dual blood supply are at risk for ischemia when torsed. The dual blood supply of the ovary also potentially complicates the imaging diagnosis since Doppler ultrasonography might detect blood flow from one pedicle even when there was significant torsion of the other vascular pedicle.

Ovarian torsion may be bilateral. Synchronous bilateral ovarian torsion is defined as simultaneous torsion of each ovary while in asynchronous or metachronous bilateral ovarian torsion the ovaries suffer torsion at different times. In either case, bilateral ovarian torsion is potentially devastating and could cause loss of future reproductive potential.

Epidemiology

Ovarian torsion is uncommon but the actual incidence is unclear. Adnexal torsion accounts for up to 2.7% of all cases of acute abdominal pain in children [11]. It is also responsible for one third of all ovarian operations in children [2]. Torsion is most common in the perimenarchal and early teenage years, but can occur at any age. The best nationwide estimate of incidence was reported from the Healthcare Cost and Utilization Project Kids' Inpatient Database (KID) that extracted data from tertiary children's hospitals. In 2006, there were over 1232 hospitalizations for ovary torsion in girls between 1 and 20 years of age. The incidence of ovarian torsion was estimated at 4.9 cases per 100,000 girls [6]. Interestingly, the incidence of ovarian torsion in this age group is roughly the same as the incidence of testicular torsion. Over 80% of cases of ovarian torsion occurred between 11 and 20 years of age and the mean age at diagnosis was 14.5 years. This study reported a lower proportion of cases in prepubertal girls (17%) than prior case series (32–68%) [3, 5, 9] probably reflecting the exclusion of infants and the different proportions of adolescents in the populations studied. When infants are included there is a bimodal age distribution with a peak incidence in infants under the age of 1 and another peak at 12 years of age (Fig. 25.1) [2].

Bilateral ovarian torsion is uncommon and can occur with or without associated underlying adnexal pathology. For example, in one large series of 76 children with ovarian torsion 5% suffered asynchronous bilateral torsion [4] while another large series of 114 patients reported no cases of bilateral ovarian torsion [12]. In the pediatric population, there have been 24 case reports of asynchronous torsion and only three cases of synchronous bilateral torsion [13].

Etiology

Ovarian torsion may occur in a normal ovary or may be associated with an abnormality of the ovary. The normal tube and ovary are mobile and may rotate 90° without any symptoms [14] and can easily twist 360° to 1080° [15]. It is now clear that torsion may occur in normal adnexa without an associated pathologic mass acting as the lead point for torsion. In the two largest case series of ovarian torsion, approximately half of the cases (46 and 48.8%) had no underlying ovarian abnormality [2, 4]. In the series reported by Oltmann et al. of 114 pathologically reviewed torsed specimens, there was no underlying etiology of torsion in one half of cases, but rather, normal tissue with hemorrhage [2]. Likewise, approximately half the cases of ovarian torsion reported in the KID database had no additional ovarian diagnoses [6, 12].

Anatomic Factors in Ovarian Torsion

The absence of a pathologic "lead point" in the setting of torsion suggests that anatomic variants of normal anatomy may predispose to torsion. The increased risk of torsion in the contralateral "normal" ovary in patients who suffer asynchronous torsions also suggests a common anatomic risk factor [16]. Anatomic variants that predispose to ovarian torsion include a long

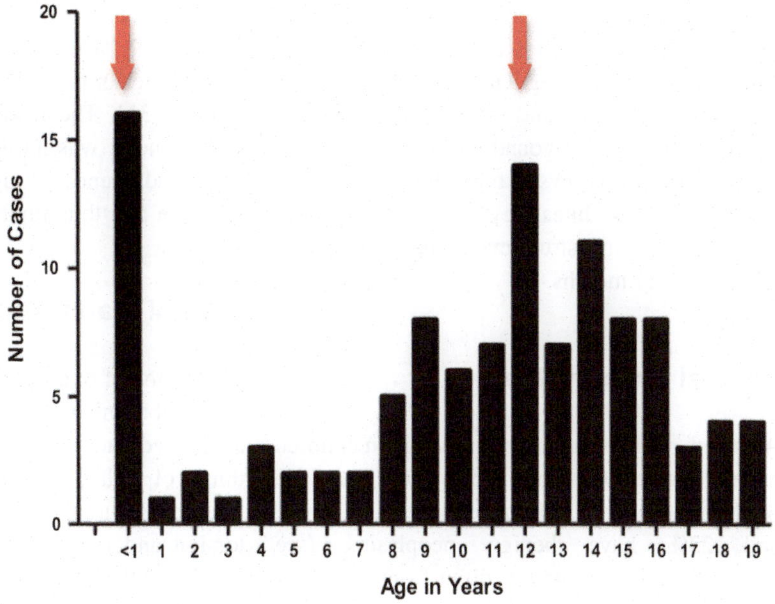

Fig. 25.1 Bimodal age distribution of ovarian torsion

fallopian tube, a long utero-ovarian ligament, such as the mesovarium and mesosalpinx, or an unusually short ovarian hilum [14, 17–19]. All the variants mentioned result in increased mobility in the ovarian suspensory ligaments. A report of familial ovarian torsion with bilateral ovarian loss in the mother and unilateral ovary loss in the daughter suggests that a genetic predisposition to torsion may exist [20]. Other factors that may contribute to hypermobility of the ovary and therefore ovarian torsion are tubal spasm, abrupt changes in intra-abdominal pressure with jarring activity, and adnexal venous congestion seen with constipation, sigmoid distension, and premenarchal or gestational hormonal changes [17, 21, 22].

A predominance of right-sided adnexal torsion has been noted with a 3:2 ratio of right to left sidedness [23]. Even most cases of asynchronous torsion first present on the right side [16]. The explanation of the right side predominance of ovarian torsion may be the associated hypermobility of the cecum and ileum compared to the relative stability of the sigmoid on the left. Alternatively, there may be an ascertainment bias because of the more likely operative intervention for right sided abdominal pain because of concern for appendicitis [14, 24].

Hormonal Factors in Ovarian Torsion

As noted, there are two peaks in the incidence of ovarian torsion—one during infancy and the other around 12 years of age [2]. The bimodal age distribution reflects peak hormonal levels seen in children—the fetal exposure to maternal hormones and the early adolescent response to the maturing reproductive hormonal axis [1]. The association between age and hormonal environment suggests that hormonal effects are a risk factor for ovarian torsion. Potentially, hormonally induced ovarian cysts and adnexal congestion could serve as "lead points" for ovarian torsion.

Ovarian cysts may form in utero in response to maternal hormones and these cysts may persist into infancy, explaining the high incidence of torsion in girls less than 1 year of age [25]. Between ages 1 and 8 years, the hypothalamic-pituitary axis resets to a baseline of low estrogen and FSH levels. As a result, the ovary is quiescent and minimal ovarian cysts are formed in this age group [26]. Around puberty, between 9 and 14 years, the reproductive hormonal axis is activated with high FSH levels long before the onset of menses [27, 28]. The high and fluctuating hormone levels in this age group prime the ovaries for cyst formation. By age 15, hormonal patterns are usually well established, and FSH and LH levels are regulated by the monthly release of estrogen and progesterone by the ovary. Changes in gonadotropin release can result in functional cysts, typically either follicular or corpus luteal cysts, which enlarge throughout the menstrual cycle and then resolve within several months.

Adnexal Abnormalities

As noted, ovaries that undergo torsion in children have no associated abnormality more than 40% of the time, while 33% have underlying cysts, and 23% have benign neoplasms (see Table 25.1). These findings differ from the adults where an underlying cyst is the most common etiology of ovarian torsion [29]. Overall at least 96% of ovaries that undergo torsion in children are normal or have associated benign conditions and only 1.7–3.5% contain a malignancy. (The categorization of serous borderline cysts as benign or malignant accounts for the variance [12].) Summation of all reported pediatric case series of ovarian torsion confirmed an even lower incidence (1.4–1.9%), of an underlying malignancy with the KID database reporting the lowest incidence (0.4%) in over 1232 cases [6, 12]. This incidence of underlying malignancy is markedly lower than the 10% risk of malignancy for all pediatric ovarian masses and is comparable to the 1–2% incidence of malignancy in adults (Table 25.2) [24, 30].

These findings, based on the pathologic analysis of surgical specimens, show a dramatic, 10–20-fold lower incidence of malignancy in ovarian torsions than found in ovarian masses and clearly refute the traditionally held tenet that an underlying malignant tumor is the most common lead point of torsion. Likewise, fewer benign and malignant tumors are found in torsed specimens compared to nontorsed ovarian masses [12]. Finally, case series show that benign ovarian etiologies cause torsion more commonly than malignant tumors. For example, Sommerville et al. reported the incidence of torsion in benign tumors was 14.3%, which was greater than the 9.7% incidence for borderline tumors and far greater than 1.1% incidence for malignant tumors [31]. The lower rate of torsion seen in malignancies was attributed to their tendency to induce adherence through inflammation and local invasion and thus limit ovarian mobility.

Clinical Manifestations

Symptoms of ovarian torsion in children include lower abdominal pain in almost all cases and associated nausea and vomiting in more than two thirds of girls [1, 8, 32]. However, this classic triad of symptoms is not specific for ovarian torsion and many causes of an acute abdomen present with similar symptoms. Although nearly all children (>97%) with ovarian torsion have abdominal pain, the classic history of an *acute onset of severe pain* is not common and the variable severity of pain is a potential diagnostic pitfall [3, 33]. There is considerable variation in the intensity, character, location, and duration of pain in patients with ovarian torsion. Often the history of recurrent pain is due to recurrent torsion and detorsion of the adnexa rather than persistent torsion [32, 34]. Torsion in infants is often not accompanied by pain since the torsion may often occur in utero, so the most common clinical presentations of an infant with ovarian torsion are positive prenatal imaging (>50%), presence of a mass (38%), or feeding tolerance (6%) (see Table 25.1) [2].

Besides the presence of pain, the location of pain is important since the symptoms of ovarian torsion commonly overlap with those of appendicitis, especially since adnexal torsion is more common on the right [29, 33]. The distinguishing features suggesting adnexal torsion rather than appendicitis include the presence of a palpable abdominal mass [3] and the synchronous onset of pain with the symptoms of nausea and vomiting, whereas in appendicitis, pain usually occurs first, followed later by nausea and vomiting [24]. Classic physical signs found in children with ovarian torsion include low-grade fever, abdominal tenderness, and an abdominal mass.

Table 25.1 Patients with ovarian torsion compared to patients with ovarian masses not associated with torsion

	Torsion	Nontorsion	*P* value
Number of cases	114 (26%)	324 (74%)	<0.0001
Mean age ± SEM	10.28 years ± 0.53	13.23 ± 0.26	<0.0001
Clinical presentation			
Abdominal mass	6%	23%	<0.0001
Abdominal pain	83%	56%	<0.0001
Prenatal diagnosis	6%	1%	0.0013
Other[a]	5%	20%	<0.0001
Size by imaging (cm)	8.1 ± 0.49 (2.9–25)	9.8 ± 0.60 (0.9–50)	0.077
WBC >12 K	56%	28%	0.0004
Pathology			
Benign, normal tissue	46 (40%)	11 (3.4%)	<0.0001
Benign cyst	38 (33%)	146 (45%)	0.0291
Benign neoplasm	26 (24%)	123 (38%)	0.0067
Malignant neoplasm	4 (3.5%)[b]	44 (13.6%)	0.0030

[a]Other clinical presentations included precocious puberty, feeding intolerance, groin hernia, incidental finding and not documented

[b]Two serous borderline cysts, a juvenile granulosa cell tumor, and a dysgerminoma (12)

Chang et al. identified that a lower Alvarado score with a paucity of pain migration, rebound pain, or fever and the presence of a palpable mass, seen in 10% cases, were the best clues to differentiate torsion from appendicitis [3, 35].

Ovarian torsion can present in an incarcerated inguinal hernia. Merriman reviewed incarcerated inguinal hernias in girls and found that 82% of incarcerated hernias in female infants contained ovaries. The median age of the girls with incarcerated hernias was 8 weeks and 15–27% contained ovarian torsions and ischemic ovaries [36, 37]. Thus, in female infants with an irreducible inguinal hernia a timely repair is important to minimize ovarian loss.

Investigations

After a history and physical examination, the evaluation of a young woman with significant abdominal pain usually continues with a complete white blood cell count (WBC), a urinalysis, and a urinary pregnancy test. Leukocytosis occurs in up to 56% of children with ovarian torsion and is more likely to occur with ovarian torsion than with ovarian masses not associated with torsion [2]. Interestingly, when ovarian torsion presents with right lower quadrant abdominal pain and a WBC elevated above 12,000 then an urgent operation is more likely to occur than when the WBC is normal, probably because the increased possibility of appendicitis compels earlier exploration [2, 3]. When an ovarian mass is suspected then serologic markers of malignancy are obtained, including alpha fetoprotein (αFP) and beta human chorionic gonadotropin (βHCG). However, even when obtained in the workup of an asymptomatic palpable ovarian mass suspected of malignancy, over 50% of the time serologic markers are not positive and thus are not conclusive [12]. In any case, during the urgent evaluation and management of ovarian torsion, serologic marker results are usually not available in time to guide management and operative decisions. Since the diagnosis of ovarian torsion is difficult to make on the basis of the history, physical examination, and laboratory investigations imaging studies are frequently obtained.

Table 25.2 Pathology of ovarian torsion—review of literature

Author	Cases ovarian torsion	Malignant neoplasms	Malignant neoplasm pathology	Benign neoplasms	Benign neoplasm pathology	Population
Meyer et al. (1995)	13	0	None	3	Cystadenoma (1) Teratoma (2)	Pediatric
Kokoska et al. (2000)	51	3	Dysgerminoma (1) Granulosa cell (2)	26	Cystadenoma (2) Teratoma (24)	Pediatric
Cass et al. (2001)	34	0	None	15	Teratoma (15)	Pediatric
Beaunoyer et al. (2004)	76	0	None	21	Cystadenoma (6) Teratoma (15)	Pediatric
Anders et al. (2005)	22	1	Granulosa cell (1)	5	Dermoid (5)	Pediatric
Servaes et al. (2007)	41	0	None	11	Cystadenoma (1) Teratoma (10)	Pediatric
Rousseau et al. (2008)	41	2	Dysgerminoma (1) Undifferentiated adenocarcinoma (1)	26	Cystadenoma (11) Teratoma (15)	Pediatric
Oltmann et al. (2010)	114	4	Dysgerminoma (1) Juvenile granulosa cell (1) Serous borderline (2)	26	Cystadenoma (7) Dermoid (2) Fibroma (1) Teratoma (16)	Pediatric
Houry et al. (2001)	87	1	Mucinous borderline (1)	30	Cystadenoma (11) Teratoma (19)	Adult
Cohen et al. (2003)	102	0	None	13	Cystadenoma (4) Dermoid (9)	Adult
White et al. (2005)	44	2	Granulosa cell (1) Serous borderline (1)	13	Cystadenoma (1) Dermoid (7) Fibrothecoma (1) Fibroma (1) Leiomyoma (1) Teratoma (2)	Adult
Göçmen et al. (2008)	18	0	None	11	Cystadenoma (7) Dermoid (4)	Adult
Shadinger et al. (2008)	39	0	None	12	Benign Spindle (1) Brenner (1) Cystadenoma (2) Dermoid (7) Fibroma (1)	Adult and pediatric (3–61 years)
Pediatric totals	431	10 (2%)	Dysgerminoma (3) Granulosa cell (3) Juvenile granulosa cell (1) Serous borderline(2) Undifferentiated adenocarcinoma (1)	133 (30.8%)	Cystadenoma (28) Dermoid (7) Fibroma (1) Teratoma (97)	Pediatric

(continued)

Table 25.2 (continued)

Author	Cases ovarian torsion	Malignant neoplasms	Malignant neoplasm pathology	Benign neoplasms	Benign neoplasm pathology	Population
Literature totals	682	13 (1.9%)	Dysgerminoma (3) Granulosa cell (4) Juvenile granulosa cell (1) Mucinous borderline (1) Serous borderline (3) Undifferentiated adenocarcinoma (1)	212 (31.0%)	Benign Spindle (1) Brenner (1) Cystadenoma (53) Dermoid (34) Fibroma (3) Fibrothecoma (1) Leiomyoma (1) Teratoma (118)	Adult and pediatric

From Oltmann SC, Fischer AC, Barber R, et al. Pediatric ovarian malignancy presenting as ovarian torsion: incidence and relevance. J Pediatr Surg. 2010;45:135–139, with permission

Imaging

Plain X-rays can show calcifications that indicate mature teratomas or they can suggest a mass effect [4, 38]. However, as with CT scanning, plain X-rays are more useful in assessing other etiologies for abdominal pain and are not recommended to diagnose torsion. Obtaining plain X-rays, a CT scan, or both may delay the definitive care of a patient with ovarian torsion [3].

The first choice in the imaging evaluation of ovarian torsion is ultrasound (US) with Doppler. In young adults, the transvaginal US approach is often advocated but in most children, the transabdominal pelvic US is preferred due to the smaller vaginal size and virginal status of children, which can limit visualization. Potential technical difficulties of using transabdominal pelvic US to diagnose ovarian pathology include a thick abdominal wall in obese patients, overlying bowel gas, and the lack of a full bladder, which is sometimes difficult to obtain in young patients in pain [39]. Also, some US exams may visualize only one ovary. When only one ovary is visualized it is more difficult to determine if it is enlarged since there is no normal "control" for comparison. In addition, the side of origin of the visualized ovary may be difficult to determine [32, 40]. When only one ovary is visualized, it is useful to estimate the expected ovarian volume based on the age and pubertal status of the patient to determine if the ovary is enlarged [41].

Even with technically adequate studies, the diagnosis of ovarian torsion requires judgment to correlate the clinical and imaging findings. Unfortunately, definitive ultrasound findings of ovarian torsion such as the *whirlpool sign* [42] and a spiral appearance of the adnexa are not found in most children with ovarian torsion [9]. The most common sonographic findings of torsion are an enlarged ovary with tissue edema or an echogenic pelvic mass with no visualization of the ipsilateral ovary [1, 4]. In particular, a unilateral enlarged ovary containing dilated, peripherally located cysts is found in 66% of patients with ovarian torsion [40, 43]. The finding most sensitive for torsion is the presence of a pelvic mass larger than 5 cm that is sonographically complex (51%) rather than purely cystic (38%) or solid (11%) [2].

The evaluation of ovarian blood flow by spectral Doppler was hoped to improve the diagnostic accuracy of US for ovarian torsion; however, this is controversial because of reports of finding ovarian flow by US but a necrotic ovary at operation [44, 45]. Pena et al. and Stark and Siegel reported that only 30–40% of patients with confirmed ovarian torsion at surgery demonstrated decreased or absent blood flow preoperatively [38, 43]. So it seems that the presence of vascularity, *even arterial flow*, does not exclude ovarian torsion and a high index of clinic suspicion is required to avoid delays in diagnosis and definitive operative treatment [16, 39]. Absent or abnormal flow in the ovarian vein has been found in 62% of cases of adnexal torsions [46].

Since the most sensitive ultrasonography finding suggesting torsion is relatively nonspecific ovarian enlargement with small cystic structures scattered around the periphery [1, 2, 4, 47], a high index of suspicion is needed to make the diagnosis and initiate treatment. It is often best to proceed with laparoscopy early to make the diagnosis and treat the torsion rather than delay until a definitive diagnosis is obtained.

Treatment

The treatment of ovarian torsion is surgical, either by resection of the involved adnexa by salpingo-oophorectomy or by detorsion. In tertiary care children hospitals, about 60% of patients with ovarian torsion had resection while the incidence of orchiectomy for testicular torsion is roughly 35% [6]. Part of these differences is related to the intrapelvic location of ovaries and difficulty in diagnosis compared to the more superficial and easily identified testicles.

In the past, resections were done frequently but it is now recognized that detorsion alone is usually preferred. There were three main reasons that resection was advocated—(1) the risk of thromboembolism, (2) the risk of an underlying malignancy or other abnormality that required resection, and (3) the judgment that the ovary was nonviable and had no potential of reproductive or hormonal function. All three reasons have been critically analyzed and not found to justify routine ovarian resection.

First, thromboembolism was thought to be potential risk after untwisting the vascular pedicle that was assumed to have thrombosed veins. McGovern reviewed the literature regarding the risk of thromboembolism in adult patients with torsion and found two cases and calculated an incidence of 0.2%. Interestingly, each case of thromboembolism occurred in patients undergoing ovarian resections, not in patients who had detorsion alone [11, 48]. Whether or not, the adult risk of thromboembolism can be extrapolated to children is debatable and the largest analysis of pediatric ovarian torsion related hospitalizations could not identify a case of pulmonary thromboembolism associated with ovarian torsion [6]. Similarly case series of ovarian torsion in children have not reported a thromboembolic complication with detorsion [15].

Second, there is often a presumption that a pathologic lead point, such as a malignancy, that requires resection, incites ovarian torsion. Unequivocally the KID database and all case series of torsions consistently report an incidence of 0.4–1.4% rate of malignancy which is 10–20-fold lower incidence than the expected 10% malignancy rate in ovarian masses in children. Thus, torsion is highly unlikely to be associated with an underlying malignancy. To maximize ovarian salvage at the time of operation, it has been advocated to either biopsy suspicious areas or simply detorse the ovary and follow the ovarian size with US and perform a 'second look' procedure, if US detects an intrinsic mass 6 weeks after detorsion [10, 49]. Intraoperative pathologic analysis by frozen section of the excised ovarian cyst or ovarian biopsied tissue can assist in deciding to proceed with ovarian salvage as opposed to resection [50]. The benefit of preserving the ovary seems worth the small risk of delaying treatment of the rare malignancy.

Thirdly, the likelihood of ovarian viability after torsion has been previously underestimated since ischemic or blackish blue ovaries were presumed to be necrotic (Fig. 25.2). However, it has been shown that the black-bluish macroscopic appearance of an ovary is not a true

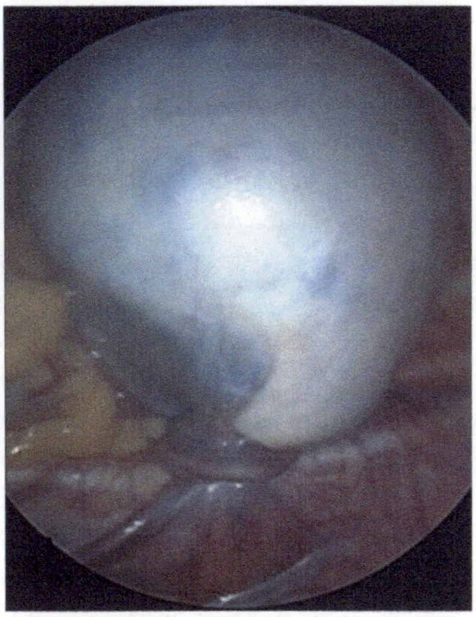

Fig. 25.2 Laparoscopic view of ovarian torsion

indicator of the degree of ischemia [10]. Even black-bluish ovaries show evidence of viable ovarian parenchyma upon pathologic review [51] and multiple case series have demonstrated that detorsion of seemingly necrotic ovaries results in viable ovarian appearance on later ultrasound [7, 8, 15]. The currently accepted treatment for ovarian torsion is detorsion and ovarian preservation regardless of macroscopic appearance of the ovary. Even ovarian cysts can be left alone at the initial operation. Functional cysts will often resolve spontaneously and cystectomy or partial resection of an ischemic edematous ovary is technically difficult because of the inability to ascertain the plane between abnormal tissue and ovarian tissue. If a large ovarian cyst is found at the initial detorsion then cyst aspiration is often done to prevent an early recurrence of torsion.

Serial ultrasonography is done beginning 6 weeks after detorsion to follow follicular return of an ischemic ovary and to assess if there is an associated ovarian mass or persistent ovarian cyst. The edema and distortion has usually resolved within 6 weeks and underlying abnormalities can be detected. If follow-up ultrasound reveals an underlying ovarian mass or persistent large cyst then a second operation can be undertaken. Persistence or recurrence of a cyst with normal tumor markers is ideally managed by an ovarian cystectomy. Persistence of an enlarged ovary and abnormal tumor markers warrants a CT scan and laparotomy to stage and resect the mass appropriately.

It has been suggested that when the ovarian mass is large then laparotomy is favored over laparoscopy [51]. However, the recommended size cutoff for laparoscopy has varied in the literature since a given size has not proven to be a significant predictor of benign versus malignant lesions. A reasonable practice is for masses less than 7.5 cm, laparoscopy is preferred to allow detorsion, aspiration of a benign cyst, and ovarian preservation, regardless of appearance and color, followed by postoperative US surveillance. However, when an ovarian mass exceeds 7.5 cm, a laparotomy is recommended to allow detorsion, protection of the peritoneal cavity to aspirate a possible cyst or perform an intraoperative biopsy with frozen section. If a malignancy is found on the frozen section further staging can be done. If a benign lesion is found then the ovary can be preserved.

Simple detorsion may predispose to recurrent torsion. It has been noted that children with torsion of normal adnexa may be at increased risk of either recurrent torsion on the same side or asynchronous bilateral ovarian torsion [16]. There is no consensus for the role of oophoropexy in treatment of ovarian torsion. Reports of ovarian atrophy in patients treated with bilateral fixation argue that the risks of recurrent torsion must be carefully balanced against the risks of oophoropexy when deciding upon the best strategy for ovarian preservation [7]. Oophoropexy is not routinely recommended at the time of detorsion because the ovary is often edematous and friable and difficult to operatively stabilize without injury to the ovary. Oophoropexy should be performed for specific indications, usually at the time of a second procedure when it is not heavy and edematous. This permits good fixation of the ovary near the fallopian tube and optimal stabilization. Indications for an oophoropexy include recurrent torsion, obviously abnormal adnexal attachments, history of a prior loss of an ovary without an underlying pathology, and bilateral synchronous torsion [52].

Fixing the ovary by plication of the utero-ovarian ligament with a nonabsorbable suture is a simple technique involving minimal interference with fallopian function or blood supply and thus may be the preferred method of fixation when needed [52].

Outcomes

The ideal outcome for a girl suffering from ovarian torsion would be an urgent presentation to medical attention, a prompt diagnostic evaluation driven by a high index of suspicion for torsion, and early operative intervention with detorsion leading to preservation of the ovary. Although diagnostic methods are improving and operative interventions are becoming less invasive, the outcomes of children with ovarian torsion are not yet ideal. Nationwide data from 2006 from tertiary care children's hospitals showed that 60% of girls with ovarian torsion had resection of the ovary [6]. This contrast to roughly 35% of boys with testicular torsion having orchiectomy. This difference is due to delay in presentation to medical attention, delay in diagnosis, delay in surgical treatment, and the perception that resection was necessary because of an underlying ovarian tumor or that the ovary was irreversibly damaged [1].

As noted in the previous sections, despite the often abnormal appearance of a torsed ovary it is rare to have an underlying tumor. Therefore, attempting ovarian salvage by detorsion alone and following the ovary by serial ultrasound exams is recommended treatment. Also, despite the common intraoperative finding of a blue or even a black ovary, simple detorsion results in a >90% ovarian salvage as defined by follicular changes suggesting folliculogenesis seen on follow-up ultrasound exam [6, 10]. Complete functional recovery of the ovaries can occur after untwisting the ischemic adnexa, regardless of their intraoperative appearance [10, 51]. Atrophy of the ovary is seen on follow-up ultrasound exam in about 5% of cases of ovarian torsion [15]. A significantly lower median time from onset of symptoms to operation [8]. This reflects the duration of ischemia although there is no clear correlation between duration of symptoms and ovarian infarction [5]. It also may represent the surgeon's inclination to resect ovaries when there has been a longer durations of symptoms.

The likelihood of ovarian salvage also varies by surgical specialty with general surgeons performing oophorectomies in 60% of cases compared to gynecologists performing oophorectomies in 40% of cases. This specialty difference may reflect a lower index of suspicion for torsion in children with lower abdominal pain who present to pediatric centers (and pediatric surgeons) compared to those who present to gynecologists. Or it may represent different indications for resection between the two specialties. It has been noted that a high index of suspicion for ovarian torsion before operative intervention is associated with an increase in the likelihood of ovarian salvage—with torsions suspected preoperatively in 94% of those who eventually underwent detorsion compared to preoperative suspicion in less than half of those who had oophorectomy [8]. Another factor effecting ovarian salvage is the age at presentation with children less than 12 years more likely to undergo oophorectomies (77–88%) [2, 6]. This may represent delays in presentation, diagnosis, and operative intervention in younger children. Or it may represent differences in the indications for resection between surgeons treating younger children and those treating older adolescents.

References

1. Kokoska ER, Keller MS, Weber TR. Acute ovarian torsion in children. Am J Surg. 2000;180:462–5.
2. Oltmann SC, Fischer AC, Barber R, et al. Cannot exclude torsion—a fifteen year review. J Pediatric Surg. 2009;44:1212–7.
3. Chan Y, Yan D, Kong M, et al. Adnexal torsion in children. Pediatr Emerg Care. 2008;24(8):534–7.
4. Beaunoyer M, Chapdelaine J, Bouchard S, et al. Asynchronous bilateral ovarian torsion. Am J Surg. 2000;180:462–5.

5. Anders JF, Powell EC. Urgency of evaluation and outcome of acute ovarian torsion in pediatric patients. Arch Pediatr Adolesc Med. 2005;159:532–5.
6. Gutherie BD, Adler MD, Powell EC. Incidence and trends of pediatric ovarian torsion hospitalizations in the United States, 2000–2006. Pediatrics. 2010;125:532–8.
7. Celik A, Ergun O, Aldemir H, et al. Long-term results of conservative management of adnexal torsion in children. J Pediatr Surg. 2005;40(4):704–8.
8. Aziz D, Davis V, Allen L, Langer J. Ovarian torsion in children: is oophorectomy necessary? J Pediatr Surg. 2004;39(5):750–3.
9. Rousseau V, Massicot R, Ahmed A, et al. Emergency management and conservative surgery of ovarian torsion in children: a report of 40 cases. J Pediatr Adolesc Gynecol. 2008;21(4):201–6.
10. Oelsner G, Bider G, Goldenberg M, et al. Long term follow-up of the twisted of ischemic adnexa managed by detorsion. Fertil Steril. 1993;60:976–9.
11. Roday A, Jackish C, Klockenbusch W, et al. The conservative management of adnexal torsion—a case report and review of the literature. Eur J Obstet Gynecol Reprod Biol. 2002;101:83–6.
12. Oltmann SC, Fischer AC, Barber R, et al. Pediatric ovarian malignancy presenting as ovarian torsion: incidence and relevance. J Pediatr Surg. 2010;45:135–9.
13. Dumont T, Caccia N, Allen L. Pediatric synchronous bilateral ovarian torsion: a case report and review of the literature. J Pediatr Surg. 2011;46:e19–23.
14. Evans JP. Torsion of the normal uterine adnexa in premenarchal girls. J Pediatr Surg. 1978;13:195–6.
15. Wang J-H, Wu D-H, Jin H, Wu Y-Z. Predominant etiology of adnexal torsion and ovarian outcome after detorsion in premenarchal girls. Eur J Pediatr Surg. 2010;20:298–301.
16. Ozcan C, Celik A, Ozok G, Erdener A, Balik E. Adnexal torsion in children may have a catastrophic sequel; asynchronous bilateral torsion. J Pediatr Surg. 2000;37:1617–29.
17. Dunnihoo DR, Wolff J. Bilateral torsion of the adnexa: a case report and a review of the world literature. Obstet Gynecol. 1984;64:55S–9S.
18. Kurzbart E, Mares AJ, Cohen Z, et al. Isolated torsion of the fallopian tube in premenarcheal girls. J Pediatr Surg. 1994;29:1384–5.
19. Sozen I, Nobel P, Nobel J. Partial tubal salvage through neosalpingostomy in a 12-year-old girl with combined ovarian and fallopian tube torsion. J Pediatr Surg. 2006;41:E17–9.
20. Crough S, Gyampoh B, Cutner AS, et al. Ovarian torsion: to pex or not to pex? Case report and revue of the literature. J Pediatr Adolesc Gynecol. 2003;16:381.
21. McCrea RS. Uterine adnexal torsion with subsequent contralateral recurrence. J Reprod Med. 1980;24:123–4.
22. Moredehai J, Mares AJ, Barki Y, et al. Torsion of uterine adnexa in neonates and children: a report of 20 cases. J Pediatr Surg. 1991;26:1195–9.
23. Descargues G, Tinlot-Mauger F, Gravier A, et al. Adnexal torsion: a report on forty-five cases. Euro J Obstet Gynecol Reprod Biol. 2001;98:91–6.
24. Cass DL. Ovarian torsion. Semin Pediatr Surg. 2005;14:86–92.
25. Bagolan P, Rivosecchi M, Giorlandino C, et al. Prenatal diagnosis and clinical outcome of ovarian cysts. J Pediatr Surg. 1992;27:879–81.
26. Helmrath MA, Shin CE, Warner BW. Ovarian cysts in the pediatric population. Semin Pediatr Surg. 1998;7:19–28.
27. Legro RS, Lin HM, Demers LM, et al. Rapid maturation of the reproductive axis during perimenarche independent of body composition. J Clin Endocrinol Metab. 2000;85:1021–5.
28. Chumlea WC, Schubert CM, Roche AF, et al. Age at menarche and racial comparisons in US girls. Pediatrics. 2003;111:110–3.
29. Houry D, Abbott JT. Ovarian torsion: a fifteen-year review. Ann Emerg Med. 2001;38:156–9.
30. Cass D, Hawkings E, Brandt ML, et al. Surgery for ovarian masses in infants, children, and adolescents: 102 consecutive patients treated in a 15-year period. J Pediatr Surg. 2001;36:693–9.
31. Sommerville M, Grimes DA, Koonings PP, et al. Ovarian neoplasms and the risk of adnexal torsion. Am J Obstet Gynecol. 1991;164:577–8.
32. Meyer JS, Harmon CM, Harty MP, et al. Ovarian torsion: clinical and imaging presentation in children. J Pediatr Surg. 1995;30:1433–6.
33. Emonts M, Doornewaard H, Admiral JC. Adnexal torsion in very young girls: diagnostic pitfalls. Eur J Obstet Gynecol Reprod Biol. 2004;1126:207–10.
34. Styaert H, Meynol F, Valla JS. Torsion of the adnexa in children: the value of laparoscopy. Pediatr Surg Int. 1998;13:384–7.
35. Alvarado A. A practical score for the early diagnosis of acute appendicitis. Ann Emerg Med. 1986;15:557–64.
36. Merriman TE, Auldist AW. Ovarian torsion in inguinal hernias. Pediatr Surg Int. 2000;16:383–5.
37. Boley SJ, Cahn D, Lauer T, et al. The irreducible ovary: a true emergency. J Pediatr Surg. 1991;26:1035–8.
38. Pena JE, Ufberg D, Cooney N, et al. Usefulness of Doppler sonography in the diagnosis of ovarian torsion. Fertil Steril. 2000;73:1047–50.
39. Schultz KA, Ness KK, Nagarajan R, et al. Adnexal masses in infancy and childhood. Clin Obstet Gynecol. 2006;49:464–79.
40. Graif M, Itzchak Y. Sonographic evaluation of ovarian torsion in childhood and adolescence. Am J Roentgenol. 1988;150:647–9.
41. Herter LD, Golendziner E, Monteiro Flores JA, et al. Ovarian and uterine sonography in healthy girls between 1 and 13 years old: correlation of findings with age and pubertal status. Am J Roentgenol. 2002;178:1531.
42. Vijayaraghavan SB. Sonographic whirlpool signs in ovarian torsion. J Ultrasound Med. 2004;23:1643–9.

43. Stark JE, Siegel MJ. Ovarian torsion in prepubertal and pubertal girls: sonographic findings. Am J Roentgenol. 1994;163:1479–82.
44. Servaes S, Zurakowski D, Laufer M, et al. Sonographic findings of ovarian torsion in children. Pediatr Radiol. 2007;37:446–51.
45. Hurh PJ, Meyer JS, Shaaban A. Ultrasound of a torsed ovary: characteristic gray-scale appearance despite normal arterial and venous flow on Doppler. Pediatr Radiol. 2002;32:586–8.
46. Nizar K, Deutsch M, Filmer S, et al. Doppler studies of the ovarian venous blood flow in the diagnosis of adnexal torsion. J Clin Ultrasound. 2009;37:436–9.
47. Albayram F, Hamper UM. Ovarian and adnexal torsion: spectrum of sonographic findings with pathologic correction. J Ultrasound Med. 2001;20:1083–9.
48. McGovern P, Noah R, Koenigsberg R, Little A. Adnexal torsion and pulmonary embolism: case report and review of the literature. Obstet Gynecol Surv. 1999;54(9):601–8.
49. Karpelowsky J, Hei E, Matthews K. Laparoscopic resection of benign ovarian tumors in children with gonadal preservation. Pediatr Surg Int. 2009;25:251–4.
50. Dolgin S, Lublin M, Shlasko E. Maximizing ovarian salvage when treating idiopathic adnexal torsion. J Pediatr Surg. 2000;35(4):624–6.
51. Galinier P, Carfagna L, Delsol M, et al. Ovarian torsion. Management and ovarian prognosis: a report of 45 cases. J Ped Surg. 2009;44:1759–65.
52. Fuchs N, Smogick N, Tovbin Y, et al. Oophoropexy to prevent torsion: How, When and for Whom? J Minim Invas Gynecol. 2010;17:205–8.

Fertility Preservation

26

Jennia Michaeli, Stephen Kennedy and Ariel Revel

There are several ways that the treatment of malignant and non-malignant diseases in children may interfere with the child's future fertility. To alleviate these adverse effects of therapy innovative methods to preserve fertility are being proposed and investigated. This chapter will focus on children who have been treated for cancer since they make up the largest and best studied group of patients with this problem.

In 2010, a total of 10,700 children and adolescents under the age of 14 were diagnosed with cancer in the United States. More than 80% will survive the disease [1]. However, survivors often face long-term sequelae of their treatment including irreversible damage to their reproductive organs that may harm pubertal development, cause infertility or lead to premature menopause, defined as cessation of ovarian function below the age of 40 [2].

The most obvious cause of fertility impairment is the surgical removal of the reproductive organs. However, chemotherapy and radiotherapy may also eliminate or severely compromise hormonal production and a patient's reproductive potential by damaging steroid-producing cells and gametes.

Both female and male gonadal tissues are very sensitive to chemotherapy [3, 4]. The degree of damage is determined by the patient's sex and age, the specific drug used and the dose administered [5, 6]. All chemotherapeutic drugs affect gonadal function although some are more harmful than others [7]. For example, alkylating agents such as cyclophosphamide and procarbazine are categorised as high risk drugs [3, 8], whereas vincristine and methotrexate have lower risks. However, because multi-drug protocols are increasingly common, it is difficult to advise patients and their parents about an individual's specific risk of future reproductive impairment.

Total-body irradiation (TBI) or radiation therapy delivered to the pelvis/abdomen may cause irreversible damage to the gonads. In both sexes, the degree of gonadal damage depends on the total radiation dose, where the radiation is directed (the field), how the radiation is delivered (the fractionation schedule) and the patient's age. In females, for a given dose of radiation, the younger the patient is at the time of treatment, the later is the onset of premature menopause [9]. A radiation dose of 2 Gy is estimated to damage 50% of ovarian follicles irreversibly, while doses of 5–20 Gy cause complete loss of ovarian function and result in sterility [10]. In males,

J. Michaeli · A. Revel (✉)
Department of Obstetrics and Gynaecology, Hadassah Medical Center and Hebrew University-Hadassah Medical School, Jerusalem, Israel
e-mail: arielrevel2@gmail.com

S. Kennedy
Nuffield Department of Obstetrics and Gynaecology, University of Oxford, Oxford, UK
e-mail: stephen.kennedy@obs-gyn.ox.ac.uk

S. Kennedy
John Radcliffe Hospital, Headley Way, Oxford OX3 9RZ, UK

D.J. Ledbetter and P.R.V. Johnson (eds.), *Endocrine Surgery in Children*,
DOI 10.1007/978-3-662-54256-9_26

radiation doses as low as 0.2 Gy cause damage to spermatogonial cells [11] and doses above 15 Gy adversely affect Leydig cell function [12].

As might be expected, combinations of chemotherapy and radiation are potentially even more injurious. Hematopoietic stem cell transplantation, which requires preparatory intensive chemotherapy (usually containing alkylating agents) and TBI, presents the greatest risk for gonadal dysfunction [13].

A variety of 'experimental' procedures, including gonadal tissue transplantation, are available to preserve fertility, especially in females, but major ethical, legal and medical issues must be addressed before they are offered [14]. For example, when a malignancy is diagnosed in a pre-pubertal child, parental consent must be obtained before harvesting gonadal tissue containing immature germ cells. However, consent to use stored tissue for fertilization or research purposes should be obtained solely from the patient [15, 16]. A multidisciplinary team including paediatric oncologists, reproductive endocrinologists, paediatric surgeons, anaesthetists and social workers, must work closely together to provide optimal counselling for patients and their parents [17].

History of Procedures to Preserve Fertility

The idea of reproductive organ transplantation has a long history. The first attempts were reported in the eighteenth century, when the Scottish anatomist and surgeon John Hunter transplanted testis into a chicken [18]. Robert Morris performed the first human ovarian transplant in 1895, and was a pioneer in the field of reproductive organ transplantation [19]. The motivation for these early attempts at ovarian transplantation was to achieve sex hormone production as a means to rejuvenate women or delay menopausal symptoms. This line of treatment was superseded when exogenous administration of sex hormones became possible, although the experiments contributed to our understanding of normal physiology [18].

In more recent times, various surgical procedures have been used to preserve ovarian function by moving the ovaries away from radiation fields in the pelvis. These procedures have included using vascular anastomoses in the abdominal cavity and microsurgical techniques for heterotopic transplantation of an ovary to the forearm [20]. Although oocytes have been retrieved from such grafts, this approach has not been widely used.

In the current era, new developments and techniques in the fields of in vitro fertilization (IVF) and tissue cryopreservation have revolutionized ovarian transplantation. Now it is possible to harvest and freeze gonadal tissue until the patient is well enough for that tissue to be transplanted back to the patient, and then later, oocytes can be retrieved for IVF treatment.

Indications and Patient Selection for Fertility Preservation

Although it is an innovative or even "experimental" procedure, cryopreservation of gonadal tissue can now be offered to patients with malignancies that require gonadotoxic therapy. Since the severity of the insult to gonadal function varies across different diseases and treatment protocols, it is important to counsel patients effectively about their individual risk of infertility. To support this goal a classification system has been developed that lists most malignant diseases and their associated treatments [21] (see Table 26.1).

In our opinion, fertility preservation procedures should be offered in specialist centres to all patients at high risk of gonadal failure. However, the precise course of any patient is never completely predictable despite the best attempts to estimate prognosis prior to treatment. For example, in a series of 58 girls less than 16 years old, Jadoul et al. [22] showed that 14% initially received treatment that placed them at low- to

Table 26.1 Estimates of infertility risk after treatment for common cancers of children and adolescents

Low risk (<20%)
Acute lymphoblastic leukaemia
Wilms' tumour
Soft-tissue sarcoma, stage 1
Germ cell tumours (with gonadal preservation and no radiotherapy)
Retinoblastoma
Brain tumour: surgery only, cranial irradiation <24 Gy
Medium risk
Acute myeloblastic leukaemia (difficult to quantify)
Hepatoblastoma
Osteosarcoma
Ewing's sarcoma: non-metastatic
Soft-tissue sarcoma, stage II or III
Neuroblastoma
Non-Hodgkin lymphoma
Hodgkin's disease: alternating treatment
Brain tumour: craniospinal radiotherapy, cranial irradiation >24 Gy
High risk (>80%)
Whole body irradiation
Localized radiotherapy: pelvic or testicular
Chemotherapy conditioning for bone marrow transplantation
Hodgkin's disease: treatment with alkylating drugs
Soft-tissue sarcoma, stage IV (metastatic)
Ewing's sarcoma: metastatic

From Wallace et al. [21] with permission

medium risk of premature ovarian failure but later needed more aggressive gonadotoxic treatment in the months following cryopreservation. Patient selection for gonadal tissue cryopreservation is further complicated by the fact that new treatment protocols are emerging that may alter the risks of infertility.

Fertility preservation procedures may also be indicated in patients receiving gonadotoxic treatments for non-malignant conditions such as haematological or autoimmune diseases and also in patients with certain genetic conditions such as Fragile-X and Turner syndrome which predispose women to premature ovarian failure. Examples of these conditions are listed in Table 26.2. In addition, patients who have multiple operations for ovarian cysts or ovarian torsion may have decreased ovarian reserve [22] and are potential candidates for fertility preservation procedures.

Fertility Preservation Procedures in Males

Harvesting

Male gonadal tissue can be harvested by orchiectomy or testicular biopsy. Both procedures can be performed in children with a low

Table 26.2 Benign diseases that may increase the risk of infertility by the need for treatment with cytotoxic agents or genetic factors

Haematological	Autoimmune	Genetic
Sickle cell anaemia	SLE	Fragile-X
Thalassaemia major	Wegener's granulomatosis	Turner syndrome
Aplastic anaemia	Behcet's disease	Klinefelter syndrome

risk of major surgical complications [23]. Due to the small size of testicles in young boys, harvesting a whole testis instead of partial orchiectomy is sometimes preferable [24].

Storage

Immature testicular tissue contains spermatogonial stem cells with reproductive potential, which can be stored in the form of cell suspensions or tissue fragments prepared from the harvested testicle or biopsy. **Cell suspensions** are prepared by disintegration of testicular tissue through enzymatic, chemical or mechanical digestion [25]. This approach has two advantages: it optimizes the cryopreservation procedure and allows the spermatogonial stem cells in suspension to be injected through the scrotal skin into the lumen of the rete testis. The drawback of this technique is that the disintegration of the testicular tissue decreases cell viability and breaks the inter-cellular microenvironment that is essential for cell differentiation and proliferation. In contrast, **testicular tissue fragments** maintain the spermatogonial stem cells and the surrounding cells in their original extracellular architecture. This preserves the stem cell niche that promotes renewal and differentiation through various signalling pathways [26, 27]. Moreover, testicular tissue fragments preserve Sertoli and Leydig cells that may restore hormonal production along with fertility functions [28].

To create viable tissue fragments the testicular tissue is dissected into millimetre size pieces and preserved with cryoprotective agents to protect the tissue from damage caused by ice formation. Dimethyl sulfoxide (DMSO) is superior to other cryoprotective agents, such as ethylene glycol, in terms of maintaining the architectural integrity of the tissue [23, 29]. Slow-programmed freezing that gradually decreases the temperature (0.5 °C/min) effectively preserves spermatogonial morphology and survival [23]. Then when the temperature reaches approximately −70 °C, the tissue can be plunged into liquid nitrogen at −196 °C for long-term storage.

Reimplantation

Successful testicular tissue transplantation has yet to be described in humans, however, in animal studies, spermatogonial survival has been demonstrated after xenotransplantation of human immature testicular tissue [30, 31]. Theoretically, autotransplantation of thawed, cryopreserved testicular tissue into the testis could be performed. Alternatively, spermatogonial stem cell suspensions could be introduced into the testis by ultrasound-guided injection into the rete testis, as described by Brook in a murine model [25]. Further optimization of cryopreservation protocols and the development of improved transplantation techniques are needed prior to the method becoming standard treatment in humans [32].

Fertility Preservation Procedures in Females

Harvesting

Oophorectomy can be performed or ovarian tissue biopsies can be collected, either at an elective laparoscopic procedure or during a laparotomy performed for other purposes. Laparoscopic ovarian procedures appear to be safe and feasible in children [33] and offer a minimally invasive approach with a low complication rate [34]. The emerging technique of single port-laparoscopy may improve patient safety further [35]. It is important to avoid using electrocoagulation on the ovarian surface so that cortical tissue that contains follicles is preserved. In the future, laparoscopic harvesting of the whole ovary including its vascular pedicle may be performed with the prospect of subsequent microvascular anastomoses of the ovarian vessels [36, 37]. When harvesting the ovary for whole ovary transplantation it is important to resect the full length of the infundibulo-pelvic ligament, as it is crucial for the cryopreservation and transplantation procedures.

The special anaesthetic challenges of paediatric surgery must be taken into consideration [38, 39] and the haematological, infectious and metabolic status of the patient assessed to fully evaluate the operative risk. Currently, there are no clear guidelines regarding the appropriate age to harvest ovarian tissue. Weintraub et al. [17] suggested that harvesting should not be performed in girls under the age of three because of anaesthetic considerations. However, Poirot et al. [40] reported a large series of paediatric patients who underwent ovarian tissue harvesting and 13 of 47 were younger than 3 years old with the youngest being only 10 months old at the time of the surgery. If possible, it is advisable to combine ovarian tissue harvesting with other imaging or surgical procedures that require anaesthesia, such as bone marrow aspiration, lumbar puncture or central line insertion [17].

Storage

After harvesting, ovarian tissue is promptly delivered to the laboratory. Aspiration of any follicles present should be performed before cryopreserving ovarian tissue since immature oocytes obtained from premenarchal girls can be matured in vitro and cryopreserved for future fertilization [41].

Ovarian tissue is traditionally cryopreserved using a “slow freezing” method [42]. First, ovarian cortex is separated from the medulla. The cortex is then dissected into small fragments, to maximize permeation of into the cells. The cryoprotective agents are necessary to protect the oocyte and surrounding stromal cells from freezing injuries [43]. The exact composition of the cryoprotective solution and the freezing protocol vary between institutions [44, 45]. Most commonly, the solutions contain permeating cryoprotectants such as DMSO, 1,2-propanediol or ethylene glycol, in combination with non-permeating substances such as sucrose and human serum albumin. Tubes containing immersed ovarian tissue fragments are gradually cooled by a programmable freezer that allows slow and stepwise decreases in temperature. When the temperature reaches −140 °C, the tubes can be plunged into liquid nitrogen at −196 °C for storage.

A recent and promising technique for cryopreservation of ovarian tissue is “rapid freezing” or vitrification. Small ovarian cortical fragments are immersed for a short period in a highly concentrated cryoprotective solution. Then, without a slow cooling delay, the ovarian tissue is plunged directly into liquid nitrogen. This induces a glass-like state that avoids the formation of ice crystals, which may harm the oocyte and stromal cells. The efficiency and safety of this technique still needs to be fully investigated before it becomes standard practice, however, it has been suggested that vitrification is superior to slow freezing in terms of follicular survival and tissue preservation in general [46, 47]. Others have reported that conventional freezing is a more suitable method for ovarian tissue cryopreservation than vitrification [48, 49]. Currently, new vitrification protocols are being developed that may achieve better results [50].

Cryopreservation of an intact ovary is challenging because cryoprotective agents cannot penetrate all cells equally. The vascular pedicle of the ovary must be harvested and carefully dissected to avoid damaging the ovarian vessels. The ovarian artery is usually perfused, via a catheter, with a heparinized physiological solution that flushes all the blood from the ovary. Thereafter, the ovary is perfused by, and immersed in, a cryoprotective solution followed by a cooling process, using a slow freezing protocol, as described above [36].

Reimplantation

The preserved ovarian tissue can be autotransplanted back into the patient once she is well enough. The autotransplantation can be either orthotopic (in the normal ovarian position) or heterotopic (at another anatomic site). Regardless of the site, the ovarian tissue fragments are sutured directly to the recipient site without any vascular anastomosis. Orthotopic transplantation is performed at laparoscopy [51] or laparotomy [52] by suturing the fragments into or onto the remaining ovary or ovarian stump, or by transplanting the tissue into a peritoneal pocket created by the surgeon in the broad ligament or pelvic peritoneum of the ovarian fossa. In the presence of intact and patent fallopian tubes, spontaneous conception has been reported after orthotopic transplantation [51]. Alternatively, oocytes can be aspirated from the transplanted tissue for IVF [53]. All live births that have resulted from ovarian tissue transplantation have arisen from orthotopic sites.

Heterotopic transplantation is placement of the ovarian fragments at any site in the body other than the ovary or the adjacent peritoneum, for example, in the subcutaneous space of the forearm or in the abdominal wall [54, 55]. Other sites that have been proposed include the uterus, the rectus abdominis muscle, and the space between the breast and superficial fascia of the pectoralis muscle [56]. Clearly, spontaneous conception is impossible at such sites, and IVF treatment is required. The advantages of using heterotopic sites are that the transplantation procedure is easier and the oocytes are more accessible for aspiration during IVF treatment. However, no clinical pregnancies have been achieved from heterotopic sites even though ovarian function has been restored [55].

The intact, whole ovary can be transplanted by microsurgical anastomosis of the ovarian vessels to vessels at orthotopic or heterotopic site. Although successful transplantation of a frozen-thawed whole ovary has not yet been described in humans, encouraging data from sheep have been reported [57]. In humans, a successful pregnancy was achieved following a microsurgical anastomosis of an intact fresh ovary [37]. Several sites for heterotopic transplantation have been proposed, including the deep inferior epigastric and the deep circumflex iliac vascular pedicles [58]. The optimal site for whole ovary transplantation remains to be determined.

Complications

The biggest drawback to ovarian tissue transplantation, carried out without a vascular anastomosis, is that the graft may not survive. In the immediate period after transplantation there may be ischaemic damage to the tissue, resulting in massive follicular death; however, most primordial follicles survive this ischaemic insult [43, 59]. Surgical manipulations have been described to encourage prompt neovascularization of the transplanted tissue by performing a two-step procedure. The first step involves creating a bed of granulation tissue one week before orthotopic transplantation. This two-step procedure is believed to decrease the ischaemic damage [51].

Transplantation of a whole ovary with its vascular pedicle clearly avoids the ischemia associated with the time for neovascularization as immediate reperfusion of the ovary should occur with reanastomosis of the arterial inflow. In sheep, hormonal function is reported to have continued for 6 years following transplantation of whole ovaries [60].

The only other major risk of transplantation is the possibility of seeding malignant cells by reintroducing ovarian tissue containing micro-metastases, as recently shown through quantitative reverse-transcribed polymerase chain reaction (RT-PCR) studies. In cryopreserved ovarian tissue from leukaemia patients, RT-PCR and long-term xenotransplantation detected malignant cells, which had been missed histologically [61]. For this reason, molecular studies are recommended prior to transplanting the tissue; long-term follow-up is also advisable to monitor for disease recurrence.

Follow-Up

Ovarian activity usually returns approximately 4 months after transplantation [62]. This period corresponds to the time it takes for primordial follicles, which are the ones that principally survive freezing and the insult of transplantation, to mature into antral follicles. Ovarian activity is confirmed by tracking follicular development with ultrasound, detecting ovulation and measuring circulating sex hormones.

Outcomes of Fertility Preservation Procedures

Outcomes of Fertility Preservation Procedures in Males

Successful transplantation of testicular tissue has not yet been described in humans.

Outcomes of Fertility Preservation Procedures in Females

Successful transplantation of ovarian tissue has not yet been described in paediatric patients, mainly because the cryopreservation and transplantation techniques are relatively new. However, we can assume that significant numbers of patients will undergo transplantation in the near future given that harvesting and cryopreservation of ovarian tissue has been performed in children for more than a decade. In adults, 14 healthy babies have been born after autotransplantation of cryopreserved ovarian tissue [62, 63]. These results suggest that the harvesting, cryopreservation, storage and transplantation procedures are both feasible and safe. Ovarian tissue in children is rich in primordial follicles that appear to survive the cryopreservation and transplantation insults well. The tissue harvested from young children is therefore expected to yield good results after transplantation.

Future Prospects

New technologies of ovarian tissue culture and in vitro follicular growth are currently being developed in animal models [64, 65]. We estimate that, in the next decade, technological advances will facilitate follicular development from the very early stage primordial follicle to the mature antral follicle. If this can be done in the laboratory then there would be no need to transplant ovarian tissue back into the human body to obtain eggs ready for fertilization.

References

1. Cancer Facts and Figures, 2010. In: Atlanta, GA: American Cancer Society, Inc.; 2010.
2. Green DM, Sklar CA, Boice JD Jr, Mulvihill JJ, Whitton JA, Stovall M, et al. Ovarian failure and reproductive outcomes after childhood cancer treatment: results from the Childhood Cancer Survivor Study. J Clin Oncol. 2009;27:2374–81.
3. Meirow D, Lewis H, Nugent D, Epstein M. Subclinical depletion of primordial follicular reserve in mice treated with cyclophosphamide: clinical importance and proposed accurate investigative tool. Hum Reprod. 1999;14:1903–7.
4. Elangovan N, Chiou TJ, Tzeng WF, Chu ST. Cyclophosphamide treatment causes impairment of sperm and its fertilizing ability in mice. Toxicology. 2006;222:60–70.
5. Larsen EC, Muller J, Schmiegelow K, Rechnitzer C, Andersen AN. Reduced ovarian function in long-term survivors of radiation- and chemotherapy-treated childhood cancer. J Clin Endocrinol Metab. 2003;88:5307–14.
6. Thomson AB, Campbell AJ, Irvine DC, Anderson RA, Kelnar CJ, Wallace WH. Semen quality and spermatozoal DNA integrity in survivors of childhood cancer: a case-control study. Lancet. 2002;360:361–7.
7. Sonmezer M, Oktay K. Fertility preservation in female patients. Hum Reprod Update. 2004;10:251–66.
8. Viviani S, Ragni G, Santoro A, Perotti L, Caccamo E, Negretti E, et al. Testicular dysfunction in Hodgkin's disease before and after treatment. Eur J Cancer. 1991;27:1389–92.

9. Wallace WH, Thomson AB, Kelsey TW. The radiosensitivity of the human oocyte. Hum Reprod. 2003;18:117–21.
10. Wallace WH, Thomson AB, Saran F, Kelsey TW. Predicting age of ovarian failure after radiation to a field that includes the ovaries. Int J Radiat Oncol Biol Phys. 2005;62:738–44.
11. Howell SJ, Shalet SM. Spermatogenesis after cancer treatment: damage and recovery. J Natl Cancer Inst Monogr. 2005;34:12–7.
12. Ogilvy-Stuart AL, Shalet SM. Effect of radiation on the human reproductive system. Environ Health Perspect. 1993;101(Suppl 2):109–16.
13. Salooja N, Szydlo RM, Socie G, Rio B, Chatterjee R, Ljungman P, et al. Pregnancy outcomes after peripheral blood or bone marrow transplantation: a retrospective survey. Lancet. 2001;358:271–6.
14. Brougham MF, Wallace WH. Subfertility in children and young people treated for solid and haematological malignancies. Br J Haematol. 2005;131:143–55.
15. Grundy R, Gosden RG, Hewitt M, Larcher V, Leiper A, Spoudeas HA, et al. Fertility preservation for children treated for cancer (1): scientific advances and research dilemmas. Arch Dis Child. 2001;84:355–9.
16. Grundy R, Larcher V, Gosden RG, Hewitt M, Leiper A, Spoudeas HA, et al. Fertility preservation for children treated for cancer (2): ethics of consent for gamete storage and experimentation. Arch Dis Child. 2001;84:360–2.
17. Weintraub M, Gross E, Kadari A, Ravitsky V, Safran A, Laufer N, et al. Should ovarian cryopreservation be offered to girls with cancer. Pediatr Blood Cancer. 2007;48:4–9.
18. Nugent D, Meirow D, Brook PF, Aubard Y, Gosden RG. Transplantation in reproductive medicine: previous experience, present knowledge and future prospects. Hum Reprod Update. 1997;3:267–80.
19. Gosden RG, Robert T, Morris MD. Appreciation of an enlightened surgeon and pioneer of ovarian transplantation. Fertil Steril. 2010;94:1960–3.
20. Leporrier M, von Theobald P, Roffe JL, Muller G. A new technique to protect ovarian function before pelvic irradiation. Heterotopic ovarian autotransplantation. Cancer. 1987;60:2201–4.
21. Wallace WH, Anderson RA, Irvine DS. Fertility preservation for young patients with cancer: Who is at risk and what can be offered? Lancet Oncol. 2005;6:209–18.
22. Jadoul P, Dolmans MM, Donnez J. Fertility preservation in girls during childhood: is it feasible, efficient and safe and to whom should it be proposed? Hum Reprod Update. 2010;16:617–30.
23. Keros V, Hultenby K, Borgstrom B, Fridstrom M, Jahnukainen K, Hovatta O. Methods of cryopreservation of testicular tissue with viable spermatogonia in pre-pubertal boys undergoing gonadotoxic cancer treatment. Hum Reprod. 2007;22:1384–95.
24. Wyns C, Curaba M, Vanabelle B, Van Langendonckt A, Donnez J. Options for fertility preservation in prepubertal boys. Hum Reprod Update. 2010;16:312–28.
25. Brook PF, Radford JA, Shalet SM, Joyce AD, Gosden RG. Isolation of germ cells from human testicular tissue for low temperature storage and autotransplantation. Fertil Steril. 2001;75:269–74.
26. Dadoune JP. New insights into male gametogenesis: what about the spermatogonial stem cell niche? Folia Histochem Cytobiol. 2007;45:141–7.
27. Oatley JM, Brinster RL. Regulation of spermatogonial stem cell self-renewal in mammals. Annu Rev Cell Dev Biol. 2008;24:263–86.
28. Kvist K, Thorup J, Byskov AG, Hoyer PE, Mollgard K, Yding Andersen C. Cryopreservation of intact testicular tissue from boys with cryptorchidism. Hum Reprod. 2006;21:484–91.
29. Goossens E, Frederickx V, Geens M, De Block G, Tournaye H. Cryosurvival and spermatogenesis after allografting prepubertal mouse tissue: comparison of two cryopreservation protocols. Fertil Steril. 2008;89:725–7.
30. Wyns C, Curaba M, Martinez-Madrid B, Van Langendonckt A, Francois-Xavier W, Donnez J. Spermatogonial survival after cryopreservation and short-term orthotopic immature human cryptorchid testicular tissue grafting to immunodeficient mice. Hum Reprod. 2007;22:1603–11.
31. Wyns C, Van Langendonckt A, Wese FX, Donnez J, Curaba M. Long-term spermatogonial survival in cryopreserved and xenografted immature human testicular tissue. Hum Reprod. 2008;23:2402–14.
32. Schlatt S, Ehmcke J, Jahnukainen K. Testicular stem cells for fertility preservation: preclinical studies on male germ cell transplantation and testicular grafting. Pediatr Blood Cancer. 2009;53:274–80.
33. Panteli C, Minocha A, Kulkarni MS, Tsang T. The role of laparoscopy in the management of adnexal lesions in children. Surg Laparosc Endosc Percutan Tech. 2009;19:514–7.
34. Davidoff AM, Hebra A, Kerr J, Stafford PW. Laparoscopic oophorectomy in children. J Laparoendosc Surg. 1996;6(Suppl 1):S115–9.
35. Ponsky TA, Krpata DM. Single-port laparoscopy: considerations in children. J Minim Access Surg. 2011;7:96–8.
36. Jadoul P, Donnez J, Dolmans MM, Squifflet J, Lengele B, Martinez-Madrid B. Laparoscopic ovariectomy for whole human ovary cryopreservation: technical aspects. Fertil Steril. 2007;87:971–5.
37. Silber SJ, Grudzinskas G, Gosden RG. Successful pregnancy after microsurgical transplantation of an intact ovary. N Engl J Med. 2008;359:2617–8.
38. Wedgewood J, Doyle E. Anaesthesia and laparoscopic surgery in children. Paediatr Anaesth. 2001;11:391–9.
39. Gupta R, Singh S. Challenges in paediatric laparoscopic surgeries. Indian J Anaesth. 2009;53:560–6.
40. Poirot CJ, Martelli H, Genestie C, Golmard JL, Valteau-Couanet D, Helardot P, et al. Feasibility of ovarian tissue cryopreservation for prepubertal

females with cancer. Pediatr Blood Cancer. 2007;49:74–8.
41. Revel A, Revel-Vilk S, Aizenman E, Porat-Katz A, Safran A, Ben-Meir A, et al. At what age can human oocytes be obtained? Fertil Steril. 2009;92:458–63.
42. Hovatta O. Methods for cryopreservation of human ovarian tissue. Reprod Biomed Online. 2005;10:729–34.
43. Nisolle M, Casanas-Roux F, Qu J, Motta P, Donnez J. Histologic and ultrastructural evaluation of fresh and frozen-thawed human ovarian xenografts in nude mice. Fertil Steril. 2000;74:122–9.
44. Rosendahl M, Schmidt KT, Ernst E, Rasmussen PE, Loft A, Byskov AG, et al. Cryopreservation of ovarian tissue for a decade in Denmark: a view of the technique. Reprod Biomed Online. 2010.
45. Gook DA, Edgar DH, Stern C. Cryopreservation of human ovarian tissue. Eur J Obstet Gynecol Reprod Biol. 2004;113(Suppl 1):S41–4.
46. Keros V, Xella S, Hultenby K, Pettersson K, Sheikhi M, Volpe A, et al. Vitrification versus controlled-rate freezing in cryopreservation of human ovarian tissue. Hum Reprod. 2009;24:1670–83.
47. Silber S, Kagawa N, Kuwayama M, Gosden R. Duration of fertility after fresh and frozen ovary transplantation. Fertil Steril. 2010;94:2191–6.
48. Gandolfi F, Paffoni A, Papasso Brambilla E, Bonetti S, Brevini TA, Ragni G. Efficiency of equilibrium cooling and vitrification procedures for the cryopreservation of ovarian tissue: comparative analysis between human and animal models. Fertil Steril. 2006;85(Suppl 1):1150–6.
49. Isachenko V, Lapidus I, Isachenko E, Krivokharchenko A, Kreienberg R, Woriedh M, et al. Human ovarian tissue vitrification versus conventional freezing: morphological, endocrinological, and molecular biological evaluation. Reproduction. 2009;138:319–27.
50. Amorim CA, David A, Van Langendonckt A, Dolmans MM, Donnez J. Vitrification of human ovarian tissue: effect of different solutions and procedures. Fertil Steril. 2011;95:1094–7.
51. Donnez J, Dolmans MM, Demylle D, Jadoul P, Pirard C, Squifflet J, et al. Livebirth after orthotopic transplantation of cryopreserved ovarian tissue. Lancet. 2004;364:1405–10.
52. Silber SJ, DeRosa M, Pineda J, Lenahan K, Grenia D, Gorman K, et al. A series of monozygotic twins discordant for ovarian failure: ovary transplantation (cortical versus microvascular) and cryopreservation. Hum Reprod. 2008;23:1531–7.
53. Meirow D, Levron J, Eldar-Geva T, Hardan I, Fridman E, Zalel Y, et al. Pregnancy after transplantation of cryopreserved ovarian tissue in a patient with ovarian failure after chemotherapy. N Engl J Med. 2005;353:318–21.
54. Callejo J, Salvador C, Miralles A, Vilaseca S, Lailla JM, Balasch J. Long-term ovarian function evaluation after autografting by implantation with fresh and frozen-thawed human ovarian tissue. J Clin Endocrinol Metab. 2001;86:4489–94.
55. Oktay K. Ovarian tissue cryopreservation and transplantation: preliminary findings and implications for cancer patients. Hum Reprod Update. 2001;7:526–34.
56. Kim SS, Hwang IT, Lee HC. Heterotopic autotransplantation of cryobanked human ovarian tissue as a strategy to restore ovarian function. Fertil Steril. 2004;82:930–2.
57. Revel A, Elami A, Bor A, Yavin S, Natan Y, Arav A. Whole sheep ovary cryopreservation and transplantation. Fertil Steril. 2004;82:1714–5.
58. Ploteau S, Rogez JM, Donnez J, Lengele B. Which are the ideal donor and recipient vessels for a whole ovarian transplantation? Fertil Steril. 2011;95:751–5.
59. Nottola SA, Camboni A, Van Langendonckt A, Demylle D, Macchiarelli G, Dolmans MM, et al. Cryopreservation and xenotransplantation of human ovarian tissue: an ultrastructural study. Fertil Steril. 2008;90:23–32.
60. Arav A, Gavish Z, Elami A, Natan Y, Revel A, Silber S, et al. Ovarian function 6 years after cryopreservation and transplantation of whole sheep ovaries. Reprod Biomed Online. 2010;20:48–52.
61. Dolmans MM, Marinescu C, Saussoy P, Van Langendonckt A, Amorim C, Donnez J. Reimplantation of cryopreserved ovarian tissue from patients with acute lymphoblastic leukemia is potentially unsafe. Blood. 2010;116:2908–14.
62. Donnez J, Silber S, Andersen CY, Demeestere I, Piver P, Meirow D, et al. Children born after autotransplantation of cryopreserved ovarian tissue. A review of 13 live births. Ann Med. 2011;43:437–50.
63. Revel A, Laufer N, Assaf BM, Lebovich M, Mitrani E. Micro organ ovarian transplantation enables pregnancy: a case report. Hum Reprod. 2011;26:1097–103.
64. Smitz J, Dolmans MM, Donnez J, Fortune JE, Hovatta O, Jewgenow K, et al. Current achievements and future research directions in ovarian tissue culture, in vitro follicle development and transplantation: implications for fertility preservation. Hum Reprod Update. 2010;16:395–414.
65. Xu J, Lawson MS, Yeoman RR, Pau KY, Barrett SL, Zelinski MB, et al. Secondary follicle growth and oocyte maturation during encapsulated three-dimensional culture in rhesus monkeys: effects of gonadotrophins, oxygen and fetuin. Hum Reprod. 2011;26:1061–72.

Part VII
Breast

Breast Embryology, Anatomy, and Physiology

27

Monica E. Lopez and Oluyinka O. Olutoye

Embryology

Normal Development

Mammary glands are considered as modified apocrine glands. Mammary gland morphogenesis may be divided into various developmental stages. The first event is the formation of bilateral milk lines, followed by the invagination of the ectoderm-derived primary mammary bud into surrounding mesoderm, leading to the proliferation and branching of the bud to form a rudimentary ductal tree (Fig. 27.1). Early in development, between the fifth and sixth week of gestation, two lateral thickened ridges of ectoderm appear along the ventral body wall between the anterior and posterior limb buds [1]. This bilateral thickening is known as the mammary ridge or "milk line," and in humans, it is transitory and recedes, except for the area on the chest wall where the mammary glands ultimately develop (Fig. 27.2). In this region, proliferation of mammary ridge ectoderm takes place to give rise to the primary mammary bud. The primary mammary bud invaginates and extends deep into the underlying mesoderm giving rise to multiple, greater than 20, secondary buds by the twelfth week of gestation. During this process, there is condensation and differentiation of the surrounding mesoderm into dense mammary mesenchyme arranged radially around the epithelial bud [2]. The secondary buds then lengthen and branch throughout the remainder of gestation until the eight month, when they become canalized forming lactiferous ducts, which come together at the site of an epidermis-lined pit, known as the mammary pit. At birth, proliferation of underlying mesenchymal elements leads to eversion of the pit to give rise to the definitive nipple [1, 3, 4]. Hormonal influences then direct the growth and development of the breast. Embryonic mammary gland development involves the activation of multiple signaling pathways to account for proper spatial and temporal cellular communication between epidermis and mesenchyme. The elucidation of some of these molecular mechanisms has demonstrated an important functional role for Wnt, fibroblast growth factor, and parathyroid protein-related protein in various processes, such as the specification of the milk line and mammary bud formation [2]. However, many more genes are likely to be involved in the control of mammary gland morphogenesis.

Two theories of embryogenesis have arisen based on the development of the breast. One is based on the vertebrate evolution sequence and the other on atavism. Since development generally follows the vertebrate evolution sequence

M.E. Lopez · O.O. Olutoye
Division of Pediatric Surgery, Texas Children's Hospital, 6701 Fannin, CC 1210, Houston, TX 77030, USA

O.O. Olutoye (✉)
Texas Children's Fetal Center, Texas Children's Hospital, 6701 Fannin, CC 1210, Houston, TX 77030, USA
e-mail: ooolutoy@texaschildrens.org

D.J. Ledbetter and P.R.V. Johnson (eds.), *Endocrine Surgery in Children*,
DOI 10.1007/978-3-662-54256-9_27

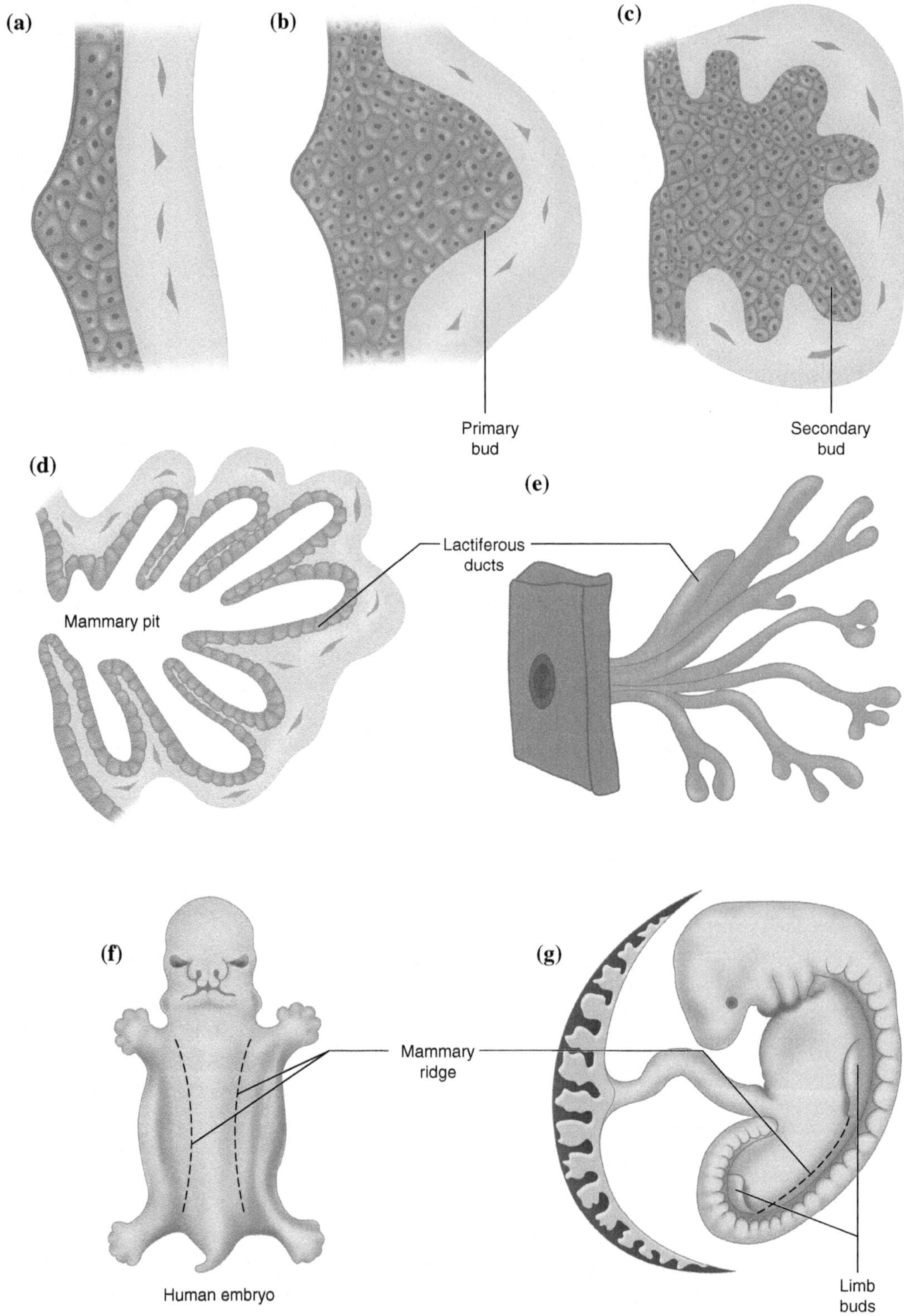

Fig. 27.1 Gross anatomic developmental embryology

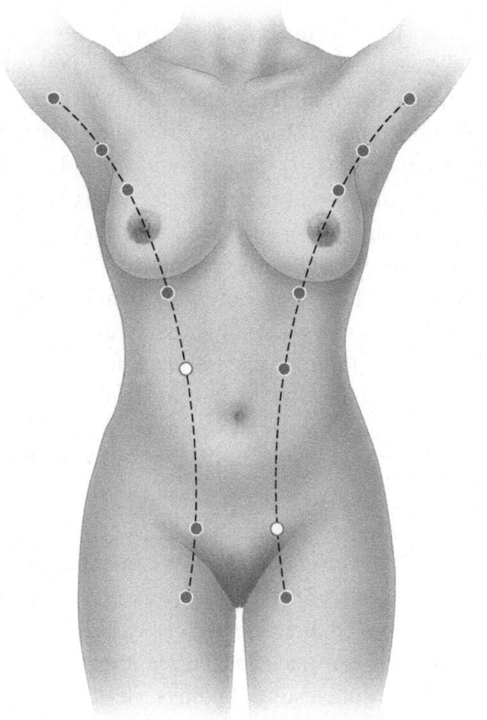

Fig. 27.2 Sites of accessory breast tissue along the embryonic milk line

and mammary glands have no precursors in reptilian predecessors, it is surprising that they appear so early in embryonic life [1]. However, atavism, the spontaneous reappearance of ancestral characteristics within a species, reminds us that important genetic and developmental information has not been lost during evolution but lies quiescent within the genome and in the process of embryonic development. Atavisms demonstrate that embryologic processes are so complex and integrated that the loss of simple information like the genetic programming for limbs would mean the loss of many other important functions at the same time. The most well-known spontaneous atavisms found in natural populations are the hind limbs in whales and extra toes in horses. An example of an atavism in humans is the appearance of supernumerary nipples, which will be discussed in the section on congenital anomalies below. Abnormal expression of *Hox* genes has been implicated in the production of atavisms, because of their effect on regulating spatial relationships and the development of structures out of time or out of place [5].

Congenital Anomalies

There are multiple abnormalities of the breast that arise from faulty embryologic mechanisms. These may involve and affect the development of the nipple, the mammary glandular tissue, or the entire breast. Multiple classification systems exist that group the types of defect according to the component of the breast that is affected or the location of these components. However, we agree with Elwood [6] that the precise description of the anatomic defect is more helpful and direct.

Congenital inversion of the nipple is a condition in which mesenchymal infiltration and proliferation beneath the mammary pit does not occur, leading to flat or inverted nipples. This may occur unilaterally or bilaterally having significant functional and aesthetic consequences. Its frequency has been estimated as 17.7 per 1000 women [7], although in a Korean series its prevalence was found to be 3.26% [8]. The majority of congenital inverted nipples can be classified as umbilicated [8, 9] and the rest as invaginated. An important clinical point is that congenital inverted nipples must be differentiated from instances of secondary or acquired nipple inversion, which may due to carcinoma, chronic ductal mastitis, macromastia, and post-breast reduction surgery [10]. Several reconstruction techniques have been described to correct inverted nipples. These range from creating tightness at the neck of the inverted nipple, to dividing the lactiferous ducts and adding soft tissue bulk, to duct-preserving operations with release of fibrosis and placement of purse string sutures [9, 10], and more recently, to a contemporary technique based on the principle of tissue expansion involving body jewelry [11].

Athelia is defined as the absence of the nipple-areola complex. It almost invariably occurs in conjunction with absence of glandular tissue, which together result in complete absence of the breast. **Amastia** or complete absence of the breast is a rare condition defined by the absence of one or both breasts and nipples. This results from failure of the mammary ridge to develop at 6 weeks of gestation. It is important to note that this condition features different patterns of familial inheritance and may be associated with other anomalies. The original classification dates back to 1965 by Trier, who reported on a series of 43 patients with congenital absence of the breast and classified them according to mode of inheritance and association with anomalies [12]. Since then, only six other cases have been reported in the literature [13, 14]. When this defect is unilateral and occurs in association with absence of pectoral muscles, it is known as Poland's syndrome. Bilateral congenital absence of the breast in association with ectodermal dysplasia is transmitted in a sex-linked recessive pattern, thus only affecting boys. Other patterns of inheritance include autosomal dominant and autosomal recessive [14].

Athelia may occur in the presence of breast tissue (isolated athelia), very rarely at the normal anatomic site but not infrequently at other accessory locations [1]. A review by Ishida, et al. [15] revealed that ectodermal dysplasia, a hereditary disease of the skin and its appendages, underscores the majority of reports of athelia in the literature. In their case report of isolated athelia, the authors make reference to deficient parathyroid hormone-related protein production as a potential causative factor. This molecule was shown to induce mammary mesenchymal cell formation, triggering morphogenesis of the nipple epidermis [16]. Athelia may also be one of the clinical features in Al-Awadi/Raas-Rothschild syndrome, choanal atresia-athelia syndrome and scalp–ear–nipple syndrome [15]. Historically, the labia minora skin graft was proposed for nipple reconstruction [12], however tattooing of the hypochromic skin is a more recently used and less deforming alternative.

Polythelia is a common abnormality of breast development in which extra-thoracic areas of the mammary ridge do not regress, leading to the formation of supernumerary nipples. These remnants can also develop into complete mammary glands, a condition known as **polymastia**. This occurs most frequently along the milk line in the axilla, followed by the submammary location. They may also be found in the groin area. However, migration of the embryonic rests [17] may account for polythelia or polymastia found in ectopic locations beyond the mammary ridge, such as the perineum [18], the vulva [19], the posterior thigh [20], and the neck [21]. The prevalence of polythelia ranges from 0.22 to 5%, varying considerably among different ethnic groups. In white European children, polythelia was least prevalent at 0.22% [22], in Black neonates, it was noted to be 1.63% [23], and in Jewish neonates 2.5% [24]. The results of a study by Jaber in 1988 [25] demonstrated a higher prevalence of supernumerary nipples in Arab children—4.7% in infants and 5% in children. This finding was attributed to differences in ethnicity, as well as to high rates of consanguinity in many of the participating families. Other interesting findings in this ethnic group included high incidence of left-side location and positioning just below the normally situated nipple, as well as same sex distribution. A large, early case series dated 1879 by Bruce reported a prevalence of 1.54% among a population of 3956 patients in London [26]. He found that supernumerary nipples occurred more than four times as frequently in men as in women. In addition, there was a remarkable preponderance of supernumerary nipples on the left side. As for the location of supernumerary nipples, the majority of the cases were found on the front of the trunk just below the normal breast near the midline. In a study by Schmidt [27], the prevalence of supernumerary nipples was reported as 5.6% in a series of 502 Caucasian infants. In this series, the higher prevalence may be explained by the fact that both supernumerary areola and supernumerary areola with nipple were ascertained in this population. In fact, supernumerary areola without nipple predominated in this series, as well as predilection for left side and male gender.

While the majority of instances of polythelia occur in sporadic fashion, familial polythelia also has been documented in sequential generations and in siblings [28]. Most pedigrees are consistent with autosomal dominant inheritance with variable expressivity, although X-linked dominant and recessive modes of inheritance are also known to occur [29]. The occurrence of left-sided pseudomammae (nipple and areola with no glandular tissue) inferomedial to the normal breast along the mammary line may be suggestive of a "hereditary" trait of familial cases of accessory mammary tissue. This finding was reported to occur in 72% of the patients in Urbani's familial series [29]. By comparison, there is a higher frequency of polythelia (nipple only) in the sporadic forms of the condition.

The association of polythelia with genitourinary anomalies has been the subject of debate for many years and still remains unclear whether such link exists. A broad spectrum of nephrourinary defects has been described, including adult polycystic kidney disease, renal agenesis, cystic renal dysplasia, familial renal cysts, and congenital stenosis of the pyeloureteral junction [29]. In one of the first studies examining this issue, Mehes demonstrated that 40% of patients with polythelia also had renal abnormalities, mostly obstructive, an 800-fold increase beyond what would be expected by chance alone [30].This association was later corroborated in a larger study of 10770 infants and children [31], as well as by other investigators [32, 33]. Nevertheless, others have found no such correlation and have challenged this view [18, 23, 24]. Based on their extensive review of the literature, Leung and others recommend at the minimum, an awareness of the possible urologic implications of polythelia, leading to a detailed family history, complete physical examination, and a screening abdominal ultrasound in patients with a definitive diagnosis of polythelia [18, 29].

Sporadic and familial polythelia may also be associated with malignancies of the genitourinary tract such as kidney, testes, prostate, and urinary bladder [34]. Cohen has advocated the inclusion of polythelia in the group of conditions known as genodermatoses with malignant potential, which are inherited disorders of mucocutaneous features predisposing to internal neoplasms [35]. This should prompt surveillance for polythelia-related urinary anomalies and malignancies in patients with supernumerary nipples.

Anatomy

Gross Structure

The anatomy of the breast and its relationship to underlying chest structures is essential in the management of benign and malignant breast diseases (Fig. 27.3a).

The mature human breast is a hemispherical eminence located toward the lateral aspect of the pectoral region, encompassing the interval of the third to sixth or seventh ribs, from the side of the sternum to the axilla as the tail of Spence [36]. Its peripheral anatomical boundaries are not precisely defined except in the deep posterior plane, as the gland lies on the pectoralis fascia on a thin layer of loose areolar tissue. Occasionally, microscopic extensions of glandular tissue and posterior suspensory attachments may traverse into the retromammary space and underlying pectoralis fascia. Clinically, infiltration of this space by neoplastic or inflammatory processes may be manifested as fixation of the breast to the chest wall [37]. The retromammary space and deep fascia over the pectoralis muscle are included with the breast in a total mastectomy specimen [38].

The breast parenchyma lies cushioned in fat and invested by the superficial and deep layers of the superficial pectoral fascia. This superficial fascia layer is contiguous with the cervical fascia superiorly and with the superficial abdominal wall fascia inferiorly. Fibrous extensions of the dermis into the glandular tissue of the breast are known as the suspensory ligaments of Cooper, which attach the skin and nipple to the breast. Clinically, distortion of Cooper's ligaments by parenchymal lesions may result in skin dimpling or nipple retraction [37]. The left breast is generally larger than the right [36]. While minor variations in breast size leading to asymmetry are considered normal and may become more prominent during puberty, breast asymmetry can be visible in 25% of the population [39]. In a

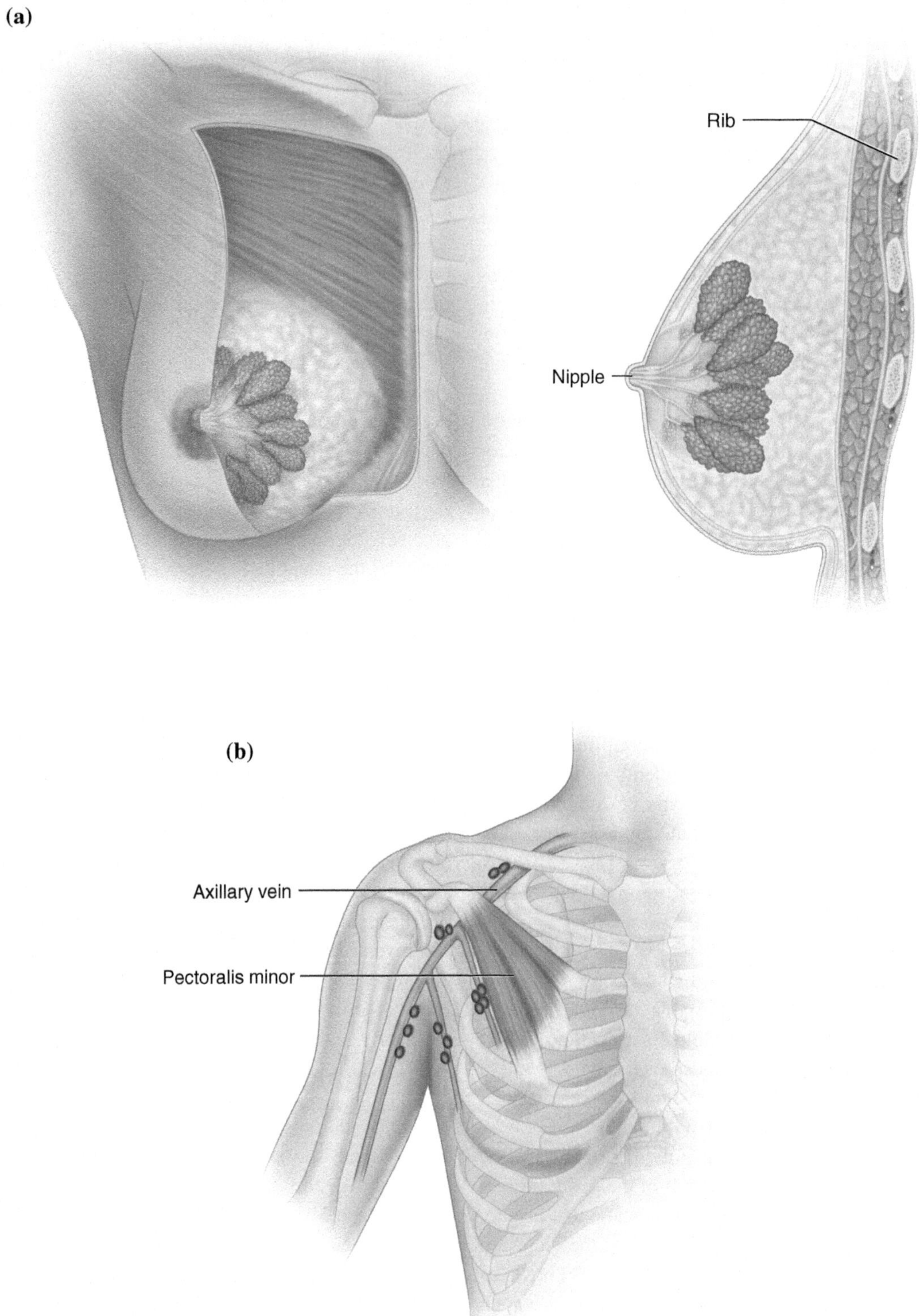

Fig. 27.3 **a** Structure of breast. **b** Lymph nodes of the axilla

series of 500 mammoplasties, severe asymmetry was observed in 5.2% of the cases [40].

The nipple is a conical prominence lined with stratified squamous epithelium and perforated by the multiple openings of the lactiferous ducts. In the prepubertal breast, the nipple is unpigmented. Melanin pigmentation causes the darkening of the nipple and surrounding areola during menarche and most prominently during pregnancy. Various degrees of pigmentation may persist beyond pregnancy and lactation. The glands of Montgomery lie beneath the areola, a specialized ring of mammary skin surrounding the nipple. These modified sebaceous glands exit onto the areola through the tubercles of Montgomery, which become enlarged during pregnancy, and are responsible for secretion of fatty substances that help lubricate the integument of the nipple during lactation [36].

Blood Supply

The arterial blood supply to the breast is derived from the thoracic branches of the axillary, internal mammary, and intercostal arteries [36]. The relative contributions of these vessels vary between individuals and the pattern of circulation may differ between the left and right breasts within an individual. Furthermore, the blood supply of the breast parenchyma does not follow its lobar architecture [41]. In many cases, the perforating branches of the internal mammary artery are the primary perfusion source. These vessels traverse the chest wall near the sternum in the first four intercostal spaces. In 30% of individuals there is no contribution from the axillary artery, while the intercostal arteries are not relevant to the arterial circulation of the breast in nearly 50% of the cases [42]. The venous drainage of the breast is more variable than its arterial supply, but generally follows an anastomotic circle around the base of the nipple, known as the circulus venosus. From there, larger branches disperse through the circumference of the gland and drain into the axillary and internal mammary veins [36].

Lymph Nodes and Nerves

The lymphatic drainage of the breast follows a centrifugal pathway in which lymphatic afferent vessels from the subareolar plexus course along the major lactiferous ducts, retromammary space, and efferent veins into the nodal basins. There are three major mammary lymphatic drainage routes. The principal site of drainage is the axilla, which receives about 75% of lymphatic flow. The central axillary lymph nodes are the major site of drainage, although the external mammary, axillary, scapular, and subclavicular groups are also in the axillary circuit. The internal mammary nodes and interpectoral or Rotter's nodes constitute the two other pathways of lymph drainage, but are rarely involved exclusively in nodal metastases from breast cancer, except in cases of advanced progression of disease [43]. In addition, there seems to be a differential pattern of lymphatic drainage between palpable and non-palpable lesions [44].

The loose areolar fat of the axilla contains a variable number of lymph nodes organized into groups. The axillary nodes are divided into three groups according to their position relative to the pectoralis minor muscle (Fig. 27.3b). This division into three levels has standardized the extent of axillary dissection. Level I defines nodes located lateral to the pectoralis minor muscle and includes those in the external mammary, scapular, axillary vein, and central axillary groups. Level II nodes are those that lie beneath the pectoralis minor muscle, which are those in the central axillary group. Level III nodes are located medial to the medial border of the pectoralis minor muscle (subclavicular nodes) and are difficult to visualize and remove unless the muscle is sacrificed as in a standard radical mastectomy [43]. The nerve supply to the breast is derived from the anterior and lateral cutaneous nerves of the fourth to sixth thoracic nerves [45]. However, more important is the knowledge of the nervous structures in the axilla to avoid their injury during axillary lymph node resection. The long thoracic nerve, or external respiratory nerve of Bell, innervates the serratus anterior and arises from the fifth, sixth, and seventh cervical nerves, descends behind the brachial plexus and axillary vein and can be seen coursing close to the chest wall on the medial aspect of the axilla. Its function is important for fixation of the scapula to the chest wall during shoulder adduction and extension of the arm, and its injury results in a winged scapula deformity [38]. The thoracodorsal nerve supplies the latissimus dorsi muscle and arises from the sixth, seventh, and eight cervical nerves making up a branch of the posterior cord of the brachial plexus. It travels with the subscapular artery along the lateral border of the axilla. Its injury results in difficulty with adduction and medial rotation of the arm.

The medial pectoral nerves wrap around the lateral border of the pectoralis minor muscle and are part of the neurovascular bundle supplying the pectoralis major muscle. As a landmark in axillary dissection, they mark the position of the axillary vein just above and below the bundle, and should be preserved. The intercostal brachial nerves provide cutaneous innervation to the inner aspect of the upper arm and anterior chest wall. These nerves are encountered during axillary dissection along the posterior margin of the axilla and should be preserved to avoid cutaneous anesthesia in that distribution and potential chronic pain syndromes [38].

Microscopic Anatomy

The human breast is made up of glandular epithelium, connective tissue stroma, and subcutaneous fat. The glandular tissue is pale reddish and firm, and is arranged into lobes, each containing many lobules, and terminating in clusters of alveoli. This system of branching ducts is organized in a radial pattern, spreading outward and downward from the nipple-areola complex [38]. The alveoli drain into the smallest of the lactiferous ductules, which in turn join to form larger ducts terminating into single canals corresponding to each of the lobes of the gland. The number of major lactiferous ducts ranges from fifteen to twenty-five and they converge near the areola, forming dilatations or lactiferous sinuses just beneath the nipple, which they then perforate in multiple orifices. The anatomic subdivision of the breast into lobes is not apparent on gross dissection or histological sections of the breast. However, this functional arrangement is relevant clinically, allowing some benign conditions of the breast to be treated by major duct excision, and some malignant processes by quadrantectomy [37].

The fibrous stroma, its supporting structures, and fatty tissue comprise the rest of the mammary gland. The relative proportions of fat and stroma vary greatly among individual women of any age. In youth, the predominant tissues are epithelium and stroma, which are replaced by fat in the breasts of older women. Fatty tissue surrounds the surface of the gland and occupies the interval between its lobes. It usually exists in considerable abundance, and determines the form and size of the gland. There is no fat immediately beneath the areola and nipple [36].

Breast Development and Physiology

Fetal mammary gland development is not dependent on steroid hormones until beyond the 15th gestational week when breast structure development takes place. In the last weeks of gestation, the fetal breast is responsive to maternal steroid hormones, which are manifested in the neonatal period by the secretion of colostrum and palpable enlargement of the breast bud [37]. This unilateral or bilateral breast enlargement and secretion of opaque fluid or "witches' milk" occurs in about 60% of normal newborns. However, both these findings resolve spontaneously during the first or second month after birth due to disappearance of maternal hormones from the infant's bloodstream and do not require treatment [46]. It can occur in both male and female infants.

The development of the alveoli and their surrounding supportive framework remains quiescent until puberty once the perinatal influence of maternal hormones subsides. During childhood, breast tissue is dormant and mainly composed of ducts lined with epithelium and surrounded by connective tissue. Before breast development is completed, surgery around the breast bud in young girls must be avoided or exercised with great care to prevent injury and potential growth disturbance [6].

Breast development (**thelarche**) is usually the first sign of puberty. At this time, female breasts change due to the influence of increasing levels of estrogen, which controls stromal and ductal development, as well as pigmentation and increase in size of the areola [39, 46]. Progesterone promotes lobular development, alveolar budding, and secretory growth of lobules and alveoli. Prolactin, thyroxine, insulin, growth hormone, and adrenal corticosteroids are also implicated in breast growth and differentiation [39, 46]. The average age for onset of thelarche is 11.2 years, with a range of 9.0–13.4 years [47]. In the United States, a recent cross-sectional study demonstrated that girls are developing pubertal characteristics at an earlier age than currently used norms. At every age for each characteristic, African-American girls were more advanced than white girls. Mean ages for onset of breast development in African-American and white girls were 8.87 (SD, 1.93) and 9.96 (SD, 1.92), respectively [48]. Thus, the definition of precocious puberty and delayed puberty may vary from expert to expert. Once it ensues, duration of breast maturation may range from 18 months to 9 years. Pubertal breast development can be classified according to the Tanner stages or Sexually Maturity Rating (SMR) stages (Fig. 27.4). These five stages described by Tanner in 1962 [49] were based on classic work by Reynold and Wines in 1948 and Stratz in 1909 [50]. There is no breast development in stage 1, a breast bud in stage 2, small breast appearance in stage 3, double-contoured appearance in stage 4 (nipple-areola complex forms mound on top of breast mound), and single-contour breast appearance in stage 5.

Benign premature thelarche is defined as isolated breast development in females from 6 months to 9 years of age [51]. The incidence of premature thelarche in white female infants and children up to 7 years old in the United States in 1980 was 20.8 per 100,000 [52]. Premature thelarche may result from aberrant levels of endogenous hormones, and serum estradiol is typically elevated [53]. If pubic hair and accelerated bone growth are also present on physical examination, precocious puberty must be excluded. If thelarche if isolated, treatment is reassurance and re-evaluation every 6–12 months. Early onset of puberty is more common in girls than boys, usually triggered by early activation of the hypothalamic-pituitary-gonadal axis [51], and may be central, peripheral, or incomplete. Central precocious puberty is most commonly idiopathic or caused by a pituitary hamartoma, trauma, or central nervous system lesion. Treatment is directed at the underlying etiology. Peripheral precocious puberty is due to sex steroid hormone secretion independent of gonadotropin release, as in McCune–Albright syndrome, administration of exogenous steroids or circulation of endogenous steroids from an ovarian or adrenal tumor [39, 46]. Sometimes premature thelarche presents as a form of incomplete precocious puberty, which is benign and only requires reassurance and observation. Histologically, the breast tissue in premature thelarche resembles gynecomastia, because it is characterized by epithelial hyperplasia in the duct system with a solid and micropapillary configuration [37].

After puberty and during adolescence, lobular and stromal units develop and alveolar cells mature into secretory cells under the influence of cyclic hormonal changes related to ovulation. These changes have clinical manifestations in the form of breast size and texture changes. Cyclical changes in breast volume involve parenchymal growth as well as fluctuations in water content [54]. During days 4–12 of the menstrual cycle, edema fluid is minimal. However, breasts may increase in size and volume by 50% during the luteal phase of the cycle [39].

However, the most glandular differentiation and breast growth occurs during pregnancy and lactation in the female. During this time, under the influence of estrogen and progesterone, the alveolar ductal epithelium proliferates to form numerous secretory alveoli. The breast lobules expand greatly at the expense of interlobal

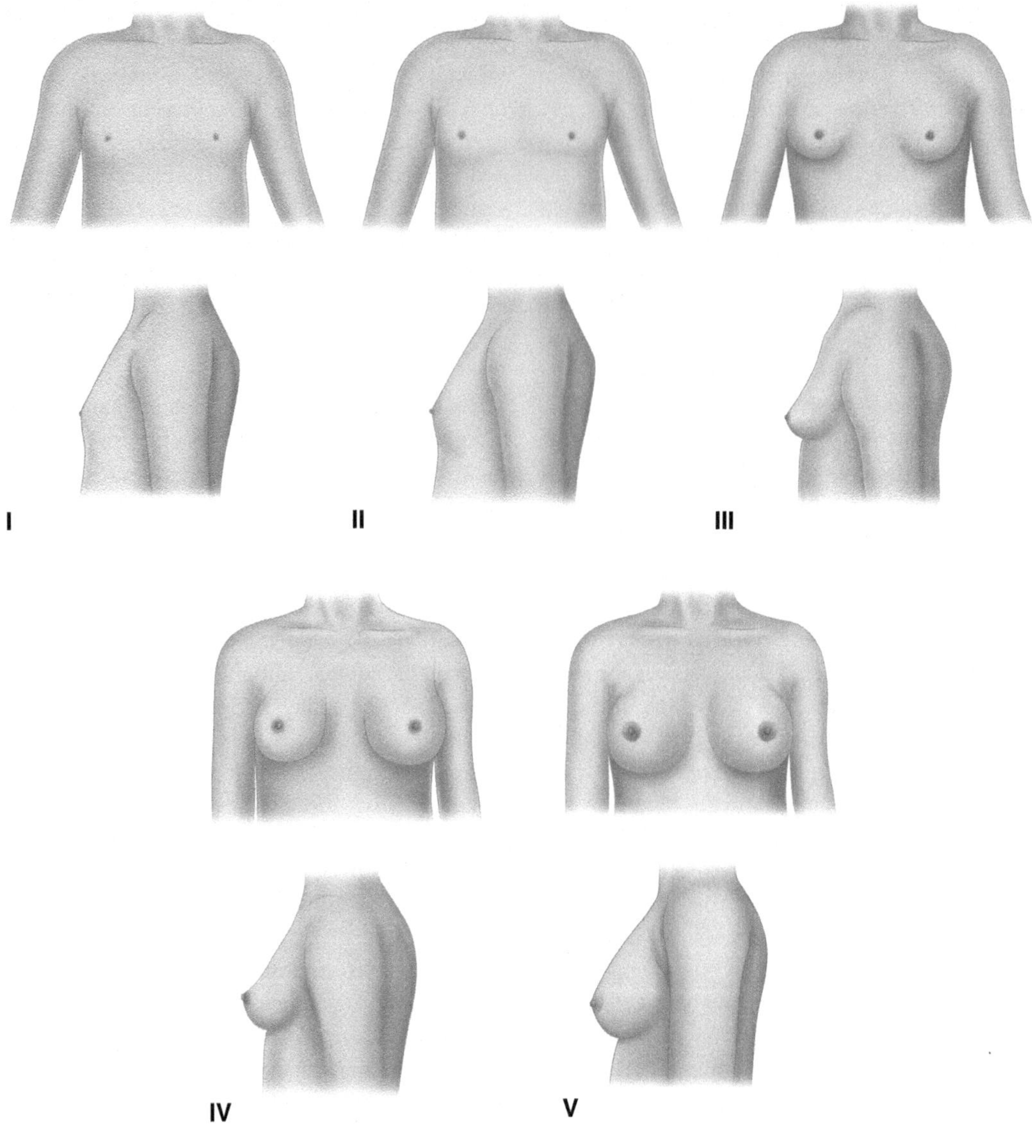

Fig. 27.4 Tanner stages of breast development

adipose tissue. With progression of pregnancy and accumulation of colostrum in the alveoli, the alveolar and duct lumina become dilated. After parturition, prolactin activity rises as circulating estrogen and progesterone fall. This stimulates milk production. In the lactating breast, the alveoli are distended with milk, the interlobular stromal tissue being reduced to thin septa between the lobules. The alveoli are filled with eosinophilic material containing clear vacuoles representing lipid droplets. Milk production proceeds for as long as suckling continues. This process is mediated by a neuro-hormonal reflex, which causes release of prolactin by nipple stimulation. Another neuro-hormonal reflex causes production of oxytocin, which causes contraction of myoepithelial cells around alveoli and ducts and leads to propelling of the milk into the lactiferous ducts. During weaning, the suckling stimulus ceases, resulting in regression of the lactating breast and resumption of the ovarian cycle [55].

References

1. Skandalakis JE, Gray SW, Ricketts R, Skandalakis LJ. Embryology for surgeons: the embryological basis for the treatment of congenital anomalies. Baltimore: Williams & Wilkins; 1994.
2. Hens JR, Wysolmerski JJ. Key stages of mammary gland development: molecular mechanisms involved in the formation of the embryonic mammary gland. Breast Cancer Res. 2005;7(5):220–4.
3. Larsen W. Essentials of human embryology. New York: Churchill Livingstone Inc; 1998.
4. Ellis H, Colborn GL, Skandalakis JE. Surgical embryology and anatomy of the breast and its related anatomic structures. Surg Clin North Am. 1993;73(4):611–32.
5. Hall BK. Atavisms and atavistic mutations. Nat Genet. 1995;10(2):126–7.
6. Elwood E, Hultman CS. Reconstruction of congenital and traumatic breast defects. Breast Dis. 2002;16:129–39.
7. Schwager RG, Smith JW, Gray GF, Goulian D Jr. Inversion of the human female nipple, with a simple method of treatment. Plast Reconstr Surg. 1974;54(5):564–9.
8. Park HS, Yoon CH, Kim HJ. The prevalence of congenital inverted nipple. Aesthetic Plast Surg. 1999;23(2):144–6.
9. Crestinu JM. Inverted nipple: the new method of correction. Aesthetic Plast Surg. 1989;13(3):189–97.
10. Han S, Hong YG. The inverted nipple: its grading and surgical correction. Plast Reconstr Surg. 1999;104(2):389–95 (discussion 396–7).
11. Scholten E. A contemporary correction of inverted nipples. Plast Reconstr Surg. 2001;107(2):511–3.
12. Trier WC. Complete breast absence: case report and review of the literature. Plast Reconstr Surg. 1965;36:431–9.
13. Tawil HM, Najjar SS. Congenital absence of the breasts. J Pediatr. 1968;73(5):751–3.
14. Lin KY, Nguyen DB, Williams RM. Complete breast absence revisited. Plast Reconstr Surg. 2000;106(1):98–101.
15. Ishida LH, Alves HR, Munhoz AM, et al. Athelia: case report and review of the literature. Br J Plast Surg. 2005;58(6):833–7.
16. Foley J, Dann P, Hong J, et al. Parathyroid hormone-related protein maintains mammary epithelial fate and triggers nipple skin differentiation during embryonic breast development. Development. 2001;128(4):513–25.
17. Hanson E, Segovia J. Dorsal supernumerary breast. Case report. Plast Reconstr Surg. 1978;61(3):441–5.
18. Leung W, Heaton JP, Morales A. An uncommon urologic presentation of a supernumerary breast. Urology. 1997;50(1):122–4.
19. Hassim AM. Bilateral fibroadenoma in supernumerary breasts of the vulva. J Obstet Gynaecol Br Commonw. 1969;76(3):275–7.
20. Camisa C. Accessory breast on the posterior thigh of a man. J Am Acad Dermatol. 1980;3(5):467–9.
21. Pellegrini JR, Wagner RF Jr. Polythelia and associated conditions. Am Fam Physician. 1983;28(3):129–32.
22. Mehes K. Association of supernumerary nipples with other anomalies. J Pediatr. 1983;102(1):161.
23. Rahbar F. Clinical significance of supernumerary nipples in black neonates. Clin Pediatr (Phila). 1982;21(1):46–7.
24. Mimouni F, Merlob P, Reisner SH. Occurrence of supernumerary nipples in newborns. Am J Dis Child. 1983;137(10):952–3.
25. Jaber L, Merlob P. The prevalence of supernumerary nipples in Arab infants and children. Eur J Pediatr. 1988;147(4):443.
26. Bruce JM. Supernumerary nipples and mammae: with an account of sixty-five instances observed. J Anat Physiol. 1879;13(Pt 4):425–48.
27. Schmidt H. Supernumerary nipples: prevalence, size, sex and side predilection—a prospective clinical study. Eur J Pediatr. 1998;157(10):821–3.
28. Toumbis-Ioannou E, Cohen PR. Familial polythelia. J Am Acad Dermatol. 1994;30(4):667–8.
29. Urbani CE, Betti R. The significance of familial polythelia. J Am Acad Dermatol. 1995;32(4):687–8.
30. Mehes K. Association of supernumerary nipples with other anomalies. J Pediatr. 1979;95(2):274–5.
31. Meggyessy V, Mehes K. Association of supernumerary nipples with renal anomalies. J Pediatr. 1987;111(3):412–3.
32. Matesanz R, Teruel JL, Garcia Martin F, Orte L, Guisasola L, Ortuno J. High incidence of supernumerary nipples in end-stage renal failure. Nephron. 1986;44(4):385–6.
33. Hersh JH, Bloom AS, Cromer AO, Harrison HL, Weisskopf B. Does a supernumerary nipple/renal field defect exist? Am J Dis Child. 1987;141(9):989–91.
34. Goedert JJ, McKeen EA, Fraumeni JF Jr. Polymastia and renal adenocarcinoma. Ann Intern Med. 1981;95(2):182–4.
35. Cohen PR, Kurzrock R. Miscellaneous genodermatoses: Beckwith-Wiedemann syndrome, Birt-Hogg-Dube syndrome, familial atypical multiple mole melanoma syndrome, hereditary tylosis, incontinentia pigmenti, and supernumerary nipples. Dermatol Clin. 1995;13(1):211–29.
36. Gray H. Anatomy, descriptive and surgical. Philadelphia, Pennsylvania: Running Press Book Publishers; 1974.
37. Rosen PP. Rosen's breast pathology. Philadelphia: Wolters Kluwer Health/Lippincott Williams & Wilkins; 2009.

38. Iglehart JD, Kaelin, CM. Diseases of the Breast. In: Townsend CM Jr, Beauchamp RD, Evers BM, Mattox KL, editors. Sabiston textbook of surgery: the biological basis of modern surgical practice. 16th ed. Philadelphia: W.B. Saunders Company; 2001.
39. Greydanus DE, Matytsina L, Gains M. Breast disorders in children and adolescents. Prim Care. 2006;33(2):455–502.
40. Gliosci A, Presutti F. Asymmetry of the breast: some uncommon cases. Aesthetic Plast Surg. 1994;18(4):399–403.
41. Cunningham L. The anatomy of the arteries and veins of the breast. J Surg Oncol. 1977;9(1):71–85.
42. Skandalakis JE, Gray SW, Rowe JS Jr. Anatomical complications in general surgery. New York: McGraw-Hill Book Company; 1983.
43. Donegan WL, Spratt JS. Cancer of the breast. 3rd ed. Philadelphia: WB Saunders; 1988.
44. Estourgie SH, Nieweg OE, Olmos RA, Rutgers EJ, Kroon BB. Lymphatic drainage patterns from the breast. Ann Surg. 2004;239(2):232–7.
45. Moore KL, Agur AM. Essential clinical anatomy. Baltimore: Williams & Wilkins; 1995.
46. Arca MJ, Caniano DA. Breast disorders in the adolescent patient. Adolesc Med Clin. 2004;15(3):473–85.
47. Neinstein LS. Adolescent health care: a practical guide. 3rd ed. Baltimore: Williams & Wilkins; 1996.
48. Herman-Giddens ME, Slora EJ, Wasserman RC, et al. Secondary sexual characteristics and menses in young girls seen in office practice: a study from the pediatric research in office settings network. Pediatrics. 1997;99(4):505–12.
49. Tanner JM. Growth at adolescence, with a general consideration of the effects of hereditary and environmental factors upon growth and maturation from birth to maturity. Oxford: Blackwell Scientific Publications; 1962.
50. Greydanus DE, Parks DS, Farrell EG. Breast disorders in children and adolescents. Pediatr Clin North Am. 1989;36(3):601–38.
51. Draznin MB. Endocrine disorders. In: Greydanus DE, Patel DR, Pratt HD, editors. Essential adolescent medicine. New York: McGraw-Hill, Medical Pub. Division; 2006.
52. Van Winter JT, Noller KL, Zimmerman D, Melton LJ 3rd. Natural history of premature thelarche in Olmsted County, Minnesota, 1940 to 1984. J Pediatr. 1990;116(2):278–80.
53. Klein KO, Mericq V, Brown-Dawson JM, Larmore KA, Cabezas P, Cortinez A. Estrogen levels in girls with premature thelarche compared with normal prepubertal girls as determined by an ultrasensitive recombinant cell bioassay. J Pediatr. 1999;134(2):190–2.
54. Christov K, Chew KL, Ljung BM, et al. Proliferation of normal breast epithelial cells as shown by in vivo labeling with bromodeoxyuridine. Am J Pathol. 1991;138(6):1371–7.
55. Burkitt HG, Young B, Heath JW, Wheater PR. Wheater's functional histology: a text and colour atlas. 3rd ed. Edinburgh: Churchill Livingstone; 1993.

Paediatric and Adolescent Breast Disorders

28

Clare M. Rees, Kokila Lakhoo and P.G. Roy

Breast disorders in children are usually benign and self-limiting and require careful clinical examination followed by reassurance only. Rarely, investigations may be required and for a few selected conditions surgical intervention may be necessary. Presenting symptoms and signs can include pain, nipple discharge, abnormal enlargement, mass or asymmetrical growth. In this chapter, we consider disorders of the paediatric and adolescent breast.

Premature Thelarche

Normal thelarche occurs at about 10 years of age in the UK [1] and earlier in the US (8.87 years in African-American girls and 9.96 in white American girls [2]). This is younger than previously described in the earlier literature (previously age 11 years in the UK [3]). If a girl has not begun thelarche by age 13, investigation for delayed development is warranted [4]. Breast development was described by Tanner [3] in five stages (Table 28.1) and usually occurs over a period of about 4 years from thelarche. These stages have typical ultrasound appearances which help to confirm normal breast development if a patient presents with asymmetry or a mass [5].

Premature thelarche may present at any age from the neonatal period (Fig. 28.1), but is commonest before the age of 2, with symmetrical or asymmetrical breast development. It should be noted that physiological breast tissue is palpable in normal children in the first few years of life. Premature breast development is usually an isolated finding but may rarely be associated with hypothyroidism [6]. It is differentiated from precocious puberty by the absence of any other signs of sexual maturation (e.g. pubic hair development) [7] and normal growth. Hormonal investigations include LH (often normal) and FSH (FSH often raised in under 2 year olds [7]). Children who present before age 2 are most likely to undergo regression, with older girls being more likely to have progression of symptoms or persistence of breast tissue [7]. In premature thelarche breast development does not progress beyond Tanner stage 3.

In normal thelarche, one breast may starts developing first (asynchronous thelarche), and this may be mistaken for a breast lump. On examination, normal breast tissue is palpated and the patient can be reassured.

Precocious puberty (Fig. 28.2) is defined as development of secondary sexual characteristics earlier than would normally be expected [2]. This condition warrants urgent investigation to exclude lesions within the pituitary-endocrine

C.M. Rees · K. Lakhoo (✉)
Department of Paediatric Surgery, Children's Hospital Oxford, Oxford Radcliffe Hospitals NHS Trust, Headley Way, Headington, UK
e-mail: mary.trinder@ouh.nhs.uk; kokila.lakhoo@orh.nhs.uk

C.M. Rees
e-mail: clare.rees@nhs.net

P.G. Roy
Churchill Hospital, Oxford OX3 9DU, UK
e-mail: Pankaj.roy@ouh.nhs.uk

D.J. Ledbetter and P.R.V. Johnson (eds.), *Endocrine Surgery in Children*,
DOI 10.1007/978-3-662-54256-9_28

system, as well as the reproductive organs (pituitary, thyroid, adrenal, ovary, testis, etc.). Precocious puberty encompasses breast and pubic hair development, and concerns that children will not reach their full adult height prompt investigation and treatment with GnRH analogues in younger children.

Table 28.1 Tanner stages of breast development

Stage	Characteristics
1	Pre-adolescent: Elevation of breast papilla/nipple
2	Breast bud stage: Elevation of the breast and papilla as small mound and enlargement of areola
3	Further enlargement of breast and areola, with no separation of contours
4	Projection of nipple and areola to form secondary mound above the level of the breast
5	Mature stage: projection of papilla only due to recession of the areola to the contour of the breast

From [3], with permission

Congenital Anomalies

Amastia and Hypomastia

Amastia (congenital absence of the breast) is rare, and may be associated with Poland's syndrome (hypoplasia or absence of the pectoralis muscle with ipsilateral syndactyly). Amastia may be unilateral or bilateral and may occur in both sexes. It is a condition where the nipple is present but the breast does not develop. Athelia is a rare condition in which breast tissue is present but the nipple is absent [8].

Amastia and hypomastia may be acquired due to iatrogenic damage to the developing breast tissue in a child during central line insertion, chest tube placement, thoracotomy, radiotherapy or burns. Due to nipple complex development only occurring in the eighth month of gestation, premature infants are more susceptible to injury to the developing breast during surgical intervention of central line and thoracic tube insertion.

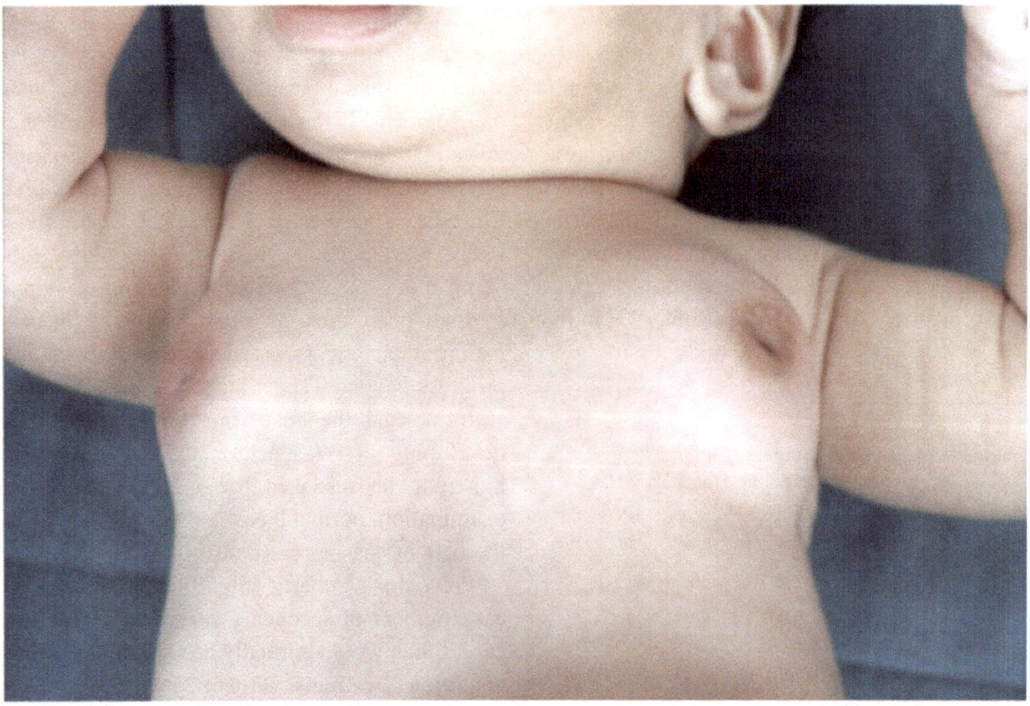

Fig. 28.1 Premature

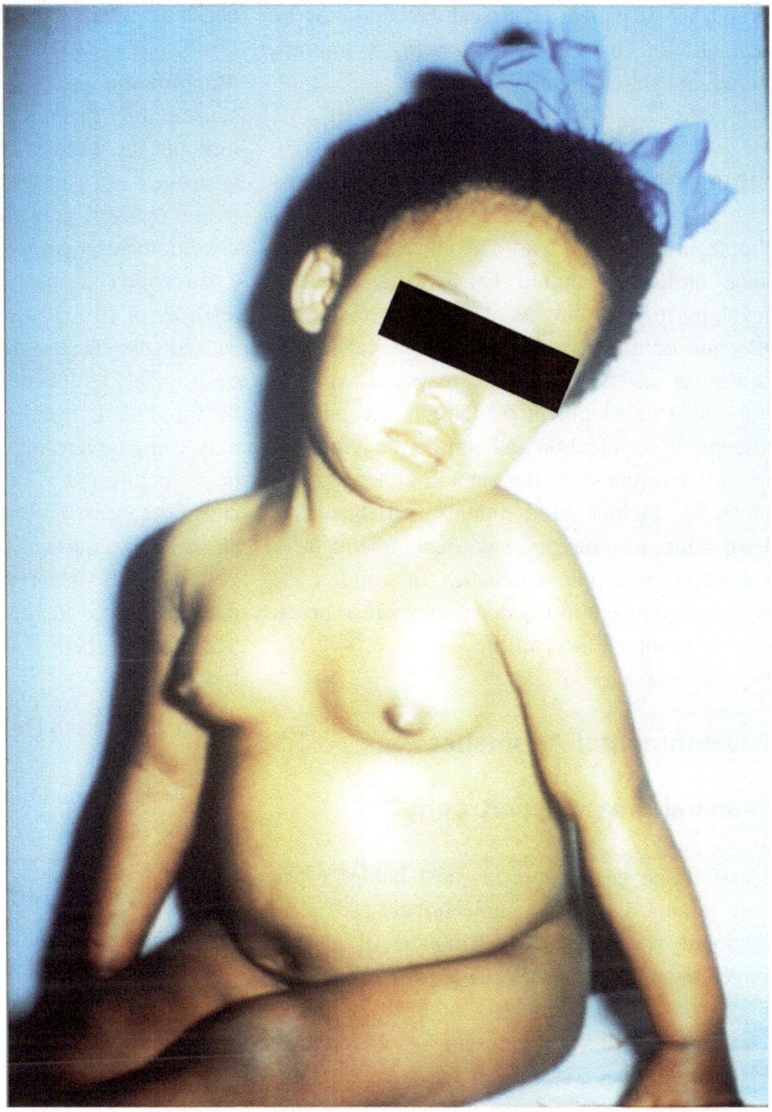

Fig. 28.2 Precocious puberty

Lack of breast development may be associated with delayed puberty, which would require investigation of ovarian failure, hypothyroidism or androgen-producing tumours.

Polymastia and Polythelia

Polythelia (accessory nipple) or polymastia (accessory breast) may occur in up to 2% of the population and breast tissue may be found anywhere along the milk line from the axilla to the groyne and very rarely in other anatomical sites [8, 9]. It is common in girls and there is an increased incidence in some geographical populations in America (black, white and Native Americans), Japan and Israel and a decreased incidence in white Europeans (0.2%) [9]. Some cases are familial, with both autosomal dominant and x-linked inheritance described. Accessory breast tissue may be mistaken for other conditions including lipoma, lymphatic disorders and sebaceous cysts [9]. Other congenital anomalies, especially urogenital anomalies are identified in up to 15% of patients. Surgical excision may be indicated for cosmetic reasons or for symptoms including cyclical pain.

Nipple Anomalies

Nipple inversion is a normal variant if present since birth, but should be investigated if it develops in later life as it may be a sign of infection or underlying tumour. It is caused by failure of eversion of the mammary pit in embryonal development [8]. Nipple inversion is susceptible to infection and can be prevented by careful hygiene to the area. Other nipple anomalies include bifid nipples and dysplastic divided nipples. Surgery is not recommended for correction of nipple anomalies in children as invariable damage to the ducts may cause breast feeding problems later in life.

Developmental Anomalies

Neonatal Breast Hypertrophy

Breast tissue is palpable in most babies (75% male infants and 84% female infants [10]) and commonly persists until 10 months of age or longer, especially in breast-fed babies. The palpable nodule is asymmetric in 63% [10], but decreases in size with increasing age. This correlates with the concept of a neonatal 'mini-puberty' where endogenous gonadotrophins and sex hormones are produced. Clear or milky fluid nipple discharge may occur. This condition is self-limiting and requires reassurance only.

Breast Asymmetry

Asymmetry is common, in normal development one side usually appears first and may present as a tender lump. Some degree of breast asymmetry is normal in the adult population. Surgery to augment or reduce the breast is not indicated until breast development is complete after puberty.

Macromastia and Breast Hypertrophy

Macromastia (excessively large breasts) may be caused by juvenile hypertrophy, pregnancy, tumours or excess endogenous or exogenous oestrogen or progesterone [11]. Reduction mammoplasty may be indicated after breast development is complete.

Juvenile (virginal) breast hypertrophy is a rare disorder of stromal hyperplasia [12] that may be caused by increased end-organ sensitivity to oestrogen [11]. It is usually symmetrical and may be familial. It usually occurs at menarche and may cause severe mastalgia. Breast growth may be controlled with progesterone or anti-oestrogens. Failure of medical management allows for reduction mammoplasty in teens or young adults when the breasts have achieved maturity. Later in life this condition may affect lactation but there is no risk for breast cancer.

Tubular Breast Deformity

This is a rare condition of skin deficiency at the base of the breast resulting in decreased horizontal and vertical breast growth [13]. The nipple areola complex may become necrosed due to the resulting breast deformity and the overlying skin may be oedematous with venous congestion. Appearance may raise concern for breast malignancy. Therefore, this clinical finding requires careful assessment and reassurance to parents. Reconstructive surgery is indicated after puberty.

Gynaecomastia

Enlargement of the glandular breast tissue in boys is termed gynaecomastia and can present at any age but is commonest in adolescents. A full discussion can be found elsewhere in this book.

Breast Infection

Infection of the breast or nipple may occur at any age and presents with pain, pyrexia, localised tenderness, erythema and induration (cellulitis)

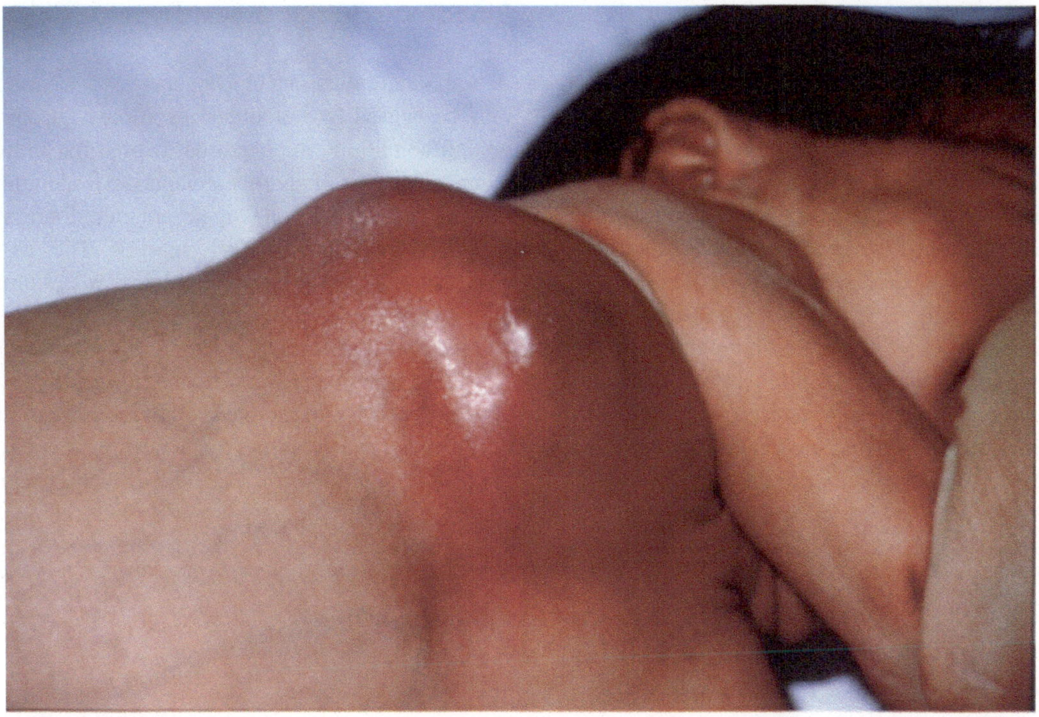

Fig. 28.3 Breast abscess

progressing to a fluctuant mass (abscess) (Fig. 28.3). The aetiology may be skin infection, nipple abrasion or mammary duct obstruction [14]. Antibiotic therapy may be sufficient, but if an abscess requires drainage, aspiration is recommended initially to prevent damage to the developing breast. If a formal incision and drainage is required, the incision should be as small as possible. Common causative organisms include *Staphylococcus Aureus*, beta-haemolytic *Streptococcus*, *E.Coli* and *Pseudomonas Aeruginosa* [15].

Mastitis

Neonatal mastitis is uncommon but affects girls more often than boys and commonly proceeds to abscess formation [16]. Certain systemic conditions such as diabetes mellitus, steroid therapy, rheumatoid arthritis could predispose to increased risk of infections. The most common organism is *Staphylococcus aureus*, less common being *Streptococci*, gram-negative enteric organisms such as *E.coli*, anaerobes. Aggressive antibiotic therapy is successful in half of cases and needle aspiration is as effective as formal incision and drainage when required [16].

Periductal mastitis associated with mammary duct ectasia presents with nipple discharge, non-cyclical pain, nipple retraction or a tender lump near the nipple [17]. It is managed with antibiotics and does not usually require surgical duct excision.

Nipple Discharge

Discharge may occur at any age, and is usually associated with benign conditions. It should be investigated if unilateral, persistent and associated with a single duct. Investigations include microbiological culture of the discharge, ultrasound and very occasionally ductogram.

Galactorrhoea

Galactorrhoea is a milky nipple discharge (Fig. 28.4). In the neonate, it is a normal response to the peak of prolactin at birth and will resolve spontaneously. Other causes in children include can be classified as endocrine (hypo or hyperthyroidism), neurogenic (disorders of the chest wall or thorax, including thoracotomy) [6], hypothalamic or pituitary (prolactin-secreting tumours such as prolactinoma), drug-induced (e.g. dopamine receptor blockers) or idiopathic. Investigations include tests of serum prolactin, FSH, LH and thyroid function tests. Treatment of the underlying disorder is required.

Bloody Discharge

A serosanguinous or bloody nipple discharge may be caused by intraductal papilloma—a rare benign condition which can be excised but may recur. Other differential diagnoses include mammary duct ectasia, nipple trauma, foreign body [17] and chronic cystic mastitis. The discharge should be sent for microbiological culture and appropriate antibiotics started.

Mammary duct ectasia is an inflammatory condition characterised by dilatation of the subareolar ducts. Bacterial overgrowth in obstructed ducts may cause abscesses. Ultrasound may confirm tubular anechoic ducts filled with debris

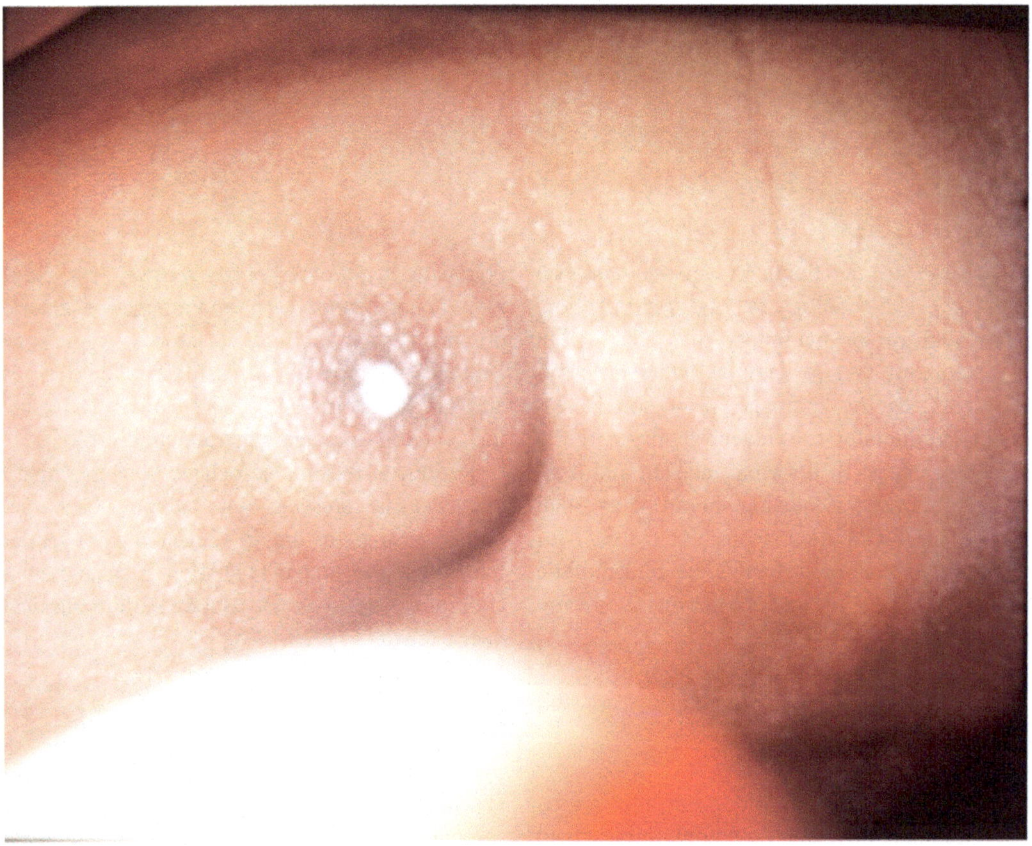

Fig. 28.4 Galactorrhea

[18]. This condition may resolve spontaneously and surgical duct excision is rarely required.

Nipple Adenoma

Nipple adenoma is a very rare benign nipple lesion, usually presenting in middle-aged women (<500 cases reported), with a few case reports in children described. It presents as an enlarging nipple lesion with induration, ulceration or bloody discharge [19]. The recommended treatment is surgical excision, but some recommend that this is deferred in asymptomatic cases until after puberty to preserve developing breast tissue.

Prepubertal Breast Masses

A breast lump in a prepubertal child should be examined carefully and investigated if there are atypical features. Atypical features include hard craggy lump, lump with bloody discharge, inverted nipple, skin changes, ulceration and associated axillary lymph nodes Usually the lump is benign and the child and parents can be reassured, and a policy of watchful waiting is appropriate. Children may present with premature or asynchronous thelarche or breast asymmetry which is mistaken for a mass. Trauma, such as from a seat-belt injury, can result in fat necrosis which may present as a solid mass. Other causes of breast lumps are described below.

Haemangioma

Haemangioma in the breast region may present as a lump. This can be diagnosed clinically and with confirmation on ultrasound or MRI. If the haemangioma grows rapidly it may require treatment with steroids [20]; excision is not usually necessary [14]. There may be associated mammary hypoplasia if the developing breast bud is involved in the haemangioma [14].

Lymphangioma

A lymphangioma is a benign congenital hamartoma or sequestration of the lymphatic system. It most commonly arises in the neck or axilla and is very rare in the breast. A few cases have been described as painless enlarging breast lumps, very rarely in children. Ultrasound may help with diagnosis but usually the definitive diagnosis is made on histological examination of a resected lump, which is curative. In other sites sclerotherapy of large lesions (e.g. with OK432, bleomycin) is used to reduce their size before excision, and this may be useful in the breast to preserve surrounding breast tissue [21].

Lipoma

Lipomas are benign adipose tumours which may occur anywhere on the trunk, neck or limbs. They present as a soft rubbery mass and are rare in the breast in paediatric patients. One case of lipoblastoma has been described in a male infant [22].

Galactocele

A galactocele is an uncommon cystic lesion containing milk or viscous material, most commonly found in women after lactation. The cause of galactocele in children is unknown [23]. It can present in male and female children as a unilateral non-tender breast lump or asymmetry. Ultrasound may show a complex mass and allows guided aspiration [18]. Aspiration of the cyst contents may be curative [24], otherwise surgical excision is recommended.

Juvenile Papillomatosis

Juvenile papillomatosis is a benign lesion that presents with a nodular mass. On ultrasound a poorly defined mass is detected. The treatment is total excision of the mass with preservation of the normal breast. Histologically the characteristics include cysts, epithelial hyperplasia, papillomatosis, apocrine metaplasia and cytological atypia. Juvenile papillomatosis is a marker for increased frequency of breast cancer [4], including juvenile secretory carcinoma.

Breast Masses in Adolescents

Cyclical breast pain and nodularity may occur with fibrocystic change. This does not require surgical treatment, as it is a normal variant. Conservative management includes non-steroidal anti-inflammatory medication, oral contraceptive pill or evening primrose oil [20].

Scarring from trauma or after a breast abscess may present as a breast lump and be mistaken for a breast malignancy [25]. In children with a family history of breast cancer the family may be concerned that a lump represents breast cancer and will require reassurance if an alternative diagnosis is made. The role of breast self-examination is adolescents is controversial.

Fibroadenoma

Fibroadenoma is the commonest cause of a breast mass in adolescents but may also occur in the prepubertal child. They consist of epithelial and stromal components, formed due to stromal hyperplasia, and are not true neoplasms. They present as a well-defined, round, smooth and mobile lump in the breast (also described as 'breast mouse'). The mass is usually non-tender, firm, discrete and mobile. It may be bilateral (10%) or multiple (10–15%) [4], and is commoner in Afro-Caribbean girls. The commonest site is the upper outer quadrant of the breast [14]. The mass arises from a single breast lobule and is now considered a disorder of breast development rather than a pathological entity [12]. If the mass is larger than 5 cm it is regarded as a disease process and termed a giant fibroadenoma (see below).

The natural history of fibroadenomas is that they slowly enlarge over time. About a third of these regress spontaneously [14]. About 15% patients have multiple fibroadenomas.

Most surgeons would recommend ultrasound to confirm the diagnosis and then watchful waiting, although if there are atypical features or concern a fine needle aspiration (FNA) biopsy may be warranted [26]. Clinical observation with repeat ultrasound at 6 monthly or yearly intervals is recommended [4]. On ultrasound, a well circumscribed, hypoechoic homogeneous mass [5] is seen.

Indications for surgery include a symptomatic mass, rapid growth or an atypical ultrasound appearance. The mass should be approached via a circumareolar incision. Normal breast tissue is not excised, only the encapsulated fibroadenoma. Most surgeons suggest surgery should be deferred until after puberty, and in older adolescents in whom malignancy is suspected [17]. Histological examination confirms epithelial and stromal components [27] and excludes other diagnoses such as phyllodes tumour.

Simple fibroadenomas are not associated with an increased risk of future invasive breast cancer; complex fibroadenomas (with features of cysts, sclerosing adenosis, epithelial calcifications and/or apocrine metaplasia) are associated with a two-fold increased risk of malignancy for more than 20 years after removal [27].

Juvenile (Giant) Fibroadenoma

These occur during puberty and are rapidly growing tumours, reaching size more than 5 cm. They should be differentiated from phyllodes tumour by biopsy and treatment involves surgical excision, and can be enucleated from inframammary crease incision. The rapid growth of these lesions often result in increased breast size and asymmetry, however, surgical excision would result in normalisation of the breast and rarely needs any further intervention.

Phyllodes Tumours (Cystosarcoma Phyllodes)

Phyllodes tumours (also known as cystosarcoma phyllodes) are stromal tumours characterised by epithelial hyperplasia [13], which may be benign, intermediate or malignant. They account for up to 35% of adolescent breast tumours. Even histologically benign lesions may metastasize (10% haematogenous metastases) and up to 25% recur locally [28]. Clinically they can be difficult to distinguish from fibroadenomas; they are usually large, non-tender and grow rapidly. There may be a serosanguinous nipple discharge. On ultrasound there may be lobulations and a heterogenous echo pattern without microcalcification [20]. It is recommended that core needle biopsy is performed for diagnosis and to assist surgical planning. Treatment is by excision with a margin of normal breast tissue if benign, or mastectomy if malignant. The prognosis is more favourable in children than adults [29]. The 5-year survival rates for benign, borderline, and malignant phyllodes tumours in adults are 96, 74 and 66%, respectively.

Hamartoma

These are rare in children and adolescents. The clinical presentation is similar to a fibroadenoma. Hamartoma refers to presence of varying amount of benign epithelial elements, fat and fibrous tissue. They are usually benign and do not necessarily need surgical excision.

Malignant Primary Breast Tumours

Primary breast cancer is very rare in children, with fewer than 100 cases described worldwide. Breast cancer in children accounts for less than 0.1% of all breast cancers and less than 1% of paediatric cancers [28, 29]. The incidence is estimated at 0.1–0.3 per 100,000 population [29, 30]. Primary breast tumours may be adenocarcinomas or sarcomas.

Breast Cancer Risk

It is important to assess the family history in adolescents with breast cancer. About 5% of breast cancers are linked to genetic predisposition. The following gene mutations are associated with breast cancer:

- BRCA mutation
- P53 mutation
- Ataxia Telangiectasia
- Cowden's Syndrome

The other risk factor is radiation exposure: Radiation exposure for girls during peak breast development, typically 10–16 years of age, is most harmful. Approximately 40% of girls treated with radiation for Hodgkin lymphoma will develop breast cancer. For women exposed to ionizing radiation before the age of 30 years, annual MRI for screening of breast cancer development is recommended from the age of 30 years or 8 years after first irradiation, whichever is later.

Breast Carcinoma

Breast carcinoma has been described in children as young as 3 years of age, with a female predominance (92%) [31]. The commonest presentation is with a enlarging, painless, firm, immobile, poorly circumscribed breast lump but nipple retraction and discharge are rare [31]. Ultrasound is useful in the investigation, but mammography is not generally helpful in children [32]. FNA may be helpful, although excision biopsy is usually required.

Due to its rarity, the treatment of primary breast cancer in children remains controversial [4, 29, 32]. Adjuvant therapy is considered for metastatic disease.

Juvenile Secretory Carcinoma

Juvenile secretory carcinoma is a type of invasive ductal carcinoma with good prognosis. It is common in girls and presents with an asymptomatic breast lump with no nipple discharge. Histologically it is characterised by intra- and extra-cellular eosinophilic secretion in cytoplasm and rudimentary ducts, is well demarcated but not encapsulated and is locally invasive [33]. These tumours may recur locally and metastasize to local lymph nodes or haematogenously. Patients have been managed with local excision (but 25% have local recurrence) [33], quadrantectomy or mastectomy. Adjuvant therapy is not required, even in the presence of axillary node metastases.

Ductal Carcinoma

Ductal carcinoma in situ (DCIS) is a premalignant condition that may be detected on histological examination of an excised breast lump, such as a fibroadenoma. It may occur secondary to previous radiotherapy for other tumours such as Hodgkin's lymphoma [34].

Infiltrating ductal carcinoma is the commonest subtype of primary breast carcinoma in some childhood series, accounting for about 30% of cases [29]. Other types identified include secretory carcinoma, lobular carcinoma and mucinous adenocarcinoma.

Secretory adenocarcinoma appears cystic on ultrasound due to its thick-walled capsule. Lymph node metastases may occur [29]. The recommended treatment is modified radical mastectomy with axillary lymph node dissection. The prognosis is good.

Medullary and inflammatory carcinoma are less common and more invasive with a poor prognosis [31].

Rhabdomyosarcoma

Rhabdomyosarcoma is the commonest solid malignancy in children and can occur in any part of the body. Metastasis is haematogenous or lymphatic and tumours are locally invasive. Sarcomas of the breast are very rare, but have occasionally been described as primary or metastatic tumours in children [34, 35]. Imaging includes ultrasound or MRI. Diagnosis is made on FNA or tissue biopsy and lump excision or radical mastectomy may be required.

Other sarcomas occasionally presenting with primary breast tumours include fibrosarcoma, malignant fibrous histiocytoma [20], leiomyosarcoma and hemangiosarcoma [29].

Malignant Secondary Breast Tumours

Secondary breast tumours are commoner than primary tumours in children. The primary can be rhabdomyosarcoma, lymphoma (Hodgkin and non-Hodgkin), melanoma, neuroblastoma, hepatocellular carcinoma [14] or adenocarcinoma [34]. FNA is required to make a cytological diagnosis and incisional or excision biopsy may be required, but mastectomy is not usually recommended. The prognosis depends on the primary tumour but is usually poor due to generalised metastatic disease.

Girls who have received chest wall radiotherapy for Hodgkin's lymphoma have an 82 times increased risk of developing breast cancer within 20 years [20].

References

1. Christensen KY, Maisonet M, Rubin C, et al. Pubertal pathways in girls enrolled in a contemporary british cohort. Int J Pediatr. 2010;2010:329261.
2. Kaplowitz PB, Oberfield SE. Reexamination of the age limit for defining when puberty is precocious in girls in the United States: implications for evaluation and treatment. Pediatrics. 1999;104:936–41 Drug and Therapeutics and Executive Committees of the Lawson Wilkins Pediatric Endocrine Society.
3. Marshall WA, Tanner JM. Variations in pattern of pubertal changes in girls. Arch Dis Child. 1969;44: 291–303.
4. Fallat ME, Ignacio RC Jr. Breast disorders in children and adolescents. J Pediatr Adolesc Gynecol. 2008;21:311–6.
5. Garcia CJ, Espinoza A, Dinamarca V, et al. Breast US in children and adolescents. Radiographics. 2000;20:1605–12.
6. De Silva NK, Brandt ML. Disorders of the breast in children and adolescents, Part 1: disorders of growth

and infections of the breast. J Pediatr Adolesc Gynecol. 2006;19:345–9.
7. de Vries L, Guz-Mark A, Lazar L, et al. Premature thelarche: age at presentation affects clinical course but not clinical characteristics or risk to progress to precocious puberty. J Pediatr. 2010;156:466–71.
8. Ellis H, Colborn GL, Skandalakis JE. Surgical embryology and anatomy of the breast and its related anatomic structures. Surg Clin North Am. 1993;73: 611–32.
9. Loukas M, Clarke P, Tubbs RS. Accessory breasts: a historical and current perspective. Am Surg. 2007;73:525–8.
10. Jayasinghe Y, Cha R, Horn-Ommen J, et al. Establishment of normative data for the amount of breast tissue present in healthy children up to two years of age. J Pediatr Adolesc Gynecol. 2010;23:305–11.
11. O'hare PM, Frieden IJ. Virginal breast hypertrophy. Pediatr Dermatol. 2000;17:277–81.
12. Hughes LE, Mansel RE, Webster DJ. Aberrations of normal development and involution (ANDI): a new perspective on pathogenesis and nomenclature of benign breast disorders. Lancet. 1987;2:1316–9.
13. Moore RL, Mungara A, Shayan K, et al. Bilaterally symmetric juvenile fibroadenomas and tubular breast deformity in a prepubescent girl. J Pediatr Surg. 2007;42:1133–6.
14. West KW, Rescorla FJ, Scherer LR III, et al. Diagnosis and treatment of symptomatic breast masses in the pediatric population. J Pediatr Surg. 1995;30:182–6.
15. Turbey WJ, Buntain WL, Dudgeon DL. The surgical management of pediatric breast masses. Pediatrics. 1975;56:736–9.
16. Efrat M, Mogilner JG, Iujtman M, et al. Neonatal mastitis–diagnosis and treatment. Isr J Med Sci. 1995;31:558–60.
17. Foxcroft LM, Evans EB, Hirst C, et al. Presentation and diagnosis of adolescent breast disease. Breast. 2001;10:399–404.
18. Weinstein SP, Conant EF, Orel SG, et al. Spectrum of US findings in pediatric and adolescent patients with palpable breast masses. Radiographics. 2000;20:1613–21.
19. Clune JE, Kozakewich HP, VanBeek CA, et al. Nipple adenoma in infancy. J Pediatr Surg. 2009;44:2219–22.
20. De Silva NK, Brandt ML. Disorders of the breast in children and adolescents, Part 2: breast masses. J Pediatr Adolesc Gynecol. 2006;19:415–8.
21. Singh O, Singh GS, Upadhyaya VD, et al. Cystic lymphangioma of the breast in a 6-year-old boy. J Pediatr Surg. 2009;44:2015–8.
22. Zani A, Cozzi DA, Uccini S, et al. Unusual breast enlargement in an infant: a case of breast lipoblastoma. Pediatr Surg Int. 2007;23:361–3.
23. Perez-Boscollo AC, Dutra RA, Borges LG, et al. Galactocele: an unusual cause of breast enlargement in children. J Pediatr Surg. 2009;44:e1–3.
24. Boyle M, Lakhoo K, Ramani P. Galactocele in a male infant: case report and review of literature. Pediatr Pathol. 1993;13:305–8.
25. Siegal A, Kaufman Z, Siegal G. Breast masses in adolescent females. J Surg Oncol. 1992;51:169–73.
26. Pacinda SJ, Ramzy I. Fine-needle aspiration of breast masses. A review of its role in diagnosis and management in adolescent patients. J Adolesc Health. 1998;23:3–6.
27. Dupont WD, Page DL, Parl FF, et al. Long-term risk of breast cancer in women with fibroadenoma. N Engl J Med. 1994;331:10–5.
28. Tea MK, Asseryanis E, Kroiss R, et al. Surgical breast lesions in adolescent females. Pediatr Surg Int. 2009;25:73–5.
29. Gutierrez JC, Housri N, Koniaris LG, et al. Malignant breast cancer in children: a review of 75 patients. J Surg Res. 2008;147:182–8.
30. Kothari AS, Beechey-Newman N, D'Arrigo C, et al. Breast carcinoma in women age 25 years or less. Cancer. 2002;94:606–14.
31. Murphy JJ, Morzaria S, Gow KW, et al. Breast cancer in a 6-year-old child. J Pediatr Surg. 2000;35: 765–7.
32. Corpron CA, Black CT, Singletary SE, et al. Breast cancer in adolescent females. J Pediatr Surg. 1995;30:322–4.
33. Karl SR, Ballantine TV, Zaino R. Juvenile secretory carcinoma of the breast. J Pediatr Surg. 1985;20: 368–71.
34. Rogers DA, Lobe TE, Rao BN, et al. Breast malignancy in children. J Pediatr Surg. 1994;29: 48–51.
35. Binokay F, Soyupak SK, Inal M, et al. Primary and metastatic rhabdomyosarcoma in the breast: report of two pediatric cases. Eur J Radiol. 2003;48:282–4.

Gynecomastia

29

Tim Goodacre and Gavin McCoubrey

Definition

The term gynaecomastia refers to the appearance of breast-like tissue in males. It is caused by a benign proliferation of the glandular component of male breast tissue [1]. It is common in infancy, adolescence, and in adulthood from middle age onward [2]. Most commonly caused by increased oestrogen, decreased androgen, or the use of numerous medications, gynaecomastia can be unilateral or bilateral and presents as a rubbery or firm mass extending concentrically from beneath the nipple–areolar complex [3–5]. Pseudogynaecomastia, often seen in obesity, refers to accumulation of fat in the breast region without the glandular proliferation [6].

The most important differential diagnosis from either of these conditions is male breast carcinoma. This is exceptionally rare, usually unilateral, eccentric and hard in consistency. It may be associated with skin dimpling, nipple retraction or discharge, and axillary lymphadenopathy [7].

T. Goodacre (✉)
Nuffield Department of Surgery, University of Oxford, Henry Wellcome Building for Molecular Physiology, Old Road Campus, Headington, Oxford OX3, UK
e-mail: tim.goodacre@nds.ox.ac.uk

G. McCoubrey
Salisbury NHS Foundation Trust, Odstock Rd, Salisbury SP2 8BJ, UK
e-mail: gavinmccoubrey@hotmail.com

The appearance of male breast enlargement requires accurate diagnosis and treatment. This is not only to rule out a rare sinister cause, but much more importantly the suggestion of a feminine habitus may have major psychosocial significance to the patient or parents in the case of a child [8, 9].

Incidence

Gynaecomastia can occur in the male at any age. However, it is more common at particular times of life [1–4, 10–17]. Pre-pubertal gynaecomastia is rare and should raise suspicion of a pathological cause.

Neonatal	60–90% of newborns
Adolescense/pubertal	Up to 65% of males
Middle age/elderly (50–80 years)	25–65% of men affected

Aetiology

Physiological

Neonatal—This is thought to result from transplacental transfer of maternal oestrogens [18]. Seen in both males and females, it usually disappears after a few weeks, and no treatment required.

Adolescent/Pubertal—This develops during puberty (mean age 13) and is thought to be caused by excess oestrogen and/or an oestrogen–

D.J. Ledbetter and P.R.V. Johnson (eds.), *Endocrine Surgery in Children*,
DOI 10.1007/978-3-662-54256-9_29

androgen imbalance [19]. Despite the presumed hormonal aetiology, the condition is frequently asymmetrical. Unilateral nodular lesions in particular can be tender. The condition may regress by the later teen years, but a considerable number may persist into adulthood and present a permanent abnormality [20].

Pathological

Pathological causes are invariably related to hormonal/endocrinological disorders.

Hypogonadism (congenital/acquired)	Klinefelters, testicular feminisation,orchitis, hermaphroditism, congenital anorchia, trauma
Endocrine	Hyperthyroidism
Metabolic	Cirrhosis, starvation, chronic renal failure
Neoplasia (ectopic hCG)	Adrenal, pituitary, testicular, bronchogenic, thyroid

Pharmacological

Drugs can cause 10–25% of all cases of gynaecomastia [21]. Some drugs act like oestrogens, some enhance endogenous oestrogen formation, some inhibit testosterone synthesis and action and others act by an unknown mechanism. All may induce gynaecomastia through hormonal imbalance.

There is an extensive list of possible drug related gynaecomastia. We have included the most common therapies involved with examples in Table 29.1.

Idiopathic/Pseudo/Obesity

Gynaecomastia developing in young adults and beyond is often multifactorial. Body fat increases relative to lean body mass as we age. Adipose

Table 29.1 Possible drug-related causes of gynaecomastia

Hormones
Anti-androgens (Prostate Cancer)
Gonadotrophin releasing hormone
Oestrogenic Agonists (diethylstilbestrol)
Anabolic steroids
Anti-ulcer therapy
Histamine 2 receptor blockers (cimetidine)
Proton pump inhibitors (omeprazole, esomeprazole)
Cardiac agents
Calcium channel blockers (verapamil, nifedipine, diltiazem, amlodipine)
Angiotensin Converting Enzyme inhibitors (captopril)
Cholesterol lowering agents (fenofibrate, simvastatin, fluvastatin)
Digoxin
Spironolactone
Neuroleptics
Wide variety of neurotransmitter agonists, antagonists and modulators
Tricyclic antdepressants
Diazepam
Phenothiazines
Antifungals
Ketoconazole
Cancer agents
Chemotheraputic agents
Alkylating agents
5 alpha reductase inhibitors
Antiretroviral therapy
Highly Active Antiretroviral Therapy (HAART)
Protease inhibitors
Nucleoside/non-nucleoside containing regimes
Recreational drugs
Alcohol
Cannabis
Heroin
Others
Methotrexate
Metronidazole
Metoclopramide
Phenytoin
Theophylline

tissue is an active site of extraglandular aromatization of testosterone to oestradiol and androstenedione to oestrone. In addition, there tends to be a gradual decrease in testosterone production by the ageing testes and an increase in sex hormone binding globulin, resulting in less free testosterone and a reciprocal increase in Luteinising hormone [22, 23]. These two factors probably account for most idiopathic gynaecomastia in the adult.

Obesity alone will also result in deposition of fat in the area of the breast. This Pseudogynaecomastia can be expected to reduce following weight loss. However, excessive weight loss following morbid obesity frequently leads to the development of a redundant, ptotic, skin fold that can only be corrected by surgery.

Familial

Aromatase excess syndrome is a rare autosomal dominant disorder resulting in severe oestrogen excess involving the p450 aromatase gene (CYP19) [24, 25]. Aromatase inhibitors may be effective in this disorder.

Differential Diagnosis

Male breast cancer, lipoma, neurofibroma, lymphangioma and vascular malformations (hamartomatous conditions), haematoma, dermoid cyst.

Pathogenesis

Gynaecomastia may be caused by a decrease in androgen production, an increase in oestrogen production, or increased availability of oestrogen precursors for peripheral conversion to oestrogen. The blockade of androgen receptors and increased binding of androgen to sex hormone binding globulin (SHBG) are other mechanisms [2]. Thus the circulating concentration of SHBG, the target cell response, and the extraglandular conversion of androgens to oestrogens are factors which might determine the development of abnormal breast tissue in the male.

SHBG is found normally in the circulation, binding the sex hormones tightly when compared with the weakly binding protein albumin. SHBG has a higher affinity for androgens than oestrogens; therefore oestrogens will be displaced more easily if an excess of hormone is present [26, 27].

Extraglandular conversion of androgens (testosterone and androstenedione) to oestrogen occurs in the liver, skin, fat, muscle, bone, and kidney. All these tissues contain an aromatase enzyme, responsible for conversion. The 17-hydroxysteroid dehydrogenase enzyme has a similar interconversion effect on androgens and oestrogens in extra glandular tissues [28, 29].

Testes and ovaries each secrete both oestrogen and androgen (testosterone). The production of these steroids or their precursors also occurs in the adrenal glands. An imbalance in the normal ratio of oestrogen to androgen causes an increase in glandular breast tissue [30].

There is no difference between the nature of male and female breast tissue hormonal response, which is individually led. By this, it is meant that breast proliferation depends on a particular individual's hormonal constitution, and the duration, sensitivity, and intensity of hormonal stimulation.

Oestrogen causes breast ductal epithelial hyperplasia, ductal elongation and branching, proliferation of periductal fibroblasts, and an increase in vascularity. Separately, in females, progesterone causes acinar development, not seen in males [28].

The transient neonatal appearance of gynaecomastia relates directly to elevated oestrogen levels in the foetal circulation. The placenta transforms dehydroepiandrosterone and dehydroepiandrosterone sulphate to oestrone and oestradiol, stimulating breast glandular proliferation.

Histopathology

Glandular proliferation in the breast depends upon the intensity and duration of stimulation and has the same histological appearance regardless of aetiology.

Firstly, there is extensive ductal epithelial hyperplasia, proliferation and lengthening of the ducts, an increase in the stromal and periductal connective tissue, and proliferation of periductal inflammatory cells and fibroblasts. This early oedematous stage lasts for approximately 6 months and the breast can be painful or tender to palpation [19].

With time (12 or more months) the inflammatory reaction subsides and discomfort usually settles. There remains an increase in the more dilated ducts with a commensurate increase in stroma that may show frank histological fibrosis at this later stage [31, 32].

This dense fibrous glandular tissue forms directly beneath the nipple–areolar complex, and is supported by a fibrofatty stroma peripherally [33]. This stroma may develop further as the BMI of the patient increases. Medical management is much more effective in the early stages before fibrosis has developed.

Diagnosis

All patients presenting with proliferation of tissue in the breast area require a detailed history and examination. Often this is all that is necessary to obtain an accurate diagnosis.

The history should include duration of symptoms, presence of discharge, pain, or skin changes. The age of the patient, the pubertal development, and presence of testicular masses should also be queried. The past medical history and general health is of great importance and may reveal evidence of liver, kidney or thyroid disease, and current medication including possible non-prescribed drugs are of considerable relevance.

A careful and sympathetic psychosocial history should also be taken. The psychological sequelae of male breast enlargement may be the main reason for presentation in children over the age of around 7–8 years, when 'visible difference' from peer groups becomes a source of possible distress [9].

Examination is general and specific. BMI calculation and the search for signs of liver, kidney, and thyroid disease is mandatory. Examination of the genitals for abnormalities and development and palpation the regional lymph nodes is also indicated.

The breast is observed for size, shape, symmetry, and skin appearance. The patient is asked to lie supine and place their hands behind their head. The breasts are then examined with thumb and forefinger, gradually moving the digits towards the nipple [1]. In true gynaecomastia a rubbery or firm, mobile, disc of tissue will be identified concentrically beneath the nipple–areolar complex. This mass can normally be detected when greater than 0.5 cm in diameter [34]. If no such mass is palpated in the enlarged male breast then a diagnosis of pseudogynaecomastia is confirmed. The presence of an eccentric, fixed, hard, or unilateral growth requires differential diagnostic consideration.

Laboratory testing, radiological studies and FNA/Core biopsy are not required on adolescents when idiopathic gynaecomastia is diagnosed. Adult males presenting without an obvious cause commonly undergo investigation. Radiological imaging in these less frequent cases should include ultrasound scan or mammogram and a FNA or core biopsy to complete the 'triple assessment', similar to the female with a breast lump.

Laboratory tests include liver, kidney and thyroid function tests. Hormonal testing measures levels of testosterone, oestradiol, prolactin, luteinising hormone, and hCG. Results can direct towards pituitary, gonadal, and extragonadal causes [6].

Further investigations in the search for a more sinister causative diagnosis can include testicular ultrasound scan, abdominal CT scan (imaging adrenal glands) or an MRI scan of the brain (imaging the sella turcica) [34].

Classification

There have been numerous classification systems; therefore we have included this in Table 29.2 [35]. In practice, clinical judgements

Table 29.2 Gynaecomastia classification systems

Authors	Classification
Nydick 1961	Gland limited to retroareolar region
	Gland extends to edge of areola
	Gland extends beyond areola
Tanner 1971	1. Nipple prominence
	2. Mammillary button stage; breast and areola slightly swollen
	3. Further swelling breast and areola
	4. Protrusive areola and nipple above the breast
	5. Protrusion of nipple only after retraction of the areola
Simon 1973	1. Small visible breast enlargement; no skin redundancy
	2a. Moderate breast enlargement without skin redundancy
	2b. Moderate breast enlargement with skin redundancy
	3. Marked breast enlargement and skin redundancy (pendulous)
Deutinger 1986	1. Thoracic wall poor in flesh; mammary tissue localised behind nipple; no skin excess
	2. Adipose thoracic wall; widespread alterations, feminine breasts
	3. Widespread alterations; excess adipose tissue, skin redundancy inframammary fold, ptosis
Cohen 1987	1. Glandular gynaecomastia
	2. Glandular gynaecomastia with ptosis
	3. Adipose gynaecomastia
	4. Adipose gynaecomastia with slight glandular component
Rohrich 2003	1. Minimal hypertrophy without ptosis
	2. Moderate hypertrophy without ptosis
	3. Severe hypertrophy with ptosis grade 1
	4. Severe hypertrophy with ptosis grade 2 or 3
Cordova 2004	1. Increase in diameter and protrusion limited to areolar region
	2. Areola–nipple complex above inframammary fold
	3. Areola–nipple complex at level of inframammary fold
	4. Areola–nipple complex below inframammary fold

are based on individual factors that include psychosocial aspects.

Treatment

Neonatal

Most babies with neonatal gynaecomastia will be identified in the immediate post natal examination, and the family reassured. Immediate investigation in this age group is usually not indicated unless the condition is accompanied by other abnormal findings suggestive of a congenital anomaly or syndrome.

First Decade

Children presenting with gynaecomastia in the first decade of life will usually have either obesity related pseudogynaecomastia, or a more specific cause (often pharmacologically induced) which will be evident from knowledge of the child's other conditions. Presentation at this age is most frequently to a General Practitioner or Paediatrician, and requires a full appraisal as described, with referral to a specialist paediatric endocrinologist in most cases if the BMI is normal. Referral to a paediatric general or plastic surgeon for an early opinion may be indicated at this time. Even if surgery is deferred until the adolescent period, careful consideration should be given to the merits of surgery to alleviate serious teasing and bullying around the common school transfer age of 11. Surgery in the first decade is uncommon, but in severe cases may be the only means to address a highly visible external deformity and be the most valuable option for management. Surgical management is described below.

Endocrine management of children in whom gynaecomastia has been the presenting sign of a more general condition is beyond the scope of this chapter. However, the need for long-term definitive management of hormonal or other disorders should not preclude the use of surgical intervention where it might prove to be the single most effective intervention in improving the child's overall health and well being.

Second Decade

Adolescents presenting with gynaecomastia frequently seek help from diverse routes. Although initial advice from a GP might be sought, many such affected young people are already deeply concerned about the developing condition and avoid contact with familiar and more conventional sources of help. Direct presentation to a plastic surgeon is common, and the proliferation of easily accessible sources of information from the internet and mass media has served to facilitate this diversification of possible sources of help. This is something of a mixed blessing; information streams are of variable quality and accuracy, and the commercial economy of much global health provision offers potential for the exploitation of vulnerable and inadequately advised young people. Many affected teenage boys become greatly distressed by what they perceive as dismissive and unsympathetic first consultations if they are merely advised that the condition will disappear and they should simply cope with their condition without skilled counselling or psychological advice.

Those presenting conventionally should be offered a sympathetic general assessment, and all possible underlying causes considered and excluded. The majority of adolescents with gynaecomastia will not have such an underlying cause. Those with painful, unilateral nodules should be considered for relatively early excision, following a period of around a year to allow the condition to either resolve or stabilise. Those with more diffuse, usually bilateral, lesions, should be offered advice on how best to approach social situations that they find difficult and embarrassing. Such advice is usually best delivered by clinical psychologists or counsellors with specific experience and training in managing young people with body image disorders or disfigurement; in the absence of such services, specialists in adolescent plastic surgery or related disorders may offer appropriate background experience.

The use of medical management for adolescent gynaecomastia is controversial. However, the best evidence suggests that if it is to be instigated that early referral for a specialist opinion offers the best hope for resolution of the developing condition. (See following paragraph)

Pseudogynaecomastia may simply require a weight loss programme in the obese male. The discontinuation of offending drugs may allow the problem to resolve spontaneously in those patients on medication or using cannabis.

Pharmacotherapy

Medical treatment options are generally more effective during the early phase of gynaecomastia before fibrotic changes to the tissues. The physician should first stop any offending drug causing gynaecomastia, once again more effective when halted in the proliferative phase. Improvement will usually be apparent within 1 month of stopping the medication. If the causative agent cannot be discontinued, there are several treatment options available.

The use of drugs in gynaecomastia treatment is supported by a very low quality of evidence due to very few randomised, double-blind, placebo controlled trials and limited long-term follow-up data. For these reasons licensing is a problem for their use in gynaecomastia treatment.

Medical therapy may be attempted in the proliferative phase. Most studies of drugs including testosterone, dihydrotestosterone, Danazol, clomiphene citrate, tamoxifen, raloxifene and testolactone have been uncontrolled and thus difficult to interpret as the condition may resolve spontaneously [36–39].

Tamoxifen and raloxifene, both selective oestrogen receptor modulators, may be most effective for patients with painful or severe gynaecomastia prior to surgery. Their use will not result in complete regression of the gynaecomastia but may relieve discomfort [40, 41].

Clinical trials to date have not demonstrated any clinical benefits in aromatase inhibitors (anastrozole) in the treatment of pubertal gynaecomastia [42].

Tamoxifen, anastrozole, and radiotherapy have all been used to reduce the incidence and extent of anti-androgen associated gynaecomastia in men with prostate cancer, but have little effect when the gynaecomastia is established in these patients [43, 44]

Fortunately, 75–90% of adolescents experience spontaneous breast tissue regression over a 1–3 year period. However, if after this period of observation there is no or insufficient regression, medical treatment is unlikely to be effective due to stromal fibrosis in long-standing gynaecomastia [19].

Surgery

Surgical techniques for gynaecomastia correction have been considerably modified in the past two decades by the introduction of a variety of liposuction methods. The value of liposuction has been its relatively scarless involvement; the disadvantages, however, relate to the difficulty in removing fibrous tissue, the incompleteness of involved tissue excision, and the inability to obtain tissue for histopathological examination.

Liposuction Alone

Liposuction can be considered a first choice method for lesions which are very soft and non-fibrous, and where complete excision is not a major consideration—especially if surgical scarring or other possible adverse effects of excisional surgery are major concerns. This situation is rare in the adolescent case, with the exception of obesity induced pseudogynaecomastia.

Consent for liposuction includes the unpredictable degree of correction, since even apparently diffusely fatty breast fullness can prove to be related to a densely fibrous lesion and be remarkably resistant to liposuction. The surrounding area will be bruised, and may resolve with permanently uneven rippling or waviness of the surface. Skin necrosis is rare, but residual firmness beneath the nipple area is almost invariable, and some alteration or loss of sensation is common. Haematoma is less common than with excisional techniques, but several small stab incision sites around the breast area might be visible and (especially in the midline) might give rise to long-standing hypertrophic irritable scars.

The procedure is usually undertaken under general anaesthetic in the adolescent, although smaller areas are amenable to local anaesthetic techniques in the cooperative patient. General pre-operative assessment is all that is required, and the procedure is often undertaken as day surgery. Post-operative care involves the use of a compression vest where the area treated is extensive, and simple analgesia.

The breast area is prepared with infiltration of saline with adrenaline and hyaluronidase. The 'pre-tunnelling' is especially necessary with firmer gynaecomastia tissue, and should be thorough and extensive. Suction itself is usually undertaken with a shorter cannula using high vacuum pressures (Fig. 29.1). Measurement of

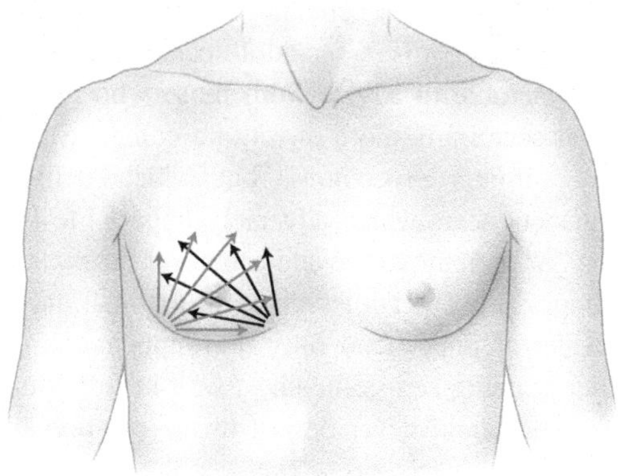

Fig. 29.1 The breast area is prepared for liposuction with infiltration of saline with adrenaline and hyaluronidase. The 'pre-tunnelling' is especially necessary with firmer gynaecomastia tissue, and should be thorough and extensive. Suction itself is usually undertaken with a shorter cannula using high vacuum pressures

the aspirated volume of fat is helpful in maintaining symmetry in bilateral cases.

Ultrasound-assisted liposuction is an additional technique functioning by emulsifying the breast fat and permitting a more efficient removal of fat in areas with a high density of fibroconnective tissue. The equipment availability and cost limits its use in many departments [45].

Excisional Surgery

Removal of the affected tissue remains the mainstay of effective surgical management of gynaecomastia. It can almost invariably be undertaken through incisions which are confined to the areolar circumference, with the major benefit that permanent potentially embarrassing scars outside the nipple area are avoided. There is no indication for the use of transverse chest wall incisions, or approaches similar to those used for female breast reduction, in the first surgical approach for such patients. If the breast is grossly enlarged, a wide excision of as much tissue as possible using a concentric ring technique should be the first procedure, with the option for a secondary or further resection or 'tidy up' of the residual chest fullness once the outcome can be fully evaluated. The use of more scar inducing and disfiguring total excisional techniques is outmoded and unacceptable at this time; the psychologically distressed adolescent and parents are vulnerable to advice from those who might proffer seemingly more direct and complete primary surgical procedures, but which deliver permanent scars which adversely impact life for many years in the future and can never be revised or improved. The adolescent is in no position to consider or understand fully the implications of major scarring across the chest wall in full adult life, and should never be put in the position of making such decisions.

Nodular Excision

Consent for excision should include the unpredictable degree of post-operative concavity or irregularity of the site following removal of all affected tissue. The child and/or parents should understand that the tissue itself has taken up the normal fatty layer beneath the nipple, and complete removal frequently leaves a residual concavity that can be difficult to address. The outer borders of the excision site can also be somewhat irregular, and liposuction as an adjunct can be employed to 'smooth' these borders if the surgeon considers it advantageous. Other side effects include loss of nipple sensation, very rarely nipple necrosis, and the need for further excision of any residual tissue following full wound healing.

Simple local nodules (one or both sides) can be excised using carefully placed incisions in the inferior half of the circumareolar line (Fig. 29.2a). Such surgery can again be undertaken under either local or general anaesthesia, with most young people preferring the latter for both comfort and psychosocial reasons. The area is infiltrated with local anaesthetic for both vasospastic and hydrodissection effects around the circumference, below the nodule, and immediately below the nipple disc to facilitate transection of the tissue. The incision is completed through dermis, and the nipple then lifted free of the firm mass of tissue below it (Fig. 29.2b, c). The depth of remaining tissue beneath the nipple is subject to surgical preference, but it is important to recognise that there is usually no remaining 'normal' or non-breast disc involved tissue between the nipple and the pectoral fascial layer. If significant permanent long-term chest wall 'dishing' or concavity is to be avoided, then judiciously leaving a wafer of fibrous tissue beneath the nipple is helpful in preventing an abnormal appearance. The remaining nodule of tissue is circumscribed by

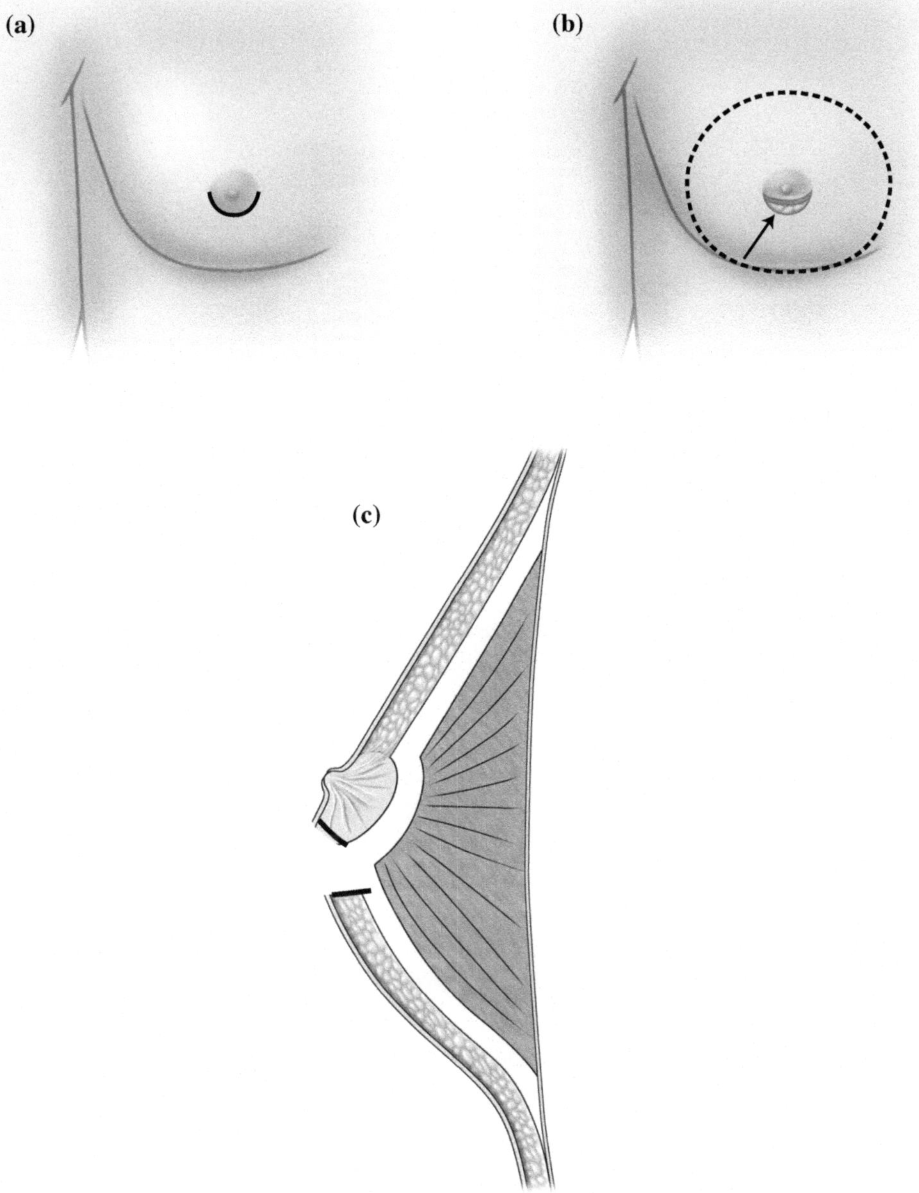

Fig. 29.2 **a** Simple local nodules (one or both sides) can be excised using carefully placed incisions in the inferior half of the circumareolar line. **b** The area is infiltrated with local anaesthetic for both vasospastic and hydrodissection effects around the circumference, below the nodule, and immediately below the nipple disc to facilitate transection of the tissue. **c** The incision is completed through dermis, and the nipple then lifted free of the firm mass of tissue below it

lifting the skin and subcutaneous fat away from its upper surface. Care should be exercised here as well to ensure that adequate normal subcutaneous fat remains to prevent further 'dishing'. The nodule is then grasped with tissue forceps and dissected free of the chest wall, starting at one

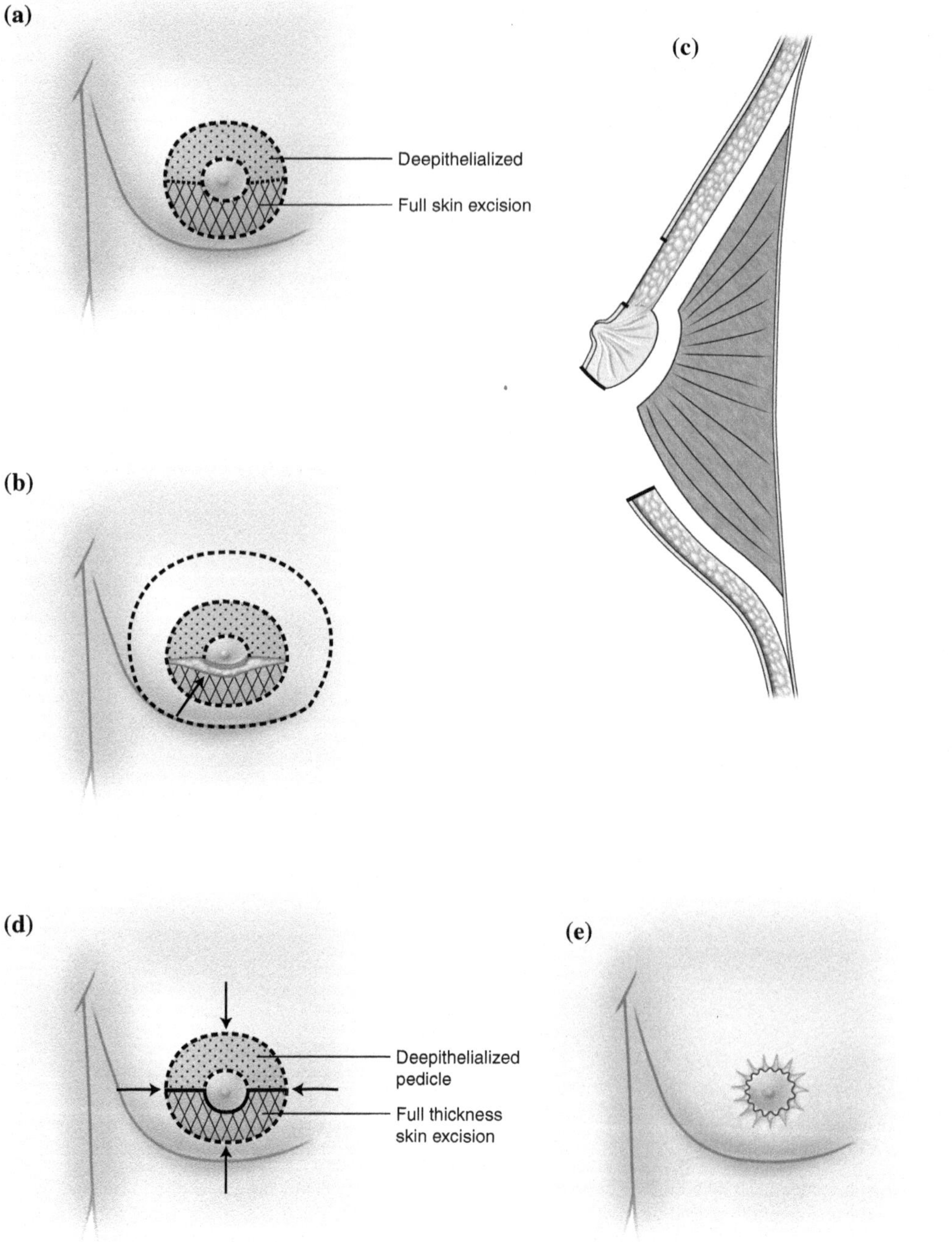
(a)
Deepithelialized
Full skin excision
(b)
(c)
(d)
Deepithelialized pedicle
Full thickness skin excision
(e)

◀ **Fig. 29.3** More major gynaecomastia requires better access than can be provided by the circumareolar incision. **a** A means of achieving this as well as reducing some of the excess skin envelope is to adopt an approach which mobilises the nipple–areolar complex on a de-epithelialised pedicle of skin around half of the circumference of a larger 'ring' of skin excision. **b** and **c** This nipple and its 'carrier' tissue is then lifted free of the underlying breast tissue, and preserved throughout the remaining excisional stage of the procedure. **d** Closure of this wound then involves matching the outer, and wider, ring of the margin of skin excision to the inner nipple–areolar ring. **e** The 'mismatch' in length of these two rings is dealt with by 'concertina-ing' the skin edges together, with the full knowledge that the wrinkling or 'pleating' effect at the wound edges will subsequently flatten and become barely perceptible with time

peripheral border. Full and careful haemostasis throughout the procedure offers the best hope of avoidance of post-operative haematoma formation —one of the most commonly encountered adverse sequelae of this site of surgery and encountered in up to a third of patients treated conventionally. Following excision, meticulous haemostasis, and saline washout of the cavity, the incision is closed with subcutaneous absorbable suture to avoid external 'tell tale' suture marks. The cavity is frequently drained and a small pressure dressing can assist in preventing early post-operative seroma or haematoma development.

Concentric Ring Approach for Larger Excision

More major gynaecomastia requires better access than can be provided by the circumareolar incision. A means of achieving this as well as reducing some of the excess skin envelope is to adopt an approach which mobilises the nipple–areolar complex on a de-epithelialised pedicle of skin around half of the circumference of a larger 'ring' of skin excision (Fig. 29.3a–e). This nipple and its 'carrier' tissue is then lifted free of the underlying breast tissue, and preserved throughout the remaining excisional stage of the procedure. The increased access that this approach offers enables even a breast of considerable volume to be completely removed from the chest wall. Full haemostasis can be obtained under direct vision, and the cavity washed out thoroughly before inserting vacuum drains and closure.

Closure of this wound then involves matching the outer, and wider, ring of the margin of skin excision to the inner nipple–areolar ring (Fig. 29.3d). The 'mismatch' in length of these two rings is dealt with by 'concertina-ing' the skin edges together, with the full knowledge that the wrinkling or 'pleating' effect at the wound edges will subsequently flatten and become barely perceptible with time (Fig. 29.3e). The huge advantage of this method is the complete avoidance of any large transverse or inferior scars across the chest wall, which carry such stigma for the patient who then has to bear them for the rest of his life. Using this method, the senior author has never had to resort to the more disfiguring approaches, even in massively enlarged male breasts, and such severe scar inducing techniques should be all but relegated to the history books. Confirmation of the value and success of such surgical methods is demonstrated by the widespread adoption of similar procedures for managing the female hypertrophied breast.

Psychosocial Considerations

Gynaecomastia is a breast disease with a strong impact on men, especially during the pubertal phase. There is a high prevalence and a need to accurately identify the cause. Treatment varies according to the cause, but correction of excessive breast tissue is surgical.

Body deformities may cause limitations and interfere in the emotional and social aspects of the patient's life. Surgical treatment can afford positive changes in patients' lives but each case must be considered, counselled, and consented preoperatively to ensure that expectations of what can be achieved by surgery are realistic [8, 46].

References

1. Braunstein GD. Gynaecomastia. N Eng J Med. 2007;357(12):1229–37.
2. Braunstein GD. Epidemiology and pathogenesis of gynaecomastia. 2010. www.uptodate.com/online/content.
3. Johnson RE, Murad MH. Gynaecomastia: pathophysiology, evaluation, and management. Mayo Clin Proc. 2009;84(11):1010–5.
4. Abaci A, Buyukgebiz A. Gynaecomastia: review. Pediatr Endocrinol Rev. 2007;5:489–99.
5. Narula HS, Carlson HE. Gynaecomastia. Endocrinol Metab Clin N Am. 2007;36:497–519.
6. American Society of Plastic Surgeons. Practice parameters: gynaecomastia. 2004. www.plasticsurgery.org/Documents/Medical_Profesionals/Gynecomastia.
7. Moore MP. Male breast cancer. In: Harris JR, Lippman ME, Morrow M, Hellman S, editors. Diseases of the breast. Philadelphia: Lippincott-Raven; 1996. p. 859.
8. Davanco RAS, Sabino Neto M, Garcia EB. Quality of life in the surgical treatment of gynaecomastia. Aesthetic Plast Surg. 2009;33(4):514–7.
9. Wassersug RJ, Oliffe JL. The social context for psychological distress from iatrogenic gynaecomastia with suggestions for its management. J Sex Med. 2009;6(4):989–1000.
10. Nordt CA, DiVasta AD. Gynaecomastia in adolescents. Curr Opin Paediatr. 2008;20(4):375–82.
11. Georgiadis E, Papandreou L, Evangelopoulou C, et al. Incidence of gynaecomastia in 954 young males and its relationshipto somatometric parameters. Ann Hum Biol. 1994;21(6):579–87.
12. Niewoehner CB, Nuttal FQ. Gynaecomastia in a hospitalised male population. Am J Med. 1984;77 (4):633–8.
13. McKiernan JF, Hull D. Breast development in the newborn. Arch Dis Child. 1981;56(7):525–9.
14. Kumanov P, Deepinder F, Robeva R, et al. Relationship of adolescent gynaecomastia with varicocele. J Adolesc Health. 2007;41:126–31.
15. Williams MJ. Gynaecomastia. Its incidence, recognition and host characterisation in 447 autopsy cases. Am J Med. 1963;34:103.
16. Nuttal FQ. Gynaecomastia as a physical finding in normal men. J Clin Endocrinol Metab. 1979;48:338.
17. Carlson HE. Gynaecomastia. N Eng J Med. 1980;303:795.
18. Bembo SA, Carlson HE. Gynaecomastia: its features, and when and how to treat it. Cleveland Clin J Med. 2004;71(6):511–7.
19. Ma NS, Geffner ME. Gynaecomastia in prepubertal and pubertal boys. Curr Opin Paediatr. 2008;20 (4):465–70.
20. Braunstein GD. Causes and evaluation of gynaecomastia. 2010. www.uptodate.com/online/content.
21. Eckman A, Dobs A. Drug-induced gynaecomastia. Expert Opin Drug Safety. 2008;7(6):691–702.
22. Smals AG. Gynaecomastia. Neth J Med. 1987;31:47.
23. Swerdloff RS, Wang C. Androgen deficiency and aging in men. Western J. Med. 1993; 159:579–585
24. Czajka-Oraniec I, Zgliczynski W, Kurylowicz A, et al. Association between gynaecomastia and aromatase polymorphisms. Eur J Endocrinol. 2008;158:721–7.
25. Berkovitz GD, Guerami A, Brown TR, et al. Famalial gynaecomastia with increased extraglandular aromatisation of plasma C19-steroids. J Clin Invest. 1985;75:1763.
26. Rose LI, Underwood RH, Newmark SR, et al. Pathophysiology of spironolactone-induced gynaecomastia. Ann Intern Med. 1977;87:398.
27. Grosso DS, Boyden TW, Pamenter RW, et al. Ketoconazole inhibition of testicular secretion of testosterone and displacement of steroid hormones from serum transport proteins. Antimicrob Agents Chemother. 1983;23:207.
28. Wilson JD, Aiman J, MacDonald PC. The pathogenesis of gynaecomastia. Adv Intern Med. 1980;25:1.
29. Weinstein RL, Kelch RP, Jenner MR, et al. Secretion of unconjugated androgens and oestrogens by the normal and abnormal human testis before and after human chorionic gonadotrophin. J Clin Invest. 1974;53:1.
30. Pensler JM, Merle JY. Gynaecomastia. 2009. www.emedicine.medscape.com/article/1273437-overview.
31. Andersen JA, Gram JB. Gynaecomastia: histological aspects in a surgical material. Acta Pathol Microbiol Immunol Scand. 1982;90:185.
32. Nicolis GL, Modlinger RS, Gabrilove JL. A study of the histopathology of human gynaecomastia. J ClinEndocrinol Metab. 1971;32:173.
33. Hammond DC. Surgical correction of gynaecomastia. Plast Reconstr Surg. 2009;124(SUPPL): 61e–8e.
34. Gikas P, Mokbel K. Management of gynaecomastia: an update. Int J Clin Pract. 2007;61(7):1209–15.
35. Cordova A, Moschella F. Alogrithm for clinical evaluation and surgical treatment of gynaecomastia. J Plast Reconstr Aesthet Surg. 2008;61(1):41–9.
36. Buckle R. Danazol therapy in gynaecomastia. Postgrad Med J. 1979;55(5):71–8.
37. Zachmann M, Eiholzer U, Muritano M, et al. Treatment of pubertal gynaecomastia with testolactone. Acta Endocrinol Suppl (Copenh). 1986;279:218–26.
38. Plourde PV, Kulin HE, Santner SJ. Clomiphene in the treatment of adolescent gynaecomastia. Am J Dis Child. 1983;137:1080–2.
39. Lawrence SE, Faught KA, Vethamuthu J, et al. Beneficial effects of raloxifene and tamoxifen in the treatment of pubertal gynaecomastia. J Pediatr. 2004;145:71–6.
40. Parker LN, Gray DR, Lai MK, et al. Treatment of gynaecomastia with tamoxifen: a double-blind crossover study. Metabolism. 1986;35:705.

41. McDermott MT, Hofeldt FD, Kidds GS. Tamoxifen therapy for painful idiopathic gynaecomastia. South Med J. 1990;83:1283.
42. Plourde PV, Reiter EO, Jou HC, et al. Safety and efficacy of anastrozole for the treatment of pubertal gynaecomastia. J Clin Endocrinol Metab. 2004;89:4428–33.
43. Dicker AP. The safety and tolerability of low-dose irradiation for the management of gynaecomastia caused by antiandrogen monotherapy. Lancet Oncol. 2004;4:30.
44. Perdona S, Autorino R, Battaglia M, et al. Efficacy of tamoxifen and radiotherapy for prevention and treatment of gynaecomastia and breast pain caused by bicalutamide in prostate cancer: a randomised controlled trial. Lancet Oncol. 2005;6:295.
45. Malata C, Rabey N. Surgery for gynaecomastia. In: Association of Breast Surgery Year Book; 2011. p. 72–76.
46. Ridha H, Colville RJI, Vesely MJJ. How happy are patients with their gynaecomastia surgery. J Plast Reconstr Aesthet Surg. 2009;62(11):1473–8.

Part VIII
Miscellaneous

30 Multiple Endocrine Neoplasia Type 1 and Type 4

Gerard V. Walls

Multiple endocrine neoplasia (MEN) syndromes are autosomal dominant disorders characterised by the combined occurrence of tumours involving two or more endocrine glands, and are categorised into four types (Fig. 30.1). Multiple endocrine neoplasia type 1 (MEN1 or Wermer) syndrome patients develop synchronous or metachronous neuroendocrine tumours (NETs) of the endocrine pancreas and anterior pituitary, with parathyroid and adrenocortical tumours [1, 2] due to germline inactivating mutations of the *MEN1* tumour suppressor gene that encodes Menin [3]. Multiple endocrine neoplasia type 2 (MEN2 or Sipple's) syndrome, is an autosomal dominant disorder characterised by the combined occurrence of medullary thyroid carcinoma (MTC) and adrenal medullary pheochromocytomas [4], due to activating germline mutations of the *RET* proto-oncogene that encodes a transmembrane tyrosine kinase receptor [5, 6]. Although MEN1 and MEN2 usually occur as distinct syndromes, tumours that are associated with both syndromes may occasionally develop in some patients [7]. For example, patients suffering from pancreatic NETs and pheochromocytoma, or from acromegaly and pheochromocytoma have been described, and MEN in these patients may represent an "overlap" syndrome. Recently, a new MEN syndrome was identified, designated MEN type 4, in which patients develop parathyroid and anterior pituitary tumours due to mutations in the *CDKN1B* gene that encodes p27, a cyclin-dependent kinase inhibitor that regulates the transition of cells from G_1 to S phase of the cell cycle [8]. To date, 13 germline *CDKN1B* mutations have been reported in patients with an MEN1-like phenotype, but who do not have *MEN1* mutations [9–11]. Finally, the Hyperparathyroidism-Jaw Tumour syndrome is another possible autosomal dominant MEN syndrome that is characterised by the occurrence of parathyroid adenomas and carcinomas, ossifying jaw fibromas, uterine and renal tumours, and associated tumours of the thyroid, testis and pancreas, due to inactivating mutations of the Cell Division Cycle 73 (*CDC73*) gene that encodes Parafibromin [12].

Multiple Endocrine Neoplasia Type 1 (MEN1)

Clinical Features

Patients with MEN1 develop parathyroid (95%), pancreatic islet (80%) and pituitary (30%) tumours (Fig. 30.1) [7]. A number of other syndromic tumours occur and include cutaneous angiofibromas (88%) and collagenomas (72%), adrenal cortical tumours (35%), multiple lipomas (33%), foregut carcinoids (15%), meningiomas (<10%) and facial ependymomas (<5%) [13, 14]. A progression of tumour development from hyperplasia

G.V. Walls (✉)
Royal Lancaster Infirmary, University Hospitals of Morecambe Bay NHS Foundation Trust, Ashton Road, Lancaster LA1 4RP, UK
e-mail: gerard.walls@nds.ox.ac.uk; gerard.walls@ndm.ox.ac.uk

D.J. Ledbetter and P.R.V. Johnson (eds.), *Endocrine Surgery in Children*,
DOI 10.1007/978-3-662-54256-9_30

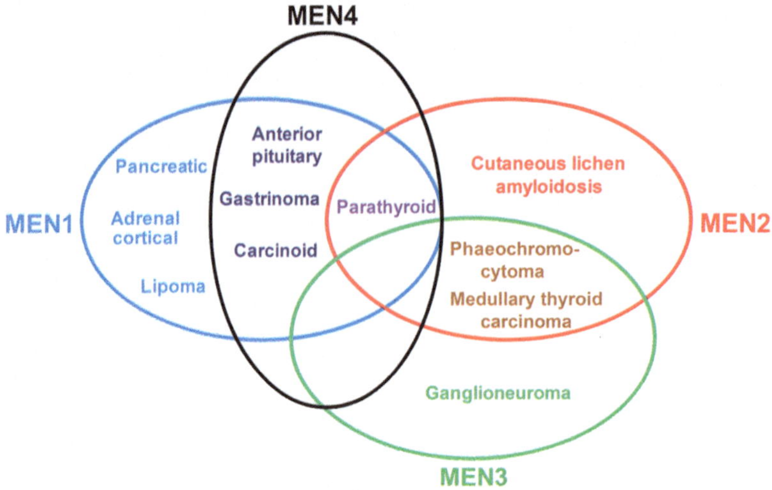

Fig. 30.1 MEN syndromes and their associated tumours. Multiple endocrine neoplasia type 1 (*MEN1*) is characterised by the combined occurrence of anterior pituitary, pancreatic islet and parathyroid tumours; MEN type 2A (*MEN2*) by parathyroid, medullary thyroid and adrenal medullary tumours; MEN type 2B (*MEN3*) by medullary thyroid, adrenal medulla and neuroma tumours; and MEN type 4 (*MEN4*) by anterior pituitary, gastroenteric neuroendocrine and parathyroid tumours

to adenoma to carcinomas occurs in MEN1 patients [1]. The prevalence of MEN1 in the UK was estimated to be ~10 per 100,000 of the population, with an equal sex distribution [15]. Amongst the pancreatic NETs, over half are gastrinomas, a third are insulinomas, and <5% are glucagonomas, vasoactive intestinal peptide (VIP)-omas or pancreatic polypeptide (PP)-omas; and amongst the pituitary NETs, two thirds are prolactinomas, a quarter are somatotrophinomas, ~5% are adrenocorticotrophinomas, and ~5% are non-functioning adenomas [15]. MEN1 has a high degree of penetrance, such that >95% of patients develop clinical symptoms by the fifth decade [15], and children as young as 5 years old have been found to have MEN1-associated tumours [16, 17]. However, most MEN1-associated tumours develop after 10 years of age [18].

Diagnosis and Treatments of MEN1-Associated Tumours

Parathyroid Tumours

Primary hyperparathyroidism is the commonest and first manifestation of MEN1 and occurs from ~20 years of age in MEN1 patients [7]. Children with primary hyperparathyroidism may often have MEN1 [19]. Patients have hypercalcaemia, hypophosphataemia and a raised or inappropriately normal parathyroid hormone (PTH) level, with normal or increased 24 h urinary calcium excretion [1]. This is often asymptomatic and discovered on biochemical screening, but patients may also present with nephrolithiasis, peptic ulceration, polyuria, polydipsia, constipation and fatigue [7]. Surgery is the treatment of choice for primary hyperparathyroidism. Subtotal (leaving half of the smallest parathyroid gland) or total parathyroidectomy with transcervical near-total thymectomy is the recommended treatment [3, 20]. Parathyroid autotransplantation may be considered, but parathyroidectomy for hyperparathyroidism in MEN1 is associated with a high failure rate, including an image-guided approach in children with MEN1 [21], with recurrent hypercalcaemia in ~50% within a decade of surgery [22]. Randomised controlled trials in MEN1 patients are lacking and guidelines are mainly based on expert opinion [3].

Pancreatic Islet Neuroendocrine Tumours (Nets)

Pancreatic islet NETs are the second commonest manifestation of MEN1, occurring in up to 80% of patients [15]. These tumours are discussed in detail in Chap. 13.

Anterior Pituitary NETs

Anterior pituitary tumours occur in 30–50% of MEN1 patients, with a higher incidence in female patients [23]. The clinical manifestations are related to hypersecretion of anterior pituitary hormones, or from compression of adjacent structures by an enlarging tumour, such as bitemporal hemianopia from compression of the optic chiasm, or hypopituitarism from compression of adjacent normal pituitary. Prolactinomas are the commonest pituitary tumour (~60% of pituitary NETs in MEN1 patients) and the excess prolactin secretion from lactotrophs results in secondary amenorrhea, infertility and galactorrhoea in female patients, and impotence in male patients [15]. Somatotrophinomas (~25%) secrete growth hormone from somatotrophs resulting in acromegaly. Least common amongst pituitary NETs in MEN1 patients are non-functioning adenomas (~5%) and adrenocorticotrophinomas (~5%), which secrete adrenocorticotrophic hormone (ACTH) and cause Cushing's disease [15]. Diagnosis relies on biochemical testing for prolactin and insulin-like growth factor-1 with magnetic resonance imaging (MRI) of the pituitary fossa. Treatment of pituitary NETs is often with dopamine agonists such as bromocriptine or cabergoline for prolactinomas, somatostatin analogues for somatotrophinomas [24] or transphenoidal hypophysectomy for enlarging tumours causing mass effects [25]. Radiotherapy is available for inoperable or recurrent tumours.

Adrenal Cortical Tumours

Cortical adrenal tumours occur in 10–30% of MEN1 patients [26]. Most adrenal tumours in MEN1 patients are benign and non-functioning, and since the prevalence of adrenal tumours is ~5% in the general population, only MEN1 patients with adrenal tumours >4 cm in diameter should be assessed for adrenalectomy, as the risk of malignant transformation increases with adrenal size [14, 27]. Adrenal tumours in MEN1 may be hyperplastic, cystic, cortical adenomas, or carcinomas [28]. However, functioning adrenocortical tumours in patients with MEN1 cause hypercortisolaemia (Cushing's syndrome) and primary hyperaldosteronism (Conn's syndrome), which necessitate adrenalectomy [14].

Thymic, Bronchopulmonary and Gastric Nets

NETs of foregut origin occur in up to 15% of MEN1 patients and are located in the thymus, the respiratory tract and the upper gastrointestinal tract [29]. Thymic NETs are particularly aggressive in male MEN1 patients and account for significantly increased mortality [23]. Tumours may be asymptomatic and metastases may be associated with symptoms of the carcinoid syndrome (facial flushing, bronchospasm and intractable diarrhoea). Curative surgery, where possible, is the treatment of choice for thymic and bronchial carcinoid tumours. Where disease is advanced and inoperable, additional therapies include somatostatin analogues, radiotherapy and chemotherapy, but prognosis remains poor for advanced tumours [30].

Treatment of NETs in Patients with MEN1 Versus NETs in Sporadic Patients

Treatment for NETs in MEN1 patients, which include pancreatic islet NETs, anterior pituitary NETs and foregut carcinoids, is more difficult than for equivalent tumours in non-MEN1 (sporadic) patients for several reasons [31]. First, MEN1 tumours, with the exception of anterior pituitary NETs, are multiple. For example, multiple submucosal duodenal and pancreatic gastrinomas develop in MEN1 patients, thereby reducing surgical cure rates, such that at 5 years ~5% in MEN1 patients, compared to ~40% in non-MEN1 patients were disease free [32]. Second, occult metastatic disease is more prevalent in MEN1 patients with NETs than in patients with sporadic endocrine tumours. For example, metastases are present in up to 50% of patients with MEN1-associated insulinomas, whereas <10% of non-MEN1 insulinomas metastasize [33]. Third, the majority (~80%) of NETs have low proliferation rates, with a Ki-67 index <2%, and may not respond to chemotherapy or radiotherapy. Fourth, NETs in MEN1 patients are larger, more aggressive, and resistant to treatment [31]. For example, ~85% of anterior pituitary NETs in MEN1 patients, as opposed to 64% in non-MEN1 patients are macroadenomas; ~30% of anterior pituitary NETs in MEN1 patients have invaded surrounding tissue, compared to 10% in non-MEN1 patients [34]; and >45% of anterior pituitary NETs in MEN1 patients had persistent hormonal over-secretion following appropriate medical, surgical and radiotherapy treatment, compared to 10–40% in non-MEN1 patients [35]. Thus, there is a clinical need for better and alternative treatments for NETs in MEN1 patients.

Molecular Genetics of MEN1

MEN1-associated tumours have loss of heterozygosity (LOH) for the *MEN1* gene located on chromosome 11q13 that encodes Menin [36, 37]. Germline mutations of the *MEN1* gene coding region are present in the majority (>90%) of patients with MEN1 and most of the *MEN1* mutations are inactivating, consistent with a tumour suppressor role for Menin [38]. The mutations are scattered throughout the 1830 base-pair (bp) coding region and splice sites of the *MEN1* gene, and there appears to be no genotype-phenotype correlation in MEN1, with members of the same pedigree developing different MEN1-associated tumours. Menin is an ubiquitously expressed nuclear protein that has been shown to have roles in transcriptional regulation; genome stability; cell division; proliferation; cell cycle control; and apoptosis [39, 40]. More recently, the three-dimentional structure of Menin has been solved and it has been shown that Menin is a molecular adaptor coordinating the functions of multiple proteins [41]. For example, Menin has been shown to regulate the expression of cyclin-dependent kinase inhibitors (p27 and p18) via MLL-1, thereby reducing cellular proliferation [42], and to induce caspase 8 expression that promotes apoptosis [39]. Thus, loss of menin function leads to endocrine tumourigenesis in MEN1 [1].

Mouse models with loss of *Men1* alleles that are representative of MEN1 in man have been developed to understand the molecular basis of tumourigenesis in MEN1 [43–45]. A conventional heterozygous knockout mouse model for MEN1 ($Men1^{+/-}$ knockout mice) [43] develops parathyroid, pancreatic islet, anterior pituitary and adrenal cortical tumours, associated with an increased mortality of 30%. Accurate assessment of proliferation and apoptosis rates in these MEN1 knockout mice have been investigated to understand MEN1-associated neuroendocrine tumourigenesis [46]. Using this data, mathematical modelling of NET growth rates (proliferation minus apoptotic rates) predicted that in $Men1^{+/-}$ mice, only pancreatic β-cells, pituitary lactotrophs and somatotrophs could develop into tumours within a murine lifespan. $Men1^{+/-}$ tumours had low proliferation rates (<2%), second-order growth kinetics, and the higher occurrence of insulinomas, prolactinomas and somatotrophinomas in MEN1 was consistent with a mathematical model for NET proliferation [46]. Translational studies of gene replacement therapy in $Men1^{+/-}$ mice generated menin expression in anterior pituitary tumours, and significantly reduced tumour cellullar proliferation. It demonstrated proof of concept for *MEN1* gene replacement therapy for inhibiting NET growth in MEN1 [44]. The development of such *MEN1* gene therapy is likely to be of use in MEN1 patients for the treatment of anterior pituitary, pancreatic islet and thymic NETs. Finally, evaluation of a new somatostatin analogue, pasireotide, was shown in conditional $Men1^{+/-}$ mice to have anti-proliferative and pro-apoptotic effects in insulinomas [47] and in conventional *Men1*$^{+/-}$ mice increased survival by ~20%, inhibited tumour growth, and reduced the number and volume of pancreatic islet and anterior pituitary tumours, thereby indicating its potential use to treat pancreatic and pituitary NETs [48]. Thus, new treatments may be developed for MEN1 patients following these recent advances in pre-clinical science.

Multiple Endocrine Neoplasia Type 4

Clinical Features of the MEN4 Syndrome

MEN4 was only recently described, and patients develop parathyroid (81%) and anterior pituitary tumours (42%) [8, 9, 11, 49]. Patients may also develop gastric and bronchial carcinoids or gastrinomas that cause Zollinger-Ellison syndrome (Fig. 30.1). A recent case report described a possible association with meningioma and papillary thyroid carcinoma in a patient with a rare *CDKN1B* gene variant [50]. MEN4 patients harbour heterozygous mutations in the *CDKN1B* tumour suppressor gene that encodes a cyclin-dependent kinase inhibitor, p27, which is involved in cellular proliferation. Parathyroid tumours have developed from 46 years of age, and pituitary tumours from 30 years old in MEN4 patients. Cases in children may be identified in known MEN4 families with genetic and biochemical screening and radiological follow-up.

Diagnosis and Treatments of MEN4-Associated Tumours

Parathyroid Tumours

Primary hyperparathyroidism occurred in 10 of 12 index MEN4 patients and parathyroidectomy was curative. Standard pre-operative localisation of symptomatic patients with concordant sestamibi and ultrasound studies permited minimally invasive parathyroidectomy in this situation [51]. No evidance of parathyroid malignancy has been described.

Anterior Pituitary NETs

In 5 of 12 index MEN4 cases, anterior pituitary tumours developed. Two patients had clinical features of acromegaly due to somatotrophinomas, one had a prolactinoma, one had Cushing's disease due to a corticotrophinoma, and one patient had a non-functioning tumour. Transsphenoidal surgery is the treatment of choice for pituitary adenomas, but is not always curative. Prolactinomas can be successfully treated with dopamine agonists, and radiotherapy may be used after surgical treatment in recurrent disease. In one MEN4 patient with a somatotrophinoma, there was local invasion, cellular atypia and a high mitotic index, indicating an aggressive tumour. However, until more cases are described, expert multidisciplinary team management is recommended.

Molecular Genetics of MEN4

MEN4 patients have inactivating mutations in the *CDKN1B* gene located on chromosome 12p13 and its 2 exons encodes a 196 amino acid cyclin-dependent kinase inhibitor referred to as p27 [8]. So far, 12 *CDKN1B* mutations have been described that are located throughout the gene and its promotor region. Furthermore, somatic mutations of *CDKN1B* have been reported in sporadic parathyroid adenomas [52]. P27 is an ubiquitously expressed nuclear protein of the cyclin-dependent kinase inhibitor family. It regulates cell cycle progression from G1 to S phase by inactivating cyclin A/E cyclin-dependent kinase (CDK) 2 complexes, so that cell division is blocked. Phosphorylation of p27 enables its export from the nucleus for cytoplasmic ubiquitination and degradation by the proteosome. Inactivating mutations of *CDKN1B* in MEN4: reduce the cellular expression of p27; alter its intracellular location; or disrupt its ability to interact with partners such as CDK2. Syndromic tumours have reduction or loss of p27 expression, indicating that loss of the tumour suppressor function of p27 causes tumourigenesis in MEN4 patients.

Conclusions

In summary, MEN syndrome types 1 and 4 are autosomal dominant disorders characterised by different combinations of pancreatic islet, anterior pituitary, parathyroid and adrenal tumours due to germline mutations of the *MEN1* and *CDKN1B* genes, which encode Menin and p27, respectively. Surgery is the principle treatment for symptomatic tumours in MEN1 and MEN4 patients, and biochemical and genetic screening of family members enables early detection of tumours to optimise individual MEN patient care.

References

1. Thakker RV. Multiple endocrine neoplasia type 1 (MEN1). Best Pract Res Clin Endocrinol Metab. 2010;24(3):355–70.
2. Newey PJ, Thakker RV. Role of multiple endocrine neoplasia type 1 mutational analysis in clinical practice. Endocr Pract. 2011;17(Suppl 3):8–17.
3. Thakker RV, Newey PJ, Walls GV, Bilezikian J, Dralle H, Ebeling PR, et al. Clinical practice guidelines for multiple endocrine neoplasia type 1 (MEN1). J Clin Endocrinol Metab. 2012;97(9):2990–3011.
4. Wells SA, Pacini F, Robinson BG, Santoro M. Multiple endocrine neoplasia type 2 and familial medullary thyroid carcinoma: an update. J Clin Endocrinol Metab. 2013;98(8):3149–64.
5. Margraf RL, Crockett DK, Krautscheid PM, Seamons R, Calderon FR, Wittwer CT, et al. Multiple endocrine neoplasia type 2 RET protooncogene database: repository of MEN2-associated RET sequence variation and reference for genotype/phenotype correlations. Hum Mutat. 2009;30(4):548–56.
6. Lakhani VT, You YN, Wells SA. The multiple endocrine neoplasia syndromes. Annu Rev Med. 2007;58:253–65.
7. Thakker R. Multiple endocrine neoplasia type 1. In: DeGroot L, Jameson J, editors. Endocrinology: adult and pediatric, vol. 1–2. 6th ed. Philadelphia: Elsevier Saunders; 2010. p. 2719–41.
8. Pellegata NS, Quintanilla-Martinez L, Siggelkow H, Samson E, Bink K, Hofler H, et al. Germ-line mutations in p27Kip1 cause a multiple endocrine neoplasia syndrome in rats and humans. Proc Natl Acad Sci U S A. 2006;103(42):15558–63.
9. Marinoni I, Pellegata NS. p27kip1: a new multiple endocrine neoplasia gene? Neuroendocrinology. 2011;93(1):19–28.
10. Molatore S, Marinoni I, Lee M, Pulz E, Ambrosio MR, degli Uberti EC, et al. A novel germline CDKN1B mutation causing multiple endocrine tumors: clinical, genetic and functional characterization. Hum Mutat. 2010;31(11):E1825–35.
11. Lee M, Pellegata NS. Multiple endocrine neoplasia syndromes associated with mutation of p27. J Endocrinol Invest. 2013;36(9):781–7.
12. Newey PJ, Bowl MR, Cranston T, Thakker RV. Cell division cycle protein 73 homolog (CDC73) mutations in the hyperparathyroidism-jaw tumor syndrome (HPT-JT) and parathyroid tumors. Hum Mutat. 2010;31(3):295–307.
13. Xia Y, Darling TN. Rapidly growing collagenomas in multiple endocrine neoplasia type I. J Am Acad Dermatol. 2007;56(5):877–80.
14. Waldmann J, Bartsch DK, Kann PH, Fendrich V, Rothmund M, Langer P. Adrenal involvement in multiple endocrine neoplasia type 1: results of 7 years prospective screening. Langenbecks Arch Surg. 2007;392(4):437–43.
15. Trump D, Farren B, Wooding C, Pang JT, Besser GM, Buchanan KD, et al. Clinical studies of multiple endocrine neoplasia type 1 (MEN1). QJM. 1996;89(9):653–69.
16. Newey PJ, Jeyabalan J, Walls GV, Christie PT, Gleeson FV, Gould S, et al. Asymptomatic children with multiple endocrine neoplasia type 1 mutations may harbor nonfunctioning pancreatic neuroendocrine tumors. J Clin Endocrinol Metab. 2009;94(10):3640–6.
17. Farrell WE, Azevedo MF, Batista DL, Smith A, Bourdeau I, Horvath A, et al. Unique gene expression profile associated with an early-onset multiple endocrine neoplasia (MEN1)-associated pituitary adenoma. J Clin Endocrinol Metab. 2011;96(11):E1905–14.
18. Goudet P, Dalac A, Le Bras M, Cardot-Bauters C, Niccoli P, Lévy-Bohbot N, et al. MEN1 disease occurring before 21 years old: a 160-patient cohort study from the Groupe d'étude des Tumeurs Endocrines. J Clin Endocrinol Metab. 2015;100(4):1568–77.
19. Romero Arenas MA, Morris LF, Rich TA, Cote GJ, Grubbs EG, Waguespack SG, et al. Preoperative multiple endocrine neoplasia type 1 diagnosis improves the surgical outcomes of pediatric patients with primary hyperparathyroidism. J Pediatr Surg. 2014;49(4):546–50.
20. Nilubol N, Weinstein LS, Simonds WF, Jensen RT, Marx SJ, Kebebew E. limited parathyroidectomy in multiple endocrine neoplasia type 1-associated primary hyperparathyroidism: a setup for failure. Ann Surg Oncol. 2016;23(2):416–23.
21. Langusch CC, Norlen O, Titmuss A, Donoghue K, Holland AJ, Shun A, et al. Focused image-guided parathyroidectomy in the current management of primary hyperparathyroidism. Arch Dis Child. 2015;100(10):924–7.

22. Goudet P, Cougard P, Verges B, Murat A, Carnaille B, Calender A, et al. Hyperparathyroidism in multiple endocrine neoplasia type I: surgical trends and results of a 256-patient series from Groupe D'etude des Neoplasies Endocriniennes Multiples Study Group. World J Surg. 2001;25(7):886–90.
23. Goudet P, Bonithon-Kopp C, Murat A, Ruszniewski P, Niccoli P, Ménégaux F, et al. Gender-related differences in MEN1 lesion occurrence and diagnosis: a cohort study of 734 cases from the Groupe d'etude des Tumeurs Endocrines. Eur J Endocrinol. 2011;165(1):97–105.
24. Melmed S. Medical progress: acromegaly. N Engl J Med. 2006;355(24):2558–73.
25. Sztal-Mazer S, Topliss DJ, Simpson RW, Hamblin PS, Rosenfeld JV, McLean CA. Gonadotroph adenoma in multiple endocrine neoplasia type 1. Endocr Pract. 2008;14(5):592–4.
26. Gatta-Cherifi B, Chabre O, Murat A, Niccoli P, Cardot-Bauters C, Rohmer V, et al. Adrenal involvement in MEN1. Analysis of 715 cases from the Groupe d'etude des Tumeurs Endocrines database. Eur J Endocrinol. 2012;166(2):269–79.
27. Zeiger MA, Siegelman SS, Hamrahian AH. Medical and surgical evaluation and treatment of adrenal incidentalomas. J Clin Endocrinol Metab. 2011;96 (7):2004–15.
28. Schaefer S, Shipotko M, Meyer S, Ivan D, Klose KJ, Waldmann J, et al. Natural course of small adrenal lesions in multiple endocrine neoplasia type 1: an endoscopic ultrasound imaging study. Eur J Endocrinol. 2008;158(5):699–704.
29. Faggiano A, Ferolla P, Grimaldi F, Campana D, Manzoni M, Davì MV, et al. Natural history of gastro-entero-pancreatic and thoracic neuroendocrine tumors. Data from a large prospective and retrospective Italian Epidemiological study: The NET management study. J Endocrinol Invest. 2011.
30. Goudet P, Murat A, Cardot-Bauters C, Emy P, Baudin E, du Boullay Choplin H, et al. Thymic neuroendocrine tumors in multiple endocrine neoplasia type 1: a comparative study on 21 cases among a series of 761 MEN1 from the GTE (Groupe des Tumeurs Endocrines). World J Surg. 2009;33 (6):1197–207.
31. Beckers A, Betea D, Valdes Socin H, Stevenaert A. The treatment of sporadic versus MEN1-related pituitary adenomas. J Intern Med. 2003;253 (6):599–605.
32. Bartsch DK, Fendrich V, Langer P, Celik I, Kann PH, Rothmund M. Outcome of duodenopancreatic resections in patients with multiple endocrine neoplasia type 1. Ann Surg. 2005;242(6):757–64, discussion 64–6.
33. Akerstrom G, Hellman P. Surgery on neuroendocrine tumours. Best Pract Res Clin Endocrinol Metab. 2007;21(1):87–109.
34. Wu ZB, Su ZP, Wu JS, Zheng WM, Zhuge QC, Zhong M. Five years follow-up of invasive prolactinomas with special reference to the control of cavernous sinus invasion. Pituitary. 2008;11(1):63–70.
35. Qu X, Wang M, Wang G, Han T, Mou C, Han L, et al. Surgical outcomes and prognostic factors of transsphenoidal surgery for prolactinoma in men: a single-center experience with 87 consecutive cases. Eur J Endocrinol. 2011;164(4):499–504.
36. Lemmens I, Van de Ven WJ, Kas K, Zhang CX, Giraud S, Wautot V, et al. Identification of the multiple endocrine neoplasia type 1 (MEN1) gene. The European Consortium on MEN1. Hum Mol Genet. 1997;6(7):1177–83.
37. Chandrasekharappa SC, Guru SC, Manickam P, Olufemi SE, Collins FS, Emmert-Buck MR, et al. Positional cloning of the gene for multiple endocrine neoplasia-type 1. Science. 1997;276(5311):404–7.
38. Lemos MC, Thakker RV. Multiple endocrine neoplasia type 1 (MEN1): analysis of 1336 mutations reported in the first decade following identification of the gene. Hum Mutat. 2008;29(1):22–32.
39. La P, Yang Y, Karnik SK, Silva AC, Schnepp RW, Kim SK, et al. Menin-mediated caspase 8 expression in suppressing multiple endocrine neoplasia type 1. J Biol Chem. 2007;282(43):31332–40.
40. Schnepp RW, Chen YX, Wang H, Cash T, Silva A, Diehl JA, et al. Mutation of tumor suppressor gene Men1 acutely enhances proliferation of pancreatic islet cells. Cancer Res. 2006;66(11):5707–15.
41. Huang J, Gurung B, Wan B, Matkar S, Veniaminova NA, Wan K, et al. The same pocket in menin binds both MLL and JUND but has opposite effects on transcription. Nature. 2012;482 (7386):542–6.
42. Milne TA, Hughes CM, Lloyd R, Yang Z, Rozenblatt-Rosen O, Dou Y, et al. Menin and MLL cooperatively regulate expression of cyclin-dependent kinase inhibitors. Proc Natl Acad Sci U S A. 2005;102(3):749–54.
43. Harding B, Lemos MC, Reed AA, Walls GV, Jeyabalan J, Bowl MR, et al. Multiple endocrine neoplasia type 1 knockout mice develop parathyroid, pancreatic, pituitary and adrenal tumours with hypercalcaemia, hypophosphataemia and hypercorticosteronaemia. Endocr Relat Cancer. 2009;16(4):1313–27.
44. Walls GV, Lemos MC, Javid M, Bazan-Peregrino M, Jeyabalan J, Reed AA, et al. MEN1 gene replacement therapy reduces proliferation rates in a mouse model of pituitary adenomas. Cancer Res. 2012;72 (19):5060–8.
45. Piret SE, Thakker RV. Mouse models for inherited endocrine and metabolic disorders. J Endocrinol. 2011;211(3):211–30.
46. Walls GV, Reed AA, Jeyabalan J, Javid M, Hill NR, Harding B, et al. Proliferation rates of multiple endocrine neoplasia type 1 (MEN1)-associated tumors. Endocrinology. 2012;153(11):5167–79.
47. Quinn TJ, Yuan Z, Adem A, Geha R, Vrikshajanani C, Koba W, et al. Pasireotide (SOM230) is effective for the treatment of pancreatic

neuroendocrine tumors (PNETs) in a multiple endocrine neoplasia type 1 (MEN1) conditional knockout mouse model. Surgery. 2012;152 (6):1068–77.
48. Walls GV, Stevenson M, Soukup B, Lines KE, Christie PT, Grossman AB, et al. Treatment with pasireotide, a somatostatin analogue, results in decreased proliferation and increased apoptosis in pancreatic and pituitary neuroendocrine tumors (NETs), in a mouse model for multiple endocrine neoplasia type 1 (MEN1). Endocr Rev. 2015;36(2): OR02–3.
49. Lee M, Pellegata NS. Multiple endocrine neoplasia type 4. Front Horm Res. 2013;41:63–78.
50. Bugalho MJ, Domingues R. Uncommon association of cerebral meningioma, parathyroid adenoma and papillary thyroid carcinoma in a patient harbouring a rare germline variant in the CDKN1B gene. BMJ Case Rep. 2016;. doi:10.1136/bcr-2015-213934.
51. Iacobone M, Carnaille B, Palazzo FF, Vriens M. Hereditary hyperparathyroidism-a consensus report of the European Society of Endocrine Surgeons (ESES). Langenbecks Arch Surg. 2015;400(8):867–86.
52. Costa-Guda J, Marinoni I, Molatore S, Pellegata NS, Arnold A. Somatic mutation and germline sequence abnormalities in CDKN1B, encoding p27Kip1, in sporadic parathyroid adenomas. J Clin Endocrinol Metab. 2011;96(4):E701–6.

Multiple Endocrine Neoplasia Type 2 31

Eduardo A. Perez and Michael Skinner

Multiple endocrine neoplasia (MEN) syndromes are rare autosomal dominant conditions which predispose affected individuals to benign and malignant tumors of the pituitary, thyroid, parathyroids, adrenals, endocrine pancreas, paraganglia, or occasionally nonendocrine organs. The classic MEN syndromes include MEN type 1 (MEN1) and MEN type 2 (MEN2).

Historically, the clinical presentation of MEN syndromes during childhood was rare and their diagnosis was based on family history. Today, thanks to advancements in genetic testing, MEN syndromes are being diagnosed more commonly in the pediatric population and may present challenging clinical management questions. This chapter will focus on the presentation and management of MEN2 in children.

Multiple endocrine neoplasia type 2 (MEN2) is an autosomal dominant disorder with an estimated prevalence of 2.5 per 100,000 in the general population. Males and females are nearly equally affected. MEN2 is often first suspected when a patient is found to have one or more of the uncommon tumors that are characteristic of the syndrome, usually medullary thyroid cancer, or when there is a family history of the same tumors, or a family history of MEN2. MEN2 is subclassified into three distinct syndromes: Multiple endocrine neoplasia type 2A (MEN2A), multiple endocrine neoplasia type 2B (MEN2B), and familial medullary thyroid cancer (FMTC). When a MEN2 kindred is identified, it is important that all family members be screened for early diagnosis, because medullary thyroid cancer can be cured or prevented by early thyroidectomy.

Multiple Endocrine Neoplasia 2A

Multiple endocrine neoplasia type 2A is a heritable predisposition to medullary thyroid cancer (MTC), pheochromocytoma (PHEO), and primary parathyroid hyperplasia (PHPT). MEN2A is the most common form of all MEN2 syndromes (55–90% of all cases) [1]. Over 90% of the patients with MEN2 develop medullary thyroid cancer, approximately 40–50% develop pheochromocytoma, and 10–20% develop multigland parathyroid hyperplasia. MTC is usually the first tumor to develop and is frequent in untreated children ages 10 years and younger [2, 3]. Most children with MEN2A have an affected parent. However, having a negative family history has to be interpreted with caution because the diagnosis of MTC in family members may be delayed until later in life [4]. Cutaneous lichen amyloidosis (CLA) is another

E.A. Perez
Division of Pediatric Surgery, The Dewitt Daughtry Family Department of Surgery, University of Miami, Miller School of Medicine, P.O. Box 016960 (R51), Miami, FL, USA
e-mail: Eperez3@med.miami.edu

M. Skinner (✉)
Department of Pediatric Surgery, University of Texas Southwestern Medical Center Children's Medical Center, 1935 Medical District Drive, Dallas, TX 75235, USA
e-mail: MICHAEL.SKINNER@childrens.com

D.J. Ledbetter and P.R.V. Johnson (eds.), *Endocrine Surgery in Children*,
DOI 10.1007/978-3-662-54256-9_31

component of the syndrome that has been described in families with the disease [5]. It can be present before the MTC, and the identification of this skin lesion should prompt an evaluation for MEN2A. Finally, a small number of families with MEN2A also have a higher risk of Hirschsprung's disease (HD) [6, 7].

Multiple Endocrine Neoplasia 2B

MEN2B shares with MEN2A the inherited predisposition to medullary thyroid cancer and pheochromocytoma but clinically significant parathyroid disease is absent. Other findings include mucosal neuromas, intestinal ganglioneuromas, and marfanoid habitus. MEN2B is the most uncommon form of MEN2 (5–10% of all cases) [8].

Medullary thyroid cancer is the most common feature of the MEN2B syndrome being present in 100% of patients. The MTC usually develops in the first several years of life [9], and is more aggressive than the MTC in MEN2A. For these reasons, early diagnosis is critical to prevent mortality and morbidity. Without prophylactic thyroidectomy at a young age, most patients with MEN2B develop metastatic MTC in childhood or adolescence [10].

The neuromas present in the tongue, lips, and eyelids with resulting characteristic facial features including enlarged lips, a "bumpy" tongue, and eversion of the eyelids [10]. The marfanoid body habitus is accompanied by increased joint mobility and decreased subcutaneous fat. Ganglioneuromatosis presents with thickening of the corneal nerves or in the gastrointestinal tract, resulting in abdominal distention, megacolon, constipation, or diarrhea. All these physical traits are usually evident in early childhood, and are sometimes present at birth.

Familial Medullary Thyroid Cancer

Familial medullary thyroid cancer (FMTC) is considered a type of MEN2A that has a strong predisposition to medullary thyroid cancer, without the other manifestations of the syndrome. It is the mildest variant of MEN2 and represents about 35–40% of all cases [1]. It can be hard to differentiate FMTC from MEN2A even in large kindreds. This potential pitfall in diagnosis is important because of the risk of missing a pheochromocytoma in a patient with MEN2 wrongly thought to have FMTC. Therefore, rigorous and strict criteria have been defined to identify a FMTC kindred [11]. These include, (1) having more than 10 carriers in the kindred, (2) multiple carriers or affected members being over the age of 50 years, and (3) an adequate medical history, particularly in older family members. It remains unclear why patients with FMTC do not develop pheochromocytomas and hyperparathyroidism, especially since many FMTC and MEN2A families carry identical RET mutations. Therefore screening for PHEO and PHPT should be done during the evaluation of these patients, because genetic testing alone cannot always predict the MEN2 phenotype and risk of developing associated tumors. MTC in FMTC families is usually less aggressive than the other MEN2 subtypes and presents at an older age [10].

Genetics

MEN2A, MEN2B, and FMTC are inherited in an autosomal dominant pattern with very high penetrance. The genetic defect in these disorders involves the RET proto-oncogene, on chromosome 10q11.2 [12]. The RET gene codes for a tyrosine kinase receptor that functions as a signal transducer upon interaction with the glial-derived neurotrophic factor family of ligands. Binding of these ligands induces dimerization of RET receptors, autophosphorylation of intracellular tyrosine residues, and ultimately cell growth and survival mediated by the mitogen-activated protein kinase intracellular signaling cascade [13]. Thus, all clinical manifestations of the MEN2 syndromes relate to a defect in transduction of growth and differentiation signals in several developing tissues that express RET, including those derived from the neural crest [14]. So far, mutation analysis in MEN2 families has identified over 50 different mutations related to the disease [15, 16].

Mutations causing FMTC and MEN2A occur predominantly in the extracellular domain cysteine residues (codons 609, 611, 618, 620, and 634) and lead to ligand independent dimerization of *RET*. Less common mutations occur in exon 13 (codons 790 and 791) [16, 17]. In contrast, MEN2B-related mutations are almost always located in the intracellular domain at codon 918 and lead to alteration of *RET* signal transduction [18]. Germline mutations in codons 768 (exon 13), 804 (exon 14) and 891 (exon 15) are found only in FMTC, but account for only a minority of cases of this disorder.

Hirschsprung's disease has been associated with exon 10 RET mutations, especially codons 620 and 618 [6]. For patients to present with both MEN2A and HD, simultaneous opposite genetic effects (dual function) are required to take place in the RET proto-oncogene, with "gain of function" mutations giving rise to MEN tumors and HD resulting from "loss of function mutations" [19]. Cutaneous lichen amyloidosis has been associated only with mutations of codon 634. Somatic RET mutations that occur later in life and are limited to C cells are present in 40–50% of sporadic MTCs [20].

Genotype–Phenotype Correlations

There are genotype–phenotype correlations regarding clinical subtype, age at onset and aggressiveness of MTC, and the presence other endocrine tumors. These relationships may be useful when planning the time for prophylactic thyroidectomy and determining if and when screening for pheochromocytoma or hyperparathyroidism is necessary (Table 31.1). Another important use of these correlations is in patients presenting with apparently sporadic MTC. The presence of specific RET mutations in these patients will impact their management. Therefore, performing genetic testing is recommended before surgical intervention in all children diagnosed with MTC [10].

Based on the recommendations from the American Thyroid Association [15] and the International Workshop on Multiple Endocrine Neoplasia [11], a risk-based stratification has been developed for MEN2 patients [1]. As seen Table 31.1, Group D patients with mutations in codon 918 and 883 are at the highest risk, and for this reason prophylactic thyroidectomy is recommended within the first months of life and screening for pheochromocytoma should start at age 8 years and continue annually. In contrast, patients in group A present with MTC an at older age and prophylactic thyroidectomy can be performed later in life. In addition, for group A patients screening for pheochromocytoma and PTH should begin in adolescence.

Genetic Screening

Historically, the diagnosis of MTC in patients with MEN2A or MEN2B depended on the demonstration of elevated plasma calcitonin levels either at baseline or after intravenous

Table 31.1 Risk-based stratification for MEN2 patients

ATA risk level	RET mutation codon(s)	MEN2 subtype	Prophylactic thyroidectomy	Screening for PHEO	Screening for PHPT
A	649, 768, 790, 791, 804, 891	FMTC	When calcitonin rises/5–10 years age	Start at 20 years age, then periodically	Start at 20 years age, then periodically
B	609, 611, 618, 620, 630, 631	FMTC and MEN2A	Before 5 years age	Start at 20 years age, then annually	Start at 20 years age, then annually
C	634	MEN2A	Before 5 years age	Start at 8 years age, then annually	Start at 8 years age, then annually
D	883, 918	MEN2B	At diagnosis	Start at 8 years age, then annually	Not needed

administration of the potent secretagogues calcium or pentagastrin. Advances in the molecular genetics underlying the MEN2 syndromes have resulted in DNA testing becoming the optimal test for their detection. Currently, genetic analysis identifies more than 95% of responsible mutations [21].

DNA testing for MEN2 is based on identification of RET mutations, and is considered the standard of care for newly identified MTC patients, regardless of age at diagnosis or family history[10]. Even in children with apparent sporadic MTC all exons should be sequenced and if no mutation is found, tumor DNA can be analyzed. Early diagnosis by screening of family members at risk in MEN2 kindreds is essential because testing can identify family members who are at risk for MTC and this life-threatening disease can be cured or prevented by early thyroidectomy. Moreover, knowledge of genotype–phenotype correlations may help estimate the chances of developing additional endocrine tumors, provide prognostic information, and plan surgical management.

Genetic testing can be useful in 3 groups of patients. First, in patients with histologically proven MTC or C-cell hyperplasia it can help differentiate between sporadic and hereditary MTC. If patients have hereditary MTC then their families should be screened. Next, in patients with familial occurrence of MTC and/or pheochromocytoma, genetic testing can differentiate between the subtypes of MEN2, identify the risk of developing other tumors, and determine when to start their screening. More importantly, genetic testing in MEN2 patients guides the timing for prophylactic thyroidectomy [11, 22]. Lastly, in first degree family members of MEN2 patients genetic testing can distinguish gene carriers from non carriers. Documentation that the RET mutation is not present eliminates the need for ongoing screening for MEN2 tumors and avoids unnecessary thyroidectomy in genetically normal subjects in MEN2 families. It is known from retrospective DNA testing, that such subjects can have falsely positive calcitonin level with pentagastrin stimulation that would suggest they have MEN2 [11].

Diagnosis and Management

Medullary Thyroid Cancer

Approximately 5% of thyroid neoplasms in children are medullary carcinomas, arising from the parafollicular C cells. MTC is usually the first tumor to develop in MEN2 patients and is the most common cause of death in this group. The malignant transformation of C cells starts early in life and C-cell hyperplasia and micro-MTC can be found as early as 2 months in some kindreds. This is especially true in MEN2B, which typically has a more aggressive form of MTC [23]. As with other thyroid neoplasms, the clinical diagnosis of MTC is often made with palpation of a thyroid nodule or after there is significant spread of the tumor to the adjacent cervical lymph nodes or to distant sites (lung, liver and bone) [24]. Also, diarrhea can be seen when there is significant hypercalcitoninemia and is usually a poor prognostic sign [25]. Less frequently, the tumor can be recognized after the diagnosis of pheochromocytoma or hyperparathyroidism. Rarely, MTC has been shown to cause Cushing's syndrome due to ectopic production of corticotropin (ACTH).

Calcitonin production is increased in C-cell hyperplasia and MTC, and measurements of plasma calcitonin are used as a tumor marker to monitor the presence and progression of MTC. Usually, serum calcitonin levels correlate with tumor mass and tend to be high (>1000 pg/m) in patients with a palpable tumor on exam. Likewise, elevated plasma calcitonin levels after tumor resection suggests persistent or recurrent disease [1].

The only effective treatment for MTC is surgical resection, underscoring the importance of early diagnosis and therapy before metastasis occurs. For this reason, current management of MTC in children from families having the MEN2 syndrome relies on the presymptomatic detection of the RET proto-oncogene mutation responsible for the disease. Affected children with MEN2A should undergo total thyroidectomy at about the age of 5 years, before the cancer spreads beyond the thyroid gland [26]. Indeed, approximately

80% of children who have thyroidectomy based on the presence of the RET mutation will already have foci of MTC within the thyroid gland [27]. As a matter of fact, almost all prophylactic thyroidectomies performed in recent years have shown that various stages of C-cell disease are present between 1 and 6 yr of age in patients of MEN2 families. Owing to the increased virulence of the MTC in children having MEN2B, it may be preferable for their thyroid glands to be removed in infancy. As discussed before, the specific RET mutation can help determine the timing of prophylactic thyroidectomy. Patients with MTC should be evaluated for possible pheochromocytoma before thyroidectomy and if the diagnosis is made, adrenalectomy should be performed first.

Because of the high incidence of bilateral disease in MTC, complete removal of the thyroid gland (total thyroidectomy) is the recommended for surgical management of MTC in children [28], as well as, for carriers of the mutation. The extent of neck lymph node dissection and the management of devascularized parathyroid glands differ depending upon the patient's MEN2 subtype, patient symptoms and whether the intervention is prophylactic or therapeutic. Also, the preoperative imaging may help determine how extensive the lymph node dissection should be. Usually, the dissection includes lymph nodes in the central compartment of the neck, medial to the carotid sheaths and between the hyoid bone and the sternum. This central lymph node dissection may be unnecessary in patients with MEN2A under the age of 11[29].

Single or combination chemotherapy has been ineffective in the treatment of unresectable or metastatic MTC. The antiangiogenesis and tyrosine kinase inhibitor drugs, such as combretastatin and imatinib mesylate, have been observed to have antineoplastic effects on MTC in vitro. Clinical trials need to be performed to determine the usefulness of these agents [21, 30–32]. Recent trials with VELF inhibitors have shown some promise in arresting MTC progression in patients with metastatic disease [33].

Palliative radiation therapy can also be used to diminish the tumor burden in the neck and to prevent local recurrence. Whether morbidity or mortality is improved remains unclear [21]. High-dose 131iodine anticarcinoembryonic antigen antibody treatment combined with posttherapy autologous hematopoietic stem cell rescue has limited toxicity, but the antitumor effect is unknown [34].

The postoperative management and monitoring of patients with MTC in the setting of MEN2 includes periodic physical exams, serial monitoring of serum calcitonin concentrations and neck ultrasound if the calcitonin is elevated. Thyroid hormone replacement is used to maintain euthyroidism and calcium supplementation is given when needed. After adolescence, yearly biochemical screening for pheochromocytoma is recommended.

Pheochromocytoma

Pheochromocytomas are rare catecholamine-secreting tumors of the adrenal medulla. It affects 40% of patients with MEN2A and MEN2B, although there is large variability of its penetrance among kindreds. In patients with MEN2 it is rare for a pheochromocytoma to be the initial manifestation and present before the development of MTC, but it has been reported [35]. Usually, pheochromocytomas become evident about 10 years after the diagnosis of C-cell hyperplasia or MTC [36]. As with MTC, the penetrance of pheochromocytoma among different MEN 2 kindreds depends on specific RET germline mutations [37].

In general, about 10% of children with pheochromocytoma have familial disease [38, 39]. Because these familial cases may include MEN2 with the risk of MCT, any child who presents with a pheochromocytoma should be screened for MEN2. Pheochromocytomas are found in an extra-adrenal location in 30% of children [39], but this is rare in MEN2 [37].

The signs and symptoms associated with pheochromocytomas in patients with MEN2 include paroxysmal hypertension which can be extreme and episodic. Also, orthostatic hypotension, when present, is suggestive of

MEN2. Occasionally, patients present with catecholamine-induced cardiomyopathy and hypertensive encephalopathy [40]. Laboratory confirmation is similar to sporadic pheochromocytomas, specifically the finding of increased plasma metanephrine [41]. Once there is biochemical confirmation of pheochromocytoma the tumor should be localized and possibility of, bilateral disease evaluated using MRI.

Pharmacologic blockade of excess catecholamines is a critical part of preoperative preparation of the patient with pheochromocytoma. The goals are to replete the intravascular volume, treat severe hypertension, control cardiac arrhythmias if present, and minimize the risk of perioperative cardiovascular instability.

The definite treatment for pheochromocytoma remains surgical removal of the lesion. Pheochromocytomas can be extraordinarily active for their size, and accurate preoperative localization of the lesions is essential. In the setting of bilateral disease, partial adrenalectomy should be considered [42]. In a series reported by Yip et al. [43], 65% of patients did not require chronic corticosteroid replacement after partial adrenalectomy in marked contrast to those who underwent total bilateral adrenalectomy. They also showed that the risk of recurrent pheochromocytoma in the adrenal gland remnant after the cortical-sparing procedure was about 10%.

Surgical management of unilateral disease is a topic of controversy. Some advocate bilateral adrenalectomy because about 30% of patients undergoing unilateral surgery may eventually develop pheochromocytoma in the remaining adrenal gland and would require resection [44]. Nevertheless, this may not happen for many years, and initial unilateral adrenalectomy would avoid the need for steroid replacement in the interval. Also favoring avoidance of initial bilateral adrenalectomy is the observation that no lethal complications from catecholamine crisis and no metastatic disease occurred in patients with MEN2 who underwent unilateral adrenalectomy and then developed contralateral disease [44].

Laparoscopic adrenalectomy is now the preferred approach for benign functioning adrenal tumors, including pheochromocytoma [45, 46]. Normalization of the blood pressure should be expected if all functioning pheochromocytoma tissue is removed. Children who have had resection of a pheochromocytoma should undergo examination with blood pressure measurements and urine catecholamine levels twice per year to monitor for recurrence. Patients with familial pheochromocytomas should be followed especially carefully for the development of disease in the opposite gland [47, 48]. For additional discussion of pheochromocytoma see Chap. 8.

Primary Hyperparathyroidism

PHPT in children is extremely rare with an incidence of 2–5 per 100,000, with most cases (80%) occurring during adolescence [49, 50]. In large series of patients with MEN2 clinically evident hyperparathyroidism was noted at a median age of 38 years (ranging from 7 to 71 years) [51–53] but it has been described in a patient as young as 5 years of age, who was found to have a pathologic parathyroid gland at time of his prophylactic total thyroidectomy [54]. In most MEN2 patients (75–80%) PHPT is diagnosed at the same time as MTC or pheochromocytoma and the rest are found at follow up after thyroidectomy [11]. Less than 5% of cases PHPT in MEN2 patients are diagnosed before the presentation of MTC or pheochromocytoma [53].

Different from the usual sporadic cases, PHPT in patients with MEN 2A is characterized by multigland hyperplasia and an increased incidence of ectopic or supernumerary glands. Signs and symptoms of hypercalcemia in PHPT tend to be more severe in children than in adults and can be associated with end-organ damage, making early diagnosis critical.

Parathyroid disease seems to develop more rarely in patients with MEN2A who undergo a total thyroidectomy at an early age [55, 56]. Some theories attribute this phenomenon to removal of normal parathyroid glands during thyroidectomy. This could decrease the incidence of parathyroid disease in two ways—either by reducing the number of parathyroid glands at risk, or by removing the stimulus for parathyroid growth after removal of C cells [55, 57].

The diagnosis of primary hyperparathyroidism is confirmed with the findings of hypercalcemia and inappropriately high-serum parathyroid hormone (PTH) concentrations. In a patient with known or presumed MEN2A, the indications for surgical intervention are similar to those in patients with sporadic primary hyperparathyroidism [58].

Although the frequency of PHPT in MEN 2A is not high, and the symptoms of hypercalcemia tend to be milder, the surgical treatment options are similar to those for patients with MEN1. Most of these patients have multiple parathyroid tumors, so bilateral exploration of previously nonoperative patients should be planned regardless of the outcome of preoperative localization studies. Such imaging studies may nonetheless be anatomically helpful to the surgeon and can therefore be indicated. These studies (ultrasonography, sestamibi imaging, or chest CT) are certainly recommended before re-operation in patients with recurrent or persistent disease.

There is some disagreement regarding the preferred surgical management with arguments and challenges similar to those for patients with hyperparathyroidism in the setting of MEN1 [52, 59, 60]. Because symptoms are milder and the likelihood of recurrent HPT is lower than in MEN1, Dotzenrath [59] and O'Riordain [60] both recommend a conservative approach with excision of only enlarged glands without transcervical thymectomy. This technique is associated with low rate of persistent and recurrent PHPT, inferring that it offers a better chance to avoid postoperative hypoparathyroidism [56]. On the other hand, it may be wise to concomitantly undertake cervical thymectomy at the initial surgery especially in patients with multiple gland involvement. For patients with more severe hypercalcemia, however, a more aggressive approach may be employed. Some surgeons recommend three and one-half-gland parathyroidectomy, (or all but one-half gland, if supernumerary glands are found), together with thymectomy, and with subtotal parathyroidectomy being repeated if the patient has a recurrence [60, 61]. On the other hand, others prefer to remove all the glands and heterotopically transplant some tissue into the nondominant forearm [62]. The latter approach has the advantage of avoiding repeated neck exploration if hyperparathyroidism should recur, and has been shown to be safe in infants and children [27, 63, 64]. Moreover, total parathyroidectomy with heterotopic autotransplantation has been shown to result in improved survival in infants with severe hypercalcemia [62]. As noted previously, patients with total parathyroidectomy and autotransplantation require a short period of vitamin D and calcium supplementation until the heterotopic tissue begins to function. If, however, the autograft does not function the patient may have permanent hypoparathyroidism.

Overall cure rates can be expected to be as high as 95%. Patients with MEN2 should have annual screening for hyperparathyroidism by serum calcium and intact parathyroid hormone level measurements.

Hirschsprung's Disease

RET mutations are responsible for up to 50% of familial cases of Hirschsprung's Disease (HD) and may also be seen in sporadic HD cases [65]. Interestingly, the clinical association between aganglionic megacolon, megaloureter, pheochromocytoma, and neuromatosis [66] was actually reported before the first MEN descriptions [65].

There are multiple publications noting the correlation of MEN2A and HD. HD was found in 57% of children in families with a C620 mutation in exon 10 with a low penetrance [67–69]. The later, as well as mutations in C618 position are the most likely to predispose to HD [69]. Even though, MEN2A and HD arise from the same gene, they act through different pathways to activate RET kinase. They arise from variations on different parts of the gene, and have both extra and intracellular targets of protein transformation [70].

The true incidence of MEN 2A in familial HD is unknown. Decker and Peacock found the HD phenotype in at least one family member in approximately 17% of their MEN2A kindreds [71]. Furthermore, 7 out of 12 patients with MEN2A and HD in their series had classic short segment disease and the rest had long segment aganglionosis indicating that the level of aganglionosis is not a reliable marker of the risk of MEN2A and need for genetic testing. They recommend MEN2A patients that are considering pregnancy be counseled about the potential risk of HD in their offspring and they also recommended alerting physicians caring for children in MEN2A families about the risk of HD and its possible occurrence in the newborn period. Finally, they recommended that all children with familial HD be considered for genetic screening for MEN2A and that children with sporadic HD have a family history inquiry for MTC [71].

In children from kindreds with the C620 mutations, symptoms of HD should be sought, and if present then rectal biopsy should be performed. It is recommended that children with HD plus RET abnormalities undergo prophylactic thyroidectomy in accordance with their risk profile as previously discussed in Sect. 33.5 [72].

Cutaneous Lichen Amyloidosis

Cutaneous lichen amyloidosis (CLA) occurs sporadically and as a familial disease. The hereditary forms are transmitted in an autosomal dominant fashion, and it has been reported in association with few syndromes. The most frequent association is with MEN2A [73]. The CLA skin lesion is usually described as intensely pruritic, red-brown hyperkeratotic papules most commonly seen in the interscapular region or on the extensor surfaces of the extremities. The first symptom is usually pruritus. The amyloid deposition is seen later and is thought to be secondary to repeated scratching. There are several different RET codon 634 mutations that have been documented in MEN2A/CLA families [55, 73, 74]. As noted previously these same mutations are common in MEN2A families who present without CLA. This implies the presence of other factors, in conjunction with the RET mutation, in the expression of the CLA phenotype.

References

1. Raue F, Frank-Raue K. Update multiple endocrine neoplasia type 2. Fam Cancer. 2010. doi:10.1007/s10689-010-9320-2.
2. Lips CJ, Landsvater RM, Hoppener JW, Geerdink RA, Blijham G, van Veen JM, van Gils AP, de Wit MJ, Zewald RA, Berends MJ, et al. Clinical screening as compared with DNA analysis in families with multiple endocrine neoplasia type 2a. N Engl J Med. 1994;331(13):828–35.
3. Machens A. Early malignant progression of hereditary medullary thyroid cancer. N Engl J Med. 2004'350(9):943. doi:10.1056/NEJM200402263500917. (350/9/943 [pii]).
4. Ponder BA, Ponder MA, Coffey R, Pembrey ME, Gagel RF, Telenius-Berg M, Semple P, Easton DF. Risk estimation and screening in families of patients with medullary thyroid carcinoma. Lancet. 1988;1(8582):397–401.
5. Donovan DT, Levy ML, Furst EJ, Alford BR, Wheeler T, Tschen JA, Gagel RF. Familial cutaneous lichen amyloidosis in association with multiple endocrine neoplasia type 2a: A new variant. Henry Ford Hosp Med J. 1989;37(3–4):147–50.
6. Mulligan LM, Eng C, Attie T, Lyonnet S, Marsh DJ, Hyland VJ, Robinson BG, Frilling A, Verellen-Dumoulin C, Safar A, et al. Diverse phenotypes associated with exon 10 mutations of the ret proto-oncogene. Hum Mol Genet. 1994;3(12):2163–7.
7. Romeo G, Ceccherini I, Celli J, Priolo M, Betsos N, Bonardi G, Seri M, Yin L, Lerone M, Jasonni V, Martucciello G. Association of multiple endocrine neoplasia type 2 and hirschsprung disease. J Intern Med. 1998;243(6):515–20.
8. Vasen HF, van der Feltz M, Raue F, Kruseman AN, Koppeschaar HP, Pieters G, Seif FJ, Blum WF, Lips CJ. The natural course of multiple endocrine neoplasia type iib. A study of 18 cases. Arch Intern Med. 1992;152(6):1250–2.
9. Iihara M, Yamashita T, Okamoto T, Kanbe M, Yamazaki K, Egawa S, Yamaguchi K, Obara T. A nationwide clinical survey of patients with multiple endocrine neoplasia type 2 and familial medullary thyroid carcinoma in japan. Jpn J Clin Oncol. 1997;27(3):128–34.
10. Callender GG, Rich TA, Perrier ND. Multiple endocrine neoplasia syndromes. Surg Clin North Am. 2008;88(4):863–95, viii. (doi:S0039-6109(08)00070-4 [pii]).
11. Brandi ML, Gagel RF, Angeli A, Bilezikian JP, Beck-Peccoz P, Bordi C, Conte-Devolx B,

Falchetti A, Gheri RG, Libroia A, Lips CJ, Lombardi G, Mannelli M, Pacini F, Ponder BA, Raue F, Skogseid B, Tamburrano G, Thakker RV, Thompson NW, Tomassetti P, Tonelli F, Wells SA Jr, Marx SJ. Guidelines for diagnosis and therapy of men type 1 and type 2. J Clin Endocrinol Metab. 2001;86(12):5658–71.
12. Donis-Keller H, Dou S, Chi D, Carlson KM, Toshima K, Lairmore TC, Howe JR, Moley JF, Goodfellow P, Wells SA Jr. Mutations in the ret proto-oncogene are associated with men 2a and fmtc. Hum Mol Genet. 1993;2(7):851–6.
13. Santoro M, Carlomagno F, Melillo RM, Fusco A. Dysfunction of the ret receptor in human cancer. Cell Mol Life Sci. 2004;61(23):2954–64.
14. Mulligan LM, Ponder BA. Genetic basis of endocrine disease: multiple endocrine neoplasia type 2. J Clin Endocrinol Metab. 1995;80(7):1989–95.
15. Kloos RT, Eng C, Evans DB, Francis GL, Gagel RF, Gharib H, Moley JF, Pacini F, Ringel MD, Schlumberger M, Wells SA Jr. Medullary thyroid cancer: Management guidelines of the american thyroid association. Thyroid. 2009;19(6):565–612.
16. Eng C, Clayton D, Schuffenecker I, Lenoir G, Cote G, Gagel RF, van Amstel HK, Lips CJ, Nishisho I, Takai SI, Marsh DJ, Robinson BG, Frank-Raue K, Raue F, Xue F, Noll WW, Romei C, Pacini F, Fink M, Niederle B, Zedenius J, Nordenskjold M, Komminoth P, Hendy GN, Mulligan LM, et al. The relationship between specific ret proto-oncogene mutations and disease phenotype in multiple endocrine neoplasia type 2. International ret mutation consortium analysis. JAMA. 1996;276 (19):1575–9.
17. Schuffenecker I, Virally-Monod M, Brohet R, Goldgar D, Conte-Devolx B, Leclerc L, Chabre O, Boneu A, Caron J, Houdent C, Modigliani E, Rohmer V, Schlumberger M, Eng C, Guillausseau PJ, Lenoir GM. Risk and penetrance of primary hyperparathyroidism in multiple endocrine neoplasia type 2a families with mutations at codon 634 of the ret proto-oncogene. Groupe d'etude des tumeurs a calcitonine. J Clin Endocrinol Metab. 1998;83 (2):487–91.
18. Berndt I, Reuter M, Saller B, Frank-Raue K, Groth P, Grussendorf M, Raue F, Ritter MM, Hoppner W. A new hot spot for mutations in the ret protooncogene causing familial medullary thyroid carcinoma and multiple endocrine neoplasia type 2a. J Clin Endocrinol Metab. 1998;83(3):770–4.
19. Toledo SP, dos Santos MA, Toledo Rde A, Lourenco DM Jr. Impact of ret proto-oncogene analysis on the clinical management of multiple endocrine neoplasia type 2. Clinics (Sao Paulo). 2006;61(1):59–70.
20. Elisei R, Cosci B, Romei C, Bottici V, Renzini G, Molinaro E, Agate L, Vivaldi A, Faviana P, Basolo F, Miccoli P, Berti P, Pacini F, Pinchera A. Prognostic significance of somatic ret oncogene mutations in sporadic medullary thyroid cancer: a 10-year follow-up study. J Clin Endocrinol Metab. 2008;93(3):682–7.
21. Gertner ME, Kebebew E. Multiple endocrine neoplasia type 2. Curr Treat Options Oncol. 2004;5(4): 315–25.
22. Simon S, Pavel M, Hensen J, Berg J, Hummer HP, Carbon R. Multiple endocrine neoplasia 2a syndrome: surgical management. J Pediatr Surg. 2002;37 (6):897–900. (doi:S0022346802200561 [pii]).
23. Samaan NA, Draznin MB, Halpin RE, Bloss RS, Hawkins E, Lewis RA. Multiple endocrine syndrome type iib in early childhood. Cancer. 1991;68(8): 1832–4.
24. Gorlin JB, Sallan SE. Thyroid cancer in childhood. Endocrinol Metab Clin North Am. 1990;19(3): 649–62.
25. Cohen MS, Moley JF. Surgical treatment of medullary thyroid carcinoma. J Intern Med. 2003;253(6):616–26.
26. Wells SA, Jr., Chi DD, Toshima K, Dehner LP, Coffin CM, Dowton SB, Ivanovich JL, DeBenedetti MK, Dilley WG, Moley JF, et al. Predictive DNA testing and prophylactic thyroidectomy in patients at risk for multiple endocrine neoplasia type 2a. Ann Surg. 1994;220(3):237–47; discussion 247–50.
27. Skinner MA, DeBenedetti MK, Moley JF, Norton JA, Wells SA, Jr. Medullary thyroid carcinoma in children with multiple endocrine neoplasia types 2a and 2b. J Pediatr Surg. 1996;31(1):177–81; discussion 172–81.
28. Telander RL, Zimmerman D, van Heerden JA, Sizemore GW. Results of early thyroidectomy for medullary thyroid carcinoma in children with multiple endocrine neoplasia type 2. J Pediatr Surg. 1986;21(12):1190–4.
29. Skinner MA, Moley JA, Dilley WG, Owzar K, Debenedetti MK, Wells SA Jr. Prophylactic thyroidectomy in multiple endocrine neoplasia type 2a. N Engl J Med. 2005;353(11):1105–13.
30. Nelkin BD, Ball DW. Combretastatin a-4 and doxorubicin combination treatment is effective in a preclinical model of human medullary thyroid carcinoma. Oncol Rep. 2001;8(1):157–60.
31. Cohen MS, Hussain HB, Moley JF. Inhibition of medullary thyroid carcinoma cell proliferation and ret phosphorylation by tyrosine kinase inhibitors. Surgery. 2002;132(6):960–6; discussion 966–7.
32. Skinner MA, Safford SD, Freemerman AJ. Ret tyrosine kinase and medullary thyroid cells are unaffected by clinical doses of sti571. Anticancer Res. 2003;23(5A):3601–6.
33. Wells SA Jr, Gosnell JE, Gagel RF, Moley J, Pfister D, Sosa JA, Skinner M, Krebs A, Vasselli J, Schlumberger M. Vandetanib for the treatment of patients with locally advanced or metastatic hereditary medullary thyroid cancer. J Clin Oncol. 2010;28 (5):767–72.
34. Juweid ME, Hajjar G, Stein R, Sharkey RM, Herskovic T, Swayne LC, Suleiman S, Pereira M,

Rubin AD, Goldenberg DM. Initial experience with high-dose radioimmunotherapy of metastatic medullary thyroid cancer using 131i-mn-14 f(ab)2 anti-carcinoembryonic antigen mab and ahscr. J Nucl Med. 2000;41(1):93–103.
35. Bethanis S, Koutsodontis G, Palouka T, Avgoustis C, Yannoukakos D, Bei T, Papadopoulos S, Linos D, Tsagarakis S. A newly detected mutation of the ret protooncogene in exon 8 as a cause of multiple endocrine neoplasia type 2a. Hormones (Athens). 2007;6(2):152–6.
36. Peppa M, Boutati E, Kamakari S, Pikounis V, Peros G, Panayiotides IG, Economopoulos T, Raptis SA, Hadjidakis D. Multiple endocrine neoplasia type 2a in two families with the familial medullary thyroid carcinoma associated g533c mutation of the ret proto-oncogene. Eur J Endocrinol. 2008;159 (6):767–71.
37. Quayle FJ, Fialkowski EA, Benveniste R, Moley JF. Pheochromocytoma penetrance varies by ret mutation in men 2a. Surgery. 2007;142(6):800–5; discussion 801–5.
38. Gross DJ, Avishai N, Meiner V, Filon D, Zbar B, Abeliovich D. Familial pheochromocytoma associated with a novel mutation in the von hippel-lindau gene. J Clin Endocrinol Metab. 1996;81(1):147–9.
39. Atiyeh BA, Barakat AJ, Abumrad NN. Extra-adrenal pheochromocytoma. J Nephrol. 1997;10(1):25–9.
40. Januszewicz P, Wieteska-Klimczak A, Wyszynska T. Pheochromocytoma in children: Difficulties in diagnosis and localization. Clin Exp Hypertens A. 1990;12(4):571–9.
41. Eisenhofer G, Walther MM, Huynh TT, Li ST, Bornstein SR, Vortmeyer A, Mannelli M, Goldstein DS, Linehan WM, Lenders JW, Pacak K. Pheochromocytomas in von hippel-lindau syndrome and multiple endocrine neoplasia type 2 display distinct biochemical and clinical phenotypes. J Clin Endocrinol Metab. 2001;86(5):1999–2008.
42. Albanese CT, Wiener ES. Routine total bilateral adrenalectomy is not warranted in childhood familial pheochromocytoma. J Pediatr Surg. 1993;28 (10):1248–51; discussion 1242–51.
43. Yip L, Lee JE, Shapiro SE, Waguespack SG, Sherman SI, Hoff AO, Gagel RF, Arens JF, Evans DB. Surgical management of hereditary pheochromocytoma. J Am Coll Surg. 2004;198(4):525–4; discussion 525–34.
44. Webb TA, Sheps SG, Carney JA. Differences between sporadic pheochromocytoma and pheochromocytoma in multiple endocrime neoplasia, type 2. Am J Surg Pathol. 1980;4(2):121–6.
45. Cheah WK, Clark OH, Horn JK, Siperstein AE, Duh QY. Laparoscopic adrenalectomy for pheochromocytoma. World J Surg. 2002;26(8):1048–51.
46. Pacak K, Linehan WM, Eisenhofer G, Walther MM, Goldstein DS. Recent advances in genetics, diagnosis, localization, and treatment of pheochromocytoma. Ann Intern Med. 2001;134(4):315–29.
47. Caty MG, Coran AG, Geagen M, Thompson NW. Current diagnosis and treatment of pheochromocytoma in children. Experience with 22 consecutive tumors in 14 patients. Arch Surg. 1990;125(8):978–81.
48. Lairmore TC, Ball DW, Baylin SB, Wells SA, Jr. Management of pheochromocytomas in patients with multiple endocrine neoplasia type 2 syndromes. Ann Surg. 1993;217(6):595–601; discussion 593–601.
49. Kollars J, Zarroug AE, van Heerden J, Lteif A, Stavlo P, Suarez L, Moir C, Ishitani M, Rodeberg D. Primary hyperparathyroidism in pediatric patients. Pediatrics. 2005;115(4):974–80.
50. Harman CR, van Heerden JA, Farley DR, Grant CS, Thompson GB, Curlee K. Sporadic primary hyperparathyroidism in young patients: a separate disease entity? Arch Surg. 1999;134(6):651–5; discussion 655–6.
51. Kraimps JL, Duh QY, Demeure M, Clark OH. Hyperparathyroidism in multiple endocrine neoplasia syndrome. Surgery. 1992;112(6):1080–6; discussion 1086–8.
52. Herfarth KK, Bartsch D, Doherty GM, Wells SA, Jr., Lairmore TC. Surgical management of hyperparathyroidism in patients with multiple endocrine neoplasia type 2a. Surgery. 1996;120(6):966–73; discussion 964–73.
53. Raue F, Kraimps JL, Dralle H, Cougard P, Proye C, Frilling A, Limbert E, Llenas LF, Niederle B. Primary hyperparathyroidism in multiple endocrine neoplasia type 2a. J Intern Med. 1995;238(4):369–73.
54. Tonelli F, Marcucci T, Giudici F, Falchetti A, Brandi ML. Surgical approach in hereditary hyperparathyroidism. Endocr J. 2009;56(7):827–41.
55. Gagel RF, Tashjian AH Jr, Cummings T, Papathanasopoulos N, Kaplan MM, DeLellis RA, Wolfe HJ, Reichlin S. The clinical outcome of prospective screening for multiple endocrine neoplasia type 2a. An 18-year experience. N Engl J Med. 1988;318 (8):478–84.
56. Kraimps JL, Denizot A, Carnaille B, Henry JF, Proye C, Bacourt F, Sarfati E, Dupond JL, Maes B, Travagli JP, Boneu A, Roger P, Houdent C, Barbier J, Modigliani E. Primary hyperparathyroidism in multiple endocrine neoplasia type iia: retrospective french multicentric study. Groupe d'etude des tumeurs a calcitonine (getc, french calcitonin tumors study group), french association of endocrine surgeons. World J Surg. 1996;20(7):808–12; discussion 803–12.
57. Mallette LE. Management of hyperparathyroidism in the multiple endocrine neoplasia syndromes and other familial endocrinopathies. Endocrinol Metab Clin North Am. 1994;23(1):19–36.
58. Brandi ML. Multiple endocrine neoplasia type i: General features and new insights into etiology. J Endocrinol Invest. 1991;14(1):61–72.
59. Dotzenrath C, Cupisti K, Goretzki PE, Yang Q, Simon D, Ohmann C, Roher HD. Long-term

biochemical results after operative treatment of primary hyperparathyroidism associated with multiple endocrine neoplasia types i and iia: Is a more or less extended operation essential? Eur J Surg. 2001;167(3):173–8.
60. O'Riordain DS, O'Brien T, Grant CS, Weaver A, Gharib H, van Heerden JA. Surgical management of primary hyperparathyroidism in multiple endocrine neoplasia types 1 and 2. Surgery. 1993;114(6):1031–7; discussion 1037–9. (doi:0039-6060(93)90319-9 [pii]).
61. Carling T, Udelsman R. Parathyroid surgery in familial hyperparathyroid disorders. J Intern Med. 2005;257(1):27–37.
62. Ross AJ 3rd, Cooper A, Attie MF, Bishop HC. Primary hyperparathyroidism in infancy. J Pediatr Surg. 1986;21(6):493–9.
63. Tonelli F, Marcucci T, Fratini G, Tommasi MS, Falchetti A, Brandi ML. Is total parathyroidectomy the treatment of choice for hyperparathyroidism in multiple endocrine neoplasia type 1? Ann Surg. 2007;246(6):1075–82.
64. Cohen MS, Dilley WG, Wells SA, Jr., Moley JF, Doherty GM, Sicard GA, Skinner MA, Norton JA, DeBenedetti MK, Lairmore TC. Long-term functionality of cryopreserved parathyroid autografts: a 13-year prospective analysis. Surgery. 2005;138 (6):1033–40; discussion 1031–40.
65. Moore SW, Zaahl MG. Multiple endocrine neoplasia syndromes, children, hirschsprung's disease and ret. Pediatr Surg Int. 2008;24(5):521–30. doi:10.1007/s00383-008-2137-5.
66. Shocket E, Teloh HA. Aganglionic megacolon, pheochromocytoma, megaloureter, and neurofibroma; co-occurrence of several neural abnormalities. AMA J Dis Child. 1957;94(2):185–91.
67. Pausova Z, Soliman E, Amizuka N, Janicic N, Konrad EM, Arnold A, Goltzman D, Hendy GN. Role of the ret proto-oncogene in sporadic hyperparathyroidism and in hyperparathyroidism of multiple endocrine neoplasia type 2. J Clin Endocrinol Metab. 1996;81(7):2711–8.
68. Butter A, Gagne J, Al-Jazaeri A, Emran MA, Deal C, St-Vil D. Prophylactic thyroidectomy in pediatric carriers of multiple endocrine neoplasia type 2a or familial medullary thyroid carcinoma: Mutation in c620 is associated with hirschsprung's disease. J Pediatr Surg. 2007;42(1):203–6.
69. Moore SW, Appfelstaedt J, Zaahl MG. Familial medullary carcinoma prevention, risk evaluation, and ret in children of families with men2. J Pediatr Surg. 2007;42(2):326–32.
70. Akhand AA, Ikeyama T, Akazawa S, Kato M, Hossain K, Takeda K, Suzuki H, Takahashi M, Nakashima I. Evidence of both extra- and intracellular cysteine targets of protein modification for activation of ret kinase. Biochem Biophys Res Commun. 2002;292(4):826–31. doi:10.1006/bbrc.2002.6731.
71. Decker RA, Peacock ML. Occurrence of men 2a in familial hirschsprung's disease: A new indication for genetic testing of the ret proto-oncogene. J Pediatr Surg. 1998;33(2):207–14.
72. Machens A, Dralle H. Multiple endocrine neoplasia type 2 and the ret protooncogene: from bedside to bench to bedside. Mol Cell Endocrinol. 2006;247(1–2):34–40.
73. Verga U, Fugazzola L, Cambiaghi S, Pritelli C, Alessi E, Cortelazzi D, Gangi E, Beck-Peccoz P. Frequent association between men 2a and cutaneous lichen amyloidosis. Clin Endocrinol (Oxf). 2003;59(2):156–61.
74. Snow KJ, Boyd AE 3rd. Management of individual tumor syndromes. Medullary thyroid carcinoma and hyperparathyroidism. Endocrinol Metab Clin North Am. 1994;23(1):157–66.

Part IX
Pituitary

Pituitary Gland Embryology, Anatomy and Physiology

32

Vaitsa Tziaferi and Mehul T. Dattani

The pituitary gland, also known as the hypophysis cerebri, is a small protrusion at the base of the brain largely encased by the sphenoid bone. Together with the immediately adjacent hypothalamus the pituitary forms the hypothalamic-pituitary system that is the body's main regulator of hormone production and is therefore intimately involved in human growth, development, reproduction, parturition, lactation, metabolism, response to stress and osmotic balance.

The pituitary gland consists of two distinct parts, the anterior pituitary, or adenohypophysis, and the posterior pituitary, or neurohypophysis. The two parts differ in origin, structure and function. The anterior pituitary derives from the oral ectoderm and produces growth hormone, prolactin, adrenocorticotropic hormone (ACTH), melanocyte-stimulating hormone (MSH), thyroid-stimulating hormone (TSH), and the gonadotrophins—follicle-stimulating hormone (FSH) and luteinising hormone (LH). The posterior pituitary originates from the neural ectoderm and consists of neurons projecting from the hypothalamus that produce antidiuretic hormone and oxytocin.

Anatomy of the Pituitary Gland

The pituitary gland is a red-grey ovoid structure that protrudes from the base of the brain. In adults it is roughly 12 mm in the transverse diameter and 8 mm in anterior-posterior diameter and it usually weighs from 500 to 1000 mg. The pituitary gland is comprised of two distinct regions or lobes, the anterior pituitary, or adenohypophysis, and the posterior pituitary, or neurohypophysis.

The pituitary lies within the *sella turcica,* the hypophyseal fossa of the sphenoid bone, which is located in the centre of the skull base [1] (Fig. 32.1a and c). The location of the pituitary gland within this fossa of the sphenoid bone permits the most common surgical approach to the pituitary to be transphenoidal. The transphenoidal approach is easier in adults than children because of the greater pneumatisation of the sphenoid bone [2] (Fig. 32.1a–d).

The pituitary gland is covered superiorly and largely separated from the brain by a circular fold of dura mater known as the diaphragmatic *sella.* The diaphragmatic sella has a central opening, or aperture, for the infundibular stalk, which connects the pituitary to the brain. Anteriorly, the diaphragmatic sella separates the anterior part of the pituitary from the optic chiasm, which lies roughly 10 mm above the diaphragmatic sella

V. Tziaferi
Department of Paediatric Endocrinology, Great Ormond Street Hospital, London WC1N 3JH, UK
e-mail: vtziaferi@yahoo.gr; vtziaferi@mail.com

M.T. Dattani (✉)
Section of Genetics and Epigenetics in Health and Disease, Genetics and Genomic Medicine Programme, UCL GOS Institute of Child Health and Great Ormond Street Hospital for Children, 30 Guilford Street, London WC1N 1EH, UK
e-mail: m.dattani@ucl.ac.uk; m.dattani@ich.ucl.ac.uk

D.J. Ledbetter and P.R.V. Johnson (eds.), *Endocrine Surgery in Children*,
DOI 10.1007/978-3-662-54256-9_32

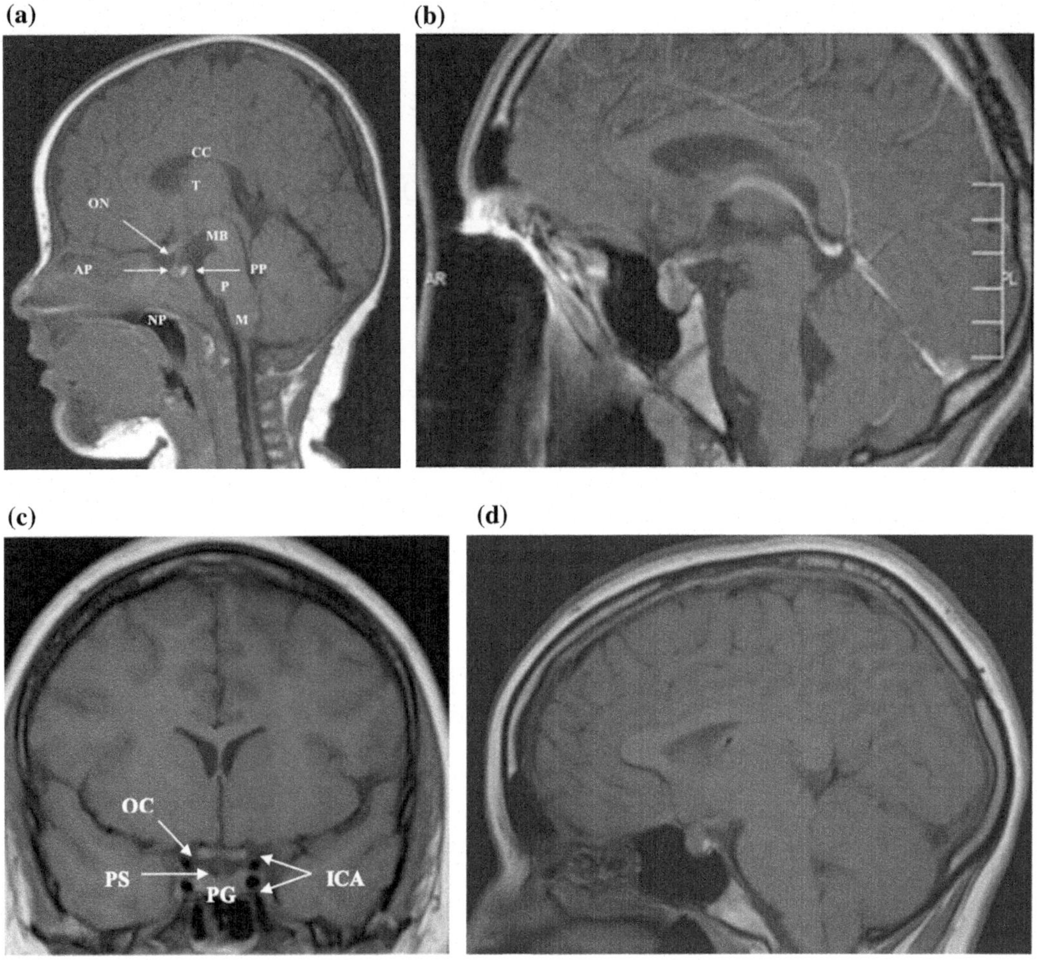

Fig. 32.1 **a** Midline sagittal section of brain MRI depicting the gross anatomical relations of anterior pituitary in a 2.5 year old infant. **b** Midline sagittal section of brain MRI in an adolescent male with Rathke's pouch cyst abutting the optic chiasm. **c** Coronal section of brain MRI at the level of pituitary. **d** Midline sagittal section of brain MRI in an adolescent female with enlarged pituitary gland. The gland appears to be moulding the optic chiasm. Follow-up MRI after 4 months showed resolution of the enlargement. This type of enlargement is not uncommon during adolescence. Sphenoid sinus is fully developed in this age rendering transphenoidal approach easier. *AP* anterior pituitary; *CC* corpus callosum; *ICA* internal carotid artery; *M* Medulla oblongata; *MB* midbrain; *NP* nasopharynx; *OC* optic chiasm; *ON* optic nerve; *P* pons; *PG* pituitary gland; *PP* posterior pituitary; *PS* pituitary stalk; *S* sphenoid sinus; *T* thalamus

[3]. The proximity of the pituitary to the optic chiasm accounts for the visual field loss that is often associated with large pituitary tumours.

When viewed from above the diaphragmatic sella may be concave, flat or convex and ranges in width from 5 to 11 mm in adults. The aperture of the sella varies in size and, if wide enough, can result in herniation of the arachnoid mater, or membrane, into the sella turcica. This herniation of the arachnoid membrane into the sella turcica enlarges the chiasmatic cistern, the subarachnoid space below the optic chiasm, and flattens the pituitary. This condition is known as the *empty sella* [4]. Herniation of the arachnoid membrane into the sella turcica increases the risk of injury to the membrane during pituitary surgery and subsequent cerebrospinal fluid (CSF) leak [2].

The walls of the sella turcica are formed by the folds of dura mater, which also form the medial walls of the cavernous sinuses, the space lateral to pituitary filled with thin walled veins [2]. The oculomotor, trochlear and the first two branches of the trigeminal nerve run in the lateral walls of the cavernous sinuses and the abducens nerve, a portion of the internal carotid artery and the sympathetic plexus are contained within the sinuses [2]. The pituitary gland is separated inferiorly from the floor of the sella turcica by a venous sinus that communicates with the circular sinus, the veins in the spaces anterior and posterior to the sella turcica that connect the two lateral cavernous sinuses [1].

Anterior Pituitary

The anterior pituitary consists of epithelial cells that derive from the oral ectoderm [5]. It consists of the *pars anterior* (or *pars distalis*), which is the anterior or distal part of the anterior pituitary, the pars *intermedia* which is the intermediate part of the pituitary between the anterior and posterior pituitary, and *pars tuberalis* which surrounds the infundibular stem of the posterior pituitary. The pars anterior and intermedia are separated by a cleft, which is a remnant of Rathke's pouch from which the anterior pituitary develops (see section on Embryology). Pathologic enlargement of the cleft may lead to a cyst known as a Rathke's cleft cyst (Fig. 32.1b). In humans, in contrast to the mouse, the *pars intermedia* largely disappears during embryogenesis and is rudimentary and ill-defined in the adult pituitary [6]. Melanocyte-stimulating hormone (MSH) is traditionally thought to be generated in the pars intermedia; however, it may actually be produced in the pars anterior [7].

Histologically distinct cells found in the anterior pituitary include chromophil cells, chromophobe cells, and folliculostellate cells. Folliculostellate cells do not produce hormones while the chromophil and chromophobe cells produce hormones. The hormone producing cells are named for the hormone(s) they produce. The anterior pituitary produces six different peptide hormones: (1) growth hormone (GH) or somatotrophin, (2) prolactin (PRL) or mammotrophin, (3) adrenocorticotropic hormone (ACTH) or corticotrophin, (4) thyroid-stimulating hormone (TSH) or thyrotrophin, (5) follicle-stimulating hormone (FSH), and (6) luteinising hormone (LH).

The chromophobe cells comprise the majority of the cells of the anterior pituitary making up about 50% of the epithelial cells. These cells are small and do not react to routine staining. This population comprises different cell types such as degranulated secretory cells and stem cells.

The chromophil cells are either acidophils or basophils. Acidophils, also known as α-cells, include somatotrophs (producing GH), mammotrophs or lactotrophs (producing prolactin), and somatomammotrophs (producing both GH and prolactin). Basophils, also known as β-cells, include corticotrophs (producing ACTH), thyrotrophs (producing TSH), and gonadotrophs (producing LH and FSH). Pituitary tumours are often characterised as basophil or acidophil depending upon the dominant cell type. The somatotrophs are the largest and most abundant making up approximately 50% of the chromophil cells in the anterior pituitary. The thyrotroph cells make up 6–10% of the chromophil cells [8]. Corticotrophs in humans are distinguished by 300 nm secretory granules [8], and account for 10% of the chromophil cells. Gonadotrophs make up another 10–15% of the chromophil cells. They are located throughout the anterior pituitary, often in close proximity to mammotrophs [6]. The majority of gonadotroph cells have granules of 200 nm but often larger—500 nm—granules are seen. All cells that produce glycoproteins (thyrotrophs and gonadotrophs) stain PAS (periodic acid-Schiff) positive [8].

The folliculostellate cells constitute the supporting and trophic network of the hormone producing cells and contain peptides with growth factor or cytokine activity. Basic fibroblast growth factor is produced in folliculostellate cells and is implicated in the control of the production of pituitary hormones in a paracrine manner.

Posterior Pituitary

The posterior pituitary arises from the diencephalon (the posterior forebrain located between the midbrain and the cerebrum) and consists primarily of axons from supraoptic and paraventricular nuclei of the hypothalamus. These neurons secrete vasopressin (or antidiuretic hormone, ADH) and oxytocin. The posterior pituitary includes the median eminence at the base of the infundibular stalk, the infundibular stalk (or infundibulum, or stalk) and the *pars posterior* (or posterior lobe, or neural lobe). The infundibulum of the pituitary is a conical process originating from the tuber cinereum of the hypothalamus that connects the posterior pituitary to brain. In the infundibulum the thin non-myelinated axons are ensheathed by typical astrocytes [1]. As the axons continue into the posterior lobe, the astrocytes are replaced by pituicytes, which are dendritic in origin.

Blood Supply of the Pituitary

The pituitary gland receives arterial supply by a single inferior and several superior hypophyseal arteries, which arise from the internal carotid artery. Branches of these arteries supply the posterior pituitary directly and supply the anterior pituitary indirectly via the hypophyseal portal venous system [1].

The inferior hypophyseal artery originates from the cavernous part of the internal carotid artery and divides into medial and lateral branches. These branches anastomose and form a ring around the infundibulum. Branches from this circular anastomosis enter the posterior lobe to supply its capillary bed [1]. The median eminence and the upper part of the infundibulum receive an arterial supply from the superior hypophyseal arteries which arise from the supraclinoid part of the internal carotid artery and the anterior and posterior cerebral arteries [1]. The lower part of the infundibulum and pars posterior receives its supply directly from the inferior hypophyseal artery and indirectly from the superior hypophyseal artery via the trabecular arteries [1].

The hypophyseal portal system that supplies the anterior lobe consists of long and short portal vessels. The long vessels arise from the external capillary plexus and the posterior part of the internal capillary plexus of the median eminence. The two plexi form a continuum with the infundibular capillary plexus which drains into the long portal veins [1]. The long portal veins allow secretions from the median eminence to reach the anterior pituitary directly. The short portal vessels come from the capillary net of the lower infundibulum. The portal system is essential for the endocrine function of the anterior pituitary, since hormone releasing and inhibiting factors secreted from the hypothalamic nuclei collect in the median eminence and infundibulum and are transferred directly to the anterior pituitary without the dilution and metabolism that would occur if they were transported via systemic venous drainage to the heart and arterial supply back to the anterior pituitary.

The venous drainage of the anterior pituitary is restricted and only a few efferent vessels connect directly to the systemic veins of the cavernous sinuses. Venous drainage of the posterior pituitary is via the inferior hypophyseal vein to the dural sinuses, via the long and short portal veins to the anterior pituitary, and via capillaries passing through the median eminence to the hypothalamus.

Embryology of the Pituitary

Studies in different species have demonstrated that pituitary development is highly conserved from lower vertebrates through to higher mammals [9]. The mature pituitary gland has a dual embryonic origin—the anterior and intermediate lobes of the pituitary derive from the oral ectoderm, while the posterior pituitary derives from the neural ectoderm.

The pituitary or adenohypophyseal placode originates from the midline of the anterior neural ridge which is the most anterior part of the neural plate in the embryo and forms the boundary between the anterior part of the ectoderm and the neuroectoderm [10]. The pituitary placode is immediately adjacent to the neural plate cells that give rise to the telencephalon, hypothalamus and posterior pituitary.

The pituitary placode is the site of an invagination of the oral ectoderm called *Rathke's pouch* which will give rise to the anterior and intermediate lobes of the pituitary (Fig. 32.2). In humans, the oral ectoderm containing the pituitary placode is formed by the third week of gestation. A week later Rathke's pouch begins to develop and by the end of the sixth gestational week the initial invagination completely disconnects from the oral ectoderm.

Pituitary development has been extensively studied in mice and the detailed description that follows refers to this species. Anterior pituitary development occurs in four stages: (1) formation of the pituitary placode, (2) development of a rudimentary Rathke's pouch, (3) formation of the definitive Rathke's pouch, and (4) terminal differentiation of various cell types [9].

At 7.5 dpc, the pituitary placode develops as a thickening of the ectoderm at the roof of the primitive oral cavity. The pituitary placode makes contact with the floor of the ventral diencephalon and this is a critical event in the development of the pituitary. At approximately 9 dpc, the oral ectoderm invaginates to form a rudimentary Rathke's pouch, the primordium of the anterior pituitary while the ventral diencephalon evaginates to form the infundibulum and the posterior pituitary (Fig. 32.2). Subsequently, the definitive Rathke's pouch is formed and the spatial and temporal differentiation of the various cell types within the mature anterior pituitary gland takes place [11]. At approximately 12.5 dpc, differentiated corticotrophs appear in the ventral region of the pouch and thyrotrophs on 13.5 dpc. Differentiated melanotrophs appear in the intermediate lobe a day later, and somatotroph, lactotroph and gonadotroph cells arise temporally between 15.5 and 16 days. By 17.5 dpc all hormone-secreting cell types have undergone terminal differentiation and are organised into distinct spatial networks within the gland [11].

The juxtaposition of the oral ectoderm forming Rathke's pouch and the neural ectoderm of the diencephalon which later develops into the hypothalamus is maintained in the early stages of pituitary organogenesis [11]. Inductive tissue interactions resulting from this contact and

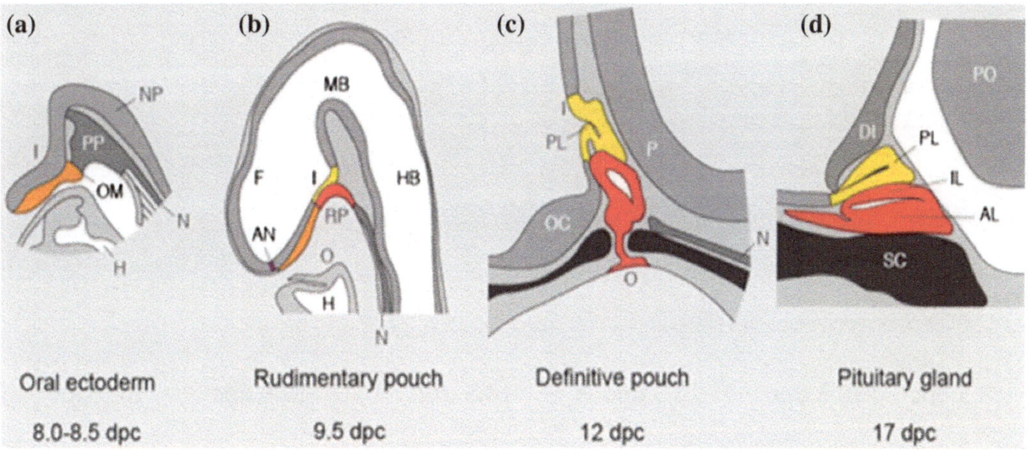

Fig. 32.2 Mouse pituitary development in sagittal section. Stages of development are indicated in dpc. *AL* Anterior lobe, *AN* anterior neural pore, *DI* diencephalon, *F* forebrain, *H* heart, *HB* hindbrain, *I* infundibulum, *IL* intermediate lobe, *MB* midbrain, *N* notochord, *NP* neural plate, *O* oral cavity, *OC* optic chiasm, *OM* oral membrane, *P* pontine flexure, *PL* posterior lobe, *P* pons, *PP* prechordal plate, *RP* Rathke's pouch, *SC* sphenoid cartilage. Adapted from Sheng and Westphal [21], with permission from Elsevier

extrinsic signalling from the neuroectoderm of the infundibulum are critical for the initial development of the pituitary gland [12]. A cascade of signalling molecules and transcription factors play crucial roles in organ commitment, cell proliferation, cell patterning and terminal differentiation events within the developing pituitary.

HESX1, PROP1, POUIF1/PIT1, LHX3, LHX4, TBX19 (TPIT), PITX1, PITX2, SF1, SOX3 and SOX2 are transcription factors implicated in pituitary organogenesis (Fig. 32.3) and mutations in these factors in humans are associated with septo-optic dysplasia, combined pituitary hormone deficiency, isolated growth hormone deficiency, or isolated adrenocorticotropic hormone deficiency (Table 32.1). This is not an exhaustive list and the roles of other transcription factors are being defined. Transcription factors act as activators or repressors and play a significant role in the cell type specification and cell fate within the pituitary gland.

Signalling molecules implicated in pituitary development are either intrinsic, emanating from the oral ectoderm such as sonic hedgehog (Shh), or extrinsic from the neuroectoderm such as Fibroblast growth factors (FGFs) and bone morphogenetic factors (BMPs) [5] (Fig. 32.3).

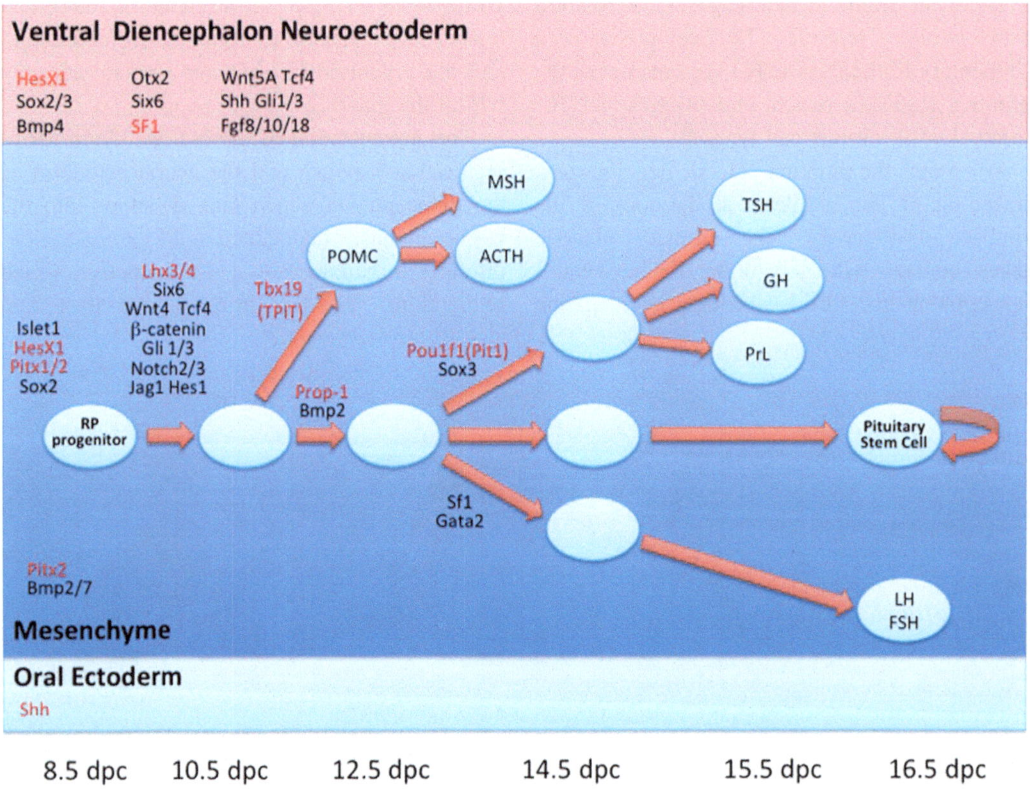

Fig. 32.3 Schematic representation of the developmental cascade of genes implicated in human pituitary development with particular reference to pituitary cell differentiation. From Kelberman et al. [5], with permission from The Endocrine Society

Table 32.1 Transcription factors and signalling molecules implicated in pituitary abnormalities and associated phenotypes

Gene	Phenotype	Inheritance
HESX1	Variable: SOD, CPHD, IGHD with EPP. APH or absent; PP: ectopic or eutopic	AD or AR
OTX2	Anophthalmia, APH, EPP, absent infundibulum	Het: haploinsufficiency
SOX2	Bilateral anophthalmia/microphthalmia, IHH, APH, Hypothalamic hamartoma, abnormal CC, Esophageal atresia, SNHL	De novo haploinsufficiency
SOX3	IGHD with LD, CPHD, APH, infundibular hypoplasia, persistent craniopharyngeal canal, EPP, midline abnormalities	X-linked recessive
GLI2	HPE, CPHD, craniofacial abnormalities, polydactyly	Haploinsufficiency
LHX3	CPHD, short rigid cervical spine, SNHL, APH or enlarged AP	AR
LHX4	CPHD, persistent craniopharyngeal canal, abnormal cerebellar tonsils, APH, EPP, absent infundibulum	AR; AD; haploinsufficiency
PROP1	CPHD, enlarged pituitary with later involution	AR
POU1F1 (PIT1)	CPHD, APH	AD or AR
TBX19/ TPIT	Isolated ACTHD	AR
SHH	HPE, cleft lip/palate	AD
FGF8	Variable: IHH, KS, cleft lip/palate, HPE	AD or AR
ARNT2	CPHD – ACTH, TSH and GHD with DI, CAKUT, progressive microcephaly with LD	AR

ACTHD ACTH deficiency, *APH* anterior pituitary hypoplasia, *CAKUT* Congenital abnormalities of the kidney and urinary tract, *CPHD* combined pituitary hormone deficiencies, *EPP* ectopic posterior pituitary, *HPE* holoprosencephaly, *IGHD* isolated GH deficiency, *IHH* isolated hypogonadotrophic hypogonadism, *KS* Kallmann syndrome, *LD* learning difficulties, *PP* posterior pituitary, *SNHL* sensorineural hearing loss, *SOD* septo-optic dysplasia
Features described here are not always present but have been variably described

These molecules may activate or repress transcription factors such as Hesx1, Lhx3 and Lhx4. They may also act as morphogens and create the appropriate environment for cell differentiation thus playing a critical role in cell fate. Such signalling molecules include members of the Shh family, FGFs, transforming growth factors (Tgfs), Bmps, Wingless (Wnts) and molecules in the Notch pathway to mention a few. To date, not many pituitary phenotypes have been reported in association with mutations in these signalling molecules (Table 32.1). However it appears that they may be implicated in pituitary tumorigenesis such as in the case of the Wnt signalling pathway [13]. A number of microarray studies have identified altered expression of Wnt inhibitors in pituitary tumours and there is clear evidence that the Wnt/β catenin pathway is involved in the pathogenesis of craniopharyngioma, a rare tumour in the hypothalamic-pituitary region.

Physiology of the Pituitary

The hypothalamic-pituitary system is the central regulator of hormone production in the body. The anterior pituitary secretes the following hormones:

(i) growth hormone (GH) or somatotropin
(ii) prolactin (PRL)
(iii) adrenocorticotropic hormone (ACTH) or corticotrophin
(iv) melanocyte-stimulating hormone (MSH) which is also produced by the intermediate lobe

(v) thyroid-stimulating hormone (TSH) or thyrotrophin
(vi) gonadotrophins: follicle-stimulating hormone (FSH) and luteinising hormone (LH)

GH and PRL are single peptides, ACTH and MSH are peptides deriving from a single precursor and TSH and the gonadotrophins are glycoproteins composed of a common α-peptide chain (89 residues) and a variable β-peptide chain.

The posterior pituitary gland secretes vasopressin or antidiuretic hormone (ADH) or AVP (arginine–vasopressin) and oxytocin. The synthesis of ADH and oxytocin takes place in the supraoptic and paraventricular hypothalamic nuclei. ADH and oxytocin reach the posterior pituitary lobe via axons of the hypothalamic neurons which project to the posterior pituitary and are secreted in the capillaries in response to hypothalamic stimuli. ADH and oxytocin share a high degree of sequence homology. ADH is activated by hyperosmolar stimuli and acts on the collecting ducts of the kidneys to facilitate water reabsorption. Oxytocin is produced at the late stage of labour both in the mother and in the baby resulting in smooth muscle contraction in the uterus and in the mammary gland.

The production of anterior pituitary hormones is regulated by a cascade system that is characterised by signal amplification and negative feedback inhibition [14]. The negative feedback systems operate when sufficient amounts of the ultimate hormone have been reached in the circulation. There are three negative feedback systems (1) long feedback; i.e. the ultimate hormone produced in the periphery back to the pituitary or brain, (2) short feedback; i.e. the anterior pituitary hormone back to the hypothalamus, and (3) ultra-short feedback; i.e. the hypothalamic releasing factor back to the hypothalamus [14].

Puberty (Fig. 32.1d) and pregnancy are two periods in human lifespan characterised by physiological enlargement of the pituitary, presumably because of the increased activity of the gland [15]. In childhood, conditions characterised by abnormal secretion of pituitary hormones are usually congenital deficiencies/insufficiencies (Table 32.2).

Growth Hormone (GH)

GH is a 22 kda peptide of 191 amino acid residues secreted by somatotroph cells. Its main effects are promotion of *growth* and *metabolism*. GH is an *anabolic hormone* promoting protein synthesis and an important *counter-regulatory hormone to hypoglycaemia*. The last action is mediated via the increase in plasma glucose concentration (diabetogenic action) and the release of free fatty acids that can serve as an alternative energy source.

The promotion of *growth* is largely mediated via GH stimulation of the liver production of Insulin-like growth factor (IGF) 1. IGF-1 acts on bone growth plates to promote linear growth. GH also has some direct action on the growth plate. Clinically, it is useful to measure IGF-1 as a surrogate marker of GH secretion or GH replacement for individuals on GH treatment.

GH is secreted in the pituitary gland following stimulation by GH-releasing hormone (GHRH) from the hypothalamus. GH production is inhibited by the hypothalamic peptide somatostatin. GH is normally secreted in a pulsatile manner. Peak levels of GH coincide with peak levels of GHRH. Trough levels of GH coincide with peak levels of somatostatin. In childhood, GH is secreted in a circadian pattern with GH peaks occurring every 1–2 h. Insufficiency of GH production is usually diagnosed using GH stimulation tests that include insulin tolerance test, glucagon provocation, exercise, dopamine, etc. However, the diagnosis of GH insufficiency is challenging as no test is perfect and the diagnosis is therefore based upon a combination of auxological (or growth), biochemical and neuroradiological data.

Table 32.2 Conditions with abnormal secretion of pituitary hormones

Hormone	Secretion	Causes
ACTH	Insufficiency	Congenital Isolated ACTHD (*TBX19/TPIT* mutations), CPHD, may be evolving (*PROP1* mutations) Acquired: tumour, surgery, trauma, radiotherapy, infiltration, autoimmune, post-infectious
	Excess	Cushing disease
TSH	Insufficiency	Congenital: Isolated (*TRHR* mutations, *TSHβ* mutations, *IGSF1* mutations), CPHD Acquired: tumour, surgery, trauma, radiotherapy, infiltration, autoimmune, post-infectious
Gonadotrophins	Insufficiency	Congenital: HH (mutations in *GPR54, GnRHR*), KS (mutations in *FGFR1, FGF8, KAL1, PROK2, PROKR2, CHD7, WDR11, NELF*); congenital forms may rarely present in adulthood Acquired: tumour, surgery, trauma, radiotherapy, infiltration, autoimmune, post-infectious
GH	Insufficiency	Congenital: IGHD (*GHRH-R, GH1* mutations), CPHD Acquired: tumour, surgery, trauma, radiotherapy, infiltration, autoimmune, post-infectious
	Excess	Adenoma: gigantism in childhood, acromegaly in adulthood
PRL	Excess	Prolactinoma
ADH	Insufficiency	Congenital: Isolated or CPHD Acquired: tumour, surgery, trauma, radiotherapy, infiltration, autoimmune, post-infectious
	Excess	SIADH –(transient) either from pituitary secretion of ADH or from ectopic production
Oxytocin	Insufficiency	CPHD, unknown clinical significance outside parturition/lactation

CPHD combined pituitary hormone deficiencies, *IGHD* isolated GH deficiency, *HH* Hypogonadotrophic Hypogonadism, *KS* Kallmann syndrome, *SIADH* syndrome of inappropriate antidiuretic hormone

Prolactin (PRL)

Prolactin is a peptide of 198 amino acid residues produced by lactotroph cells. It has considerable structural homology to GH. The classic endocrine action of this hormone is the promotion of growth and maturation of the mammary gland during pregnancy in order to achieve lactation. The exact mechanism of the mammotrophic effect of PRL in humans is largely unknown and our knowledge is based on animal studies.

Apart from its classic endocrine action, PRL has other autocrine–paracrine actions as a growth factor, neurotransmitter, and immunoregulator [16]. In males of most animal species, PRL stimulates testicular function [16]. Other actions ascribed to PRL include effects on metabolism, salt and water balance, sexual function and reproduction, and brain and behaviour.

The mechanism of PRL secretion is largely unknown and it is thought to be under the influence of a PRL-releasing factor that is not well defined and a PRL-inhibiting factor, also not well defined but it may be dopamine or a peptide controlled by dopamine [14]. Additionally, hypothalamic thyrotrophin releasing hormone (TRH) may stimulate PRL production.

Adrenocorticotropic Hormone (ACTH)

ACTH is a relatively small peptide of only 39 amino acid residues which derives along with α-MSH, β-lipotropin and β-endorphin from a single common precursor, the pre-pro-opiomelanocortin. ACTH regulates the production of glucocorticoids. Cortisol is the major glucocorticoid in humans and is released in the circulation both in a circadian and in a pulsatile manner. Circadian secretion of cortisol is subject to the circadian production of corticotrophin releasing hormone (CRH) by the hypothalamus. The highest ACTH production is at 0800 in the morning.

Glucocorticoid secretion in response to stress is crucial for homeostasis and deficiency of ACTH is life-threatening. ACTH binds to the melanocortin 2 receptors (MC2-R) which are widely distributed throughout the body [17]. Additionally, ACTH regulates the production of adrenal androgens androstenedione and dehydroepiandrosterone by the zona reticularis of the adrenal cortex. Glucocorticoids inhibit the production of ACTH in a classic model of hormonal negative feedback.

Melanocyte-Stimulating Hormone (MSH)

MSH derives from the same precursor as ACTH. Its action in humans is unclear but it may have a role in skin pigmentation. ACTH has some MSH activity that is evident by the increased skin pigmentation often seen in patients with high ACTH levels including those with Addison's disease. However, MSH does not appear to exert any ACTH-like action.

Thyroid-Stimulating Hormone (TSH)

TSH is a 28 kda glycoprotein which regulates the production of thyroxine and triiodothyronine by thyroid follicular cells [8]. TSH secretion is stimulated by hypothalamic thyrotropin-releasing hormone (TRH). There is a negative feedback mechanism with thyroxine (T4) and triiodothyronine (T3) suppressing TSH secretion. Thyroid hormones exhibit complex metabolic effects with the increased thyroid hormone concentrations in hyperthyroidism causing an increase in the basal metabolic rate, tachycardia, excess growth, sweating, poor concentration and weight loss. Low concentrations of thyroid hormone in hypothyroidism are classically associated with poor growth and short stature, weight gain, fatigue, lethargy and bradycardia. Features of hypothyroidism may be subtle in childhood.

Gonadotrophins—Follicle-Stimulating Hormone (FSH) and Luteinising Hormone (LH)

The gonadotrophins are glycoproteins consisting of α and β subunits. The β subunit confers specific biological activity and consists of 121 amino acids in LH and 118 amino acids in FSH. Gonadotrophin production is stimulated when hypothalamic gonadotrophin releasing hormone (GnRH) binds to specific receptors on the gonadotroph cells of the anterior pituitary. LH and FSH produced by the anterior pituitary bind to their receptors in the gonads stimulating steroidogenesis and gametogenesis, respectively. The synthesis of LH and FSH is dependent on the pattern of GnRH secretion such that an increased frequency of pulsatile hypothalamic GnRH release favours LH β gene transcription over FSH β gene transcription while a decreased frequency of pulsatile GnRH release, such as occurs in the luteal and early follicular phase of the female menstrual cycle, favours FSH β gene transcription [18].

Sex steroids feed back to the hypothalamus and pituitary suppressing the production of GnRH and LH and FSH, respectively, and form a classic negative feedback circuit. However, by some poorly understood mechanism, in females prior to ovulation the feedback is positive instead of negative and the result is a surge in LH resulting in ovulation [19].

Before birth, the hypothalamic–pituitary–gonadal (HPG) axis is hyperactive in a sexually dimorphic manner that is essential for the sexual differentiation of the brain [20]. This activity gradually declines over a period of 3–4 months postnatally and a long period of inactivity follows until adolescence.

Lack of gonadotrophins due to either GnRH deficiency or reduced action leads to hypogonadotrophic hypogonadism, with delayed or absent puberty and impaired fertility (Table 32.2).

References

1. Crossman AR. Neuroanatomy: diencephalon: pituitary gland. In: Standring S, editors. Gray's anatomy. St. Louis: Elsevier; 2008.
2. Cappabianca P, Cavallo LM, de Divitiis O. Pituitary surgery. In: Jamieson JL, De Groot LJ, editors. Endocrinology. Philadelphia: Elsevier-Saunders; 2006.
3. Melmed S, Kleinberg D, Anterior pituitary. In: Kronenberg HM, Melmed S, Polonsky KS, Reed Larsen P, editors. Williams textbook of endocrinology. Philadelphia: Saunders-Elsevier; 2008.
4. Busch W. Morphology of sella turcica and its relation to the pituitary gland. Virchows Arch. 1951;320: 437–58.
5. Kelberman D, Rizzoti K, Lovell-Badge R, Robinson IC, Dattani MT. Genetic regulation of pituitary gland development in human and mouse. Endocr Rev. 2009;30:790–829.
6. Ooi GT, Tawadros N, Escalona RM. Pituitary cell lines and their endocrine applications. Mol Cell Endocrinol. 2004;228:1–21.
7. Evans VR, Manning AB, Bernard LH, Chronwall BM, Millington WR. Alpha-melanocyte-stimulating hormone and N-acetyl-beta-endorphin immunoreactivities are localized in the human pituitary but are not restricted to the zona intermedia. Endocrinology. 1994;134:97–106.
8. Childs GV. Pituitary gland (cell types, mediators, development). In: Squire L, editors. The new encyclopedia of neuroscience. London: Elsevier; 2009.
9. Dattani M, Hindmarsh PC. Pituitary. In: Jameson JL, De Groot LJ, editors. Endocrinology: adult and pediatric. Philadelphia: Saunders; 2010.
10. Mehta A, Dattani MT. Developmental disorders of the hypothalamus and pituitary gland associated with congenital hypopituitarism. Best Pract Res Clin Endocrinol Metab. 2008;22:191–206.
11. Kelberman D, Dattani MT. The role of transcription factors implicated in anterior pituitary development in the aetiology of congenital hypopituitarism. Ann Med. 2006;38:560–77.
12. Takuma N, Sheng HZ, Furuta Y, Ward JM, Sharma K, Hogan BL, Pfaff SL, Westphal H, Kimura S, Mahon KA. Formation of Rathke's pouch requires dual induction from the diencephalon. Development (Cambridge, England). 1998;125: 4835–40.
13. Elston MS, Clifton-Bligh RJ. Identification of Wnt family inhibitors: a pituitary tumor directed whole genome approach. Mol Cell Endocrinol. 2010;326: 48–54.
14. Litwack G, Schmidt T. Biochemistry of hormones I: polypeptide hormones. In: Devlin TM, editors. Textbook of biochemistry with clinical correlations. New York: Wiley-Liss; 2002.
15. Argyropoulou M, Perignon F, Brunelle F, Brauner R, Rappaport R. Height of normal pituitary gland as a function of age evaluated by magnetic resonance imaging. Pediatr Radiol. 1991;21:247–9.
16. Bole-Feysot C, Goffin V, Edery M, Binart N, Kelly PA. Prolactin (PRL) and its receptor: actions, signal transduction pathways and phenotypes observed in PRL receptor knockout mice. Endocr Rev. 1998;19:225–68.
17. Papadimitriou A, Priftis KN. Regulation of the hypothalamic-pituitary-adrenal axis. NeuroImmunoModulation. 2009;16:265–71.
18. Ciccone NA, Kaiser UB. The biology of gonadotroph regulation. Curr Opin Endocrinol Diabetes Obes. 2009;16:321–7.
19. Maffucci JA, Gore AC. Hypothalamic neural systems controlling the female reproductive life cycle gonadotropin-releasing hormone, glutamate, and GABA. Int Rev Cell Mol Biol. 2009;274:69–127.
20. Gore AC. Developmental programming and endocrine disruptor effects on reproductive neuroendocrine systems. Front Neuroendocrinol. 2008;29:358–74.
21. Sheng HZ, Westphal H. Trends Genet. 1999;15:236–240 (317).

Surgical Considerations of the Pituitary

33

Toba Niazi and Samuel R. Browd

Pituitary surgery includes the excisional treatment of lesions within or adjacent to the sella turcica, the hypophyseal or pituitary fossa of the sphenoid bone which contains the pituitary gland. These pituitary lesions are not rare in children and include a variety of tumors, the most common of which are craniopharyngiomas. This chapter reviews the evaluation of and the surgical approach to pituitary lesions.

Pituitary Lesions

In the pediatric population almost 90% of lesions in the sellar and parasellar region are craniopharyngiomas. The remaining 10% include a variety of other pathological entities including pituitary adenomas, Rathke's cleft cysts, germinomas, hamartomas, lipomas, teratomas, dermoid cysts, epidermoid cysts, lymphocytic hypophysitis, and Langerhans cell histiocytosis [1–5]. Craniopharyngiomas are slow-growing, biologically benign tumors that arise from the primitive pituitary epithelium of Rathke's pouch. Craniopharyngiomas have a bimodal age distribution with the adamantinomatous variant typically presenting in the first and second decade of life and the papillary variant typically presenting in the fifth decade [6]. Although craniopharyngiomas are histologically benign and do not spread to other body areas their location at the base of the brain and close proximity to critical structures present formidable treatment challenges (Fig. 33.1).

Pituitary adenomas are the second most common lesion in the sellar and parasellar region in children and account for 3% of the total. Prolactinomas and adrenocorticotropic hormone (ACTH) secreting tumors are the most common pituitary adenomas requiring treatment and non-secretory adenomas are less frequent [4, 7] (see Fig. 33.2).

Preoperative Evaluation

Except in emergency cases of pituitary apoplexy with visual compromise or cases of acute obstructive hydrocephalus, a complete medical evaluation by a multidisciplinary team is performed before surgical intervention. Specifically, detailed endocrine and ophthalmological evaluation must be performed.

Preoperative endocrine evaluation should include measurement of prolactin, growth hormone, thyroid stimulating hormone (TSH), follicle stimulating hormone (FSH), leutinizing hormone (LH), cortisol, triiodothyrinone (T3),

T. Niazi
Department of Clinical Neurological Surgery and Pediatrics, University of Miami, Clinical Research Building, 1120 N.W. 14th St. 4th Floor, Miami, FL 33136, USA
e-mail: toba.n.niazi@gmail.com

S.R. Browd (✉)
Department of Neurological Surgery, University of Washington, 1959 NE Pacific St, Seattle, WA 98195, USA
e-mail: samuel.browd@seattlechildrens.org

D.J. Ledbetter and P.R.V. Johnson (eds.), *Endocrine Surgery in Children*,
DOI 10.1007/978-3-662-54256-9_33

(a) (b)

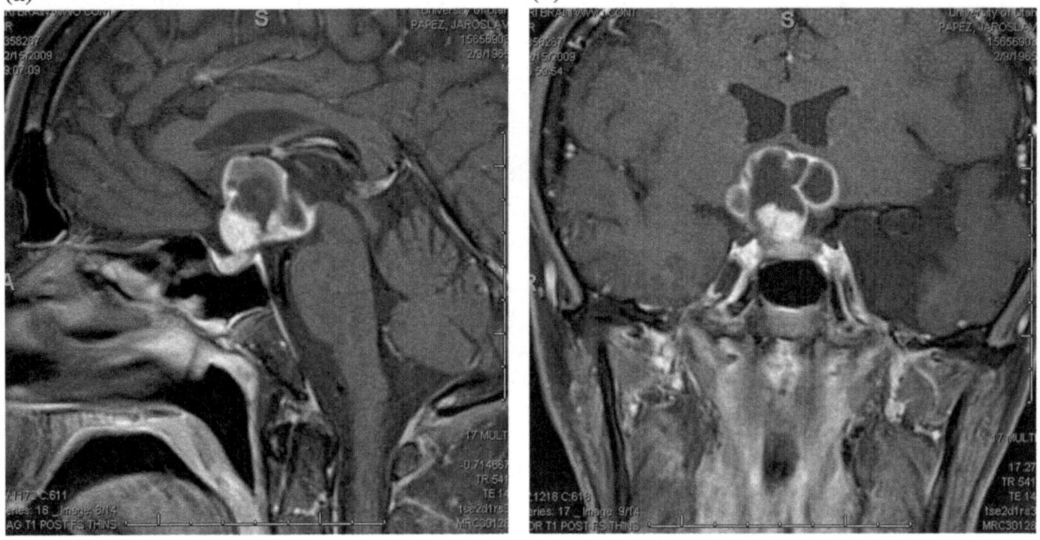

Fig. 33.1 **a** and **b** Suprasellar craniopharyngioma (sagittal and axial projections) demonstrating the common appearance of this lesion with solid and cystic components. CT imaging (not shown here) commonly demonstrates peripheral calcification

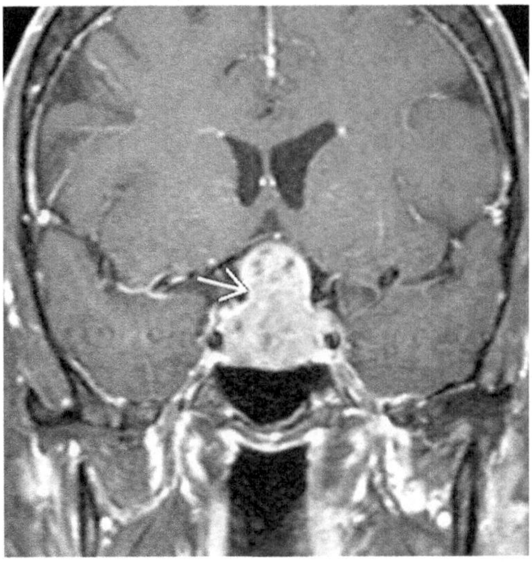

Fig. 33.2 Macroadenoma with suprasellar extension. Classic "snowman" appearance on imaging as the lesson violates the diaphrama sella superiorly. Laterally, the lesion appears to have cavernous sinus invasion with tumor around the carotid arteries bilaterally

and thyroxine (T4). This evaluation will reveal secretory lesions such as prolactinomas that might be amenable to medical therapy. In addition, baseline hormonal deficits that could cause perioperative problems will be identified and replacement therapy can be instituted. Mild hyperprolactinemia (<200 ng/mL) may occur with suprasellar lesions that do not secrete prolactin but only compress the pituitary stalk (the "stalk effect") [8, 9].

Baseline ophthalmological evaluation is necessary to assess for preoperative vision deficits that may be caused by the tumors. Although a major goal of pituitary surgery is to preserve vision, sometimes transsphenoidal and transcranial procedures may adversely affect visual acuity. The careful preoperative and postoperative assessment of vision allows for appropriate counseling of patients and families [8, 9].

All patients with sellar pathology typically undergo computed tomography (CT) and should also undergo magnetic resonance imaging (MRI) with and without contrast. The CT helps to define pneumatization of the sinuses and determines if special instrumentation is required to access the sellar region through the nonpneumatized sinuses. CT also delineates the anatomy of the sphenoid sinus including the septa that may be present and their relationship to the carotid impression on either side of the sella.

Recognition of these relationships is important to help avoid injury to the carotid arteries. MRI provides better definition of the neural structures and the relationship of the tumor to the optic chiasm, optic nerves, carotid arteries, and the cavernous sinus. The degree of tumor extension into surrounding regions is assessed and can determine which nares is used for transsphenoidal access or from which side of the head the tumor is approached during transcranial resection. High resolution MRI may also better identify the sphenoid septa and their relationship to the cavernous carotid arteries than CT. Identification of the carotid arteries is critical because some patients have paramedian or "kissing" cavernous carotid arteries that prevent the transsphenoidal approach [10]. Not recognizing this variant on preoperative imaging could lead to vascular injury, severe neurovascular morbidity and even mortality.

Redo transsphenoidal surgical procedures require a precise preoperative definition of anatomy since the normal landmarks that allow safe access through this trajectory are no longer present and the risk of injury to the cavernous carotid is higher. This imaging is essential for the computer-assisted, image-guided techniques that are especially valuable in redo cases to allow for a safe operative approach.

Surgical Goals

The aims of surgical resection of sellar and parasellar masses are to relieve compression on surrounding structures, such as the optic chiasm, to attain gross total resection to minimize recurrence and eliminate hormonal hypersecretion, to minimize brain retraction, and to preserve pituitary function [8]. The majority of children with sellar lesions present to medical attention with acute hydrocephalus due obstruction of third and lateral ventricular outflow tracts [2, 11, 12]. Resection of the mass relieves the obstruction and in some cases may obviate the need for long-term CSF diversion by either ventriculoperitoneal shunting and or endoscopic third ventriculostomy. Lesions with rapid growth, necrosis, or hemorrhage may compress the optic chiasm causing precipitous loss of vision and may also impair the blood supply to the pituitary causing "pituitary apoplexy" with loss of normal hormonal function [13–15]. Emergent medical evaluation and surgical decompression is essential to preserve visual acuity and prevent the ensuing hormonal deficiencies such as acute adrenal insufficiency [13–15].

Failure of pharmacologic management of sellar masses with continued growth and mass effect, specifically pituitary adenomas such as prolactinomas warrants surgical intervention [16]. In addition, some patients do not tolerate medical management of their sellar masses and may need surgical intervention. Recurrence of disease after prior radiation and medical management is also an indication for surgical extirpation to prevent further disease progression and neurological decline [15–19].

History of Surgical Treatment of Sellar Tumors

In 1866, Pierre Marie described two adult patients with acromegaly and an enlarged sella and sparked investigations into neuroendocrinology and surgical treatment of pituitary lesions [20]. Initially, the surgical approaches were transcranial, but high mortality rates from infection in the era before antibiotics led surgeons to pursue extracranial access to the sella turcica [21–26]. In 1907, Schloffer performed the first successful transsphenoidal resection of a pituitary lesion without complication [27]. Cushing later used the transnasal transsphenoidal approach to resect 231 pituitary tumors with a 5.6% mortality rate [28]. Cushing later abandoned the transsphenoidal procedures and advocated transcranial approaches to the pituitary, but Dott and Guiot continued to champion the transsphenoidal route [29] The morbidity and mortality rates of patients undergoing transnasal transsphenoidal surgery continued to decrease with advances in anesthesia, medical support, and surgical instrumentation [30]. A major advance was the introduction of the surgical microscope in 1971 by Hardy which markedly improved visualization and the precision of excision through the small access corridor [31].

Surgical Approaches to the Pituitary

The choice of transsphenoidal or transcranial approaches to pituitary lesions is influenced by the extent of tumor invasion within the suprasellar and parasellar space as defined by preoperative neuroimaging and by the experience of the surgeon [9, 32]. The transnasal transsphenoidal is usually the preferred route and is the mainstay of surgical treatment of lesions of the sella turcica [8, 15, 16, 19, 32–35]. Technological advancements such as computer-assisted, image-guided surgery, frameless stereotaxy, fluoroscopy, endoscopy, and extended transsphenoidal approaches allow for less invasive methods to access and attain complete tumor resection. Many series of transnasal transsphenoidal resections report mortality rates of less than 1% [17, 18, 34, 36, 37].

However, some sellar and parasellar masses are not amenable to the transsphenoidal approach due to the intimate association with neurovascular structures, the optic apparatus, and the hypothalamus. Such lesions require transcranial approaches for safe gross total resection. Transsphenoidal resections in children may be more challenging than similar resections in adults because of the lack of pneumatization of the sphenoid sinus and the smaller size of the nares and operative corridor. In these circumstances, surgeon experience is of paramount importance for optimal outcomes.

Transsphenoidal Approaches

Transsphenoidal resection of sellar tumors spaces may be done via sublabial or transnasal, also known as endonasal, approaches (Fig. 33.3). In 1910, Harvey Cushing was the first neurosurgeon to adopt the sublabial transsphenoidal approach to the sella [28]. Typically the patient is supine with the face parallel to the ceiling and the head approximately 15° above the heart to encourage venous drainage. Flexion of the head can allow for visualization of lesions that extend inferiorly along the clivus while extension of the head

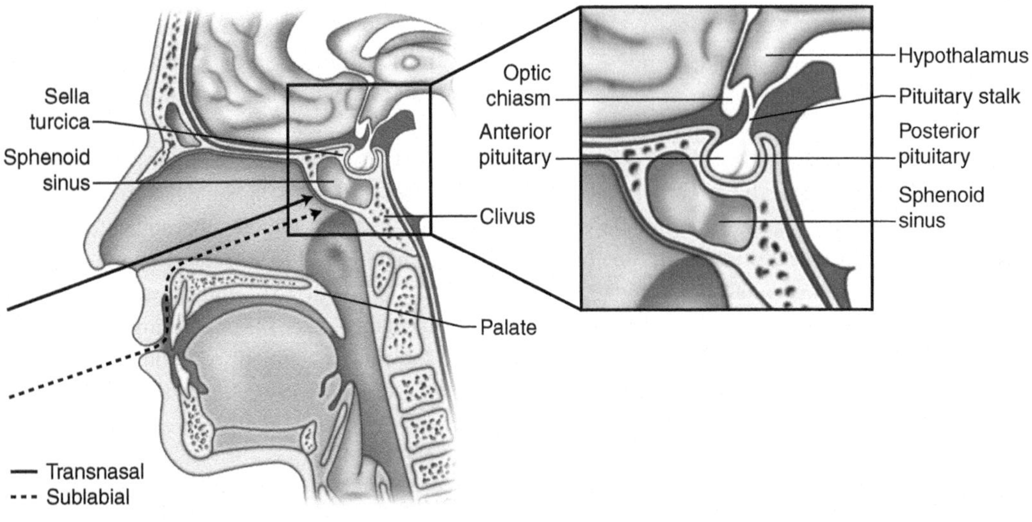

Fig. 33.3 The transphenoidal approach to the suprasellar region is accomplished through either a transnasal or sublabial trajectory. In young children, the translabial approach is preferred as it offers a larger working channel to access the sellar region

allows better visualization of lesions with suprasellar extension. The patient's head is placed on a horseshoe or Mayfield three point fixation if frameless stereotaxy and intraoperative navigation is used. The endotracheal tube is gently placed to the left of midline and the oropharynx is packed to prevent aspiration of blood. The thigh or the abdomen is also prepared as a donor site for possible fat and fascia grafts. Topical and injection of lidocaine with epinephrine promotes hemostasis and shrinks the nasal turbinates. The upper lip is everted and a sublabial incision is made from one canine fossa to the other down to the maxilla and a subperiosteal dissection superiorly exposes the piriform aperture and rostrum of the maxilla. The floor of the nasal cavity is identified and the mucosa is dissected from the floor with great care along the mesial aspect and carried posteriorly and superiorly to free the mucosa from side of the nasal septum. The quadrangular cartilage is visualized and disarticulated from the vomer and perpendicular plate and mobilized away from the midline. The rostrum and ostia of the sphenoid sinus is identified. The ostia of the sphenoid sinus mark the superior extent of bone removal. A self-retaining Hardy speculum is inserted into this opening in the sphenoid and the operative microscope is brought in. The rostrum or face of the sphenoid is then removed with a combination of ronguers and kerosene punches until the sphenoid septa and mucosa are well visualized. The mucosa is removed to help with hemostasis and prevent postoperative mucocele formation. In children whose sinus is not pneumatized, the bone must be drilled out and intraoperative navigation or fluoroscopy will be necessary to gain access through the sphenoid bone and to the sella.

Once the sella is identified, the sellar floor is removed posterosuperiorly with microronguers or a drill. Often times, the tumor has already eroded through the floor of the sella and dura may be readily appreciated. The boundaries of the bony removal of the sella are marked by the cavernous sinus laterally and the circular sinus superiorly. The dura is then incised and the mass is resected in a methodical fashion with microinstuments, starting with the floor of the sella first, followed by the lateral extent of the sella. This sequence of resection allows the superior most portion of the tumor to drop into the operative field, driven by pulsations of the intact arachnoid. Care must be taken with resection of the lateral regions of tumor to avoid carotid artery injury. It is important to understand the relationship between the tumor, the normal pituitary gland, and suprasellar arachnoid in order to minimize the risk of a cerebrospinal fluid (CSF) leak and long-term CSF fistula. If a CSF leak with violation of the arachnoid is identified, an autologous fat and fascia graft is harvested from either the abdomen or leg and the fascia graft is placed against the dural opening and the sphenoid sinus is packed with fat to hold the fascia graft in position. A Valsalva maneuver is used to ensure that the graft is in good position. The sublabial incision is then closed with plain catgut sutures, nasal tampons are inserted to aid with hemostasis, and a mustache dressing is applied.

The sublabial approach offers a wider exposure for direct view of the sella and medial portion of both cavernous sinuses [38, 39] while maintaining normal nasal anatomy with retention of the fully intact nasal mucosa and middle turbinates [40, 41]. This can be especially important in Cushing's disease when extensive inspection of the entire sella may be required to find the typical causative microadenoma [38, 39]. Children also have smaller nasal apertures and the sublabial route provides a wider corridor to access the sella than through the endonasal route [38, 39]. Great caution must be taken opening the Hardy nasal speculum within the sphenoid sinus in children because the thin surrounding bone and narrowness of the sphenoid sinus makes the carotid arteries more vulnerable to injury [2, 9]. Depending on the degree of mucosal injury and the extent of bony resection, there can be postoperative perforations within the nares and associated cosmetic concerns such as a saddle nose-deformity. The biggest disadvantage of the sublabial approach is the resulting paresthesia of the upper lip and incisors [39].

Due to the associated paresthesias experienced with the sublabial approach, the endonasal transsphenoidal approach has been used with greater frequency in those patients whose nares will allow placement of an endonasal speculum [9, 17, 39]. An incision in the posterior nasal septum or a relaxing alar incision may be made in the floor of the nasal cavity to allow easier introduction of the nasal speculum [17]. The patient is positioned and prepped as previously described. A handheld speculum is placed in the nares and the microscope is brought in. The floor of the nasal cavity, the inferior turbinate, and the middle turbinate are identified. An incision is made in the mucosa medial to the middle turbinate abutting the nasal septum and the nasal septum is disarticulated and retracted laterally. A submucosal dissection is then performed on either side of the keel of the nasal septum until the superior sphenoid ostia are identified. The Hardy speculum is then inserted into the nare and the face of the sphenoid is removed along with the mucosa with microronguers and kerosene punches. The remainder of the tumor resection proceeds as previously described.

The endonasal approach has gained widespread favor because it reduces the incidence of numbness of the upper teeth associated with the sublabial approach and avoids potential scarring of the vestibule [17, 39]. The major limitation of this approach is reduced exposure which is a more common issue in children because of their small size [9, 17]. The relaxing alar incision used to gain adequate exposure can cause postoperative bleeding and mucosal irregularity which can bother the patient. This endonasal approach may also result in septal perforations and deviation of the bony septum [9, 17].

Improvements in neuroimaging and intraoperative navigation coupled with technological advances in operative instrumentation allow access to regions of the skull base such as the cavernous sinus, suprasellar cistern, and clivus that were once thought to be accessible only by transcranial approaches. These "extended" transsphenoidal approaches are only useful in patients who have small tumors with limited intradural extension [9, 17]. The rich network of perforators that reside in this region increase the risk of bleeding for larger tumors due to the lack of proximal control and direct visualization [17, 18, 32, 42–50].

Bushe and Halves first reported the use of the endoscope in transsphenoidal surgery in 1978 [51]; however, this technique did not gain widespread acceptance until the mid-1990s when it was used extensively by otolaryngologists in sinus surgery [52]. This approach typically involves only one nostril. The endoscope can be held by either an assistant or can be held in the surgeon's nondominant hand, and surgical instruments can be held in the surgeon's dominant hand [53]. Once the anterior sphenoidectomy is performed the endoscope is introduced, or it can be introduced to perform the sphenoidectomy depending on the surgeon's preference. At this point the endoscope is mounted freeing both hands of the surgeon to proceed ahead with resection of the tumor. Others introduce the microscope when tumor resection ensues. The endonasal endoscopic approach also offers a less traumatic route for the resection of sellar and parasellar lesions, especially in the pediatric population [2, 52]. The microscope offers stereoscopic three-dimensional visualization, illumination, and magnification of the operative field. Endoscopy allows for a larger and closer view of the surgical field, particularly providing better anatomical detail and visualization of any residual pathology, and a lower complication rate. The microscope and endoscope can be used to complement each other to provide superior results than either method alone. The use of the endoscope is technically challenging, especially in the pediatric population with a small pituitary fossa and the absence of sphenoid sinus aeration. This technique provides a narrower working corridor and avoids the resection of the nasal turbinates and septum. Transcranial Approaches.

Although Cushing was a pioneer in transsphenoidal surgery, he later preferred transcranial approaches and his influence made this a common approach through the 1950s [54, 55]. As transsphenoidal approaches came into favor later in the twentieth century, indications for transcranial approaches to the sellar region became limited. Cases where the transsphenoidal approach is contraindicated include presence of sphenoid sinusitis and paramedian carotid arteries. Patients who have extensive suprasellar and parasellar extension of tumor are also good candidates for transcranial approaches that reduce the risk of injury and associated morbidity [56]. The two most common transcranial approaches to gain access to the sellar, parasellar, and suprasellar regions are the pterional (fronto-temporal) and the anterior subfrontal approach.

The pterional approach was first described by Yasargil [57] as the ideal approach to access the circle of Willis for treating anterior circulation aneurysms. This approach allows for the shortest transcranial trajectory to the suprasellar cistern [9]. It involves a craniotomy of the fronto-temporal bones and entails resection of the sphenoid wing and provides excellent visualization of the parasellar structures with minimal brain retraction. This is the favored approach for removing sellar masses that extend into the parasellar and suprasellar compartments [9]. This method also allows access to and resection of tumors adjacent to an optic chiasm that is not immediately above the pituitary, i.e., a prefixed optic chiasm. It also allows for the direct visualization of the pituitary stalk [11, 56]. Occasionally an extension of the pterional approach, the orbitozygomatic approach, is used where the orbital bar and part of the zygoma are removed in addition to the frontal and temporal regions in order to gain a better trajectory superiorly to gain access to lesions that extend above the suprasellar regions and into the ventricular system [58, 59].

An alternative to gaining access to the sellar, parasellar, and suprasellar regions described by Suzuki [60–62] and Shibuya [63] is the fronto-basal interhemispheric approach. This approach minimizes brain retraction, and the major vessels on the surface of the exposed brain in the frontal and basal regions, specifically on the medial surface of the frontal lobe and over the corpus callosum can be spared [12, 60, 61, 63]. This approach also allows for a straight frontal trajectory with direct visualization of the tumor as it is being removed between the optic nerves. This approach, however, is contraindicated in those patients with a prefixed chiasm [12, 56, 60, 61, 63]. The surgical technique is complex and postoperative psychological problems due to bilateral frontal lobe retraction and olfactory tract damage have been reported [12, 56, 60, 61, 63]. Violation of the frontal sinus is also possible and could result in CSF leak and mucocele formation [12].

Some sellar and suprasellar tumors pose unique challenges for neurosurgeon to achieve optimal resection of tumor while limiting the neurologic complications. This is particularly true in patients who have retrochiasmatic craniopharyngiomas [11, 56]. Retrochiasmatic craniopharyngiomas are often hidden behind the optic chiasm and may extend upward into the third ventricle or down in front of the brainstem. Hakuba and colleagues in 1985 first described the use of the transpetrosal-transtentorial approach now known as the posterior petrosal approach, to expose and remove retrochiasmatic craniopharyngiomas in five adult patients [64]. It was further modified by Al-Mefty and applied specifically to children [65–68]. This approach involves a more extensive craniotomy and exposes the retroclival area, the lower surface of the chiasm, the floor of the third ventricle, the tuber cinereum, pituitary stalk, and the interpeduncular cistern. This approach allows for mobilization of the sigmoid sinus medially, and allows an upward projection which facilitates dissection of the tumor under direct visualization with a wide exposure extending from the pituitary stalk and hypothalamus up to the third ventricle, so that a the tumor can be removed from below [56, 65–68]. In experienced hands, this method has the advantage of maintaining the integrity of the hypothalamus. This approach requires a mastoidectomy to gain access to the presigmoid space and there was initial concern that this would limit its utility in children because the mastoid sinus is not fully developed and pneumatized. However, Al-Mefty used the technique successfully in two children with lack of pneumatization of the mastoid to successfully expose and resect large retrochiasmatic craniopharyngiomas.

Complications

In addition to the previously mentioned complications that are specific to each surgical approach, there are complications that can occur with all the approaches. Most notably, there can be significant morbidity that results from trauma to surrounding brain, especially the hypothalamus. The hypothalamus is an important regulator not only allowing the linkage of the central nervous system to the endocrine axis via the pituitary gland, but also by regulating key metabolic processes and other activities of the autonomic nervous system. The hypothalamus is exceedingly sensitive to manipulation and even minor surgical maneuvers can disrupt its homeostasis. Hyperphagia is a significant postoperative concern in these patients, not only because of long-term health consequences but also because of the significant social implications that can in turn affect the patient's mental well-being. Temperature regulation may also be a problem postoperatively. In addition, significant damage or manipulation of the hypothalamus can result in prolonged or even permanent impairment of a patient's level of alertness. The exact mechanism that is responsible for the disruption of arousal not fully understood but revolves around disruption of the major input and output of the reticular activating system. This interference with arousal is usually the result of bilateral injury to the hypothalamus.

As previously noted, rapid correction of the compression of the optic nerves and optic chiasm produced by sellar masses can result in a catastrophic loss of vision. The normal vascular homeostasis is altered with the presence of the mass and autoregulation is disrupted. Abrupt decompression disrupts this newfound vascular homeostasis and can significantly alter blood flow to the optic nerves and can cause irreversible loss of vision. Endocrine abnormalities are common after resection of sellar tumors. Anterior pituitary dysfunction can range from minor hormonal deficits to complete loss of function of all hormonal output necessitating postoperative hormone replacement therapy. Posterior pituitary dysfunction, such as diabetes insipidus is also common and must be anticipated and treated to prevent catastrophic dehydration with resultant venous sinus thrombosis.

References

1. Bunin GR, Surawicz TS, Witman PA, Preston-Martin S, Davis F, Bruner JM. The descriptive epidemiology of craniopharyngioma. J Neurosurg. 1998;89:547–51.
2. Frazier JL, Chaichana K, Jallo GI, Quinones-Hinojosa A. Combined endoscopic and microscopic management of pediatric pituitary region tumors through one nostril: technical note with case illustrations. Childs Nerv Syst. 2008;24:1469–78.
3. Jagannathan J, Dumont AS, Jane JA Jr. Diagnosis and management of pediatric sellar lesions. Front Horm Res. 2006;34:83–104.
4. Jagannathan J, Dumont AS, Jane JA Jr, Laws ER Jr. Pediatric sellar tumors: diagnostic procedures and management. Neurosurg Focus. 2005;18:E6.
5. Mehrazin M, Yavari P. Morphological pattern and frequency of intracranial tumors in children. Childs Nerv Syst. 2007;23:157–62.
6. Sklar CA. Craniopharyngioma: endocrine abnormalities at presentation. Pediatr Neurosurg. 1994;21 (Suppl 1):18–20.
7. Blackwell RE, Younger JB. Long-term medical therapy and follow-up of pediatric-adolescent patients with prolactin-secreting macroadenomas. Fertil Steril. 1986;45:713–6.
8. Laws ER Jr. Pituitary surgery. Endocrinol Metab Clin North Am. 1987;16:647–65.
9. Liu JK, Weiss MH, Couldwell WT. Surgical approaches to pituitary tumors. Neurosurg Clin N Am. 2003;14:93–107.
10. Karnaze MG, Sartor K, Winthrop JD, Gado MH, Hodges FJ 3rd. Suprasellar lesions: evaluation with MR imaging. Radiology. 1986;161:77–82.
11. Klimo P Jr, Browd SR, Pravdenkova S, Couldwell WT, Walker ML, Al-Mefty O. The posterior petrosal approach: technique and applications in pediatric neurosurgery. J Neurosurg Pediatr. 2009;4:353–62.
12. Shirane R, Hayashi T, Tominaga T. Fronto-basal interhemispheric approach for craniopharyngiomas extending outside the suprasellar cistern. Childs Nerv Syst. 2005;21:669–78.
13. Davis DH, Laws ER Jr, Ilstrup DM, Speed JK, Caruso M, Shaw EG, et al. Results of surgical treatment for growth hormone-secreting pituitary adenomas. J Neurosurg. 1993;79:70–5.
14. Ebersold MJ, Laws ER Jr, Scheithauer BW, Randall RV. Pituitary apoplexy treated by transsphenoidal surgery. A clinicopathological and

immunocytochemical study. J Neurosurg. 1983;58:315–20.
15. Laws ER Jr, Trautmann JC, Hollenhorst RW Jr. Transsphenoidal decompression of the optic nerve and chiasm. Visual results in 62 patients. J Neurosurg. 1977;46:717–22.
16. Laws ER Jr, Fode NC, Redmond MJ. Transsphenoidal surgery following unsuccessful prior therapy. An assessment of benefits and risks in 158 patients. J Neurosurg. 1985;63:823–9.
17. Couldwell WT. The transnasal transphenoidal approach. In: Apuzzo MLJ, editors. Surgery of the third ventricle. Baltimore: Williams & Wilkins; 1998. p. 553–574.
18. Couldwell WT, Sabit I, Weiss MH, Giannotta SL, Rice D. Transmaxillary approach to the anterior cavernous sinus: a microanatomic study. Neurosurgery. 1997;40:1307–11.
19. Laws ER Jr, Piepgras DG, Randall RV, Abboud CF. Neurosurgical management of acromegaly. Results in 82 patients treated between 1972 and 1977. J Neurosurg. 1979;50:454–61.
20. Marie P. Sur deux cas d'acromegalie: hypertrophie singulire non congenitale des extremities superieures, inferieures et cephalique. Rev Med. 1886;6:297–333.
21. Caton RPF. Notes of a case of acromegaly treated by operation. BMJ. 1893;2:1421–3.
22. Elsberg C. Tumor of the hypophysis. Ann Surg. 1914;59:454–5.
23. Frazier C. An approach to the hypophysis though the anterior cranial fossa. Ann Surg. 1913;47:145–50.
24. Heuer G. The surgical approach and the therapy of tumors and other lesions about the optic chiasm. Surg Gynecol Obstet. 1931;53:489–518.
25. Horsley V. On the technique of operations on the central nervous system. BMJ. 1906;2:411–23.
26. Krause F. Hirnchirugie (freilegung do hypophyse). Deutsche Klin. 1905;8:953–1024.
27. Schloffer H. Erfolgreiche operation eines hypophysentumor auf nasalem wege. Wein Klin Wochenschr. 1907;20:621–4.
28. Cushing H. The Weir Mitchell Lecture. Surgical experiences with pituitary disorders. JAMA. 1914;63:1515–25.
29. Dott NMPB. A consideration of the hypophyseal adenomata. Br J Surg. 1925;13:314–66.
30. Guiot G: Transphenoidal approach in surgical treatment of pituitary adenmas: general principles and indicatios in nonfunctioning adenomas. In: Kohler GR, editors. Diagnosis and treatment of pituitary tumors. New York: American Elsevier; 1973. p. 159–78.
31. Hardy J. Transsphenoidal hypophysectomy. J Neurosurg. 1971;34:582–94.
32. Liu JK, Das K, Weiss MH, Laws ER Jr, Couldwell WT. The history and evolution of transsphenoidal surgery. J Neurosurg. 2001;95:1083–96.
33. Baskin DS, Wilson CB. Surgical management of craniopharyngiomas. A review of 74 cases. J Neurosurg. 1986;65:22–7.
34. Wilson CB. A decade of pituitary microsurgery. The Herbert Olivecrona lecture. J Neurosurg. 1984;61:814–33.
35. Wilson CB, Dempsey LC. Transsphenoidal microsurgical removal of 250 pituitary adenomas. J Neurosurg. 1978;48:13–22.
36. Black PM, Zervas NT, Candia GL. Incidence and management of complications of transsphenoidal operation for pituitary adenomas. Neurosurgery. 1987;20:920–4.
37. Laws ER Jr, Kern EB. Complications of trans-sphenoidal surgery. Clin Neurosurg. 1976;23:401–16.
38. Jagannathan J, Sheehan JP, Jane JA Jr. Evaluation and management of Cushing syndrome in cases of negative sellar magnetic resonance imaging. Neurosurg Focus. 2007;23:E3.
39. Kerr PB, Oldfield EH. Sublabial-endonasal approach to the sella turcica. J Neurosurg. 2008;109:153–5.
40. Das K, Spencer W, Nwagwu CI, Schaeffer S, Wenk E, Weiss MH, et al. Approaches to the sellar and parasellar region: anatomic comparison of endonasal-transsphenoidal, sublabial-transsphenoidal, and transethmoidal approaches. Neurol Res. 2001;23:51–4.
41. Jagannathan J, Smith R, DeVroom HL, Vortmeyer AO, Stratakis CA, Nieman LK, et al. Outcome of using the histological pseudocapsule as a surgical capsule in Cushing disease. J Neurosurg. 2009;111:531–9.
42. Fraioli B, Esposito V, Santoro A, Iannetti G, Giuffre R, Cantore G. Transmaxillosphenoidal approach to tumors invading the medial compartment of the cavernous sinus. J Neurosurg. 1995;82:63–9.
43. Hashimoto N, Handa H, Yamagami T. Transsphenoidal extracapsular approach to pituitary tumors. J Neurosurg. 1986;64:16–20.
44. Hashimoto N, Kikuchi H. Transsphenoidal approach to infrasellar tumors involving the cavernous sinus. J Neurosurg. 1990;73:513–7.
45. Kaptain GJ, Vincent DA, Sheehan JP, Laws ER, Jr. Transsphenoidal approaches for the extracapsular resection of midline suprasellar and anterior cranial base lesions. Neurosurgery. 2001;49:94–100; discussion 100–1.
46. Kato T, Sawamura Y, Abe H, Nagashima M: Transsphenoidal-transtuberculum sellae approach for supradiaphragmatic tumours: technical note. Acta Neurochir (Wien). 1998;140:715–8; discussion 719.
47. Kitano M, Taneda M. Extended transsphenoidal approach with submucosal posterior ethmoidectomy for parasellar tumors. Technical note. J Neurosurg. 2001;94:999–1004.
48. Kouri JG, Chen MY, Watson JC, Oldfield EH. Resection of suprasellar tumors by using a modified transsphenoidal approach. Report of four cases. J Neurosurg. 2000;92:1028–35.
49. Mason RB, Nieman LK, Doppman JL, Oldfield EH. Selective excision of adenomas originating in or

extending into the pituitary stalk with preservation of pituitary function. J Neurosurg. 1997;87:343–51.
50. Sabit I, Schaefer SD, Couldwell WT. Extradural extranasal combined transmaxillary transsphenoidal approach to the cavernous sinus: a minimally invasive microsurgical model. Laryngoscope. 2000;110: 286–91.
51. Halves E, Bushe KA. Transsphenoidal operation on craniopharyngiomas with extrasellar extensions. The advantage of the operating endoscope [proceedings]. Acta Neurochir Suppl (Wien). 1979;28:362.
52. Alfieri A. Endoscopic endonasal transsphenoidal approach to the sellar region: technical evolution of the methodology and refinement of a dedicated instrumentation. J Neurosurg Sci. 1999;43:85–92.
53. Yaniv E, Rappaport ZH. Endoscopic transseptal transsphenoidal surgery for pituitary tumors. Neurosurgery. 1997;40:944–6.
54. Luft R, Olivecrona H. Experiences with hypophysectomy in man. J Neurosurg. 1953;10:301–16.
55. Rosegay H. Cushing's legacy to transsphenoidal surgery. J Neurosurg. 1981;54:448–54.
56. Al-Mefty O, Ayoubi S, Kadri PA. The petrosal approach for the total removal of giant retrochiasmatic craniopharyngiomas in children. J Neurosurg. 2007;106:87–92.
57. Yasargil M. Microsurgical anatomy of the basilar cisterns and vessels of the brain, diagnostic studies, general operative techniques, and pathological considerations of intracranial aneurysms. In: Veriag GT, editors. Microneurosurgery. Vol. 1. Stuttgart: Thieme; 1984.
58. Golshani KJ, Lalwani K, Delashaw JB, Selden NR. Modified orbitozygomatic craniotomy for craniopharyngioma resection in children. J Neurosurg Pediatr. 2009;4:345–52.
59. Pontius AT, Ducic Y. Extended orbitozygomatic approach to the skull base to improve access to the cavernous sinus and optic chiasm. Otolaryngol Head Neck Surg. 2004;130:519–25.
60. Suzuki J, Katakura R, Mori T. Interhemispheric approach through the lamina terminalis to tumors of the anterior part of the third ventricle. Surg Neurol. 1984;22:157–63.
61. Suzuki J, Mizoi K, Yoshimoto T. Bifrontal interhemispheric approach to aneurysms of the anterior communicating artery. J Neurosurg. 1986;64:183–90.
62. Suzuki J, Yoshimoto T, Mizoi K. Preservation of the olfactory tract in bifrontal craniotomy for anterior communicating artery aneurysms, and the functional prognosis. J Neurosurg. 1981;54:342–5.
63. Shibuya M, Takayasu M, Suzuki Y, Saito K, Sugita K. Bifrontal basal interhemispheric approach to craniopharyngioma resection with or without division of the anterior communicating artery. J Neurosurg. 1996;84:951–6.
64. Hakuba A, Nishimura S, Inoue Y. Transpetrosal-transtentorial approach and its application in the therapy of retrochiasmatic craniopharyngiomas. Surg Neurol. 1985;24:405–15.
65. Al-Mefty O, Fox JL, Smith RR. Petrosal approach for petroclival meningiomas. Neurosurgery. 1988;22:510–7.
66. Hakuba A, Nishimura S. Total removal of clivus meningiomas and the operative results. Neurol Med Chir (Tokyo). 1981;21:59–73.
67. Horgan MA, Anderson GJ, Kellogg JX, Schwartz MS, Spektor S, McMenomey SO, et al. Classification and quantification of the petrosal approach to the petroclival region. J Neurosurg. 2000;93:108–12.
68. Nishimura S, Hakuba A, Jang BJ, Inoue Y. Clivus and apicopetroclivus meningiomas—report of 24 cases. Neurol Med Chir (Tokyo). 1989;29:1004–11.

Index

Note: Page numbers followed by *f* and *t* indicate figures and tables, respectively

D.J. Ledbetter and P.R.V. Johnson (eds.), *Endocrine Surgery in Children*,
DOI 10.1007/978-3-662-54256-9

E

F

G

H

Q

R

Printed by Printforce, the Netherlands